ANTICANCER DRUGS FROM ANIMALS, PLANTS, AND MICROORGANISMS

ANTICANCER DRUGS FROM ANIMALS, PLANTS, AND MICROORGANISMS

GEORGE R. PETTIT
FIONA HOGAN PIERSON
CHERRY L. HERALD

Cancer Research Institute and Department of Chemistry
Arizona State University
Tempe, AZ 85287-1604

A Wiley-Interscience Publication
JOHN WILEY & SONS, INC.
New York • Chichester • Brisbane • Toronto • Singapore

This text is printed on acid-free paper.

Library of Congress Cataloging in Publication Data:

Pettit, George R.
Anticancer drugs from animals, plants and microorganisms / George R. Pettit, Fiona Hogan Pierson, Cherry L. Herald.
p. cm.
Includes bibliographical references and index.
ISBN 0-471-03657-9 (cloth : alk. paper)
1. Antineoplastic agents—Tables. 2. Pharmacognosy—Tables.
I. Pierson Hogan, Fiona. II. Herald, Cherry L. III. Title.
[DNLM: 1. Antineoplastic Agents—pharmacology—tables.
2. Carcinogens—pharmacology—tables. QV 16 P511a 1994]
RC271.C5P46 1994
616.99'4061—dc20
DNLM/DLC
for Library of Congress 93-46997
CIP

Printed in the United States of America

10 9 8 7 6 5 4 3 2 1

Dr. Michael R. Boyd, Eleanor Waddell Libby, Virginia G. Piper,
and in memory of Herbert K. Cummings (1924–1992)
Dr. Jonathan L. Hartwell (1906–1991), and Dr. Julius A. Rippel (1901–1990).

For their splendid achievements and commitment to
discovery of new naturally occurring anticancer drugs.

PREFACE

The relentless attack by cancer continues to exact a devastating price. Even the most conservative estimates of the predicted 1991 United States death rate from cancer are in excess of 560,000 people with a one-year dollar cost of over 80 billion plus incalculable human costs. On a world-wide basis the devastation caused by cancer is staggering to contemplate. Fortunately the increasing use of well-established anticancer drugs and the introduction of new anticancer drugs combined with overall advances in cancer treatment has markedly increased survival time for most cancer patients. Best of all the number of cancer patients considered cured by expert application of anticancer drugs in the United States may be approaching 100,000 per year. The U.S. National Cancer Institute (NCI) and its approved comprehensive cancer treatment centers have been most responsible for these vital advances. Presently the NCI recognizes the following 26 comprehensive treatment centers:

Arizona Cancer Center
Cancer Center of Wake Forest University/Bowman Gray School of Medicine
Columbia University Comprehensive Cancer Center
Dana–Farber Cancer Institute
Duke Comprehensive Cancer Center
Fox Chase Cancer Center
Fred Hutchinson Cancer Research Center
Illinois Cancer Council
Johns Hopkins Oncology Center
Jonsson Comprehensive Cancer Center
Kenneth Norris Comprehensive Cancer Center
Lineberger Cancer Research Center
Mayo Comprehensive Cancer Center
M. D. Anderson Cancer Center
Memorial Sloan–Kettering Cancer Center
Meyer Prentis Comprehensive Cancer Center of Metropolitan Detroit
Norris Cotton Cancer Center
Ohio State University Comprehensive Cancer Center
Pittsburgh Cancer Institute
Roswell Park Cancer Institute
Sylvester Comprehensive Cancer Center
University of Alabama at Birmingham
University of Pennsylvania Cancer Center
University of Southern California
University of Wisconsin Clinical Cancer Center
Yale Comprehensive Cancer Center

The majority of most useful and curative anticancer drugs continue to be derived from plant and animal sources. Doubtlessly, anticancer drugs of biosynthetic origin will continue to be of accelerating importance in improving cancer treatment and overall survival rates. Illustrated here are the rapidly expanding clinical applications (e.g., small cell lung cancer) of etoposide[90, 708] (a podophyllotoxin glycoside) for human solid tumors and taxol for ovarian cancer.[951] Even some halogen derivatives of adenosine are now proving remarkably effective. For example, a single seven-day infusion of 2-chlorodeoxyadenosine (2-CdA) led to complete remission (7 to 46 months without relapse so far) of hairy cell leukemia in 11 of 12 patients with this generally fatal (3 to 5 years) disease. Prior to the recent clinical introduction of 2-CdA, treatment for the some 6000 U.S. hairy cell leukemia patients (usually males over 50 years old) was primarily limited to alpha-interferon (partial remissions and frequent relapses when the use of the interferon is stopped) and deoxycoformycin (pentostatin, a high remission rate but less than with 2-CdA). But both of these treatments are accompanied by severe toxicity that limits their utility. Analogously, the 2-fluoro analog, fludarabine monophosphate, in a series of four clinical trials with or without prednisone proved to be considerably more effective (now the best single drug) for treating chronic lymphocytic leukemia (CLL, mean survival about five years) than the currently accepted chlorambucil/prednisone drug therapy. Patients with Rai stages 0–II CLL gave a 90 percent remission rate and those with stage IV a 67 percent rate. Only 20 percent of stage IV CLL patients gain complete remissions using chlorambucil/prednisone. With fludarabine toxic side effects are generally reduced but an increase in infections due to immunosuppression have been observed. Perhaps use of the immunostimulants bryostatin 1 and/or levamisole, a well-known antihelminthic, with fludarabine would ameliorate this shortcoming. Indeed, the combination of 5-fluorouracil/levamisole is presently the most promising therapy for Dukes' stage C (involving regional lymph nodes with ~21,000 patients per year in the U.S.) colon cancer (some 110,000 patients per year),[947] affording a 31 percent and 32 percent increase respectively in five year disease-free and overall survival rate. Within five years of surgery (without chemotherapy) nearly 60 percent of Dukes' C patients will have a recurrence of colon cancer. In the United States the number of such patients alive at five years could now be increased by 2,500 using the 5-fluorouracil/levamisole adjuvant therapy.

Discovery and development of new anticancer drugs for improving cancer treatment requires a major financial and personnel strengthening of our government's cancer conquest program. Over the past decade while total deaths from cancer have continued to increase there has been a determined decrease in funding and personnel for the U.S. NCI. In 1980 the NCI funds amounted to about $960 million and in the 1991 fiscal year only some $900 million in 1980 dollars. That's a 6 percent reduction and the situation is much more severe when considering the diversion of NCI money and personnel to coping with the AIDS problem. Indeed if funding to the NCI for AIDS is subtracted the total reduction from 1980 is 18.5 percent. Currently, the NCI 1992 bypass budget requests $2,612,230,000 but the President's 1992 budget recommends only $1,810,230,000, a slim 5.6 percent increase over the 1991 appropriation of $1,714,000,000. Of the President's budget figure $846,147,000 (7.2% increase) would be expended for research project grants, $89,242,000 (2% increase) for special grants (clinical, etc.), $37,670,000 (1.1% increase) for training grants, $112,772,000 for cancer centers (2.4% increase), $348,873,000 (6% increase) for NCI intramural research (includes National Institutes of Health clinical center), $191,395,000 (2.2% increase) for research and development contracts, $89,786,000 (4.8% increase) for cancer prevention and control, $4,800,000 ($\sim$30% decrease) for construction, and $92,295,000 (13.9% increase due to congressional mandate) for research management and support. In the past 10 years the NCI funding for research and development contracts necessary to developing NCI anticancer drug leads has decreased 50 percent. At least over the same period the overall U.S. NIH appropriation has increased 27 percent in 1980 dollars. Clearly the conquest of cancer requires a much greater deployment of personnel and financial support.

The potential of animal, microorganism, and plant constituents as sources for new and potentially useful anticancer, antiviral, and other necessary drugs for solving severe medical problems forms the focus of this book. In the oncogenic virus field the current AIDS pandemic is only one symptom of what is surely to be a continuum of new and lethal human viral diseases.[634,641] Because of the rapidly increasing interactions of formerly isolated human populations, animals (e.g., primates), and insects (e.g., mosquitoes), formerly localized viruses have been given global opportunities to infect, mutate, and reproduce. Chapter 1 of this volume updates (to January 1991) the corresponding section of *Biosynthetic Products for Cancer Chemotherapy*, Volume 6[883] devoted to cancer-causing and related human viruses. Again, major emphasis was placed on HIV-1 infections.

Chapter 2 provides a summary of the better known tumor promoters and carcinogens. Here the intention was to point out the sometimes fine line between antineoplastic and carcinogenic activity and especially the obvious need to eliminate from human consumption those food and drug constituents with proven tumor promoting and/or carcinogenic properties.

The present referrence book continues the general style of *Biosynthetic Products for Cancer Chemotherapy,* Volumes 3–6.[883] The tabular survey of new antineoplastic and/or cytotoxic plant and animal constituents continues the literature coverage from January 1986 to January 1989. The marine animal and marine plant biosynthetic products, Sections C and D, also cover the period January 1986 to January 1989. The discovery of antineoplastic and other biological activities among the marine animal and plant constituents has been rapidly increasing. Because of their outstanding potential, the marine animal and marine plant surveys were continued and include all such substances isolated and characterized in the January 1986 to January 1989 period, including those currently lacking biological study. Presumably many of these substances where biological activity is still unknown will prove to be potentially important. As before we expect these summaries of potentially useful plant, microorganism, and marine organism antineoplastic and/or cytotoxic constituents along with the other marine animal and plant substances of known structure will be very useful to chemists, biologists, and clinicians concerned with the discovery and development of new anticancer drugs.

Grateful thanks and appreciation are extended to Ms. Christine H. Duplissa for exceptionally helpful contributions to the preparation of the final manuscript. We also thank Mrs. Georgia Reimus, Mrs. Mary A. Link, and Ms. Stacey L. Butler for their very capable assitance.

GEORGE R. PETTIT

Paradise Valley, Arizona
January, 1993

CONTENTS

ANTICANCER DRUGS FROM ANIMALS, PLANTS, AND MICROORGANISMS

Chapter 1 CANCER CAUSING AND RELATED LETHAL VIRAL DISEASES

The lethal threat posed by RNA-type viruses has been rapidly increasing. The death toll not only in the United States but world-wide has been rising rapidly. In *Biosynthetic Products for Cancer Chemotherapy*, Volume 6[883], we reviewed the HIV family of retroviruses and the rapidly increasing lethal and medical consequences. Hence, this chapter will continue the review from that period. The latter part of this summary will include a current synopsis of the RNA togaviruses and arenaviruses that constitute objectives for high priority research. Because of the intensive research effort now underway in the United States directed at HIV-1 it serves as a very useful illustration of potentially successful approaches to other lethal RNA viral diseases, especially those leading to human cancer.[208,458,862,974]

From evidence now in hand it appears that HIV-1 evolved into a pathogenic virus and/or spread into human populations about 30 years ago.[719] The original genesis of this virus still remains unknown.[719] But the consequences are certainly well-known in the United States. As of June, 1992, 230,179 Americans had been diagnosed with AIDS and over 152,153 (66%) had died. Present estimates of people in the U.S. infected with AIDS run to three million with a 1989 medical cost of 3.3 billion and by 1993 rising to 7.8 billion. By 1987 the World Health Organization estimated up to 10 million people world-wide (over six million in Africa) were infected with HIV[171] and by the year 2000 the very conservative estimate of some 40 million for the AIDS pandemic.[172] Obviously actual numbers will be much higher. Recent estimates have indicated that perhaps up to 40% of sexually active people throughout Central Africa are now infected.[225,354,812] Furthermore, some incubation periods have been shown to exceed ten years.[120] Already in the two-year period ending December 1988 some 513[861] active-duty U.S. Navy personnel seroconverted from HIV negative to HIV positive.[341] In the general population transmission of HIV-1 into the heterosexual population by bisexual men,[58] intravenous drug users[160,296] blood transfusions,[351] prostitutes[861] and the high-risk student[682] age population continues to increase[549,920,993]. A study of homosexual men in Kingston, Jamaica indicated that the frequency of bisexuality (65/125 men) among homosexual men and the large frequency (11%) of HIV infection among this population suggests that secondary infection of female sexual partners is a very serious problem.[785] Some estimation of the medical consequences can also be ascertained by considering that HIV-1 infection in high risk homosexual[560] males probably occurs at least 35 months prior to when HIV-1 antibodies can be detected.[454] In short this very long period of latency may be more common than earlier recognized.

The number of HIV-1 infections from events other than sexual transmission is on the increase and is now most obvious among research and medical[744] (5,096 doctors, 336 surgeons, 9,592 nurses, and 1,248 dentists and dental hygienists now HIV-1 infected in the U.S.) personnel. Most of these transmissions have occurred among health personnel (the U.S. Centers for Disease Control reported at the end of 1990 46,520 now infected in the U.S. and of these 5,815 have active AIDS) principally from needle sticks, other sharp objects, biopsies, concentrated virus on skin, and via mucous membrane and cutaneous routes.[346,698] The possibility of transmission of HIV by arthropods and by possible mutations of the HIV series with other more easily transmitted viruses persists. For example, bed bug infestations are common throughout Africa and in one study 4,000 bed bugs were collected per hut in a rural village.[681] Bites from such HIV-carriers upon a malnourished or, for example, immunosuppressed host might be a mode of transmission. Other evolving aspects of the HIV epidemic with lethal consequences include the fact that related viruses can be transmitted with the HIV-1 infection. For example, HIV-1 and HIV-2 have been isolated simultaneously from an Ivory Coast HIV patient.[277] Kaposi's sarcoma, a seemingly characteristic consequence of HIV infection, provides another unnerving example. By March 1989 15% of AIDS patients had Kaposi's sarcoma. In the United States this sarcoma is at least 20,000 times more common in HIV-1 infected people.[277] If a woman's sexual partner was found to be a bisexual male rather than an IV drug user, they were more likely to have Kaposi's sarcoma. In accord with that observation only 1% of men with haemophilia and HIV-1 advance to Kaposi's sarcoma whereas the level was 21% in homosexual or bisexual men. Such statistical evidence suggests that Kaposi's sarcoma may actually be caused by an infectious agent (virus?) transmitted with HIV by sexual contact.[61] In this regard Epstein Barr virus transformed B lymphocytes have been found sensitive to productive HIV infections.[81] In June 1990 reports appeared that nearly 10% of advanced HIV patients had developed a virulent form of non-Hodgkin's lymphoma, a cancer of the B-cells (formed in the lymph nodes). In San Francisco, Kaposi's sarcoma cases grew at a 2% annual rate in 1987 while in the same period the lymphoma cases increased 48%. Whether this rapidly increasing lymphoma is due to treatment with

AZT (*1*), infection[734] and/or general deterioration of the immune system is presently unknown. In general the survival of HIV patients has been improving, particularly that of those with *Pneumocystis carinii* pneumonia, as the use of AZT has increased.[207,635,651] Interestingly, the immune system stimulator inosine pranobex (3:1, N,N-dimethylamino-2-propanol:inosine p-acetamidobenzoic acid salt) appears to delay progression to AIDS in HIV infected patients.[456,871]

Implications of the preceding summary for the future strongly indicate a series of catastrophic events for the U.S. and world-wide unless we can discover generally curative drugs for HIV and other RNA-virus type infections. Presently AZT (*1*) is the only anti-AIDS drug in general use in the U.S.[987] Attempts, with questionable success to date, have been made to increase the utility of AZT by using r-human erythropoietin (to reduce bone marrow suppression and anemia).[297] By April 1989 ddC (*2*) was in phase 1 human trial and phase 1 human trials were underway for ddI (*3*) and ddA (*4*) (the IND was discontinued by the U.S. NCI in January, 1991 due to rapid in vivo conversion of ddA to ddI).[860] A year later (April 1990) 8,000 HIV patients were receiving ddI but the death rate among these patients from all causes in these expanded trials was much higher than among those receiving ddI in more carefully controlled clinical trials. Indeed 290 of these patients had died in the expanded access program compared with 15 enrolled in the more normal clinical trial.[860] More recent clinical trials of ddI at 12 mg/kg indicate antiretroviral activity in patients with AIDS and in early 1992 ddI trials were expanded.[195,632] In 1990 carbovir (*5*) was scheduled to begin clinical trial in the U.S. National Cancer Institute's programs.[705] Clinical trials of phosphonoformate (*6*) have continued, but renal function impairment limits the use of this drug in AIDS patients.[284,343] While major attempts at discovery of new anti-HIV and other antiviral drugs remain focused on synthetic modification (including computer-assisted SAR studies)[804] of nucleosides,[2,56,492,957,1023] increasing emphasis is being placed on discovery of naturally occurring antiviral drugs bearing unprecedented structures.[747] Even tannins and some of their structural components have been found to inhibit HIV replication.[824] Clinical trials are now underway with (+)-castanospermine (*7*) from the seeds of *Castanospermum australe*[921] and a derivative designated SC-48334.[705] Both compounds inhibit viral maturation and castanospermine has also been reported[1084] to inhibit growth of human cytomegalovirus. The nucleoside derivatives noted above are reverse transcription inhibitors that suppress viral

DNA synthesis. The protein CD4 obtained via a recombinant DNA technique apparently operates by inhibiting viral entry into cells and is now in clinical trials.[705]

Among newly discovered naturally occurring anti-HIV substances in the U.S. National Cancer Institute's program is the sulfolipid VIII (*8*) isolated from a blue-green alga.[381] The lipid was active against HIV-1 in the CEM (cultured human lymphoblastoid), C3-44, LDV-7 and MT-2 cell lines using the tetrazolium reagent assay.[1170] Other recent anti-HIV-1 actives among naturally occurring substances include a sulfate derivative of glycyrrhizin (reverse transcriptase inhibition activity)[802], a sulfate derivative of a branched (1→3)-β-D-glucan[403] and a high molecular weight sulphonated carbohydrate polymer.[813] The number of terrestrial plant constituents known to have antiviral activity has been growing rapidly,[685,1136] and the same observation applies to microorganisms and constituents from the lower plants and marine animals. For example, β-lactam antibiotics of the cephalosporin-type inhibit replication of herpes simplex 1 and vaccinia.[202] Such naturally occurring antiviral agents can also occur as very small molecules such as epoxide *9* isolated from culture broths of *Streptomyces abikoensis*.[746] Thioamide *10* known as R82150 is an exceptionally potent in vitro anti-HIV-1 substance related to some of the recently discovered marine animal constituents.[213,883]

The explosive growth in travel by our civilian population combined with requirements for extensive military travel world-wide has greatly increased the risk of exposure to other deadly RNA-type viral diseases. Unfortunately the rapidly increasing risk from non-HIV viral diseases continues largely unrecognized. Discovery and development of new drugs are urgently required to treat viral infections emanating from the togaviruses family illustrated in the alphavirus genus (group A) by Venezuelan equine encephalomyelitis[709] and in the genus flavivirus (group B) by Japanese encephalitis,[433,683,760] dengue,[178,623,948,1103] and yellow fever.[93,573,733] In the family Bunyaviridae the genus phlebovirus contains Rift Valley fever,[774,1112] and the genus nairovirus contains Crimean-Congo hemorrhagic fever (carried by ticks),[300] and Sicilian sandfly fever.[701] Crimean-Congo hemorrhagic fever is widespread in the Middle East. When transmitted to hospital personnel from patients in Iraq, the United Arab Emirates and, e.g., Pakistan the death rate ranges from 40% to 100%.

In November 1989 a serious member of the family Filoviridae, namely, ebola virus entered the United States via a shipment of cynomolgus monkeys from the Philippines.[252,493] The outbreak of ebola virus fever in Zaire recently provides a grim illustration of how such devastating and deadly viruses attack a human host. Everyone infected began with sudden onset of high fever and chills, anorexia, nausea, abdominal pain, sore throat, headache, prostration, and an expressionless face. Some of these cases proceeded on the fifth day to the hemorrhagic phase that began with rash on the trunk. Bleeding was clearly evident from ulcerations in the mouth, on the lips, gingival areas, from the ear, and all of these patients died within about one week.[1052] Interestingly, 381 adults from five areas in the Malagasy Republic (Madagascar) were tested for antibodies against ebola virus and 4.5% proved positive. But no hemorrhagic syndrome was found associated with this virus in these patients and it may represent a less pathogenic strain.[710]

Clinical control of the lethal hemorrhagic fever viruses requires discovery of new and very effective antiviral drugs. So far best results have been obtained with ribavirin (*11*) and this approach has been nicely developed by Huggins and colleagues.[443] Ribavirin has proved useful against Crimean-Congo hemorrhagic fever virus in the mouse. In the Peoples' Republic of China this drug significantly reduced mortality in hemorrhagic fever patients with renal syndrome.[443] In general ribavirin (*11*) is active against hemorrhagic fever viruses except for the ebola virus.[443] Nucleoside analog *11* was also found to inhibit replication of Rift Valley fever in the mouse and monkey.[1165] With the pichinde virus, an experimental model not pathogenic for humans,[878] chloroquine has been found to effectively inhibit its replication.[350] Obviously there remains a great need for discovery and development of new drugs against the RNA viral diseases. Successes here will contribute greatly to improving the treatment of, e.g., HIV-1 patients and those whose cancer has a viral origin. Further insights into the magnitude and urgency of these new antiviral and anticancer drug discovery problems can be ascertained from the fact that the rapid mutability of viruses will continue to produce new and lethal human viral diseases[557] such as AIOS. Just consider that HIV-1 mutates some one million times faster than eukaryotic DNA genomes.[831] Expressed another way, the HIV-1 reverse transcriptase appears to make up to ten errors during replication of the HIV genome as an important strategy for avoiding destruction by the human immune system. Certainly, plant and animal antiviral/anticancer constituents offer the best prospects for completely new structural leads and the actual new drugs necessary to combat the related attacks on our species by viruses and cancer.

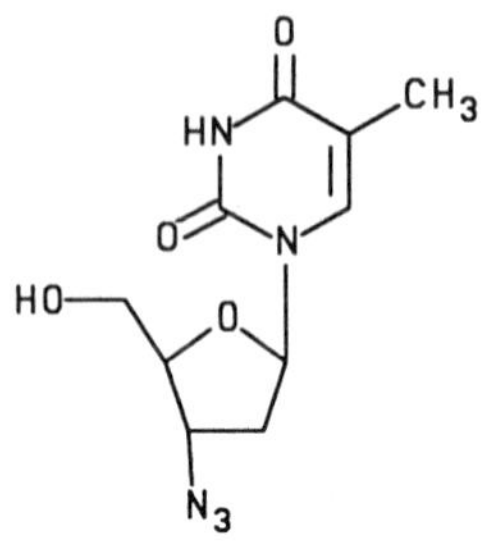

AZT

1

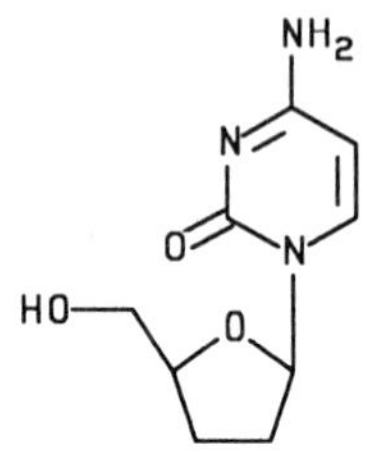

ddC

2

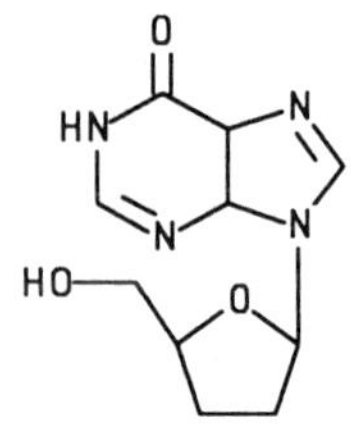

ddI

3

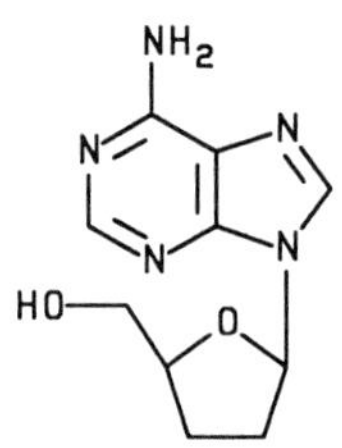

ddA

4

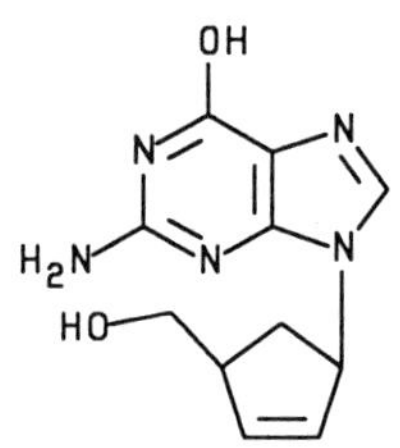

CARBOVIR

5

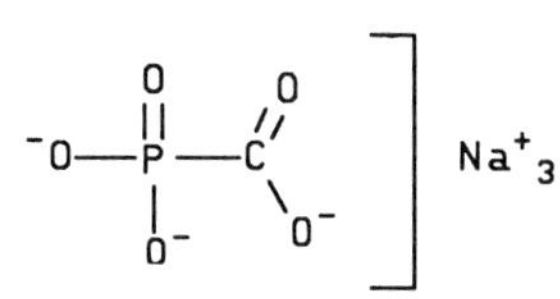

FOSCARNET

6

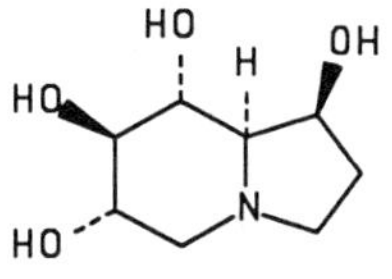

(+)-CASTANOSPERMINE

7

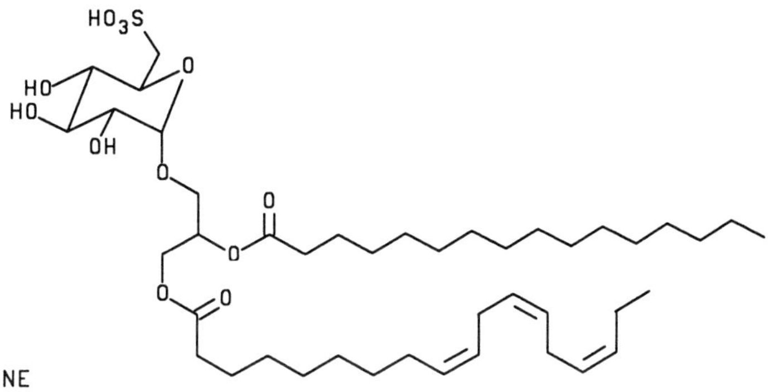

8

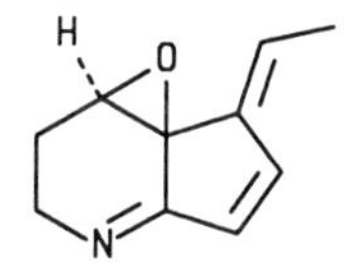

ABIKOVIROMYCIN

9

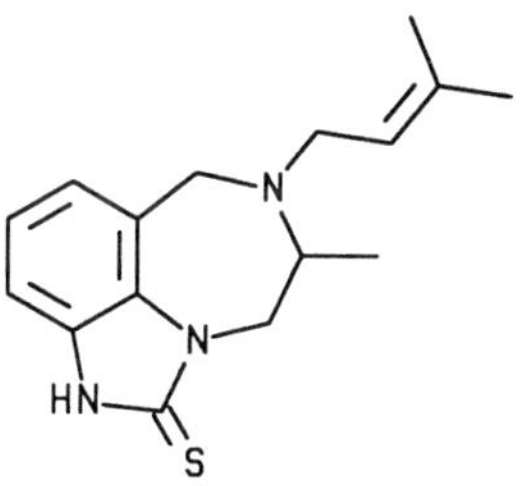

R82150

10

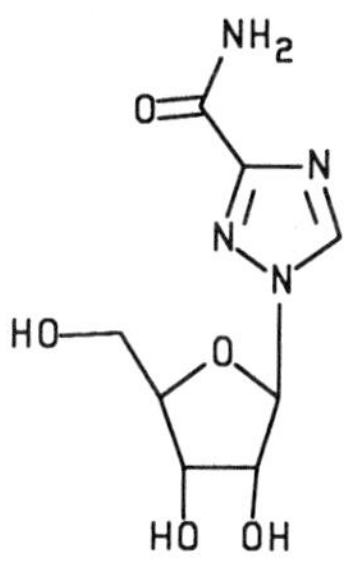

RIBAVIRIN

11

Chapter 2 TUMOR PROMOTERS AND CARCINOGENS

Environmental exposure to various tumor promoters and carcinogens constitutes a rapidly increasing public health hazard. The tables of this chapter summarize a substantial number of such substances and the carcinogenic properties of radiation. The purpose of this chapter is to illustrate the risks involved in various environmental exposures, certain cancer and/or radiation treatments and the need for more effective and safer anticancer drugs.

The historic, and still current, initial treatment course for the majority of cancer patients with life-threatening disease involves surgery and/or radiation. Most of these treatments employing radiation have not been subjected to carefully controlled clinical trials such as used to assess the value of new anticancer drugs. Hence, the real risk of exposing cancer patients to the carcinogenic and other destructive effects of radiation[544] versus potential benefits remains largely unknown.

The cancer-causing[263] properties of x-rays have been known (or suspected) for nearly a century and radiation from radioisotopes for nearly as long. Recent studies of medical x-ray technicians, e.g., in China from 1950-85 have revealed excess risk of skin cancer and leukemia as well as the possibility of breast and thyroid cancer due to occupational x-ray exposure.[1156] Furthermore, the obvious excess of leukemia in Southern Utah from 100 above ground nuclear weapons tests (50 of these deposited detectable radioactive fallout in Utah and Nevada) between 1951-58 has been well-established.[1033] In fact, the average bone marrow dose to residents of Kane County, Utah was 9.1 mGy and 19 mGy in the next county west (Washington). In general, the leukemias (possibly excepting CLL) are a predictable consequence of radiation exposure. Among Japanese atomic bomb survivors the risk of acute leukemia was about twice that for chronic granulocytic leukemia. For a series of irradiated cervical cancer patients the sequel was an excess of chronic myelogenous leukemia.[85] Skin cancer (including melanoma) from ultraviolet radiation is also well-established.[110] Here high peak and lifetime cumulative exposures combined with genetic susceptibility appear most important. Presumably mutations caused by ultraviolet radiation may reside in stem cells for decades and as the immune system becomes less effective (or already damaged by UV) over time the basal cell or squamous cell carcinomas and/or melanoma may proceed unchecked.

For several decades evidence has been accumulating that human exposure to strong magnetic fields can have serious medical consequences and lead to premature death.[811] The magnetic fields near high voltage lines have been implicated most often. Clusters of leukemia have been attributed to such fields in residential areas. Recently, evidence has been assembled that suggests certain types of household appliances (unshielded television sets, hair dryers, electric shavers, etc.) are causing an increased risk of leukemia.

The risk of developing a secondary cancer from cancer treatment is not limited to radiation. Some (cf. Table 2) of the first generation synthetic anticancer drugs and one (the nitrosoamine, streptozotocin) from a microorganism have been found to be human carcinogens.[153,161,360,777,918,1014] To date the clinically useful anticancer drugs isolated from plants or animals offer the most promise of generally avoiding carcinogenic side-effects. Illustrative here is the potent antitumor promoter bryostatin 1[413,880] now in human clinical trial. Interestingly, in a series of in vitro cell irradiation experiments the marine bryozoan constituent bryostatin 1 has been found to markedly increase the radioprotective properties of GM-CSF toward bone marrow progenitor cells.[722] In addition, the well-known plant anticancer drug etoposide (a glycoside derivative of podophyllotoxin)[1197] has displayed a protective (8.26 Gy without vs 10.35 Gy with etoposide) effect against radiation-induced bone marrow death when given to mice the day before whole-body irradiation.

Clearly, accelerating the discovery and development of naturally occurring anticancer drugs will dramatically increase prospects for greatly improving cancer treatment while reducing serious side-effects.

TABLE 1

SYNTHETIC CARCINOGENS

Compound:	**Methapyrilene**	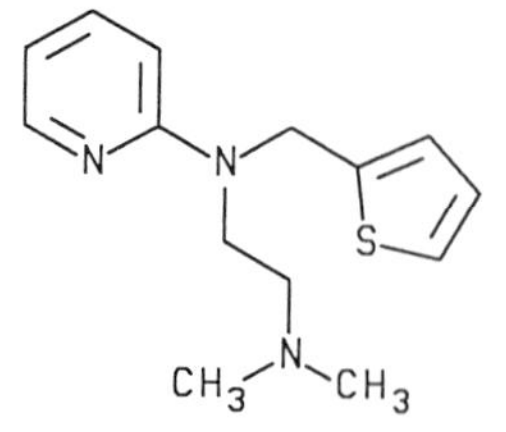
Animal Model:	Rat	
Organ Site:	Liver	
Reference:	137, 657	

Compound:	**Diethylstilbestrol** (in utero)	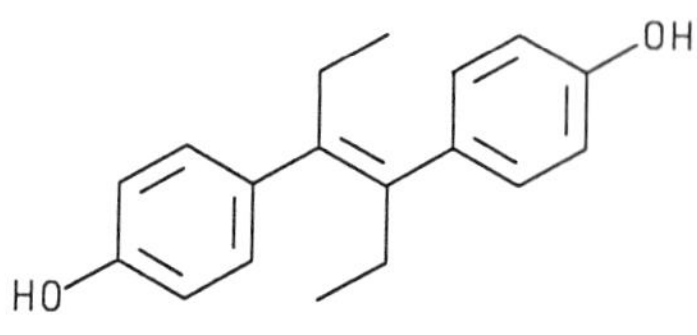
Human Site:	Cervix and vagina	
Reference:	639, 664, 665, 807	

Compound:	**Estrogens**
Animal Model:	Rodent
Organ Site:	Breast
Human Site:	Endometrium
Reference:	242, 410, 639, 664, 665, 919, 1032

Compound:	**Phenacetin**	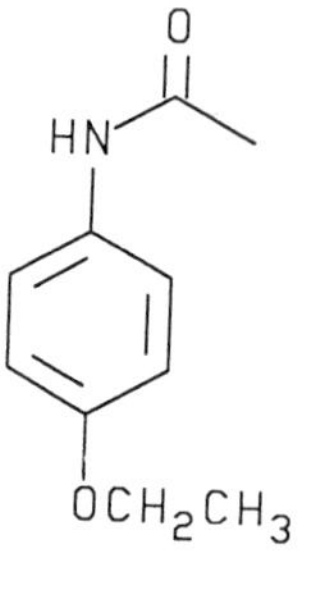
Animal Model:	Rodent	
Organ Site:	Kidney, renal pelvis, liver	
Human Site:	Renal pelvis, bladder suspect	
Reference:	194, 1098	

Compound: **Polycyclic aromatic hydrocarbons (PAH)**

Human Site: Skin, scrotum, lung, bladder

Reference: 35, 88, 242, 266, 559, 656, 990, 1028, 1029, 1088, 1139, 1157

Compound: **Benzo[a]pyrene**

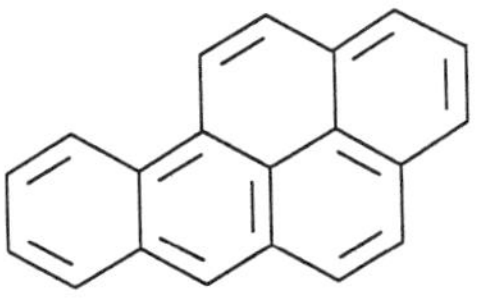

Human Site: Skin, lung, bladder, scrotum

Reference: 35, 83, 266, 656, 990, 1028, 1029, 1088, 1139

Compound: **Aromatic amines**

Animal Model: Rats, hamsters and dogs

Organ Site: Bladder, liver

Human Site: Bladder

Reference: 656, 936, 986

Compound: **β-Naphthylamine**

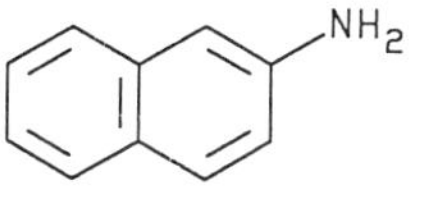

Human Site: Bladder

Reference: 936, 986, 990

Compound: **4-Methoxy-m-phenylenediamine**

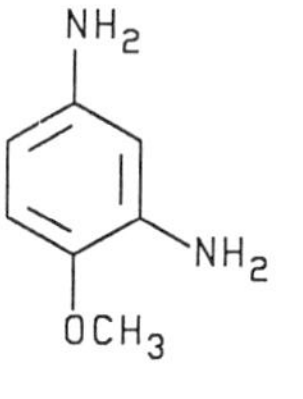

Animal Model: Mouse and rat

Organ Site: Skin, lymph, thyroid

Reference: 139

Compound: **Glu-P-1 (2-amino-6-methyl-dipyrido[1,2-a:3',2'-d]imidazole)**

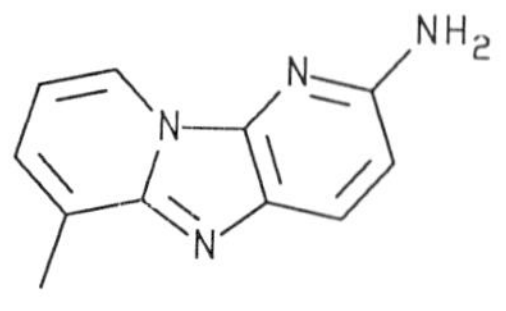

Animal Model: a) Mouse, b) rat

Organ Site: a) Liver, blood vessel
b) liver, intestines, zymbal gland, clitoral gland

Reference: 1042

Compound: **Glu-P-2 (2-aminodipyrido-[1,2-a:3',2'-d]imidazole)**

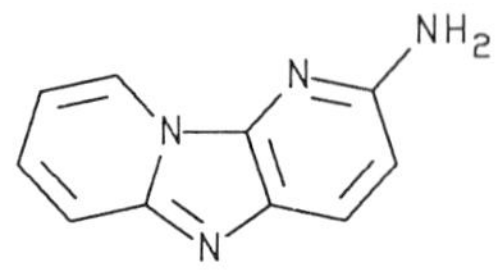

Animal Model: a) Mouse, b) rat

Organ Site: a) Liver, blood vessel
b) liver, intestines, zymbal gland, clitoral gland

Reference: 1042

Compound: **AαC (2-amino-α-carboline)**

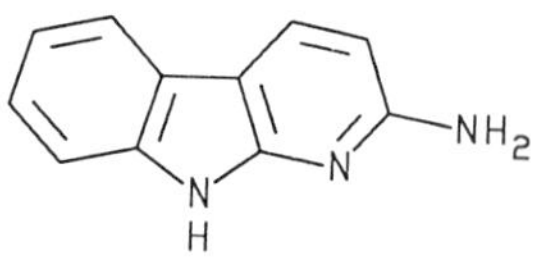

Animal Model: a) Mouse, b) rat

Organ Site: a) Liver, blood vessel
b) liver

Reference: 1042

Compound: **MeAαC (2-amino-3-methyl-α-carboline)**

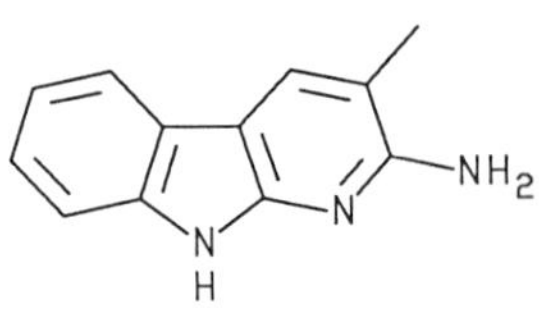

Animal Model: Mouse

Organ Site: Liver, blood vessel

Reference: 1042

Compound: **Trp-P-1 (3-amino-1,4-dimethyl-5H-pyrido[4,3-b]indole)**

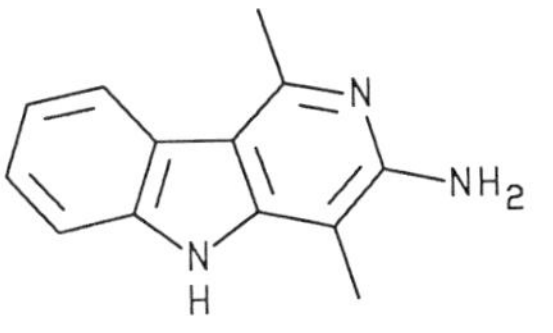

Animal Model: a) Mouse, b) rat

Organ Site: a) Liver, bladder
b) liver

Reference: 306, 402, 609, 625, 917, 1042

Compound: **Trp-P-2 (3-amino-1-methyl-5H-pyrido[4,3-b]indole)**

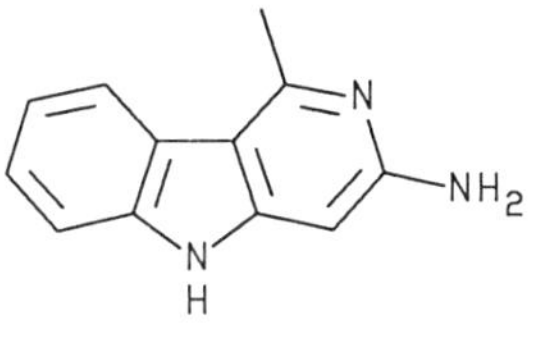

Animal Model: a) Mouse, b) rat

Organ Site: a) Liver, bladder
b) liver

Reference: 402, 609, 625, 917, 1042

Compound: **IQ (2-amino-3-methylimidazo-[4,5-f]quinoline)**

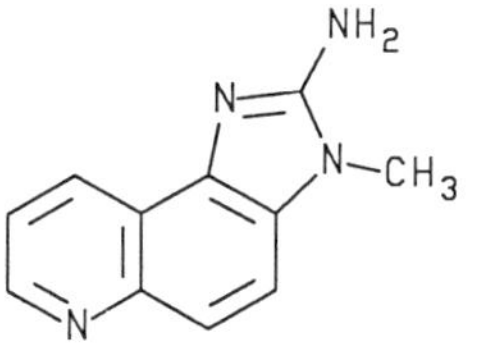

Animal Model: a) Mouse, b) rat

Organ Site: a) Liver, forestomach, lung
b) liver, intestines, zymbal gland, clitoral gland, skin, oral cavity

Reference: 517, 611, 625, 817, 917, 1030, 1042

Compound: **Me-IQ (2-amino-3,4-dimethylimidazo-[4,5-f]quinoline)**

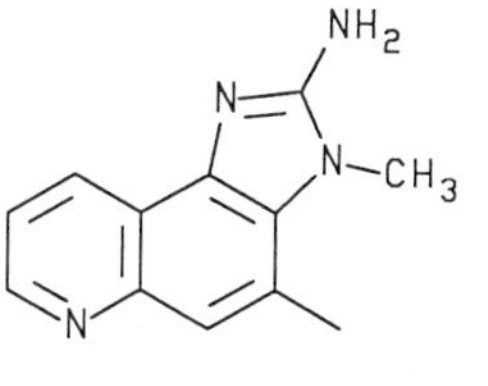

Animal Model: Mouse

Organ Site: Liver, forestomach, intestines

Reference: 518, 625, 817, 917, 1042

Compound: **N-Methyl-N-nitrosourea**

Animal Model: Many species

Organ Site: Various organs; oropharynx and esophagus in monkey

Reference: 415, 559, 899, 900, 1015, 1154, 1205

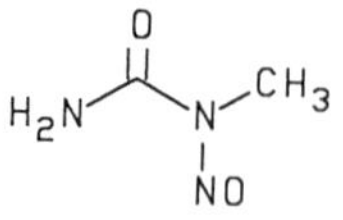

Compound: **1-Butyl-1-nitrosourea (BNU)**

Animal Model: a) Mouse, b) rat, c) dog

Organ Site:
a) Lung, liver, lymph, blood, nervous system
b) blood, breast, ovary, brain, kidney, nervous system
c) stomach

Reference: 310, 900

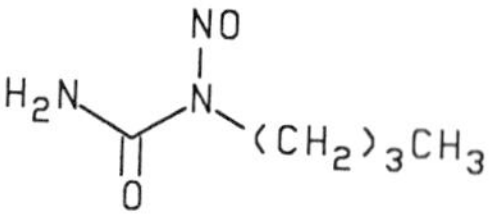

Compound: **N-Nitrosodiethanolamine**

Animal Model: Rat

Organ Site: Liver (weakly)

Reference: 281, 899, 981

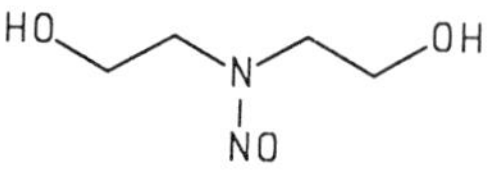

Compound: **Tris(2,3-dibromopropyl)phosphate**

Animal Model: Mouse and rat

Organ Site: Kidney, colon, skin, forestomach, oral

Human Site: Kidney

Reference: 80, 922, 1138

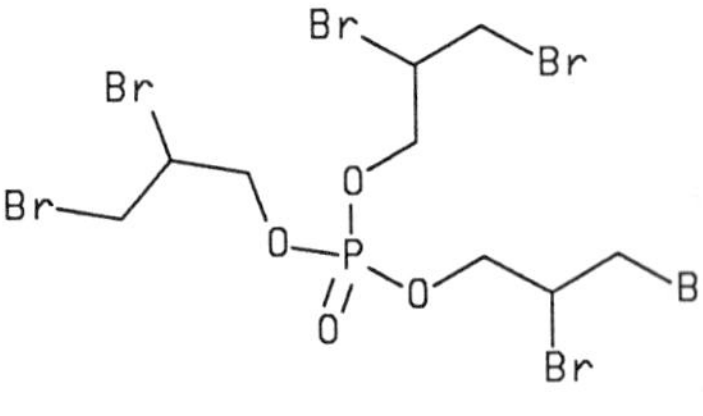

Compound: **Bis(chloromethyl)ether and chloromethyl methyl ether**

$ClCH_2-O-CH_2Cl$,

$ClCH_2-O-CH_3$

Human Site: Lung

Reference: 192, 361, 1098

Compound: **Organochlorine pesticides**

Human Site: Brain (glioma)

Reference: 197

Compound: **Pesticides**

Human Site: Lung, blood (childhood leukemia), brain

Reference: 77, 138

Compound: **Toxaphene**

Animal Model: a) Rat, b) mouse

Organ Site: a) Thyroid, follicles
b) liver, pituitary gland (female)

Reference: 361, 805

Compound: **Herbicides**

Human Site: Lymph (non-Hodgkin's lymphoma)

Reference: 76, 430

Compound: **2,4-Dichlorophenoxyacetic acid**

Human Site: Lymph (non-Hodgkin's lymphoma)

Reference: 76, 430

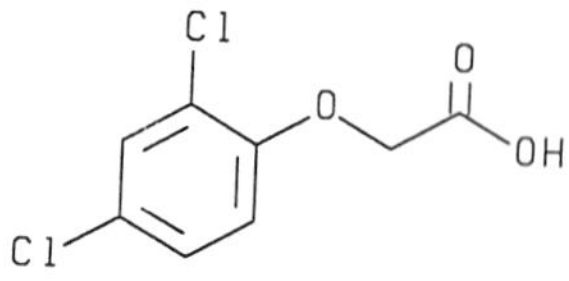

Compound: **1,2-Dichloroethane [ethylene dichloride]**

Animal Model: a) Mouse, b) rat

Organ Site: a) Forestomach, circulatory system, breast (female), skin (male)
b) respiratory tract, breast (female), endometrium

Reference: 806, 1169

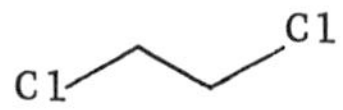

Compound: **Chloroform**

Animal Model: a) Male rat, male Swiss mouse
b) B6C3F1 mouse

Organ Site: a) Kidney
b) liver

Reference: 140, 361, 637, 1186

$CHCl_3$

Compound: **Vinyl chloride**

Human Site: Liver (angiosarcoma)

Reference: 815, 990

$CH_2{=}CHCl$

Compound: **Polyvinyl chloride**

Human Site: Mouth (site of exposure)

Reference: 159

Compound: **Vinylidene chloride (1,1-Dichloroethylene)**

Animal Model: Mouse

Organ Site: Kidney

$ClCH{=}CHCl$

Reference: 361, 1143

Compound: **Bis(2-chloroethyl)sulfide [mustard gas]**

Animal Model: Mouse

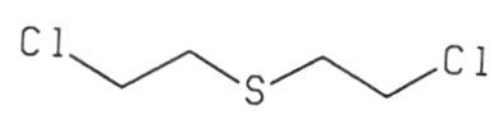

Organ Site: Lung

Human Site: Upper respiratory tract

Reference: 251, 637

Compound: **Acrylonitrile**

Animal Model: Rat

Organ Site: Stomach, central nervous system, ear canal

$CH_2{=}CHCN$

Reference: 3, 111

Compound:	**CFC 11**	
Human Site:	Skin (via depletion of ozone layer)	CCl_3F
Reference:	501	

Compound:	**CFC 12**	
Human Site:	Skin (via depletion of ozone)	CCl_2F_2
Reference:	501	

Compound:	**CFC 113**	
Human Site:	Skin (via ozone depletion)	$C_2Cl_3F_3$
Reference:	501	

Compound:	**Carbon tetrachloride**	
Animal Model:	Mouse and rat	
Organ Site:	Liver	CCl_4
Human Site:	Skin (via ozone depletion)	
Reference:	361, 501	

Compound:	**1,1,1-Trichloroethane (methyl chloroform)**	
Human Site:	Skin (via ozone depletion)	CH_3CCl_3
Reference:	501	

Compound: **Halones 1211**

Human Site: Skin (via ozone depletion)

Reference: 501

Compound: **Halones 1301**

Human Site: Skin (via ozone depletion)

Reference: 501

Compound: **Nitric oxide**

Human Site: Skin (via ozone depletion)

Reference: 501

Compound: **Silicone gel (used in breast implants)**

Animal Model: Rats

Organ Site: "Solid-state" tumors

Reference: 956

Compound: **2-Nitropropane**

Animal Model: Rat

Organ Site: Liver

Reference: 1132

20

Compound: **Ethyl oxide**

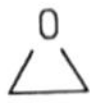

Human Site: Blood (leukemia)

Reference: 432

Table 2

CARCINOGENIC ANTITUMOR DRUGS

Compound: **Dacarbazine (DTIC)**

Animal Model: Rat, mouse

Organ Site: Lymph, blood, breast, lung, uterus

Human Site: Blood (leukemia)

Reference: 898, 1168

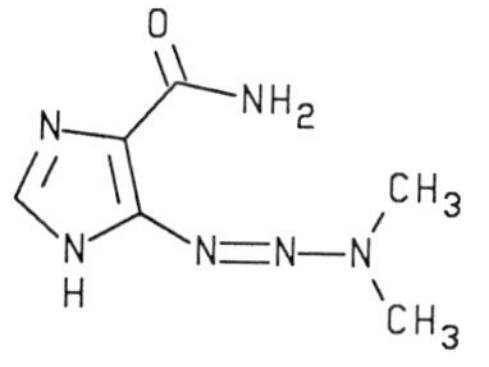

Compound: **6-Mercaptopurine**

Animal Model: Rat, mouse

Organ Site: Pituitary, breast, skin, blood, lymph, lung, testis

Reference: 1168

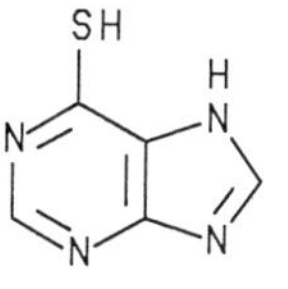

Compound: **Streptozotocin**

Animal Model: Rat, mouse

Organ Site: Kidney, lung

Reference: 1168

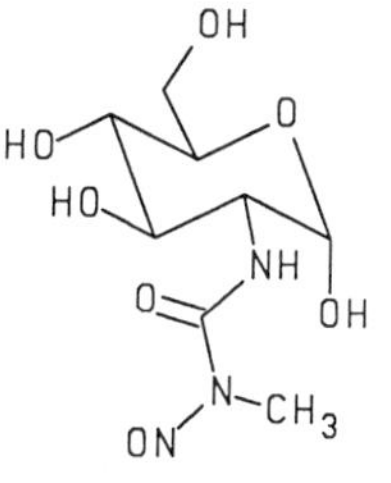

Compound: **Melphalan**

Animal Model: Mouse

Organ Site: Lymph, lung

Human Site: Blood (leukemia)

Reference: 360, 1014, 1168

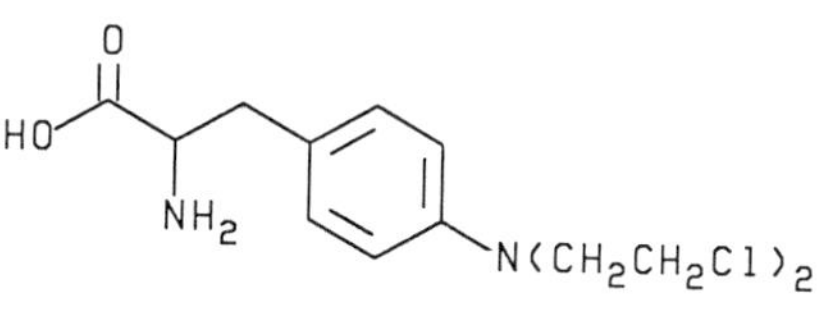

Compound: **Chlorambucil**

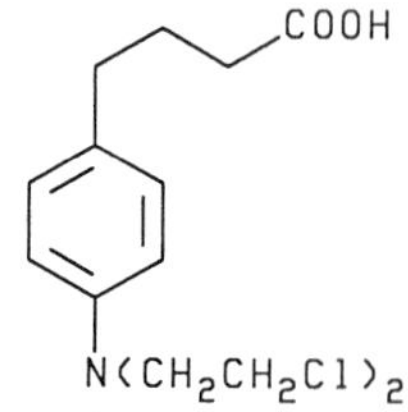

Animal Model: a) Mouse, b) rat

Organ Site: a) Lung, lymph, ovary
b) lymph, blood

Human Site: Blood (leukemia)

Reference: 194, 1098

Compound: **Chlornaphazine**

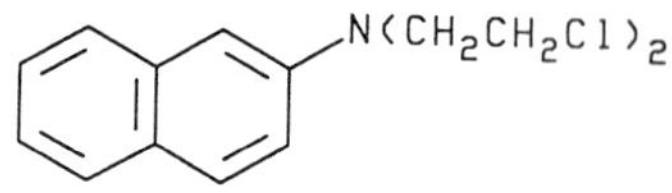

Human Site: Bladder

Reference: 1168

Compound: **Uracil mustard**

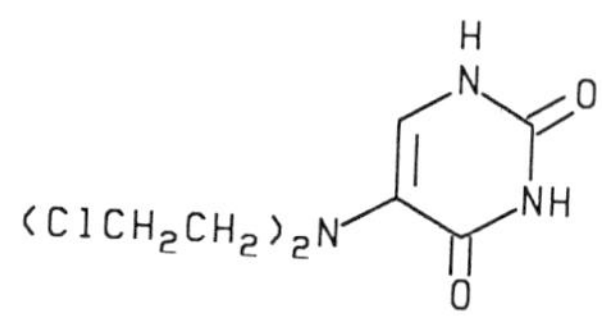

Animal Model: Mouse

Organ Site: Lung

Reference: 637

Compound: **Procarbazine**

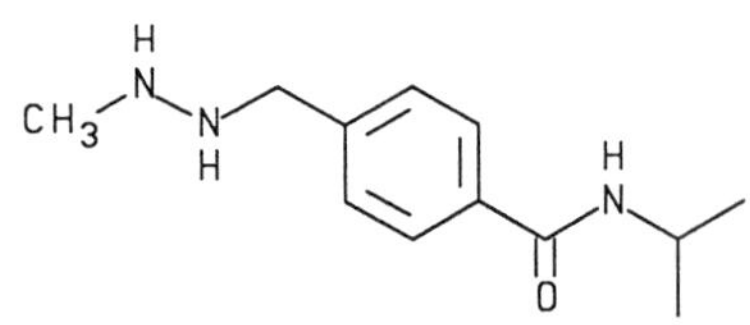

Animal Model: Monkey, mouse, rat

Organ Site: Blood (leukemia), lung,
lymph, breast

Reference: 1015, 1168

Compound: **Cisplatin**

Animal Model: Mouse, rat

Organ Site: Lung, skin, blood (leukemia)

Reference: 414

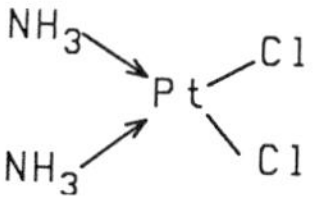

Compound: **Cyclophosphamide (cytoxan)**

Animal Model: Rat, mouse

Organ Site: Bladder, others, lung, breast, others

Human Site: Blood (leukemia), bladder

Reference: 194, 428, 637, 898, 1014

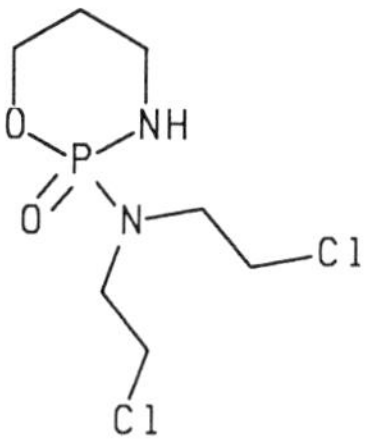

Compound: **Methyl-CCNU (semustine)**

Animal Model: Rat

Organ Site: Nervous system, forestomach, lung

Human Site: Blood (leukemia)

Reference: 86, 153, 900, 1168

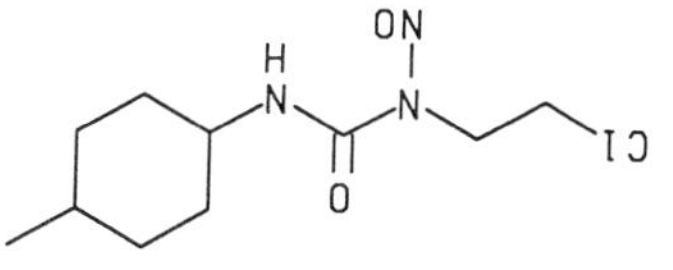

Compound: **AZT (zidovudine)**

Animal Model: Rodent

Organ Site: Vagina

Reference: 1150

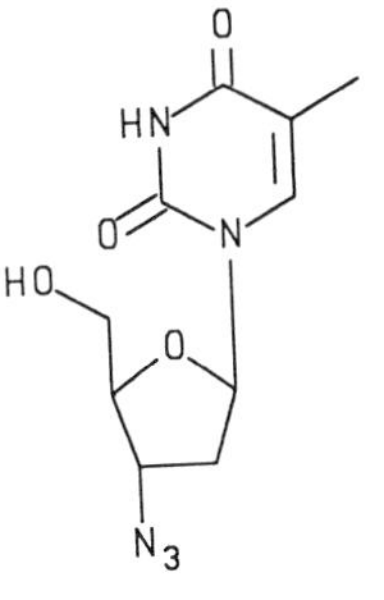

Compound: **Combination chemotherapy**

Human Site: Blood (leukemia)

Reference: 86, 153, 161, 360, 367, 396, 412, 879, 898, 1014, 1168

TABLE 3

ENVIRONMENTAL AND OTHER NATURALLY OCCURRING CARCINOGENS

Compound: **Formaldehyde**

Animal Model: Rat

Organ Site: Nasopharynx

Reference: 1, 16, 78, 294, 358, 388, 408, 949, 990

Compound: **Reserpine**

Animal Model: Mouse

Organ Site: Breast (female), seminal vesicle

Reference: 194, 665

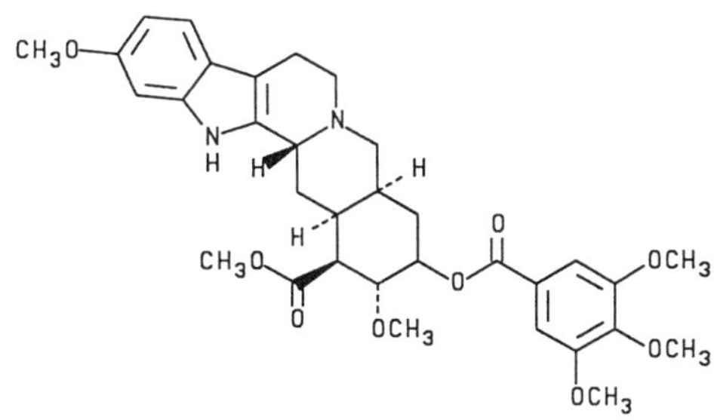

Compound: **Methyl testosterone**

Human Site: Liver

Reference: 106

Compound: **Cadmium**

Animal Model: Rat

Organ Site: Lung

Human Site: Inconclusive

Reference: 40, 62, 387, 990, 1076

Compound: **Lead**

Animal Model: Rat

Organ Site: Kidney

Reference: 763

Compound: **Arsenic**

Human Site: Skin, lung

Reference: 810, 990

Compound: **Beryllium**

Human Site: Lung

Reference: 990

Compound: **Nickel (refining)**

Human Site: Sinonasal area, lung

Reference: 273, 919, 990, 1101

Compound: **Chromium (hexavalent compounds)**

Human Site: Lung

Reference: 242, 826, 990

Compound: **Asbestos**

Human Site: Lung, pleura, peritoneum

Reference: 242, 597, 815, 826, 919, 990

Compound: **Tobacco/cigarette smoking**

Animal Model: Rat, hamster

Organ Site: Respiratory tract

Human Site: Lung, mouth, pharynx, larynx, esophagus, bladder, pancreas

Reference: 44, 119, 169, 242, 283, 308, 419, 504, 919, 1088, 1098, 1129, 1142, 1196

Compound: **Nicotine**

Animal Model: Hamster

Organ Site: Cheek pouch

Reference: 169

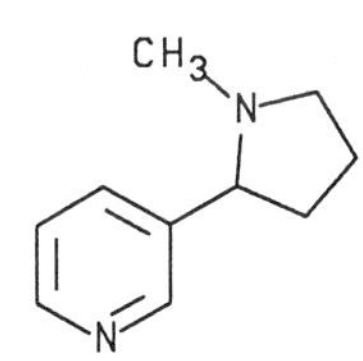

Compound: **Betel nut extract**

Animal Model: Hamster

Organ Site: Buccal pouch

Human Site: Oral cavity; esophagus

Reference: 1053, 1172

Compound: **Diet**

Human Site: Stomach

Reference: 190, 231, 357, 676, 724, 1104, 1214

Compound: **Fat/cholesterol**

Human Site: Breast, endometrium, colon, lung

Reference: 242, 729, 919, 990, 1184, 1195

Compound: **Pyrrolizidine alkaloids**

Animal Model: Laboratory animals

Organ Site: Liver

Reference: 226, 359

Compound: **Alcohol**

Human Site: Mouth, pharynx, esophagus, larynx, breast, liver

Reference: 119, 242, 308, 309, 400, 505, 636, 652, 721, 919, 977, 1099, 1113, 1114, 1142, 1178, 1183

Compound: **Aflatoxins B_1 and G_1**

Animal Model: Various vertebrate spp.

Organ Site: Liver, other organs in certain spp.

Human Site: Liver

Reference: 16, 54, 121, 242, 359, 873

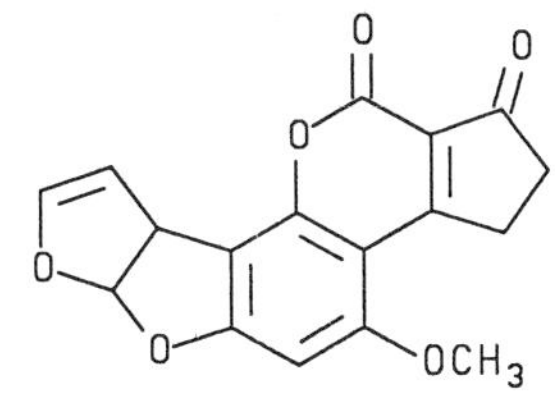

Aflatoxin B_1

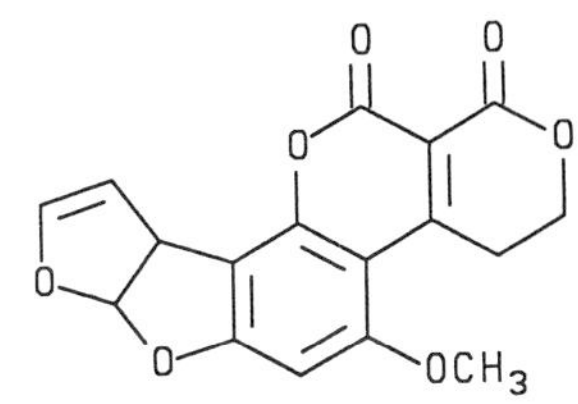

Aflatoxin G_1

Compound: **N'-Nitrosonornicotine (NNN)**

Animal Model:
a) Rat
b) Mouse
c) Golden hamster

Organ Site:
a) Esophagus, pharynx, nasal cavity
b) Lung
c) Trachea, nasal cavity

Reference: 420

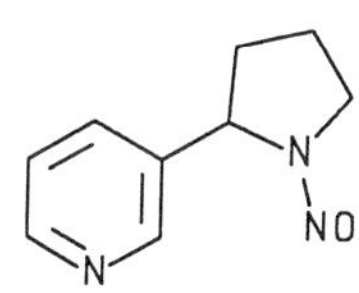

Compound: **N'-Nitrosoanabasine (NAB)**

Animal Model: Rat

Organ Site: Esophagus, pharynx, nasal cavity

Reference: 420

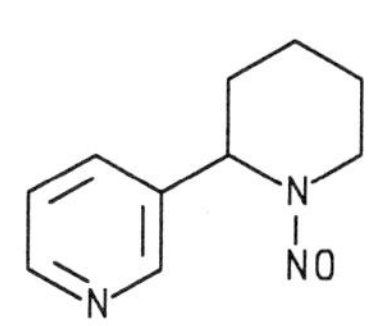

Compound: **Diethylnitrosamine (DENA)**

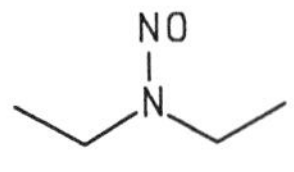

Animal Model:
a) Rat
b) Mouse
c) Chinese hamster
d) Monkey

Organ Site:
a) Liver, esophagus
b) Esophagus
c) Esophagus
d) Liver

Reference: 349, 653, 678, 899, 1015, 1082, 1148, 1154

Compound: **Dimethylnitrosamine (DMNA)**

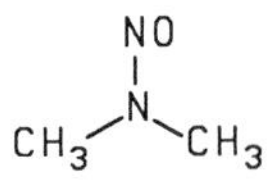

Animal Model: Various spp.

Organ Site: Liver, lung, kidney, others in several spp.

Human Site: Liver suspect

Reference: 349, 359, 653, 678, 899, 900, 1082, 1148

Compound: **Methylbenzylnitrosamine (MBNA)**

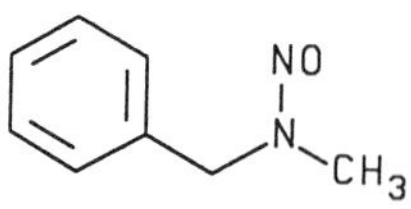

Animal Model: Rat, mouse

Organ Site: Esophagus

Reference: 349, 653

Compound:	**1,1-Dimethylhydrazine**
Animal Model:	a) Rat; b) mouse
Organ Site:	a) Colon, liver, kidney b) Lung, blood vessel, kidney and liver
Reference:	936, 981, 1219

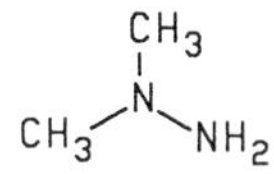

Compound:	**Benzene**
Human Site:	Bone marrow, lymph nodes, blood (leukemia)
Reference:	154, 358, 726

Compound:	**Methylglyoxal**
Animal Model:	Rat
Organ Site:	Subcutaneous tumors (injection site)
Reference:	788

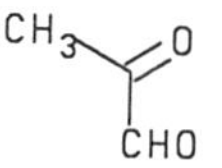

Compound:	**Ptaquiloside**
Animal Model:	a) Rat; b) sheep; c) cow
Organ Site:	a) Ileum, bladder, breast (female) b) Intestine, bladder c) Digestive tract, bladder
Reference:	276, 424, 554, 844, 845

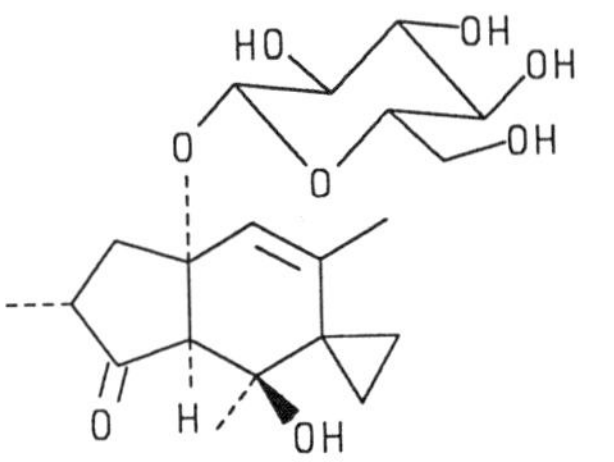

Compound: **Cyclosporine/Cyclosporin A**

Human Site: Skin (squamous cell)

Reference: 692, 901

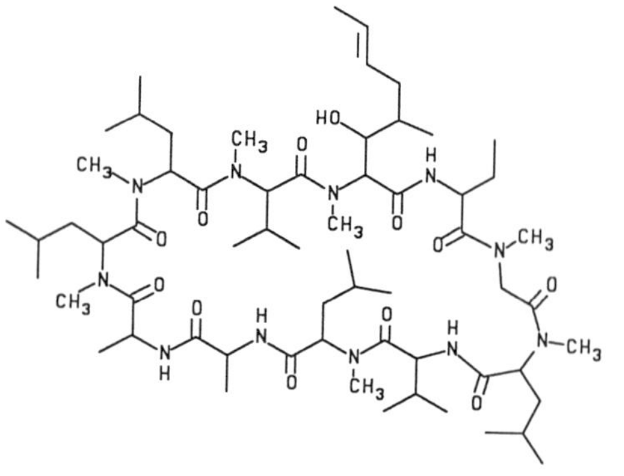

Compound: **Safrole (1-Allyl-3,4-methylenedioxybenzene)**

Animal Model: Rat

Organ Site: Liver

Reference: 992

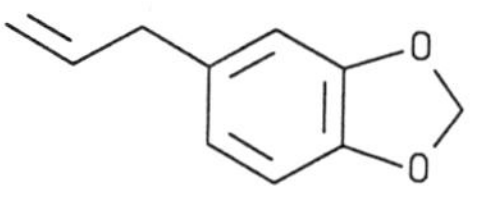

Compound: **Gasoline**

Animal Model: Male rat

Organ Site: Kidney

Reference: 342

Compound: **Diesel fumes, coal dust**

Human Site: Lung

Reference: 442

Compound: **Vulcanization**

Human Site: Esophagus

Reference: 825

Compound: **Presence of gallstones**

Human Site: Gallbladder

Reference: 677

Compound: **Urogenous contact**

Human Site: Bladder

Reference: 109

Compound: **ras Oncogene**

Human Site: Pancreas, colon/rectum, lung, skin

Reference: 23, 156, 976, 1102

TABLE 4

CARCINOGENIC IRRADIATION

Type:	**U.V. + pigmentation**
Human Site:	Skin: basal cell carcinoma; squamous cell carcinoma (and solar keratoses)
Reference:	23, 59, 203, 700, 750, 771, 1051, 1131, 1174, 1175, 1176, 1177
Type:	**U.V. + pigmentation + age at and type of exposure**
Human Site:	Skin: malignant melanoma; Eyes: intraocular malignant melanoma
Reference:	22, 59, 155, 203, 239, 265, 421, 642, 689, 743, 1051, 1111, 1131, 1174, 1175, 1176, 1177
Type:	**Electromagnetic fields**
Human Site:	Blood (leukemia) and brain suspect
Reference:	299, 811
Type:	**γ-Radiation, neutrons (nuclear fallout)**
Human Site:	Blood (leukemia), lung, thyroid, breast, colon, urinary tract
Reference:	89, 131, 212, 594, 792, 914, 1097, 1128, 1129, 1130

Type:	**Uranium mining, radon daughters**
Human Site:	Lung
Reference:	34, 394, 622, 675, 775, 912, 973, 1128

Type:	**Radium/α-particles, plutonium**
Animal Model:	Beagle, mouse
Organ Site:	Bone
Human Site:	Bone
Reference:	34, 674, 775, 911, 914, 1128

Type:	**X-ray, internal α-particles, radium**
Human Site:	Blood (leukemia), breast, soft tissue, thyroid, mouth, bone, skin
Reference:	112, 149, 212, 222, 328, 399, 775, 808, 857, 1016, 1017, 1128, 1129, 1130, 1155

Type:	**Irradiation/radium implant (in pelvis)**
Human Site:	Bladder, kidneys, rectum, ovaries, corpus uteri and non-Hodgkin's lymphoma
Reference:	572

Type:	**Cobalt-60 irradiation**
Human Site:	Site of therapeutic irradiation (angiosarcoma)
Reference:	168

Type:	**Irradiation + chemotherapy**
Human Site:	Breast, blood (leukemia), esophagus, stomach, skin, cervix
Reference:	115, 149, 352, 367, 699, 808, 977, 1089

TABLE 5

SYNTHETIC TUMOR PROMOTERS

Compound:	**Benzoyl peroxide**	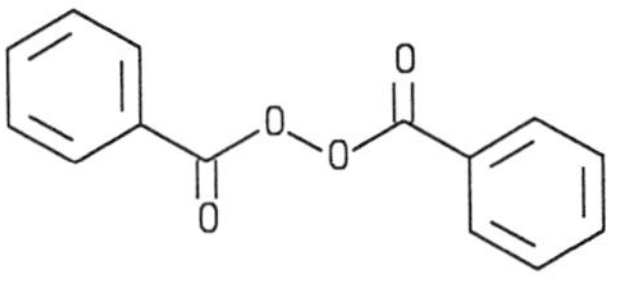
Animal Model:	Mouse	
Organ Site:	Skin [initiated with dimethylbenz[a]-anthracene (DMBA)]	
Reference:	500	

Compound:	**Chrysarobin (1,8-Dihydroxy-3-methoxy-19-anthrone)**	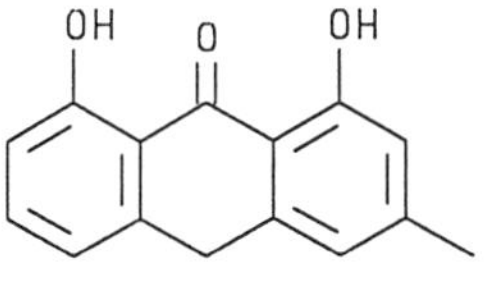
Animal Model:	Mouse	
Organ Site:	Skin (initiated with DMBA)	
Reference:	612	

TABLE 6

NATURALLY OCCURRING TUMOR PROMOTERS

Compound:	**Caffeine + unsaturated fat**
Animal Model:	Rat
Organ Site:	DMBA-induced breast cancer promotion
Reference:	742, 980

Compound:	**L-Isoleucine**
Animal Model:	Rat
Organ Site:	Bladder [initiated with N-butyl-N-(4-hydroxybutyl)nitrosamine (BHBN)]
Reference:	820

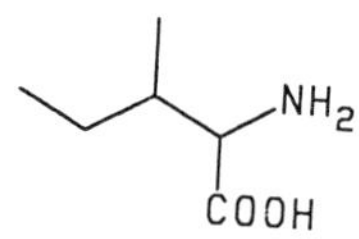

Compound:	**L-Leucine**
Animal Model:	Rat
Organ Site:	Bladder (initiated with BHBN)
Reference:	820

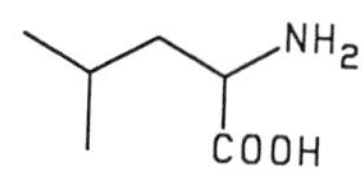

Compound:	**$\underline{N}^{13}$-Desmethylteleocidin A-1**
Animal Model:	Mouse
Organ Site:	Skin
Reference:	462, 980

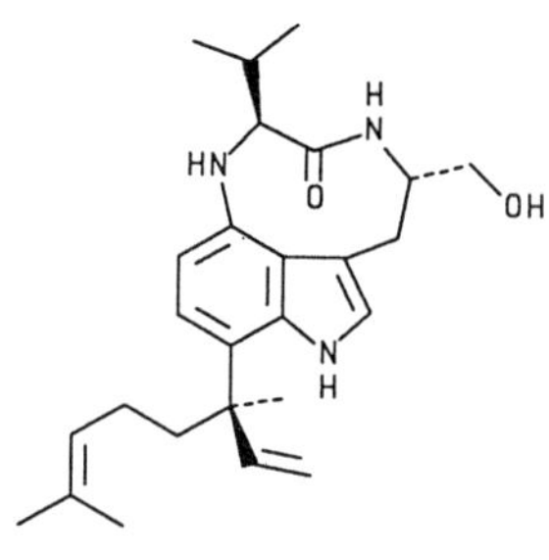

Compound: **$\underline{N}^{13}$-Desmethylteleocidin B-4**

Animal Model: Mouse

Organ Site: Skin

Reference: 462, 967

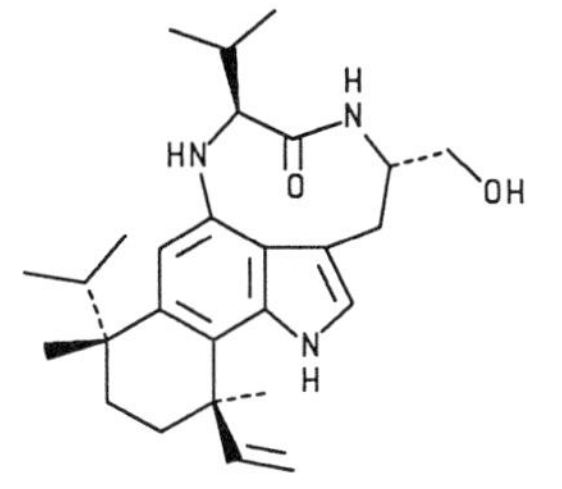

Compound: **Phorbol 12,13-dibutyrate**

Animal Model: Mouse

Organ Site: Skin and others

Reference: 246, 440

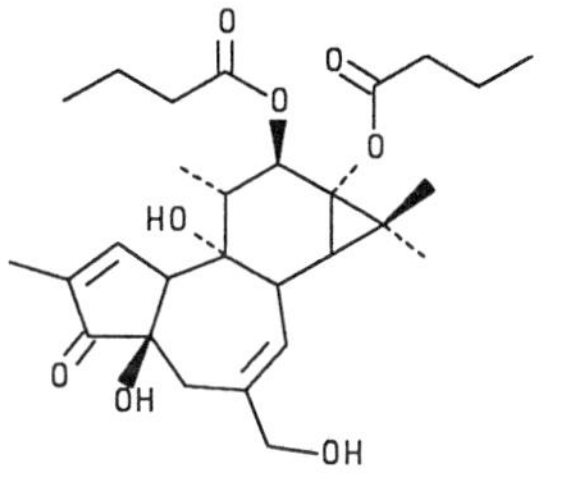

Compound: **TPA (12-$\underline{O}$-Tetradecanoylphorbol-13-acetate)**

Animal Model: Mouse, hamster

Organ Site: Skin (initiated with DMBA)

Reference: 311, 790, 980, 1019, 1096, 1167

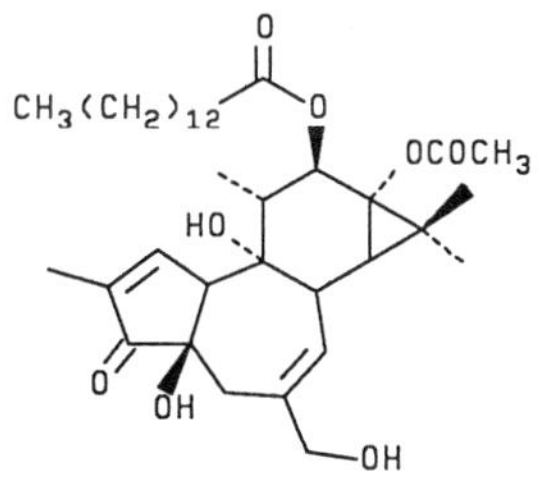

Compound: **Teleocidin A-1 (Lyngbyatoxin A)**

Animal Model: Mouse

Organ Site: Skin (initiated with DMBA)

Reference: 311, 966, 967

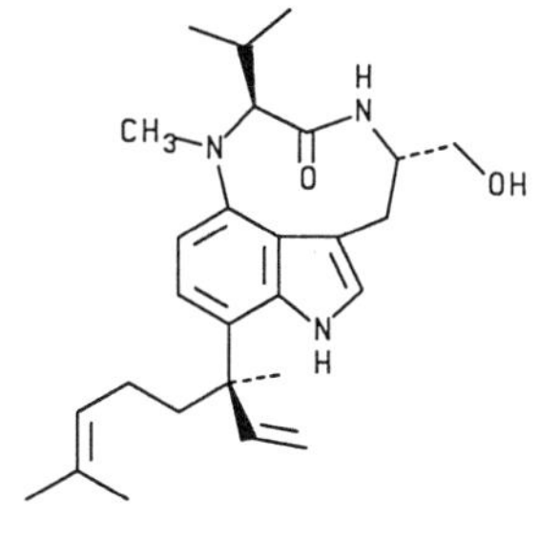

Compound: **Teleocidin A-2**

Animal Model: Mouse

Organ Site: Skin (initiated with DMBA)

Reference: 311, 966, 967

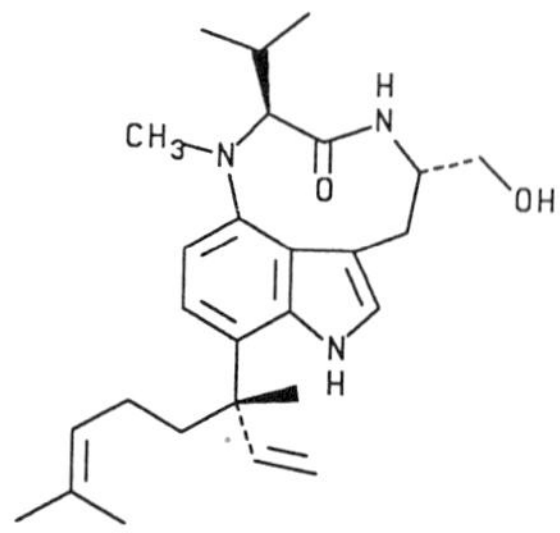

Compound: **Teleocidin B-1 (Des-O-methylolivoretin B)**

Animal Model: Mouse

Organ Site: Skin (initiated with DMBA)

Reference: 311, 429, 1096

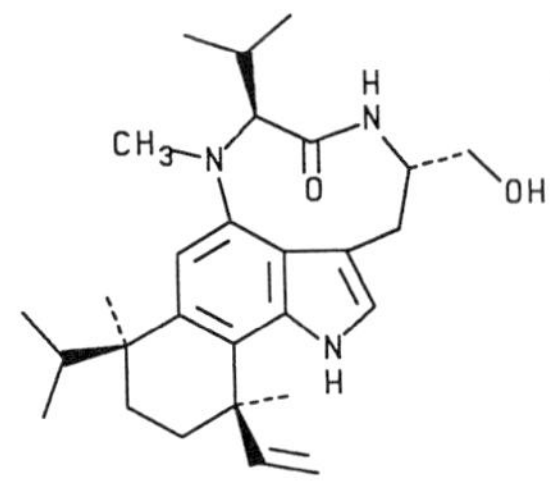

Compound: **Teleocidin B-2**

Animal Model: Mouse

Organ Site: Skin (initiated with DMBA)

Reference: 311, 429

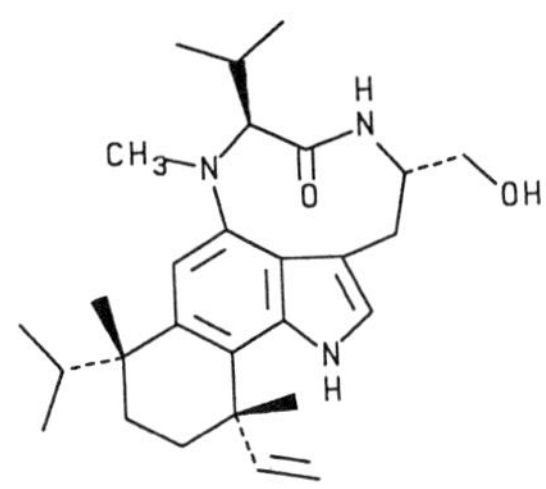

Compound: **Teleocidin B-3**

Animal Model: Mouse

Organ Site: Skin (initiated with DMBA)

Reference: 311, 429

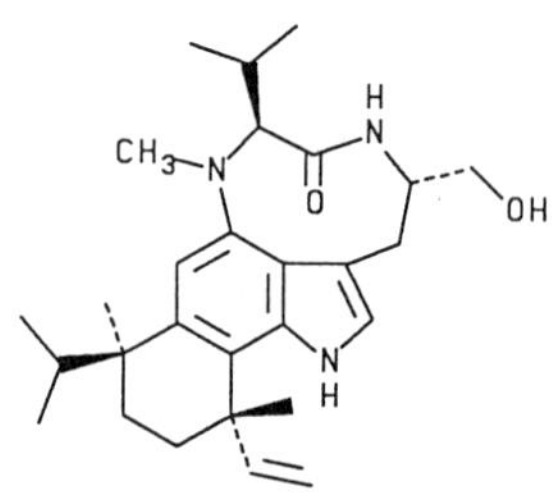

Compound: **Teleocidin B-4 (Olivoretin D)**

Animal Model: Mouse

Organ Site: Skin (initiated with DMBA)

Reference: 311, 429

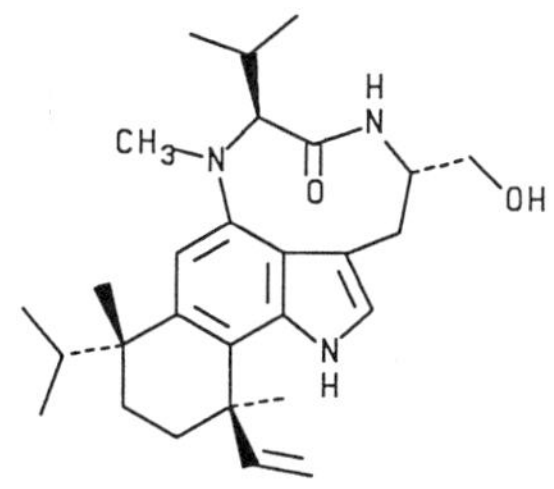

Compound: **Des-O-methylolivoretin C**

Animal Model: Mouse

Organ Site: Skin (initiated with DMBA)

Reference: 311

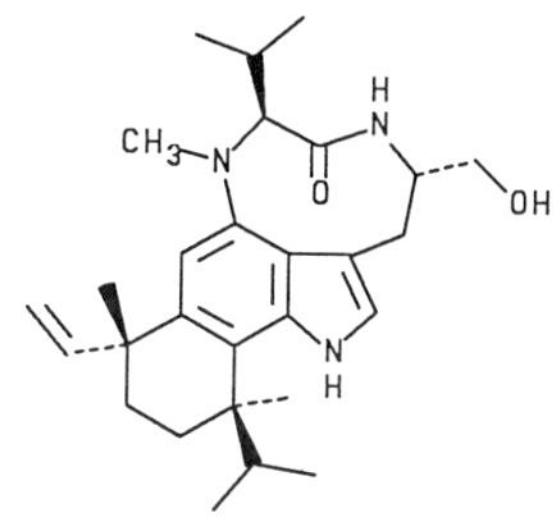

Compound: **(-)-Indolactam-V**

Animal Model: Mouse

Organ Site: Skin (initiated with DMBA)

Reference: 311

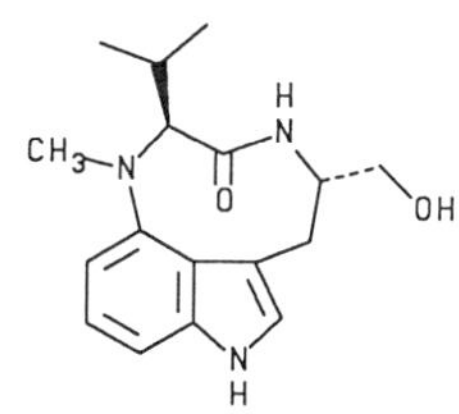

Compound: **Staurosporine**

Animal Model: Mouse

Organ Site: Skin (initiated with DMBA)

Reference: 311

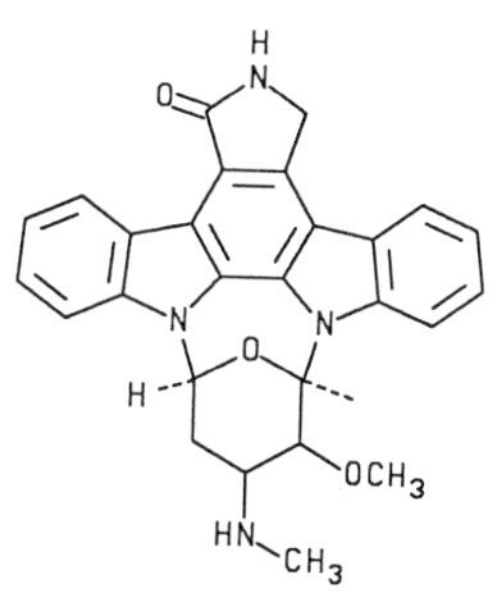

Compound: **Thapsigargin**

Animal Model: Mouse

Organ Site: Skin (initiated with DMBA)

Reference: 311

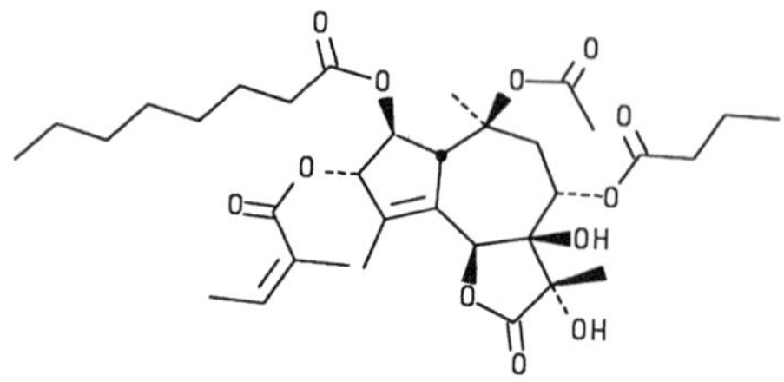

Compound: **DHPB**

Animal Model: Mouse

Organ Site: Skin (initiated with DMBA)

Reference: 311, 425

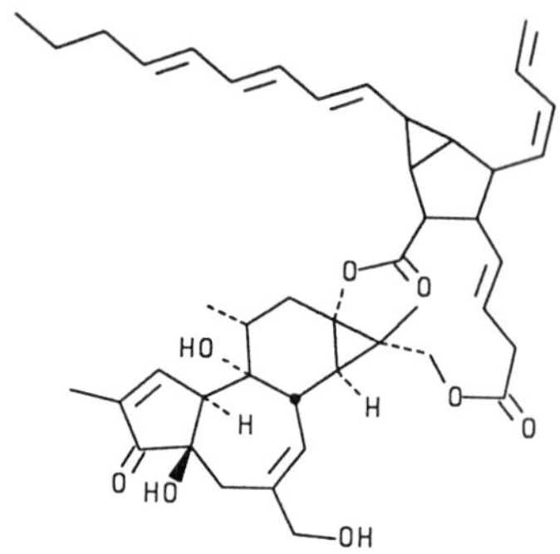

Compound: **Debromoaplysiatoxin**

Animal Model: Mouse

Organ Site: Skin (initiated with DMBA)

Reference: 311, 461, 864

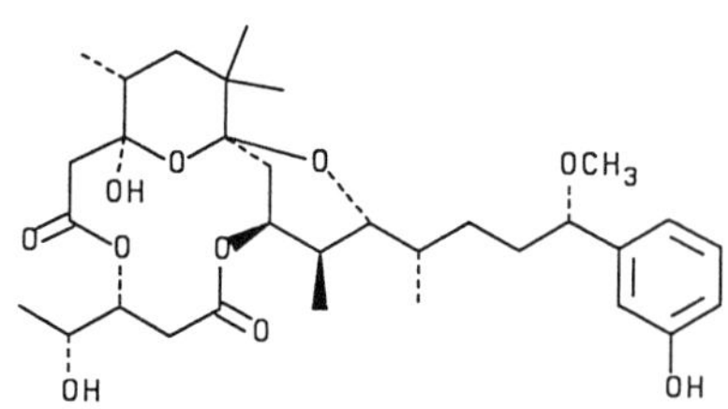

Compound: **Aplysiatoxin**

Animal Model: Mouse

Organ Site: Skin (initiated with DMBA)

Reference: 311, 461, 864

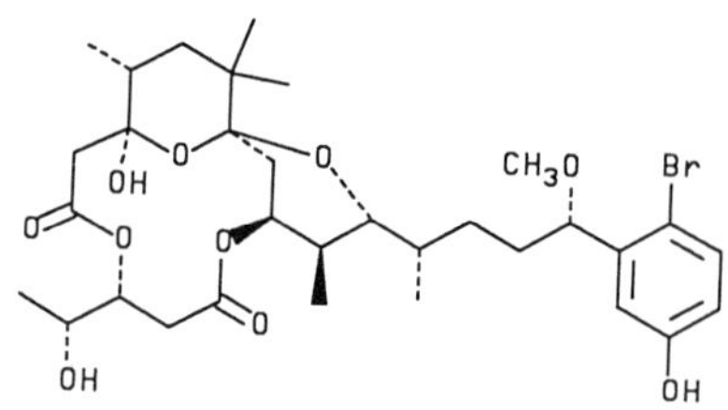

Compound: **Bromoaplysiatoxin**

Animal Model: Mouse

Organ Site: Skin (initiated with DMBA)

Reference: 311

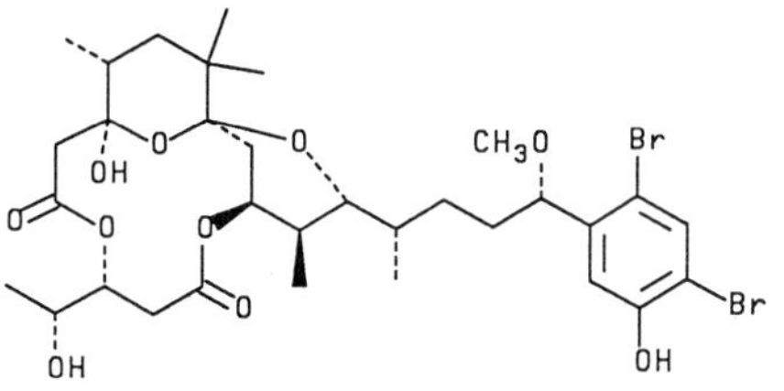

Compound: **Dibromoaplysiatoxin**

Animal Model: Mouse

Organ Site: Skin (initiated with DMBA)

Reference: 311

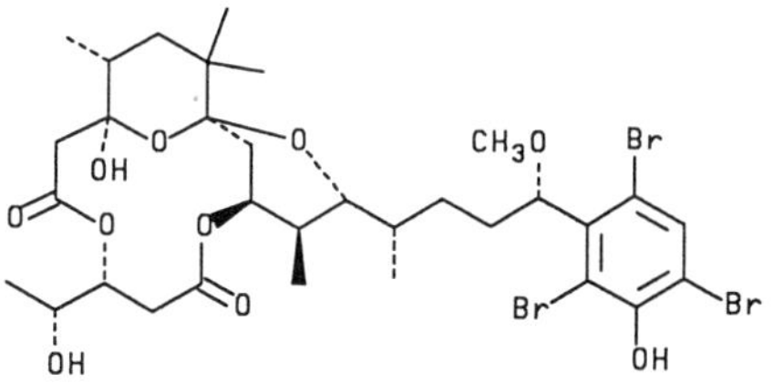

Compound: **Oscillatoxin A**

Animal Model: Mouse

Organ Site: Skin (initiated with DMBA)

Reference: 311

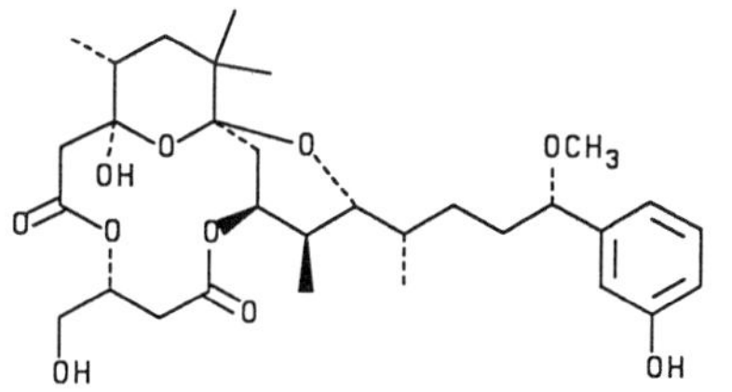

Compound: **Palytoxin**

Animal Model: Mouse

Organ Site: Skin (initiated with DMBA)

Reference: 311

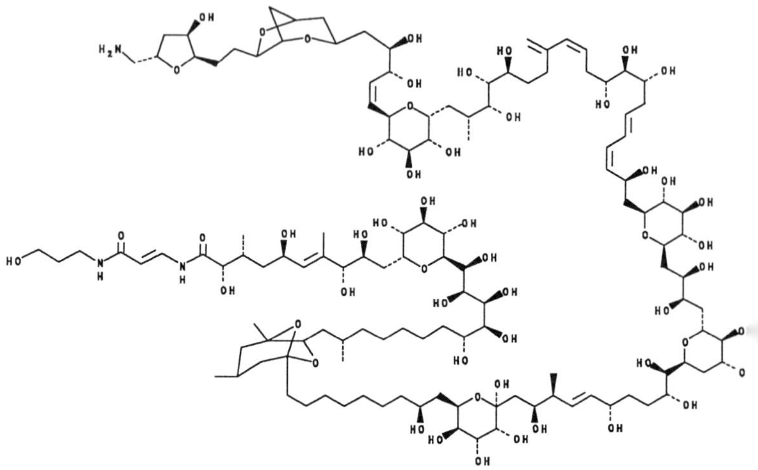

Compound: **Okadaic acid**

Animal Model: Mouse

Organ Site: Skin (initiated with DMBA)

Reference: 311, 1039, 1067, 1206

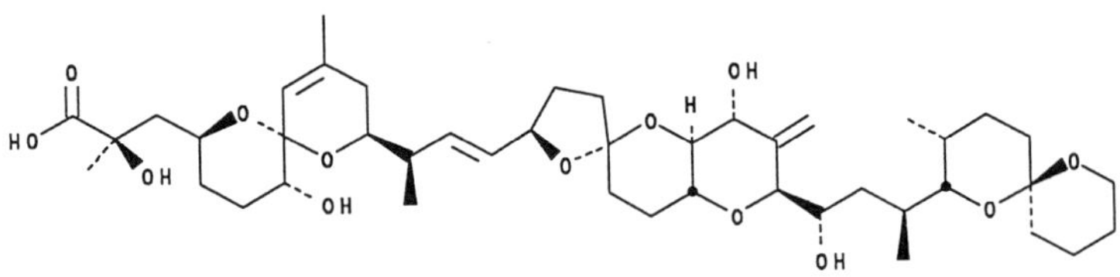

Compound: **Dinophysistoxin**

Animal Model: Mouse

Organ Site: Skin (initiated by DMBA)

Reference: 311, 1039

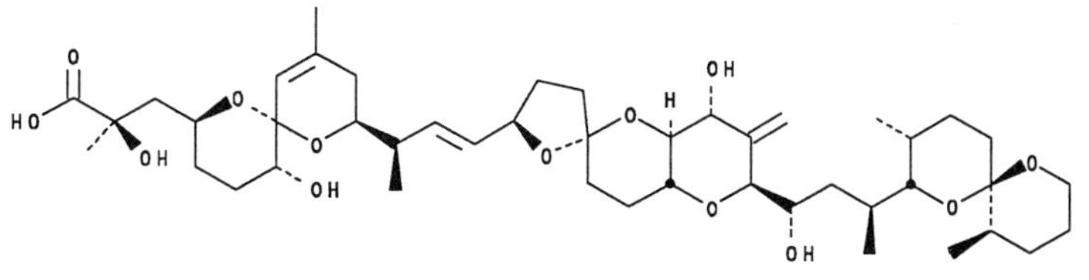

Compound: **Calyculin A**

Animal Model: Mouse

Organ Site: Skin (initiated with DMBA)

Reference: 311

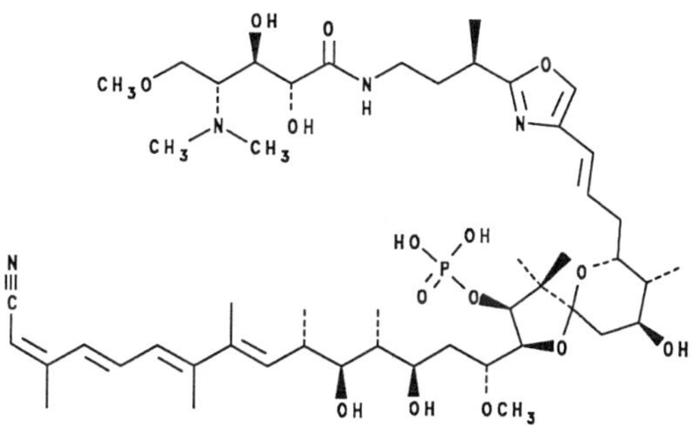

Compound: **5β-Hydroxyresiniferonol-6α,7α-oxide-9,13,14-ortho-(2E-hexadecenoate)**

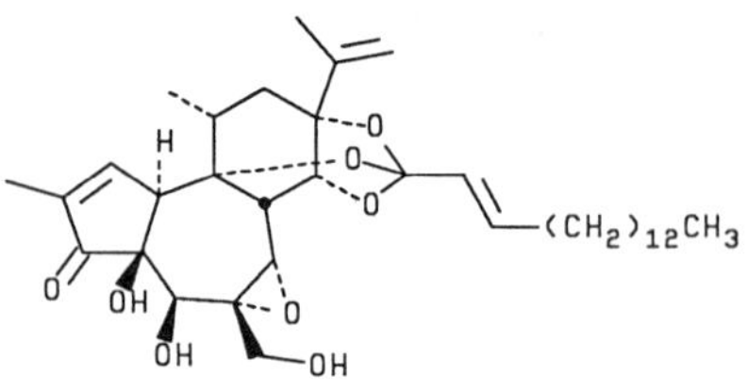

Animal Model: Mouse

Organ Site: Skin (initiated with DMBA)

Reference: 5

Compound:

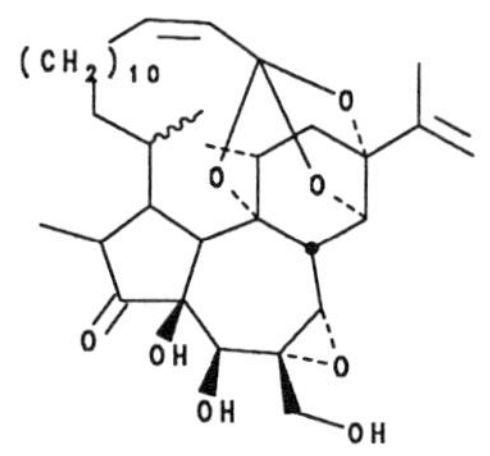

Animal Model: Mouse

Organ Site: Skin (initiated with DMBA)

Reference: 5, 1218

Compound:

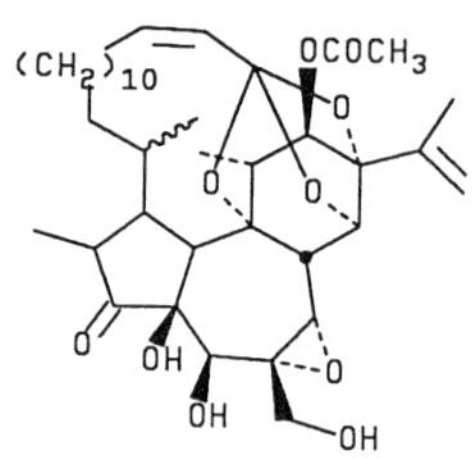

Animal Model: Mouse

Organ Site: Skin (initiated with DMBA)

Reference: 5

Chapter 3 TABULAR SURVEY

The tabular surveys of this book follow those of *Biosynthetic Products for Cancer Chemotherapy*, Volume 6.[883] Again we have attempted to include all (pure substances) animal and plant antineoplastic and/or cell growth inhibitory constituents recorded in the literature from January 1986 to January 1989. The marine animal and marine plant constituents cover the same period and include all such substances of known structure regardless of whether biological activity was available. We believe many of these substances will eventually be found to possess potentially useful antineoplastic, cytotoxic or other biological activity. The tabular survey should continue to be very useful to a broad selection of chemists and biologists. As before, we extend our apologies to anyone who might be affected by inadvertent omissions or errors.

Section A

NEW BIOSYNTHETIC ANTINEOPLASTIC AND/OR CELL GROWTH INHIBITORY AGENTS

Chapter 4 HIGHER PLANT TERPENOIDS

$C_{19}H_{20}O_6$ **Isodeoxyelephantopin**
(previously known)

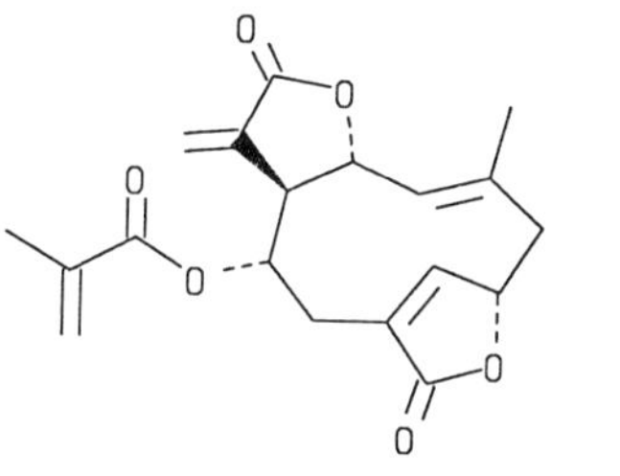

Mol. Wt.: 344
Bioactivity: KB: ED_{50} 2.5 μg/ml
Melting Point: 160-161°C
$[\alpha]_D$: +180.7 Solvent: Chf
Spectral Data: IR, PMR, Mass Spec, x-ray c.s.
Organism: *Elephantopus carolinianus* Willd. (Compositae)
Location: Chapel Hill, N.C.
Reference: 84, 236, 356, 1221

$C_{19}H_{22}O_7$ **Tomenphantopin-B**

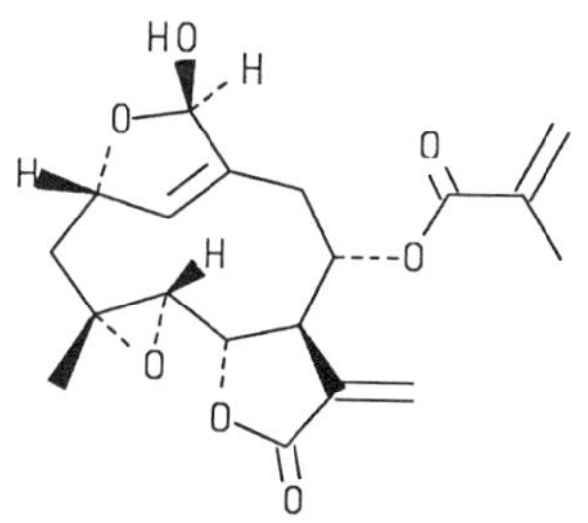

Mol. Wt.: 362
Bioactivity: KB: ED_{50} 5.0 μg/ml
Melting Point: 114-116°C
$[\alpha]_D$: -11.1 Solvent: Chf
Spectral Data: IR, PMR, x-ray c.s.
Organism: *Elephantopus tomentosus* (Compositae)
Location: Chapel Hill, N.C.
Reference: 406

$C_{20}H_{24}O_4$ **Ovatodiolide**

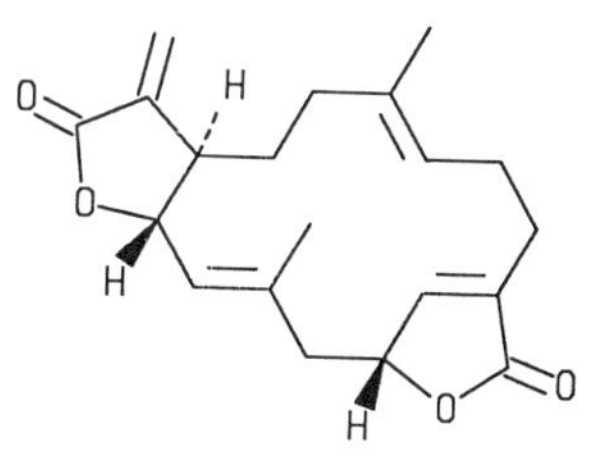

Mol. Wt.: 328
Bioactivity: KB: IC_{50} 0.6 μg/ml
Melting Point: 150-151°C
$[\alpha]_D^{23}$: +21.8 Solvent: Chf
Spectral Data: UV, IR, CMR, PMR, Mass Spec.
Organism: *Anisomeles indica* (L.) O.Ktze. (syn. *A. ovata* R.Br.) (Labiatae)
Location: China
Reference: 38, 39

$C_{20}H_{24}O_6$ **Sculponeatin C**

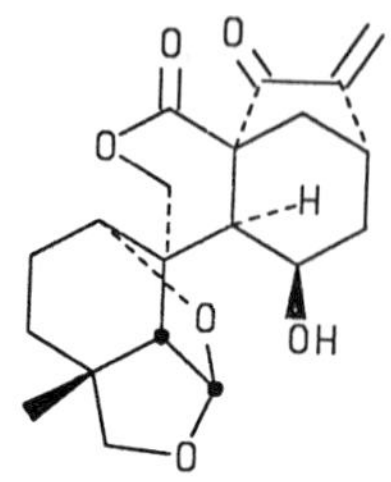

Mol. Wt.:	360
Bioactivity:	HeLa: ED_{50} 0.50 μg/ml Ehrlich ascites carcinoma: T/C >221 (30 mg/kg/day)
Melting Point:	292-294°C
$[\alpha]_D^{24}$:	-163 Solvent: Py
Spectral Data:	UV, IR, CMR, PMR
Organism:	*Rabdosia sculponeata* (Labiatae)
Location:	Yunnan, China
Reference:	316, 1046

$C_{20}H_{24}O_7$ **Tomenphantopin-A**

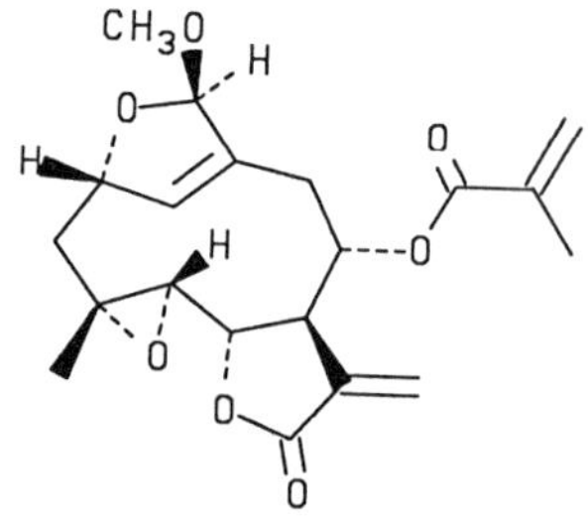

Mol. Wt.:	376
Bioactivity:	KB: ED_{50} 2.5 μg/ml
$[\alpha]_D$:	-8.6 Solvent: Chf
Spectral Data:	IR, CMR, PMR
Organism:	*Elephantopus tomentosus* (Compositae)
Location:	Chapel Hill, N.C.
Reference:	406

$C_{20}H_{26}O_4$ **Anisomelic acid**
(previously known)

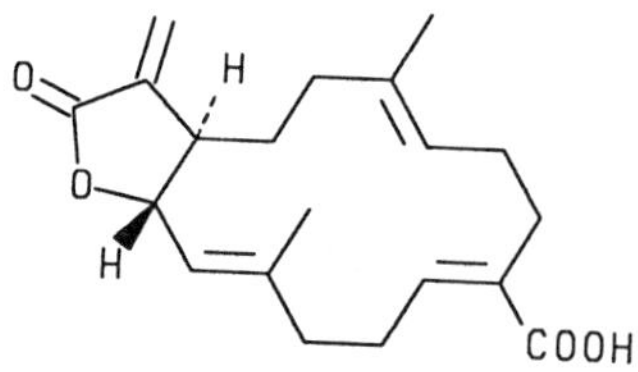

Mol. Wt.:	330
Bioactivity:	KB: IC_{50} 6.7 μg/ml
Melting Point:	148-150°C
$[\alpha]_D^{23}$:	-24.7 Solvent: Chf
Spectral Data:	UV, IR, CMR, PMR, Mass Spec. x-ray c.s. (of methyl ester)
Organism:	*Anisomeles indica* (L.) O.Ktze. (syn. *A. ovata* R.Br.) *A. malabauia* R.Br. (Labiatae)
Location:	China; South India
Reference:	38, 39, 702, 903

$C_{20}H_{26}O_5$ **4,7-Oxycycloanisomelic acid**

Mol. Wt.: 346
Bioactivity: KB: IC_{50} 1.6 μg/ml
Melting Point: 213-215°C
$[\alpha]_D^{23}$: -22.4 Solvent: Chf
Spectral Data: UV, IR, CMR, PMR, Mass Spec.
Organism: *Anisomeles indica* (L.) O.Ktze. (syn. *A. ovata)* (Labiatae)
Location: China
Reference: 38, 39

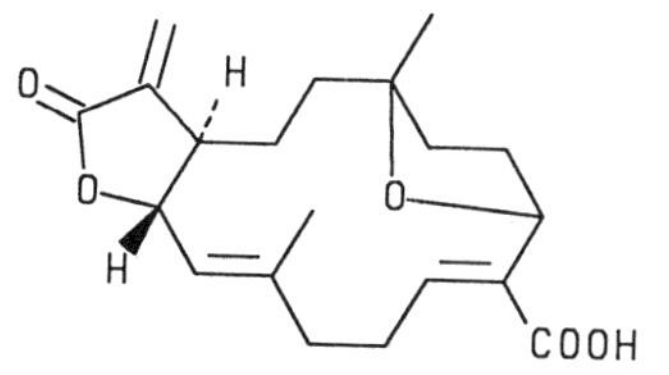

$C_{20}H_{28}O_2$ **Coronarin A**

Mol. Wt.: 300
Bioactivity: V-79: IC_{50} 1.65 μg/ml
Melting Point: 100-101°C
$[\alpha]_D$: +25.4 Solvent: Chf
Spectral Data: UV, CD, IR, CMR, PMR, Mass Spec.
Organism: *Hedychium coronarium* Koeng (Zingiberaceae)
Location: Sao Paulo
Reference: 480

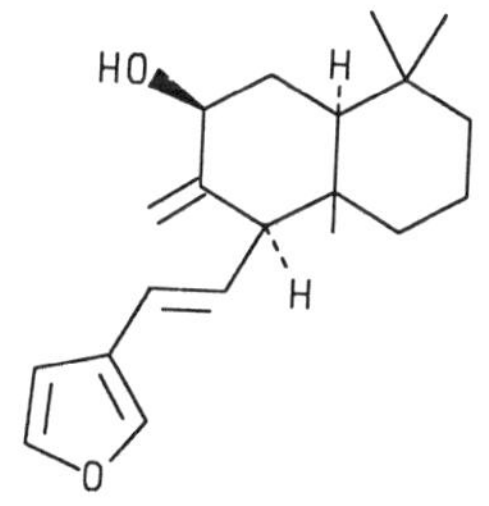

$C_{20}H_{28}O_3$ **14-Dehydroagrostistachin**

Mol. Wt.: 316
Bioactivity: P-388: ED_{50} 2.8 μg/ml
Melting Point: 132-134°C
$[\alpha]_D$: +170 Solvent: Chf
Spectral Data: UV, IR, CMR, PMR, Mass Spec.
Organism: *Agrostistachys hookeri* Benth. and Hook. f. (Euphorbiaceae)
Location: Sri Lanka
Reference: 176

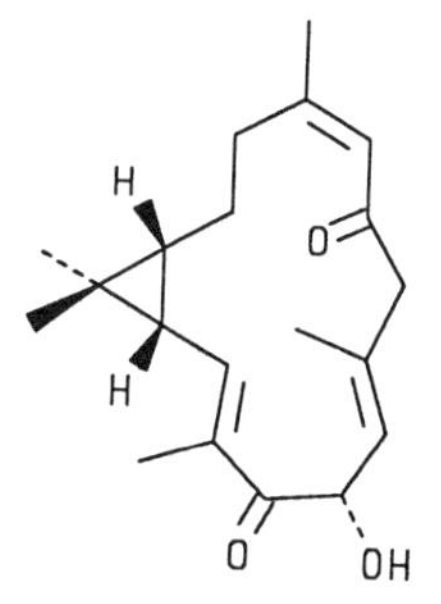

$C_{20}H_{28}O_5$ **Effusanin A**

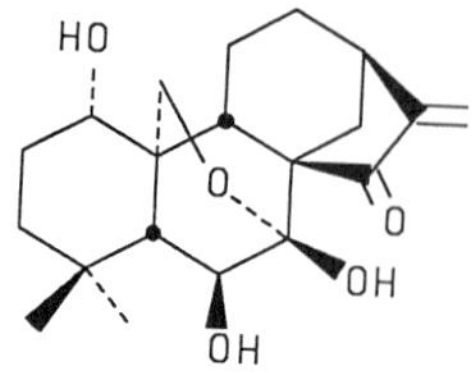

Mol. Wt.: 348
Bioactivity: HeLa: ED_{50} 0.09 μg/ml
Ehrlich ascites carcinoma:
T/C >221 (30 mg/kg/day)
Organism: *Rabdosia effusa*
(Labiatae)
Reference: 316, 318

$C_{20}H_{28}O_5$ **Longikaurin A**

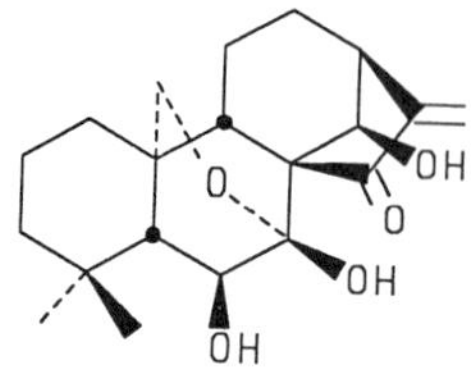

Mol. Wt.: 348
Bioactivity: HeLa: ED_{50} 0.33 μg/ml
FM 3A/B: 74% inhibition (1 μg/ml)
Antibacterial activity
Melting Point: 223-225°C
$[\alpha]_D^{25}$: -91.1 Solvent: Py
Spectral Data: UV, CD, IR, CMR, PMR
Organism: *Rabdosia longituba*
(Labiatae)
Location: Japan
Reference: 316, 317

$C_{20}H_{30}O_2$ **(E)-Labda-8(17),12-diene-15,16-dial**

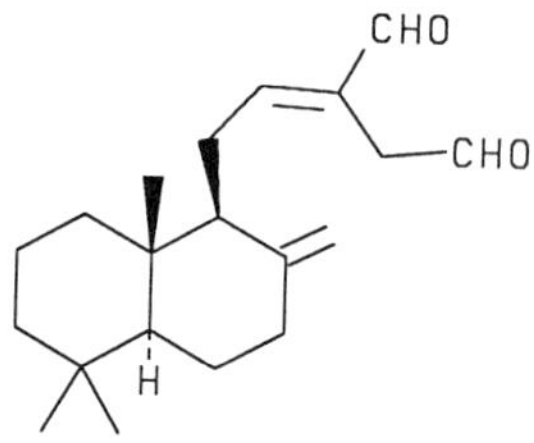

Mol. Wt.: 302
Bioactivity: V-79: IC_{50} 18.5 μg/ml
Antifungal activity
Melting Point: Oil
$[\alpha]_D$: +15.8 Solvent: Chf
Spectral Data: UV, CD, IR, CMR, PMR, Mass Spec.
Organism: *Hedychium coronarium* Koeng
Alpinia galanga
(Zingiberaceae)
Location: Sao Paulo; China
Reference: 480, 772

$C_{20}H_{30}O_3$ **Agroskerin**

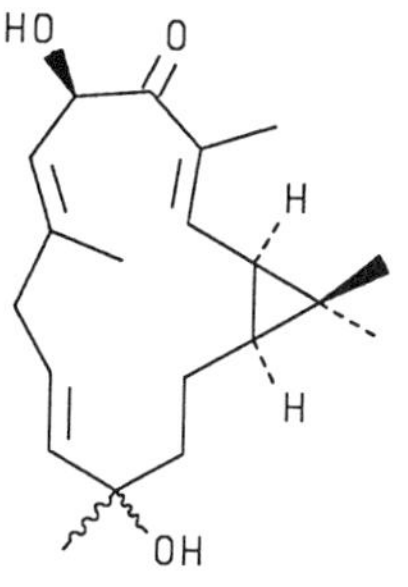

Mol. Wt.: 318
Bioactivity: P-388: ED_{50} 1.4 μg/ml
Melting Point: Resin
$[\alpha]_D$: -54 Solvent: Chf
Spectral Data: UV, IR, CMR, PMR, Mass Spec.
Organism: *Agrostistachys hookeri* Benth. and Hook. f. (Euphorbiaceae)
Location: Sri Lanka
Reference: 176

$C_{20}H_{30}O_3$ **Agrostistachin**

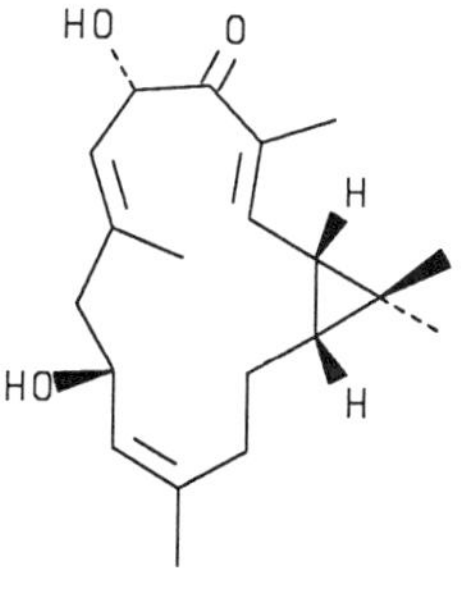

Mol. Wt.: 318
Bioactivity: P-388: ED_{50} 1.4 μg/ml
Melting Point: 155-157°C
$[\alpha]_D$: +248 Solvent: Chf
Spectral Data: IR, CMR, PMR, Mass Spec. x-ray c.s.
Organism: *Agrostistachys hookeri* Benth. and Hook. f. (Euphorbiaceae)
Reference: 175

$C_{20}H_{30}O_3$ **Coronarin C**

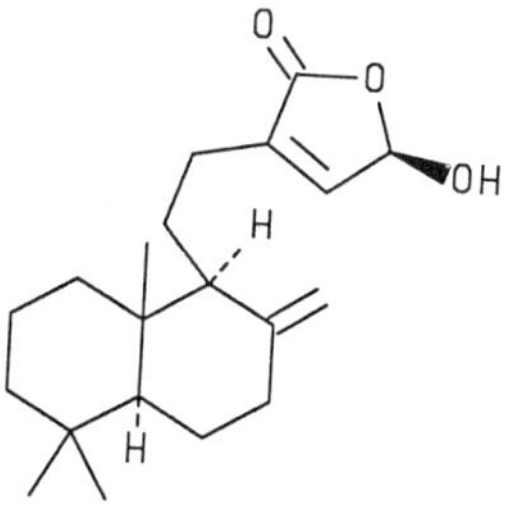

Mol. Wt.: 318
Bioactivity: V-79: IC_{50} 17.5 μg/ml
Melting Point: Oil
$[\alpha]_D$: +34.9 Solvent: Chf
Spectral Data: UV, CD, IR, CMR, PMR, Mass Spec.
Organism: *Hedychium coronarium* Koeng (Zingiberaceae)
Location: Sao Paulo
Reference: 480

$C_{20}H_{30}O_3$ **Coronarin D**

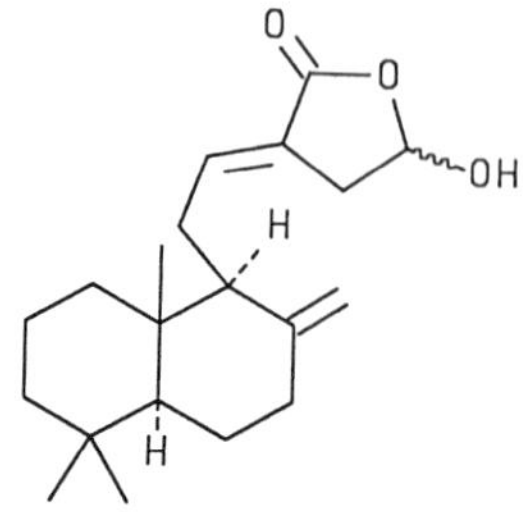

Mol. Wt.: 318
Bioactivity: V-79: IC_{50} 17.0 μg/ml
[α]$_D$: +10 Solvent: Chf
Spectral Data: UV, IR, CMR, PMR, Mass Spec.
Organism: *Hedychium coronarium* Koeng (Zingiberaceae)
Location: Sao Paulo
Reference: 480

$C_{20}H_{30}O_4$ **Coronarin B**

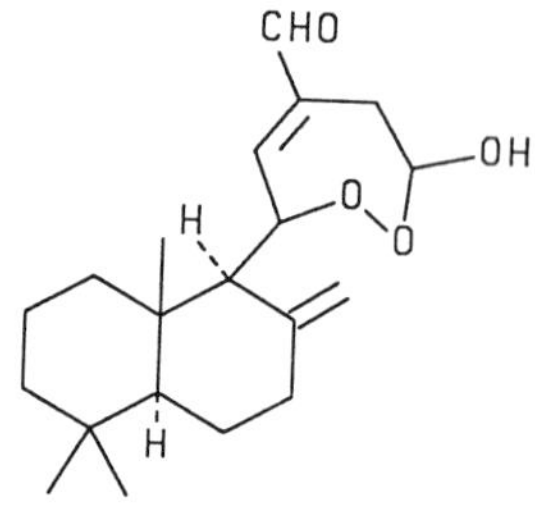

Mol. Wt.: 334
Bioactivity: V-79: IC_{50} 2.70 μg/ml
Melting Point: Oil
[α]$_D$: -43.1 Solvent: Chf
Spectral Data: UV, IR, CMR, PMR, Mass Spec.
Organism: *Hedychium coronarium* Koeng (Zingiberaceae)
Location: Sao Paulo
Reference: 480

$C_{20}H_{30}O_4$ **17-Hydroxyagrostistachin**

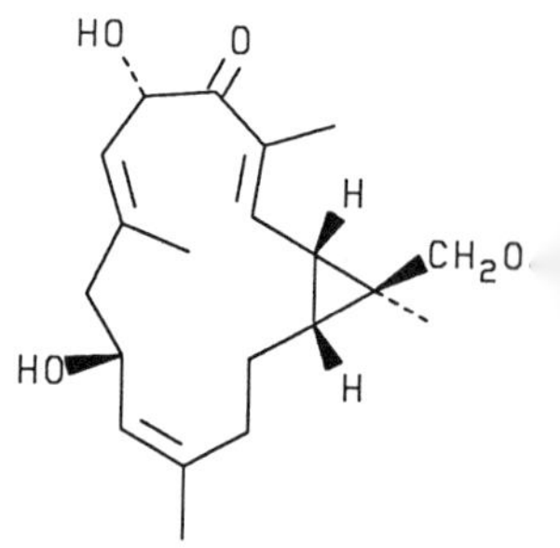

Mol. Wt.: 334
Bioactivity: P-388: ED_{50} 0.8 μg/ml
Melting Point: Resin
[α]$_D$: +167 Solvent: Chf
Spectral Data: UV, IR, CMR, PMR, Mass Spec.
Organism: *Agrostistachys hookeri* Benth. and Hook. f. (Euphorbiaceae)
Location: Sri Lanka
Reference: 176

$C_{20}H_{30}O_4$ **Kamebanin**

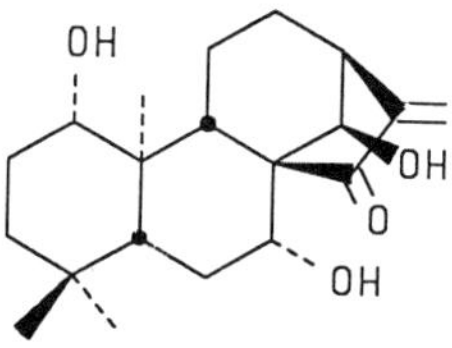

Mol. Wt.: 334
Bioactivity: HeLa: ED_{50} 0.05 μg/ml
Ehrlich ascites carcinoma:
T/C >226 (30 mg/kg/day)
Melting Point: 264-265.5°C
$[\alpha]_D^{24}$: -89 Solvent: Me
Spectral Data: UV, IR, PMR, Mass Spec.
Organism: *Rabdosia umbrosa* var. *leucantha* f. Kameba
(Labiatae)
Location: Miyagi, Japan
Reference: 316, 1075

$C_{20}H_{30}O_4$ **Umbrosin A**

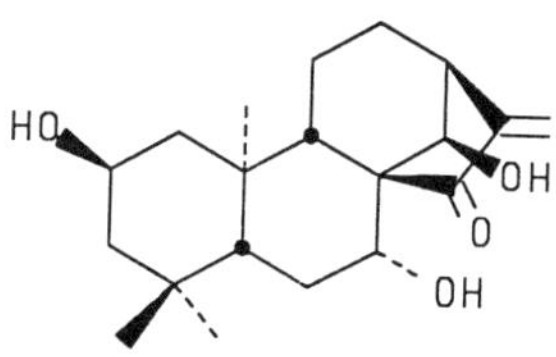

Mol. Wt.: 334
Bioactivity: HeLa: ED_{50} 0.08 μg/ml
Antibacterial activity
Melting Point: 225-228°C (dec.)
$[\alpha]_D$: -126 Solvent: Py
Spectral Data: UV, IR, PMR, Mass Spec.
Organism: *Rabdosia umbrosa*
(Labiatae)
Location: Shizuoka, Japan
Reference: 316, 619

$C_{20}H_{30}O_5$ **Excisanin A**

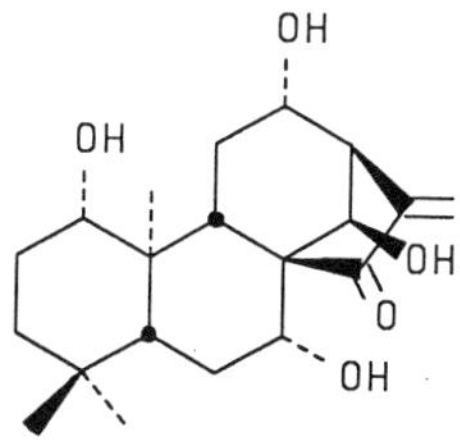

Mol. Wt.: 350
Bioactivity: HeLa: ED_{50} 0.20 μg/ml
Melting Point: 262-264°C
$[\alpha]_D^{20}$: -27.7 Solvent: Py
Spectral Data: UV, IR, CMR, PMR, Mass Spec.
Organism: *Rabdosia excisa*
(Labiatae)
Location: Anshan, China
Reference: 316, 1047

$C_{20}H_{30}O_5$ **Kamebakaurin**

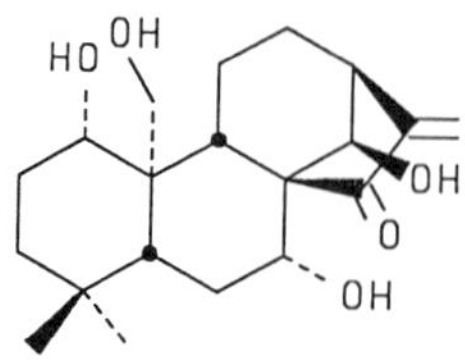

Mol. Wt.: 350
Bioactivity: HeLa: ED_{50} 0.14 μg/ml
Ehrlich ascites carcinoma:
T/C >206 (10 mg/kg/day)
Melting Point: 232-234°C
$[\alpha]_D^{21.5}$: -107 Solvent: Me
Spectral Data: UV, IR, CMR, PMR, Mass Spec.
Organism: *Rabdosia umbrosa* var. *leucantha* f. Kameba and *R. longituba* (Labiatae)
Location: Miyagi, Japan
Reference: 316, 317, 1075

$C_{20}H_{34}O_2$ **α-2,7,11-Cembratriene-4,6-diol (α-CBT)**

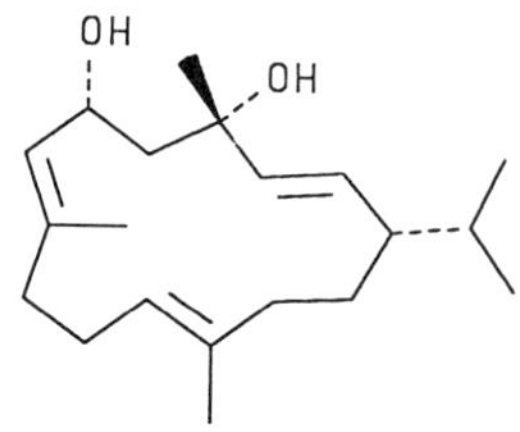

Mol. Wt.: 306
Bioactivity: Inhibition of TPA-induced EBV-EA activation in Raji cells: IC_{50} 7.7 μg/ml
Inhibition of ornithine decarboxylase activity
Plant growth inhibition
Spectral Data: CMR, PMR
Organism: *Nicotiana tabacum* (Solanaceae)
Reference: 960, 1031

$C_{20}H_{34}O_2$ **β-2,7,11-Cembratriene-4,6-diol (β-CBT)**

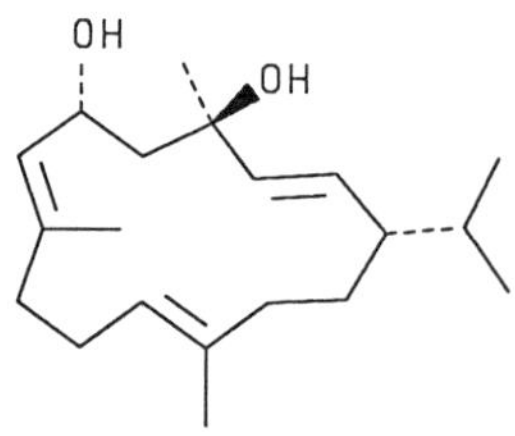

Mol. Wt.: 306
Bioactivity: Inhibition of TPA-induced EBV-EA activation in Raji cells: IC_{50} 6.7 μg/ml
Inhibition of ornithine decarboxylase activity
Plant growth inhibition
Melting Point: 123°C
Spectral Data: UV, IR, PMR, x-ray c.s.
Organism: *Nicotiana tabacum* (Solanaceae)
Reference: 703, 960, 1031

$C_{21}H_{22}O_4$ **Taxamairin A**

Mol. Wt.: 338
Bioactivity: Inhibition of hepatoma cells: IC_{50} 30 μg/ml
Melting Point: 223-224°C
Spectral Data: UV, CD, IR, PMR, Mass Spec., x-ray c.s.
Organism: *Taxus mairei* (Lemeé et Lévl.) (Taxaceae)
Location: Fujiang, China
Reference: 654

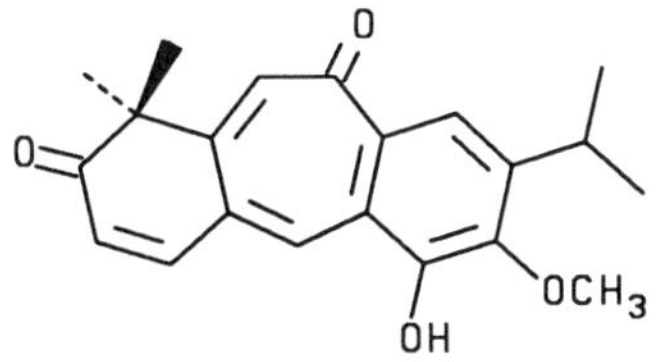

$C_{22}H_{24}O_4$ **Taxamairin B**

Mol. Wt.: 352
Bioactivity: Inhibition of hepatoma cells: IC_{50} 27 μg/ml
Spectral Data: UV, CD, IR, PMR, Mass Spec.
Organism: *Taxus mairei* (Lemeé et Lévl.) (Taxaceae)
Location: Fujiang, China
Reference: 654

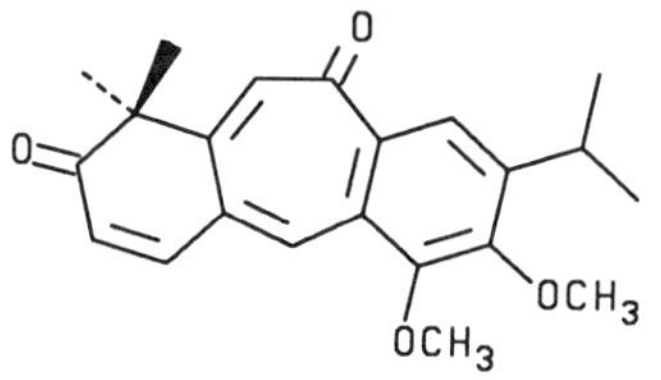

$C_{22}H_{30}O_7$ **Longikaurin B**

Mol. Wt.: 406
Bioactivity: HeLa: ED_{50} 0.16 μg/ml
Antibacterial activity
Melting Point: 238-239.5°C
$[\alpha]_D^{25}$: -115.9 Solvent: Py
Spectral Data: UV, IR, CMR, PMR
Organism: *Rabdosia longituba* (Labiatae)
Location: Japan
Reference: 316, 317

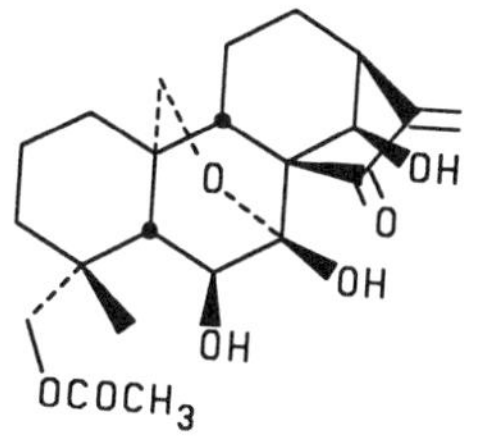

$C_{22}H_{32}O_6$ **Excisanin B**

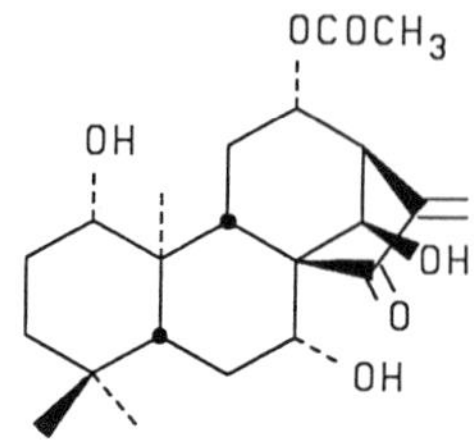

Mol. Wt.: 392
Bioactivity: HeLa: ED_{50} 0.09 μg/ml
Ehrlich ascites carcinoma:
T/C 183 (15 mg/kg/day)
Melting Point: 240-243°C
$[\alpha]_D^{20}$: -13.9 Solvent: Py
Spectral Data: UV, IR, CMR, PMR, Mass Spec.
Organism: *Rabdosia excisa*
(Labiatae)
Location: Anshan, China
Reference: 316, 1047

$C_{22}H_{32}O_6$ **Leukamenin A**

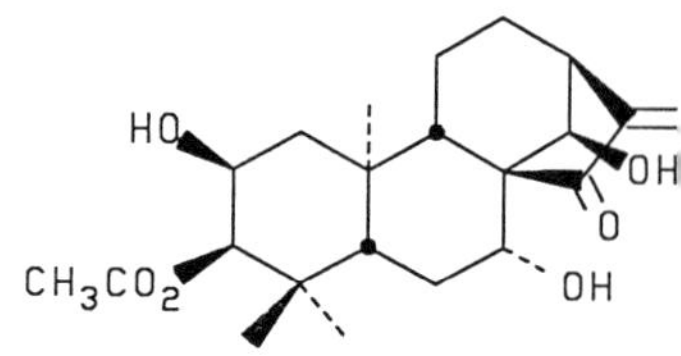

Mol. Wt.: 392
Bioactivity: HeLa: ED_{50} 0.15 μg/ml
Melting Point: 228-230°C
$[\alpha]_D^{21}$: -63.8 Solvent: Me
Spectral Data: UV, IR, CMR, PMR
Organism: *Rabdosia umbrosa* var. *leucantha* f.
Kameba
(Labiatae)
Location: Japan
Reference: 316, 1074

$C_{24}H_{34}O_7$ **Leukamenin B**

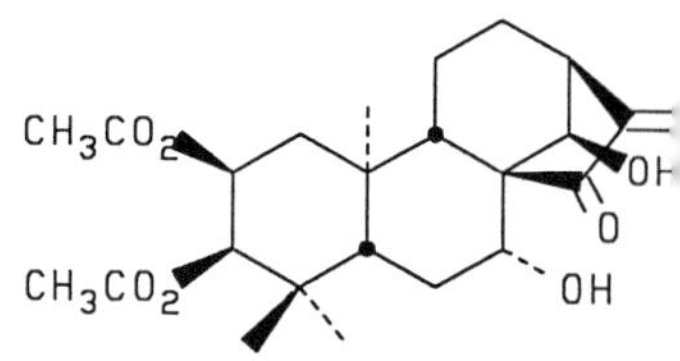

Mol. Wt.: 434
Bioactivity: HeLa: ED_{50} 0.09 μg/ml
Ehrlich ascites carcinoma:
T/C >240 (30 mg/kg/day)
Melting Point: 240-241°C
$[\alpha]_D^{21}$: -32.5 Solvent: Chf
Spectral Data: UV, IR, PMR
Organism: *Rabdosia umbrosa* var. *leucantha* f.
Kameba
(Labiatae)
Location: Japan
Reference: 316, 1074

$C_{25}H_{32}O_9$ **13,18-Dehydro-6α-senecioyloxychaparrin**

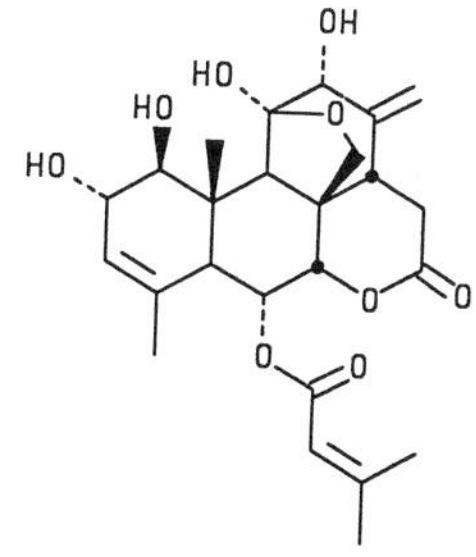

Mol. Wt.: 476
Bioactivity: PS: ED_{50} 1.7 μg/ml
Melting Point: 241-244°C
$[\alpha]_D^{22}$: +332 Solvent: Py
Spectral Data: UV, IR, CMR, PMR, Mass Spec.
Organism: *Simaba multiflora* A. Juss (Simaroubaceae)
Location: French Guiana
Reference: 767

$C_{27}H_{36}O_{11}$ **Bruceanol B**

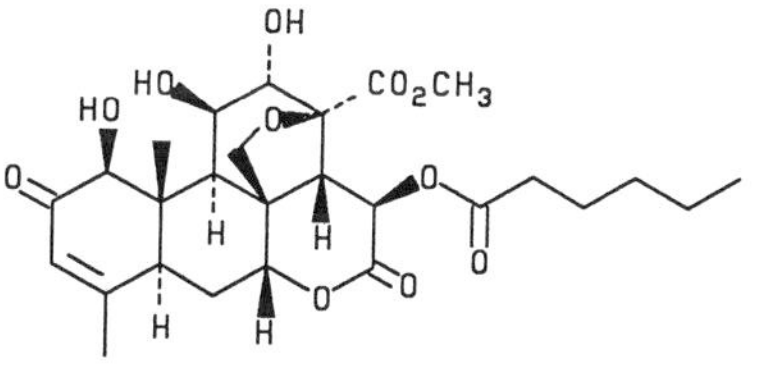

Mol. Wt.: 536
Bioactivity: P-388: T/C 123 (0.5 mg/kg, 3 day dosing)
Melting Point: 170-172°C
$[\alpha]_D^{25}$: +32 Solvent: Me
Spectral Data: UV, IR, CMR, PMR, Mass Spec.
Organism: *Brucea antidysenterica* Mill. (Simaroubaceae)
Location: Ethiopia
Reference: 849

$C_{28}H_{30}O_{11}$ **Bruceanol A**

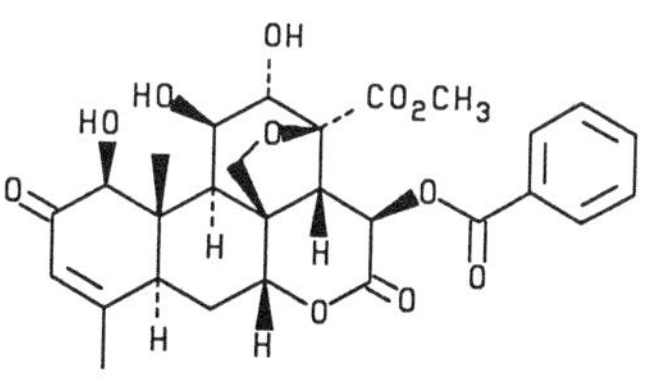

Mol. Wt.: 542
Bioactivity: P-388: T/C 134 (2mg/kg, 3 day dosing)
Melting Point: 174-177°C
$[\alpha]_D^{25}$: +60 Solvent: Alc
Spectral Data: UV, IR, CMR, PMR, Mass Spec.
Organism: *Brucea antidysenterica* Mill. (Simaroubaceae)
Location: Ethiopia
Reference: 849

$C_{29}H_{40}O_{10}$ **Baccharinoid B1**

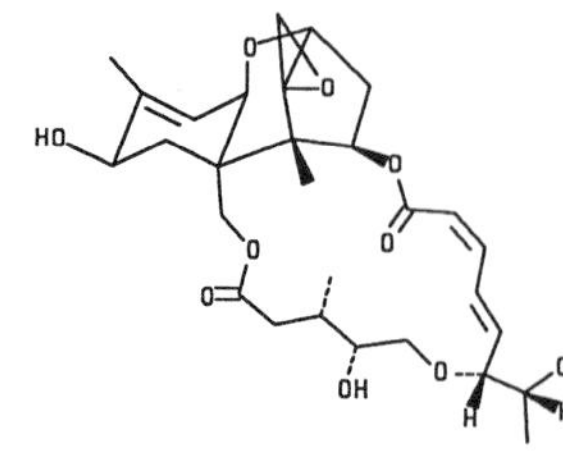

Mol. Wt.: 548
Bioactivity: P-388: T/C 175 (0.8 mg/kg)
Melting Point: 162-164°C
$[\alpha]_D^{24}$: +100 Solvent: Dcm
Spectral Data: UV, CMR, PMR, Mass Spec.
Organism: *Baccharis megapotamica* Spreng. (Compositae)
Location: Brazil
Reference: 495

$C_{29}H_{40}O_{10}$ **Baccharinoid B2**

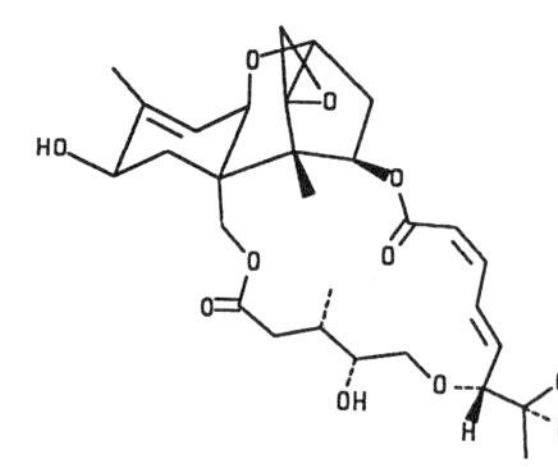

Mol. Wt.: 548
Bioactivity: P-388: T/C 203 (1.0 mg/kg)
Melting Point: 177-180°C
$[\alpha]_D^{24}$: +116 Solvent: Dcm
Spectral Data: UV, CMR, PMR, Mass Spec., x-ray c.s.
Organism: *Baccharis megapotamica* Spreng. (Compositae)
Location: Brazil
Reference: 495

$C_{29}H_{40}O_{10}$ **Baccharinoid B3**

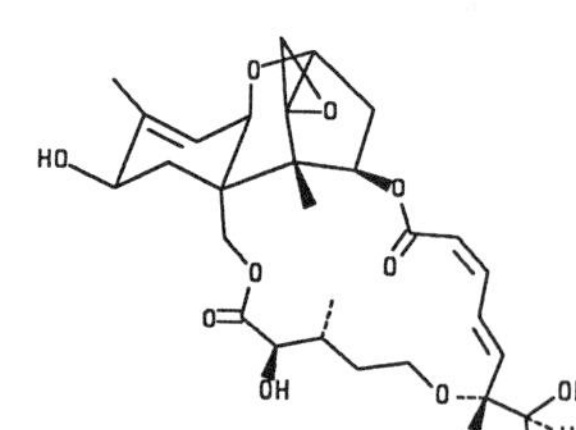

Mol. Wt.: 548
Bioactivity: P-388: T/C 250 (5.0 mg/kg)
Melting Point: 172-180°C
$[\alpha]_D^{25}$: +164 Solvent: Dcm
Spectral Data: UV, IR, CMR, PMR, Mass Spec.
Organism: *Baccharis megapotamica* Spreng. (Compositae)
Location: Brazil
Reference: 495

$C_{29}H_{40}O_{10}$ **Baccharinoid B7**

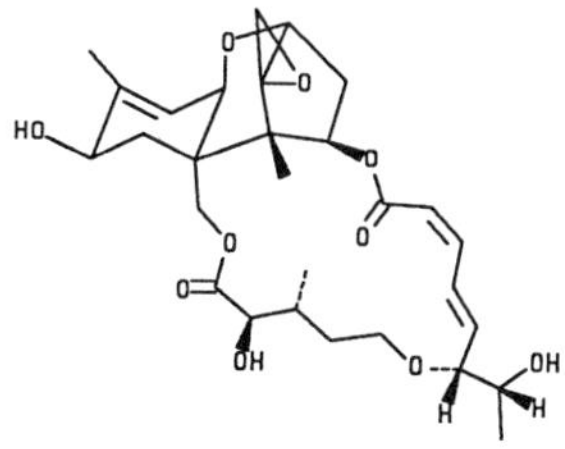

Mol. Wt.: 548
Bioactivity: P-388: T/C 196 (0.62 mg/kg)
Melting Point: 229-231°C
$[\alpha]_D^{25}$: +150 Solvent: Dcm
Spectral Data: UV, IR, CMR, PMR, Mass Spec., x-ray c.s.
Organism: *Baccharis megapotamica* Spreng. (Compositae)
Location: Brazil
Reference: 495

$C_{29}H_{42}O_9$

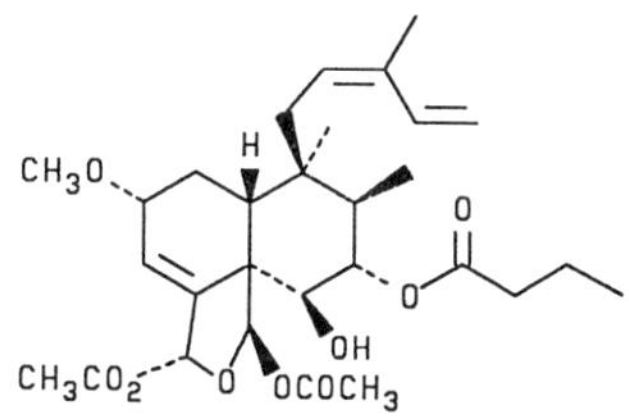

Mol. Wt.: 534
Bioactivity: Sarcoma 180: growth ratio 3.97% (15 mg/kg/day)
V-79: LD_{50} $1.0x10^{-3}$ mmol/l
Melting Point: 82-83°C
$[\alpha]_D$: +4.1 Solvent: Alc
Spectral Data: UV, CD, IR, CMR, PMR, Mass Spec.
Organism: *Casearia sylvestris* Sw. (Flacourtiaceae)
Location: Paraguay
Reference: 482

$C_{30}H_{38}O_{13}$ **Bruceanol C**

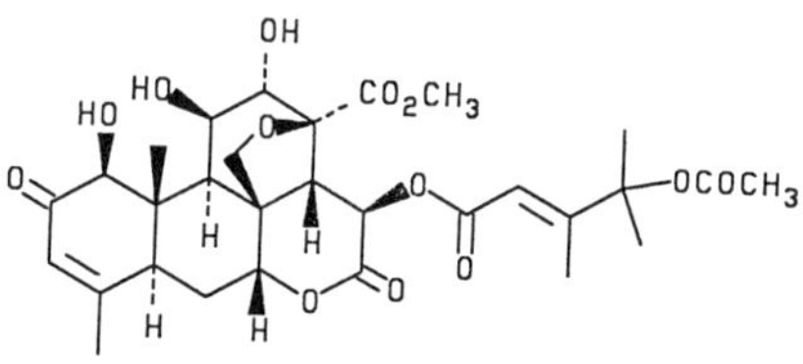

Mol. Wt.: 606
Bioactivity: KB: ED_{50} <0.04 μg/ml
A-549 lung carcinoma: ED_{50} 0.48 μg/ml
HCT-8 colon tumor: ED_{50} <0.40 μg/ml
P-388: ED_{50} 0.56 μg/ml
Melting Point: 125-127°C
$[\alpha]_D^{25}$: +38 Solvent: Alc
Spectral Data: UV, IR, CMR, PMR, Mass Spec.
Organism: *Brucea antidysenterica* Mill. (Simaroubaceae)
Location: Ethiopia
Reference: 322

$C_{30}H_{48}O_3$	**Ursolic acid** (previously known)
Mol. Wt.:	456
Bioactivity:	P-388: ED_{50} 3.15 μg/ml L-1210: ED_{50} 4.00 μg/ml A-549: ED_{50} 4.00 μg/ml (marginal activity against MCF-7, KB, and HCT-8 cells)
Melting Point:	238-240°C
$[\alpha]_D$:	+78.3 Solvent: Alc
Spectral Data:	PMR
Organism:	*Prunella vulgaris* L. (Labiatae) *Psychotria serpens* (Rubiaceae) *Hyptis capitata* (Labiatae)
Location:	Taiwan
Reference:	644, 1109

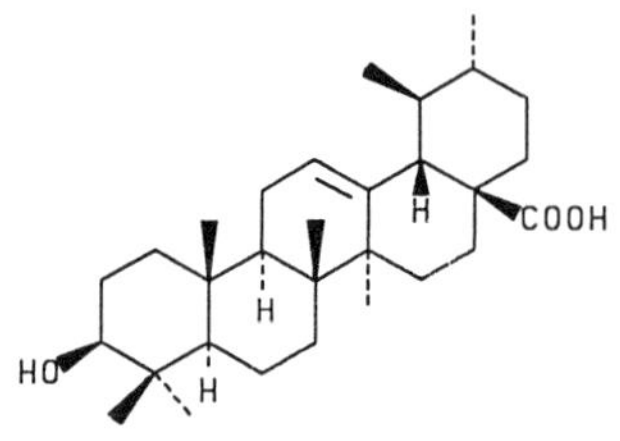

$C_{30}H_{48}O_4$	**2α-Hydroxyursolic acid** (previously known)
Mol. Wt.:	472
Bioactivity:	A-549: ED_{50} 4.9 μg/ml HCT-8: ED_{50} 2.7 μg/ml P-388: ED_{50} 6.1 μg/ml
Melting Point:	244-246°C
$[\alpha]_D$:	+49 Solvent: Me
Spectral Data:	IR, PMR, Mass Spec.
Organism:	*Hyptis capitata* (Labiatae)
Location:	Taiwan
Reference:	218, 838, 1199

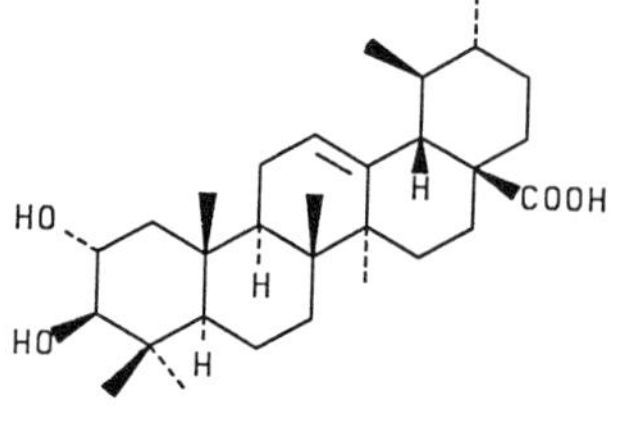

$C_{30}H_{48}O_5$ **Hyptatic acid-A**

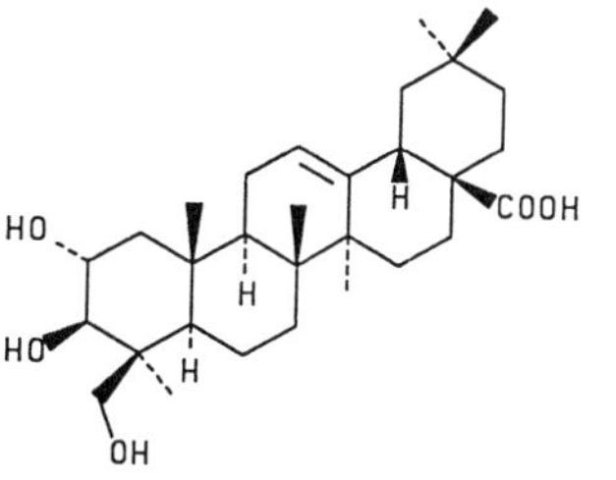

Mol. Wt.: 488
Bioactivity: A-549: ED_{50} 5.9 μg/ml
HCT-8: ED_{50} 4.2 μg/ml
P-388: ED_{50} 6.7 μg/ml
Melting Point: 298-304°C
$[\alpha]_D$: +57 Solvent: Me
Spectral Data: IR, PMR, Mass Spec., x-ray c.s.
Organism: *Hyptis capitata* (Labiatae)
Location: Taiwan
Reference: 1199

$C_{30}H_{50}O_3$ **Maytenfoliol**
(previously known)

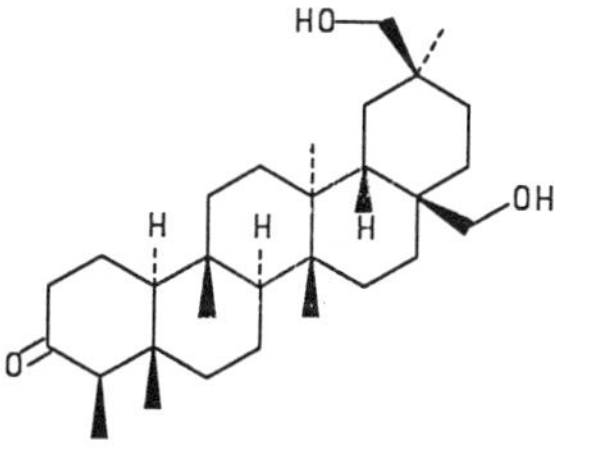

Mol. Wt.: 458
Bioactivity: P-388: T/C 120 (10 mg/kg/day)
KB: ED_{50} 4.56 μg/ml
Melting Point: 290-291°C
$[\alpha]_D$: -12.8 Solvent: Chf
Spectral Data: IR, CMR, PMR, Mass Spec., x-ray c.s.
Organism: *Maytenus diversifolia* (Gray) Hou (Celastraceae)
Location: Mt. Li-Long, Taiwan
Reference: 832, 833

$C_{30}H_{50}O_4$ **iso-Iridogermanal**
(previously known)

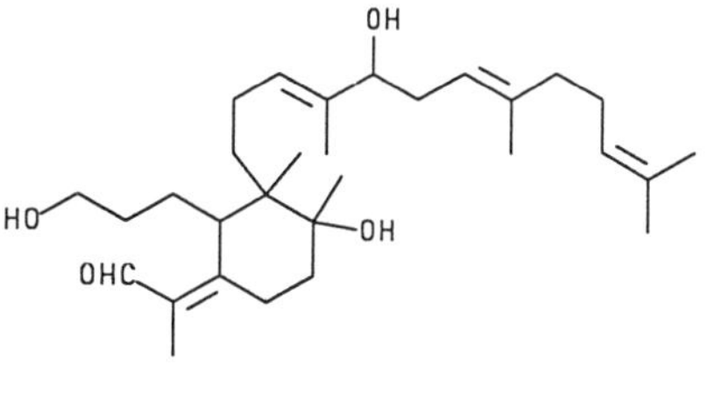

Mol. Wt.: 474
Bioactivity: P-388: ED_{50} 0.1 μg/ml
$[\alpha]_D^{25}$: +51 Solvent: Dcm
Organism: *Iris missouriensis* Nutt (Iridaceae)
Location: Nevada
Reference: 610, 1187

$C_{30}H_{52}O_2$ **Zeorin**
(previously known)

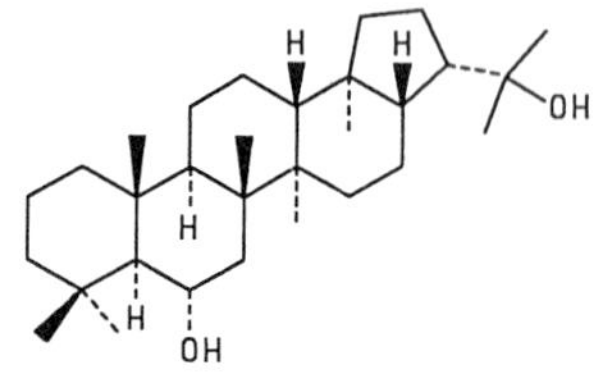

Mol. Wt.: 444
Bioactivity: P-388: ED_{50} 1.1 μg/ml
Melting Point: 223-226°C
$[\alpha]_D^{25}$: +54 Solvent: Chf
Spectral Data: CMR (acetate), PMR
Organism: *Iris missouriensis* Nutt
(Iridaceae)
Location: Nevada
Reference: 445, 1187

$C_{31}H_{40}O_{13}$ **Yadanzioside O aglycone**

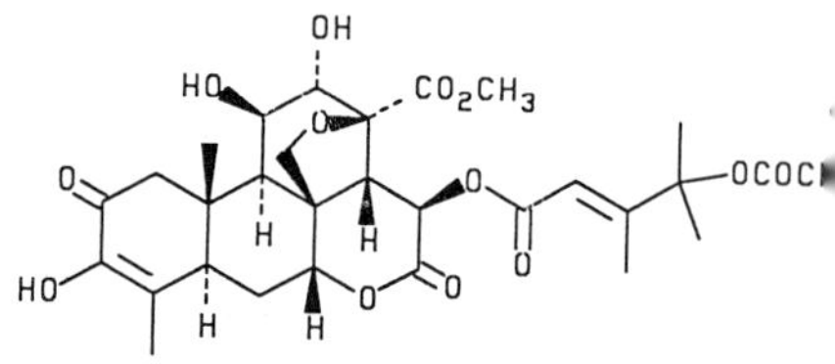

Mol. Wt.: 620
Bioactivity: P-388: T/C 147
(4 mg/kg/day)
Melting Point: 138-143°C
$[\alpha]_D^{27}$: +23 Solvent: Alc
Spectral Data: UV, IR, CMR, PMR, Mass Spec.
Organism: *Brucea javanica*
(isolated as the glycoside)
(Simaroubaceae)
Location: China
Reference: 969, 970

$C_{31}H_{48}O_4$ **Regelin**

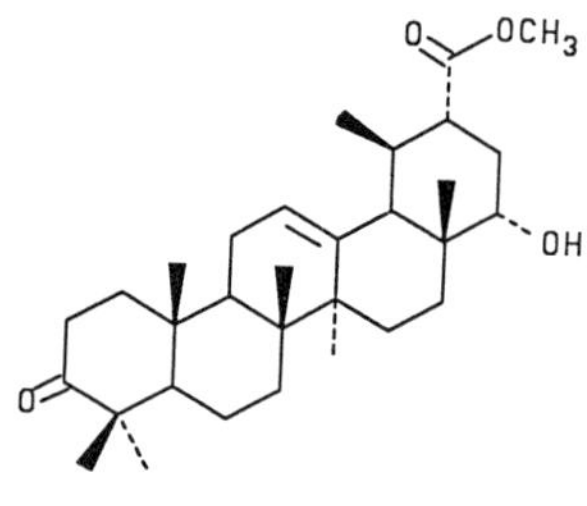

Mol. Wt.: 484
Bioactivity: KB: ED_{50} 4.2 μg/ml
Melting Point: 221-223°C
$[\alpha]_D^{27.6}$: +20 Solvent: Chf
Spectral Data: IR, PMR, Mass Spec., x-ray c.s.
Organism: *Tripterygium regelii*
Sprague et Tak.
(Celastraceae)
Location: Jilin, China
Reference: 436

$C_{31}H_{48}O_5$ **Regelinol**

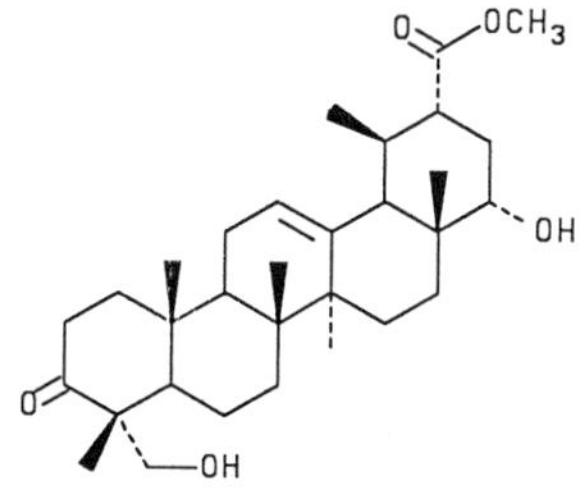

Mol. Wt.: 500
Bioactivity: KB: ED_{50} 10 μg/ml
Melting Point: 210-212°C
$[\alpha]_D^{26}$: +14 Solvent: Chf
Spectral Data: IR, CMR, PMR, Mass Spec.
Organism: *Tripterygium regelii* Sprague et Tak. (Celastraceae)
Location: Jilin, China
Reference: 436

$C_{32}H_{50}O_4$ **3-O-Acetyloleanolic acid**

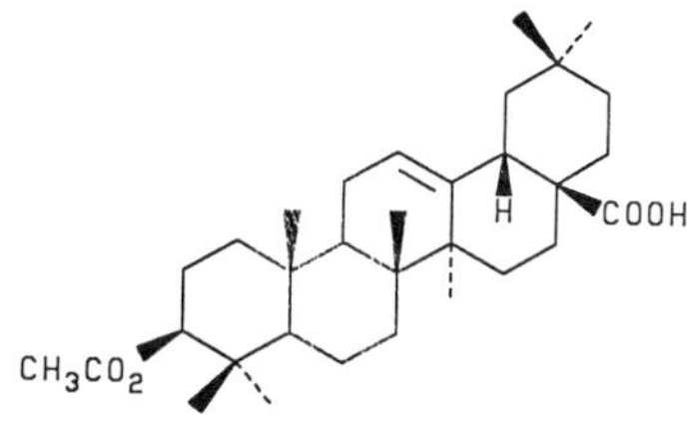

Mol. Wt.: 498
Bioactivity: Inhibition of TPA-induced EBV-EA activation in Raji cells
Organism: *Euptelea polyandra* (Eupteleaceae)
Location: Kyoto
Reference: 606, 608

$C_{34}H_{46}O_{16}$ **Yadanzioside N**

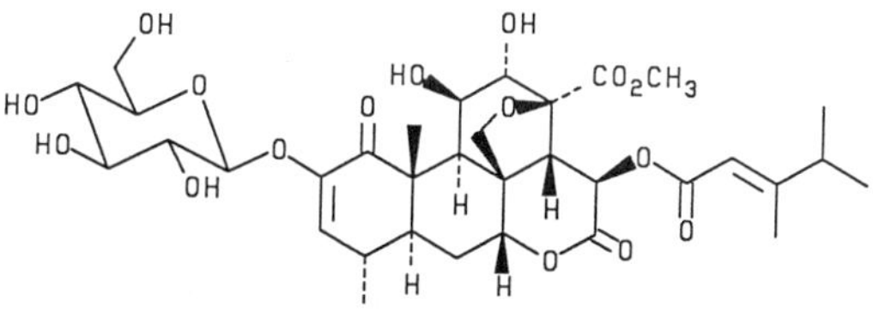

Mol. Wt.: 710
Bioactivity: P-388: ED_{50} 2.2 μg/ml
L-1210: ED_{50} 4.5 μg/ml
Melting Point: 175-180°C
$[\alpha]_D^{14}$: +7.7 Solvent: Alc
Spectral Data: UV, IR, CMR, PMR, Mass Spec.
Organism: *Brucea antidysenterica* Mill.
B. javanica (Simaroubaceae)
Location: Ethiopia; China
Reference: 323, 970

$C_{34}H_{46}O_{16}$

Yadanzioside P
(structure previously assigned to **Bruceantinoside B**)

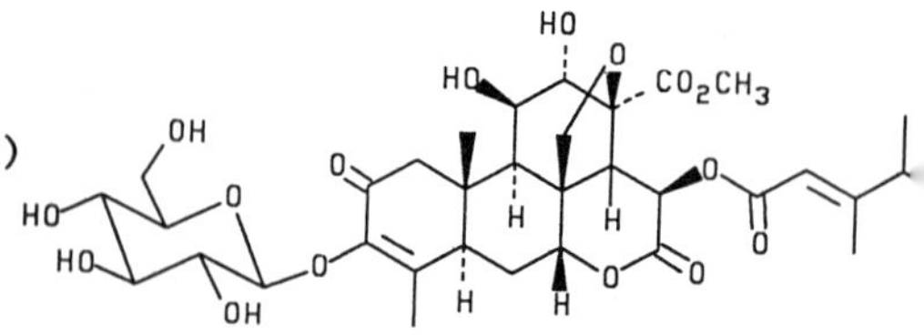

Mol. Wt.: 710
Bioactivity: P-388: T/C 129 (10 mg/kg/day)
Melting Point: 193-198°C
$[\alpha]_D^{23}$: +7.0 Solvent: Alc
$[\alpha]_D^{22}$: -45 Solvent: Py
Spectral Data: UV, IR, CMR, PMR, Mass Spec.
Organism: *Brucea javanica* (L.) Merr. (Simaroubaceae)
Location: China
Reference: 968

$C_{35}H_{56}O_6$

Barringtogenol-C21-angelate
(previously known)

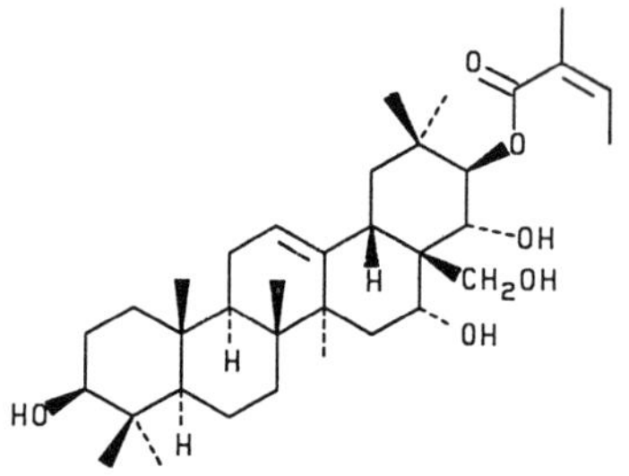

Mol. Wt.: 572
Bioactivity: KB: ED_{50} 3.0 μg/ml
Melting Point: 242-244°C
$[\alpha]_D$: +31 Solvent: Me
Spectral Data: IR, CMR, PMR, Mass Spec.
Organism: *Aesculus hippocastanum* L. (Hippocastanaceae) <u>via</u> hydrolysis of the extract
Location: U. S.
Reference: 604, 1212

$C_{36}H_{48}O_{18}$

Bruceantinoside C

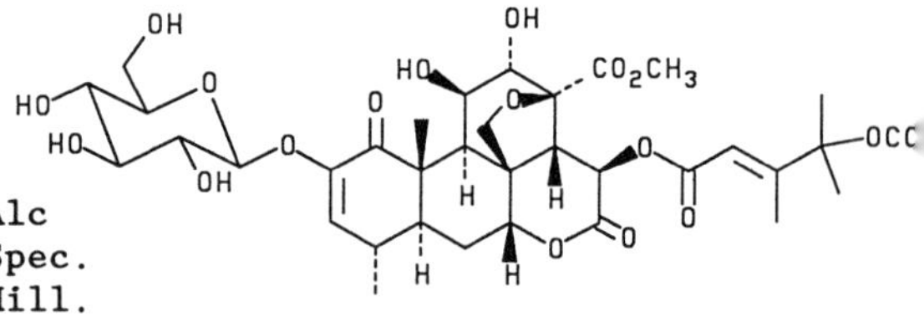

Mol. Wt.: 768
Bioactivity: P-388: ED_{50} 2.1 μg/ml
L-1210: ED_{50} 3.5 μg/ml
Melting Point: 153-155°C
$[\alpha]_D^{23}$: +12.7 Solvent: Alc
Spectral Data: UV, IR, CMR, PMR, Mass Spec.
Organism: *Brucea antidysenterica* Mill. (Simaroubaceae)
Location: Ethiopia
Reference: 323

$C_{36}H_{54}O_{10}$

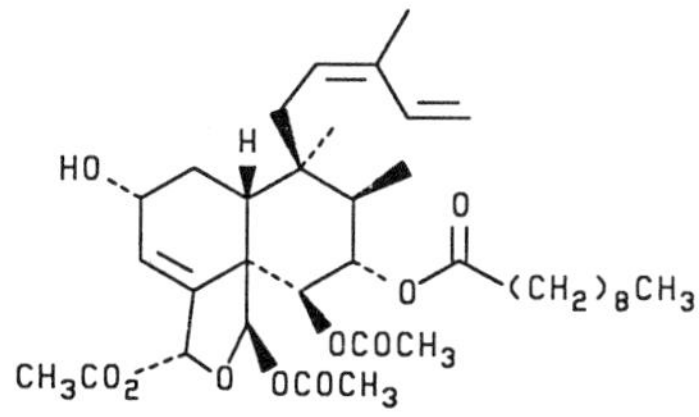

Mol. Wt.:	646
Bioactivity:	Sarcoma 180: growth ratio 1.89% (15 mg/kg/day)
	V-79: LD_{50} $7.7x10^{-4}$ mmol/l
Spectral Data:	CD (derivative), CMR
Organism:	*Casearia sylvestris* sw. (Flacourtiaceae)
Location:	Paraguay
Reference:	482

$C_{40}H_{56}O_7$ **3β-Hydroxy-24-<u>cis</u>-ferulyloxyurs-12-en-28-oic acid**

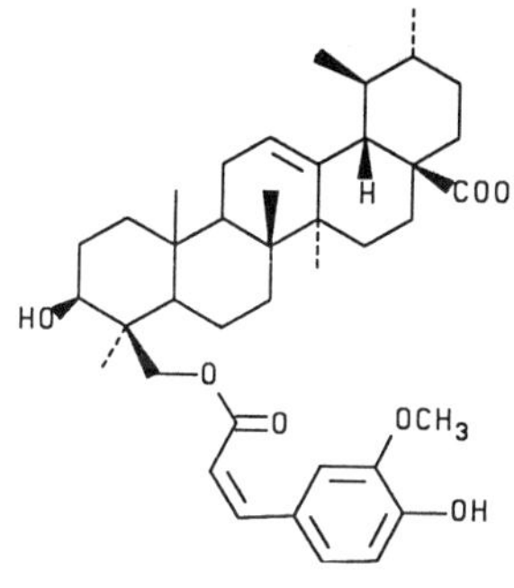

Mol. Wt.:	648
Bioactivity:	P-388: ED_{50} 1.0 μg/ml
Melting Point:	178-180°C
$[\alpha]_D^{25}$:	+33.3 Solvent: Chf
Spectral Data:	UV, IR, CMR, PMR, Mass Spec.
Organism:	*Stizophyllum riparium* (H.B.K.) Sandw. (Bigoniaceae)
Location:	Peru
Reference:	249

$C_{40}H_{56}O_7$ **3β-Hydroxy-24-<u>trans</u>-ferulyloxyurs-12-en-28-oic acid**

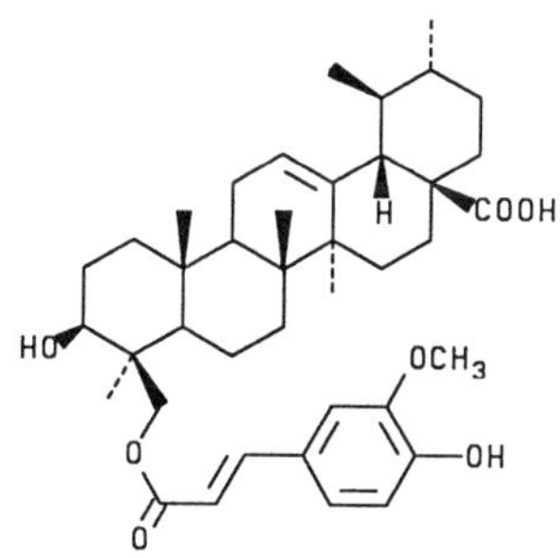

Mol. Wt.:	648
Bioactivity:	P-388: ED_{50} 1.2 μg/ml
Melting Point:	200-202°C
$[\alpha]_D^{25}$:	+28.2 Solvent: Chf
Spectral Data:	UV, IR, CMR, PMR, Mass Spec.
Organism:	*Stizophyllum riparium* (H.B.K.) Sandw. (Bigoniaceae)
Location:	Peru
Reference:	249

$C_{40}H_{62}O_8$ **Hippocaesculin**

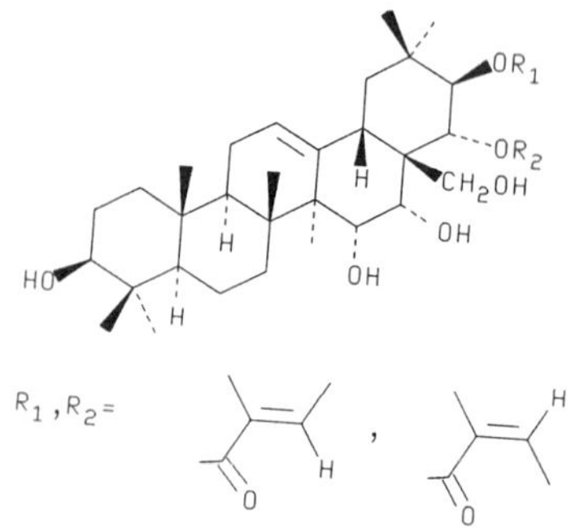

Mol. Wt.: 670
Bioactivity: KB: ED_{50} 3.6 μg/ml
Melting Point: 254-256°C
[α]D: +25 Solvent: Me
Spectral Data: IR, CMR, PMR, Mass Spec.
Organism: *Aesculus hippocastanum* L. (Hippocastanaceae)
Location: U. S.
Reference: 604

$C_{47}H_{51}NO_{14}$ **Taxol ≡ Taxol A**
(previously known)

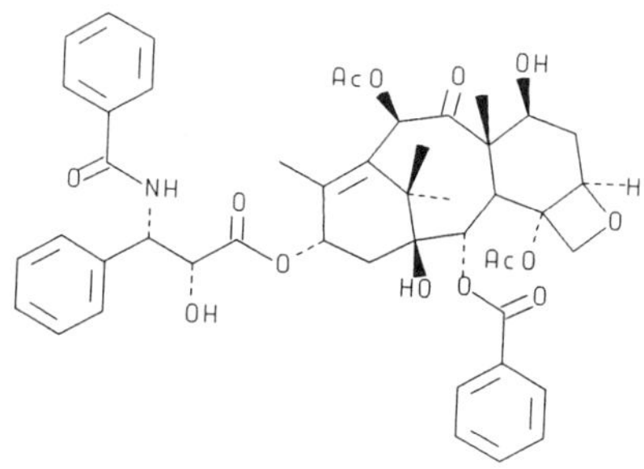

Mol. Wt.: 854
Bioactivity: P-388: T/C 164
B-16: T/C 283
L-1210: T/C 139
CX-1 colon: T/C 3
LX-1 lung: T/C 8
MX-1 mammary: T/C 77
KB: ED_{50} $3.5x10^{-5}$ μg/ml
Reduction in volume and weight of ovarian tumor
Melting Point: 213-216°C
[α]D: -49 Solvent: Chf
[α]D: -54 Me
[α]D: -21 Py
Spectral Data: UV, IR, PMR, Mass Spec.
Organism: *Taxus brevifolia*
T. baccata L.
(Taxaceae)
Location: Pacific Northwest; France
Reference: 206, 439, 937, 995, 1160

$C_{63}H_{98}O_{29}$ **Tubeimoside**

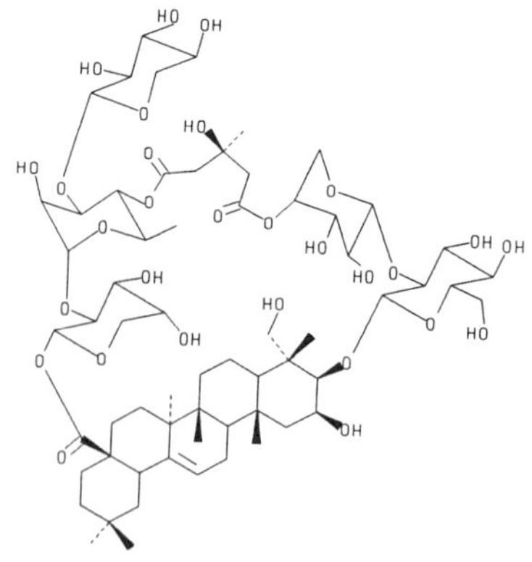

Mol. Wt.: 1320
Bioactivity: Antitumor activity
Melting Point: 250-252°C
[α]D: +14.6 Solvent: Me
Spectral Data: CMR, PMR, Mass Spec.
Organism: *Bolbostemma paniculatum* [Maxim.] Franquet (Cucurbitaceae)
Location: China
Reference: 519, 603

Semi-Syntheses or Synthetic Modifications

Compound	Activity	Reference
2'-Acetyltaxol	KB: ED_{50} $2x10^{-5}$ μg/ml P388: T/C 140 (20 mg/kg)	691
7-Acetyltaxol	KB: ED_{50} $4x10^{-3}$ μg/ml P388: T/C 130 (26 mg/kg)	691
3-O-Acetylursolic acid	KB: ED_{50} 3.7 μg/ml	644
2'-(β-Alanyl)taxol formate	KB: ED_{50} $2x10^{-4}$ μg/ml P388: T/C 153 (40 mg/kg)	691
Bis[helenalinyl] adipate	53% Inhibition of anti-inflammatory activity at 2.5 mg/kg x 2 P388: T/C 173 (8 mg/kg)	385, 643
Bis[helenalinyl] glutarate	P388: T/C 195 (8 mg/kg)	643
Bis[helenalinyl] malonate	P388: T/C 261 (15 mg/kg)	643
Bis[helenalinyl] succinate	P388: T/C 168 (8 mg/kg)	643
Bis[plenolinyl] succinate	P388: T/C 194 (15 mg/kg)	643
Erythrodiol	81.1% Inhibition of TPA-induced ^{32}P incorporation into HeLa cells	608, 819
$\Delta^{3(4)}$-5-Hydroxyovatodiolide	KB: IC_{50} 1.4 μg/ml	38

Compound	Activity	Reference
Methyl 3-O-acetyl-ursolate	P388: ED_{50} 3.1 μg/ml L1210: ED_{50} 3.5 μg/ml	644
Methyl 3-O-crotonyl-ursolate	P388: ED_{50} 3.2 μg/ml L1210: ED_{50} 2.1 μg/ml	644
Methyl 3-O-myristoyl-ursolate	P388: ED_{50} 2.6 μg/ml L1210: ED_{50} 2.8 μg/ml	644
Methyl 3-O-propionyl-ursolate	P388: ED_{50} 2.6 μg/ml L1210: ED_{50} 2.4 μg/ml	644
Methyl 3-O-senecioyl-ursolate	P388: ED_{50} 2.8 μg/ml L1210: ED_{50} 2.7 μg/ml	644
Methyl ursolate	P388: ED_{50} 4.2 μg/ml L1210: ED_{50} 5.0 μg/ml	644
18α-Olean-12-ene-3β,23,28-triol	Inhibition of TPA-induced ^{32}P incorporation: HeLa: 100% C3H10T1/2: 80% Swiss 3T3: 89% Reduction of TPA-promoted skin tumors on mice	819
18β-Olean-12-ene-3β,23,28-triol	Inhibition of TPA-induced ^{32}P incorporation: HeLa: 100% C3H10T1/2: 50% Swiss 3T3: 59% Reduction of TPA-promoted skin tumors on mice	819
18α-Olean-12-ene-3β,28-diol	100% Inhibition of TPA-induced ^{32}P incorporation into HeLa cells	819
$\Delta^{3(4),5(6)}$-Ovatodiolide	KB: IC_{50} 1.2 μg/ml	38

Chapter 5 HIGHER PLANT STEROIDS

$C_{21}H_{28}O_3$ **12β-Hydroxypregna-4,16-diene-3,20-dione** (previously known)

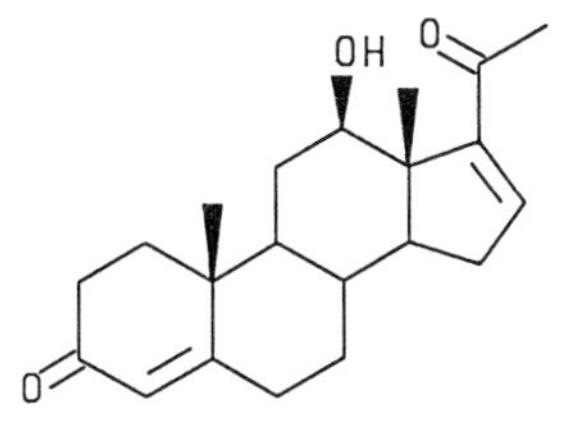

Mol. Wt.:	328
Bioactivity:	P-388: ED_{50} 0.7 μg/ml KB: ED_{50} 2.0 μg/ml
Melting Point:	232-233°C
$[\alpha]_D$:	+115 Solvent: Me
Spectral Data:	UV, IR, CMR, PMR, Mass Spec.
Organism:	*Gelsemium sempervirens* (L.) Jaume St.Hilaire (Loganiaceae)
Location:	Texas
Reference:	1203, 1208

$C_{21}H_{28}O_4$ **Stizophyllin (2α,3β,12β-Trihydroxypregna-4,7,16-trien-20-one)**

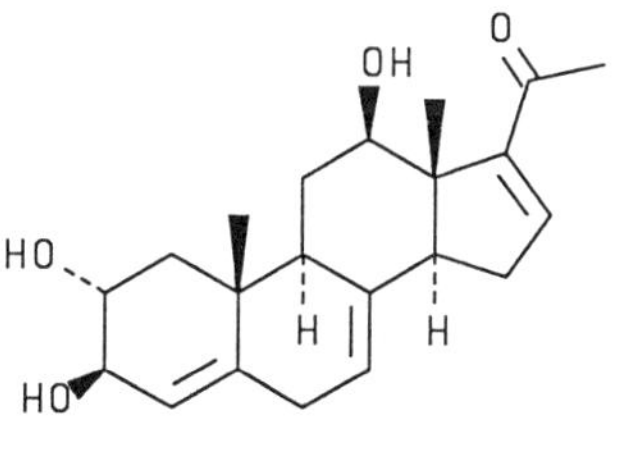

Mol. Wt.:	344
Bioactivity:	P-388: ED_{50} 0.07 μg/ml
Melting Point:	194-197°C
$[\alpha]_D^{25}$:	+60.5 Solvent: Chf
Spectral Data:	UV, IR, CMR, PMR, Mass Spec.
Organism:	*Stizophyllum riparium* (H.B.K.) Sandw. (Bignoniaceae)
Location:	Peru
Reference:	249

$C_{21}H_{30}O_3$ **12β-Hydroxy-5α-pregn-16-ene-3,20-dione**

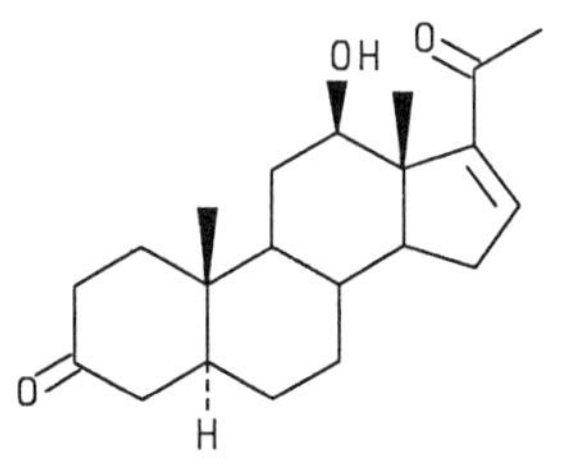

Mol. Wt.:	330
Bioactivity:	P-388: ED_{50} 0.9 μg/ml KB: ED_{50} 2.8 μg/ml
Melting Point:	231-233°C
$[\alpha]_D$:	+27 Solvent: Me
Spectral Data:	UV, IR, CMR, PMR, Mass Spec.
Organism:	*Gelsemium sempervirens* (L.) Jaume St.Hilaire (Loganiaceae)
Location:	Texas
Reference:	1208

$C_{26}H_{32}O_8$ **Bryophyllin-A**

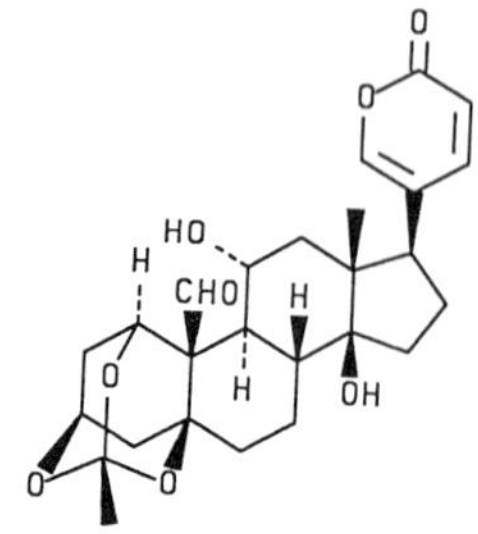

Mol. Wt.: 472
Bioactivity: KB: ED_{50} 14 ng/ml
A-549: ED_{50} 10 ng/ml
HCT-8: ED_{50} 30 ng/ml
Melting Point: 267-270°C (dec.)
$[\alpha]_D^{20}$: +14.4 Solvent: Chf
Spectral Data: UV, IR, PMR, Mass Spec., x-ray c.s.
Organism: *Bryophyllum pinnatum* (Crassulaceae)
Location: Taiwan
Reference: 1198

$C_{29}H_{42}O_{11}$ **Ghalakinoside**

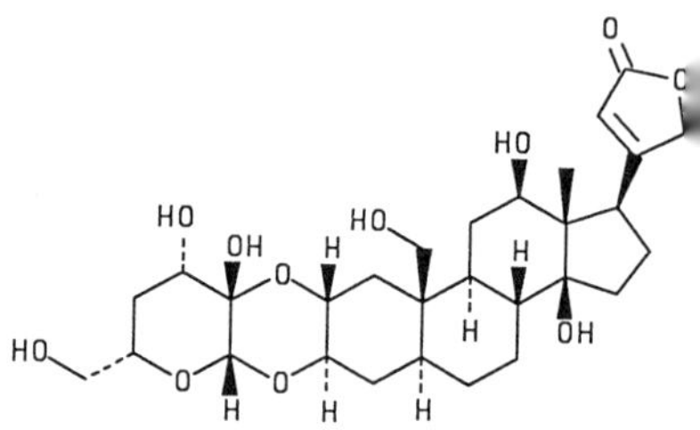

Mol. Wt.: 566
Bioactivity: 9KB: ED_{50} 2.9×10^{-2} μg/ml
Melting Point: 215-220°C
$[\alpha]_D^{25}$: +60
Spectral Data: UV, IR, CMR, PMR, Mass. Spec., x-ray c.s.
Organism: *Pergularia tomentosa* L. (Asclepiadaceae)
Location: Saudi Arabia
Reference: 15

$C_{30}H_{46}O_4$ **Manwuweizic acid**

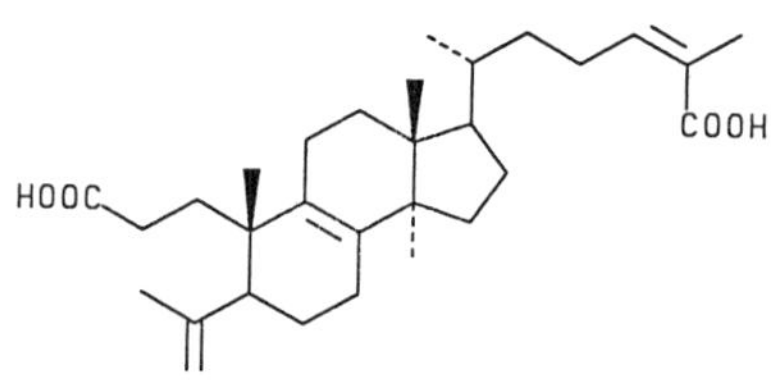

Mol. Wt.: 470
Bioactivity: Inhibition of Lewis lung cancer, brain tumor-22 and solid hepatoma
Melting Point: 191-193°C
$[\alpha]_D^{15}$: +54.3 Solvent: Chf
Spectral Data: IR, CMR, PMR, Mass Spec.
Organism: *Schisandra propinqua* (Wall) Hook. f. et Thoms
Location: Yunnan, China
Reference: 668

$C_{30}H_{46}O_8$ **Maquiroside A**

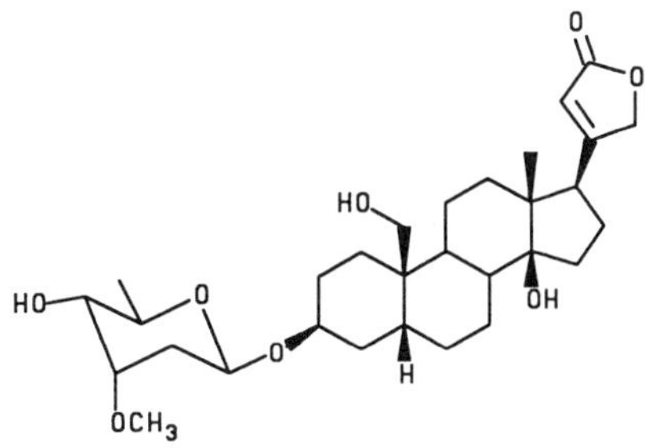

Mol. Wt.: 534
Bioactivity: KB: ED_{50} 0.013 μg/ml
Melting Point: 123-125°C
$[\alpha]_D^{25}$: +17.9 Solvent: Chf
Spectral Data: UV, IR, CMR, PMR, Mass Spec.
Organism: *Maquira calophylla* (P. & E.) C. C. Berg. (Moraceae)
Location: Peru
Reference: 950

$C_{30}H_{50}O_2$ **Inotodiol**
(previously known)

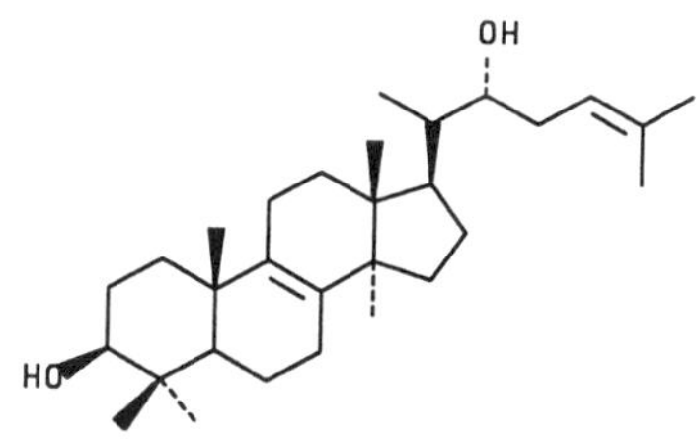

Mol. Wt.: 442
Bioactivity: Cytotoxic to HTC cells (cultured hepatoma cells)
Organism: *Inonotus obliquus* (syn. *Poria obliqua*) (Polyporaceae)
Reference: 1133

$C_{31}H_{46}O_{10}$ **Mansonin**
(previously known)

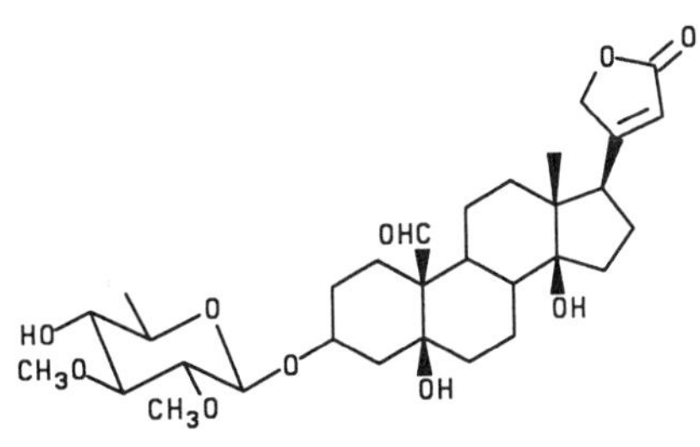

Mol. Wt.: 578
Bioactivity: KB: ED_{50} 0.04 μg/ml
Melting Point: 160°C
$[\alpha]_D^{20}$: +2.3 Solvent: Chf
Spectral Data: UV, IR, CMR, PMR, Mass Spec.
Organism: *Streblus asper* Lour. (Moraceae)
Location: Thailand
Reference: 13, 295

$C_{31}H_{46}O_{10}$ **Strebloside**
(previously known)

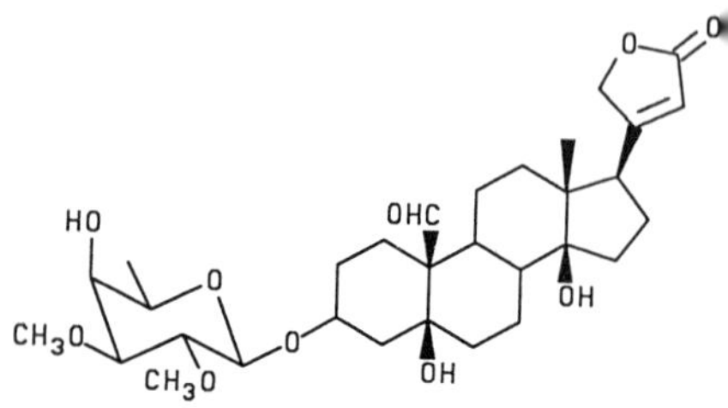

Mol. Wt.: 578
Bioactivity: KB: ED_{50} 0.035 μg/ml
Melting Point: 151°C
$[\alpha]_D^{20}$: +11.1 Solvent: Chf
Spectral Data: UV, IR, CMR, PMR, Mass Spec.
Organism: *Streblus asper* Lour.
(Moraceae)
Location: Thailand
Reference: 295, 550

$C_{32}H_{50}O_4$ **Methyl dehydrotumulosate**

Mol. Wt.: 498

$C_{32}H_{52}O_4$ **Methyl tumulosate**

Mol. Wt.: 500
Bioactivity: Cytotoxic to hepatoma cells
$[\alpha]_D$: +26 (mixture)
Spectral Data: UV, PMR, MS (mixture)
Organism: *Poria cocos*
via methylation of the extract
(Polyporaceae)
Location: China
Reference: 1133

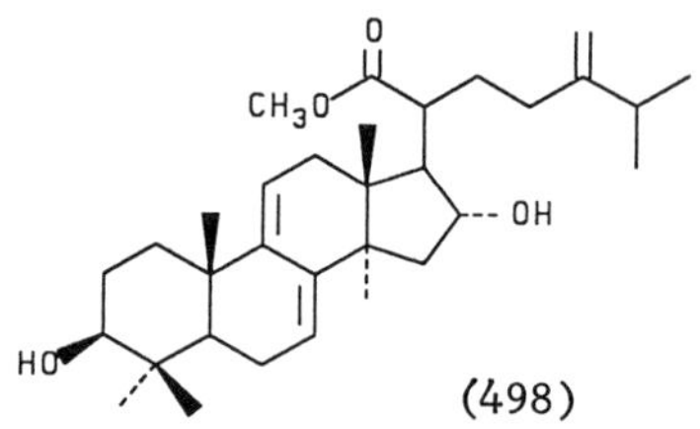

(498)

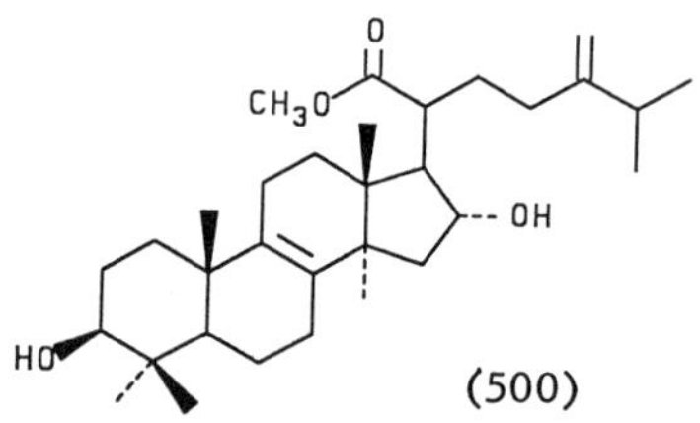

(500)

$C_{32}H_{52}O_4$ **Methyl dehydro-24-dihydrotumulosate**

Mol. Wt.: 500

$C_{32}H_{54}O_4$ **Methyl 24-dihydrotumulosate**

Mol. Wt.: 502
Bioactivity: Cytotoxicity to hepatoma cells
Spectral Data: Mass Spec.
Organism: *Poria cocos* (via methylation and reduction of the extract) (Polyporaceae)
Location: China
Reference: 1133

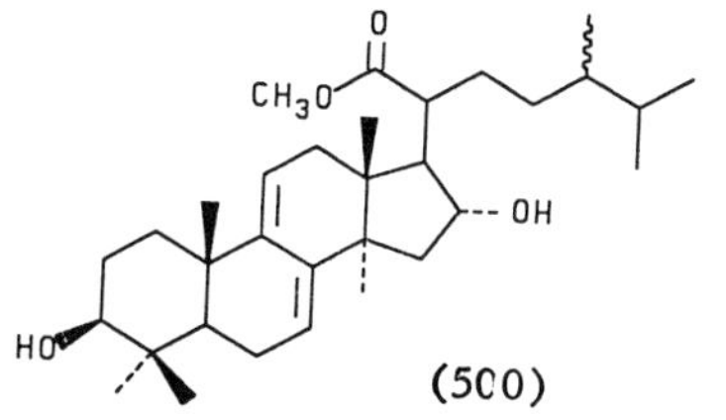

(500)

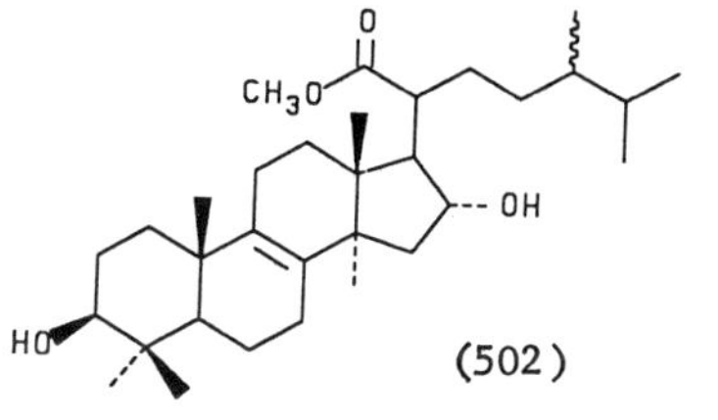

(502)

$C_{35}H_{60}O_6$ **Schottenol-3-O-β-D-glucoside**

Mol. Wt.: 576
Bioactivity: KB: ED_{50} 2.7 μg/ml
Melting Point: 260°C
Spectral Data: IR, CMR, PMR, Mass Spec.
Organism: *Baccharis coridifolia* (Compositae)
Ipomopsis aggregata (Polemoniaceae)
Location: Brazil and Idaho
Reference: 37

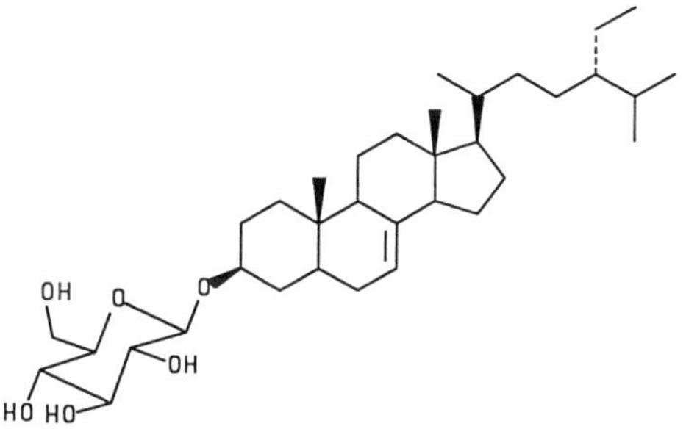

$C_{72}H_{114}O_{27}$ **Periplocoside A**

Mol. Wt.: 1412
Bioactivity: Sarcoma 180
Melting Point: 174-176°C
$[\alpha]_D^{20}$: -1.2 Solvent: Chf
Spectral Data: CMR, PMR, Mass Spec.
Organism: *Periploca sepium* (Asclepiadaceae)
Location: China
Reference: 484, 485, 486

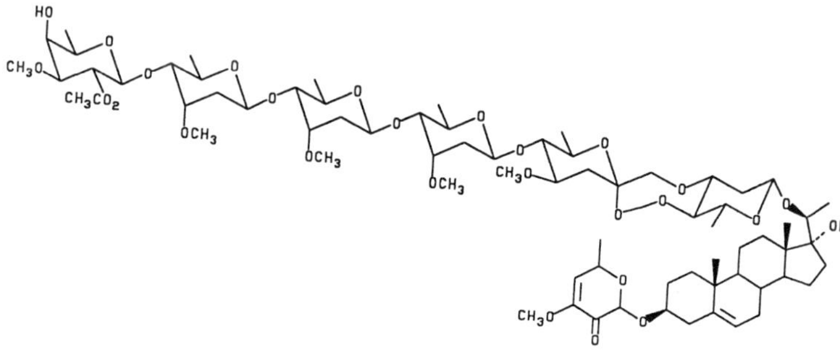

Chapter 6 HIGHER PLANT LIGNANS AND OTHER AROMATIC COMPOUNDS

$C_{20}H_{24}O_6$ **(±)-Lariciresinol**
(previously known)

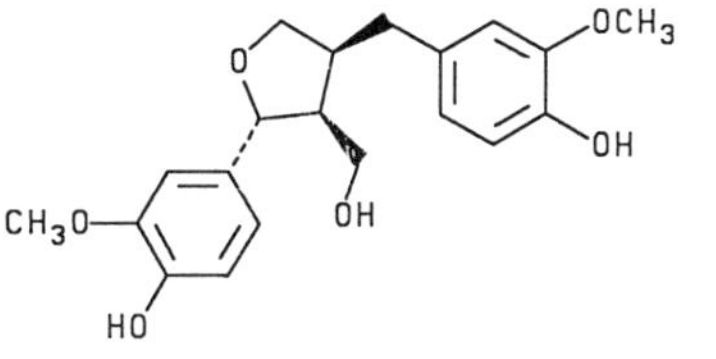

Mol. Wt.: 360
Bioactivity: P-388: ED_{50} 0.38 μg/ml
$[\alpha]_D^{25}$: -0.2 Solvent: An
Spectral Data: CMR, PMR, Mass Spec.
Organism: *Wikstroemia elliptica* Merrill (Thymelaeaceae)
Location: Hawaii
Reference: 45, 250, 404

$C_{21}H_{16}O_6$ **Justicidin B**
(previously known)

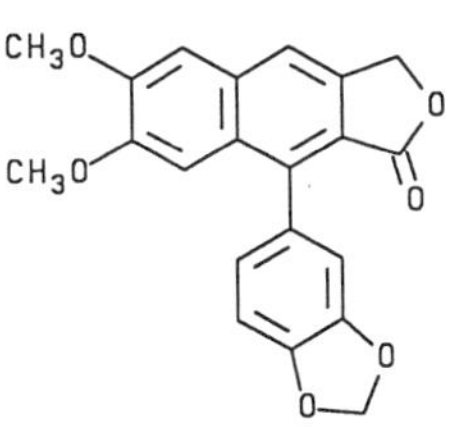

Mol. Wt.: 364
Bioactivity: P-388: ED_{50} 3.3 μg/ml
9KB: ED_{50} $7.3x10^{-2}$ and $1.2x10^{-2}$ μg/ml
Brine shrimp: LC_{50} 1.1 μg/ml
Melting Point: 263-265°C
Spectral Data: IR, PMR, Mass Spec.
Organism: *Sesbania drummondii* (Fabaceae)
Justicia pectoralis (Acanthaceae)
Phyllanthus acuminatus (Euphorbiaceae)
Location: Texas; French Guiana; Costa Rica
Reference: 444, 503, 881

$C_{21}H_{26}O_7$ **(±)-5'-Methoxylariciresinol**

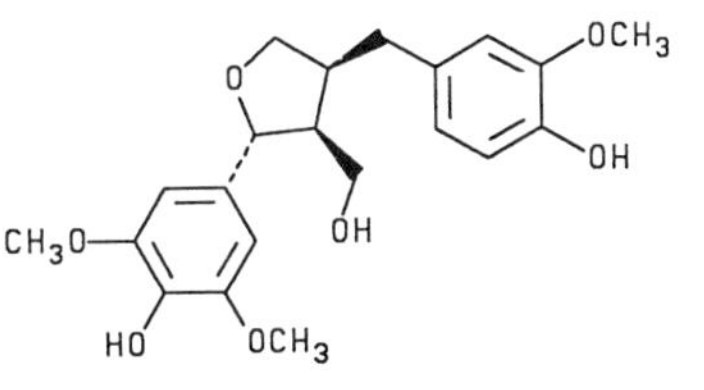

Mol. Wt.: 390
Bioactivity: P-388: ED_{50} 0.33 μg/ml
Melting Point: Resin
$[\alpha]_D^{25}$: +0.3 Solvent: An
Spectral Data: UV, IR, CMR, PMR, Mass Spec.
Organism: *Wikstroemia elliptica* Merrill (Thymelaeaceae)
Location: Hawaii
Reference: 250

$C_{22}H_{18}O_7$ **Justicidin A**
(previously known)

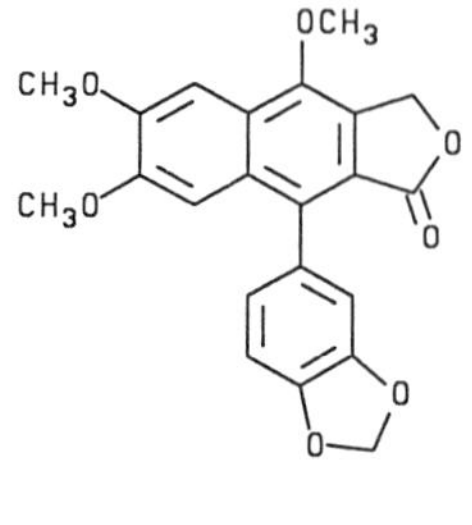

Mol. Wt.: 394
Bioactivity: KB: ED_{50} <1.0 μg/ml
Ichthyotoxicity (*Oryzias latipes*): TLm 0.049 ppm
Melting Point: 261-263°C
Spectral Data: UV, IR, PMR
Organism: *Justicia procumbens* L.
J. hayatai var. *decumbens*
(Acanthaceae)
Location: Taiwan
Reference: 319, 686, 778, 850, 851

$C_{22}H_{26}O_8$ **(±)-Syringaresinol**
(previously known)

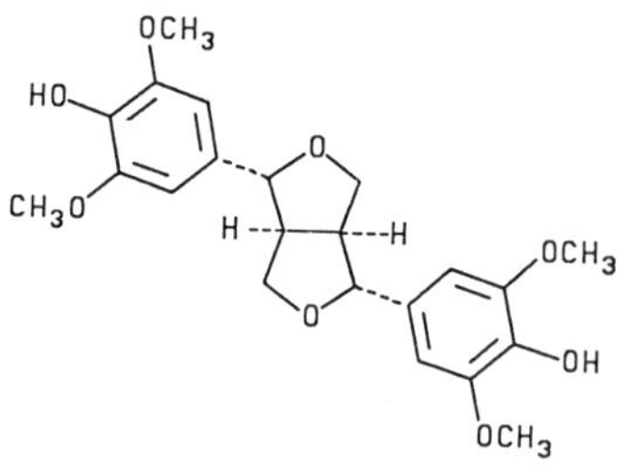

Mol. Wt.; 418
Bioactivity: P-388: ED_{50} 0.56 μg/ml
Melting Point: 174-176°C
$[\alpha]_D^{24}$: -2.1 Solvent: Chf
$[\alpha]_D^{25}$: +5.9 Solvent: Chf
Special Data: UV, IR, PMR
Organism: *Wikstroemia elliptica* Merrill
(Thymelaeaceae)
Location: Hawaii
Reference: 250, 1222

$C_{29}H_{30}O_{13}$ **Phyllanthostatin A**

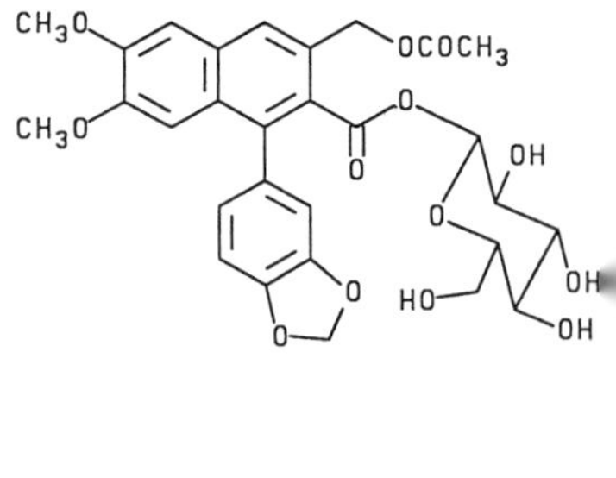

Mol. Wt.: 586
Bioactivity: P-388: ED_{50} 4 μg/ml
Melting Point: 127-130°C
$[\alpha]_D^{26}$: +24.5 Solvent: Chf
Spectral Data: UV, IR, CMR, PMR, Mass Spec.
Organism: *Phyllanthus acuminatus*
(Euphorbiaceae)
Location: Costa Rica
Reference: 891

Semi-Syntheses and Other Synthetic Modifications

Compound	Activity	Reference
1-O-(2-Amino-2-deoxy-4:6-O-ethylidene-β-D-glucopyranosyl)-4'-O-demethyl-1-epipodophyllotoxin	L1210: T/C 272 (25 μg/mouse)	958
1-O-(3-Amino-3-deoxy-4:6-O-ethylidene-β-D-glucopyranosyl)-4'-O-demethyl-1-epipodophyllotoxin	L1210: T/C 361 (25 μg/mouse)	958
4'-Demethyldehydropodophyllotoxin	KB: ED_{50} 2.2 μg/ml	57
4'-Demethylepipodophyllotoxin 4-ethyl ether	Topoisomerase II: 89% inhibition at 0.05-0.4 mM	1091
3',4'-Didemethylepipodophyllotoxin	Topoisomerase II; 75% Inhibition at 0.05-0.4 mM	1091
1-O-(2-Dimethylamino-2-deoxy-4:6-O-ethylidene-β-D-glucopyranosyl)-4'-O-demethyl-1-epipodophyllotoxin	L1210: T/C 438 (25 μg/mouse)	959
Etoposide (VP 16-213) (VP 16)	Ehrlich (ascites, ip): T/C 424 (20 mg/kg/day) Ehrlich (solid, iv): 88% inhibition at 40 mg/kg/day Sarcoma 180 (ascites, ip): T/C 228 (5 mg/kg/day) Sarcoma 180 (solid, po): 54% inhibition at 200/mg/kg/day P388 (ip-ip): T/C 242 (10 mg/kg/day) EL-LP-12 (iv): T/C 179 (40 mg/kg/day) B16 (ip-ip): T/C 223 (20 mg/kg/day) Lewis lung (iv): T/C 222 (40 mg/kg/day) Colon 26 (ip): T/C 204 (20 mg/kg/day) Colon 38 (iv): 91% inhibition at 40 mg/kg/day L1210: T/C 184 (25 μg/mouse) KB: ED_{50} 0.1 μg/ml Topoisomerase II: 85% inhibition at 0.05-0.4 mM	773, 540 686, 958 1091, 57

Chapter 7 QUINONES, FLAVANS, AND OTHER NONNITROGENOUS HIGHER PLANT PRODUCTS

$C_6H_8O_7$ **Citric acid**

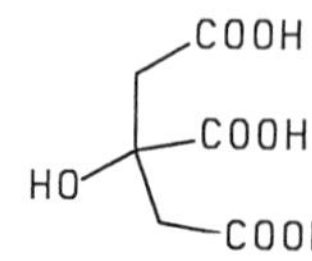

Mol. Wt.: 192
Bioactivity: Ehrlich ascites carcinoma: T/C 162 (8.4 mg/0.2 ml)
Melting Point: 153°C
Spectral Data: Mass Spec.
Organism: *Physalis alkekengi* L. var. *franchetii* Mast. (Solanaceae)
Reference: 244

$C_8H_{10}O_3$ **Halleridone**
(syn. **Rengyolone**)
(previously known)

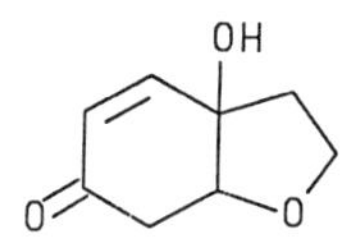

Mol. Wt.: 154
Bioactivity: P-388: IC_{50} 2.1 μg/ml
HeLa-S3: IC_{50} 2.8 μg/ml
$[\alpha]_D^{25}$: -1.5 Solvent: Me
Spectral Data: Mass Spec.
Organism: *Cornus controversa* (Cornaceae)
Location: Japan
Reference: 269, 728, 818

$C_9H_6O_3$ **Umbelliferone**
(previously known)

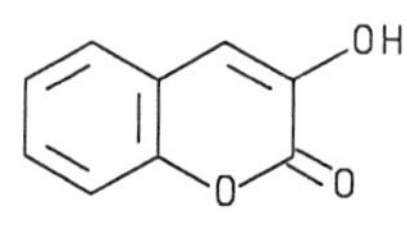

Mol. Wt.: 162
Bioactivity: P-388: ED_{50} 3.1 μg/ml
Melting Point: 245-247°C
Organism: *Wikstroemia elliptica* Merrill (Thymelaeaceae)
Location: Hawaii
Reference: 250, 392

$C_{11}H_{14}O_3$ **2,4,5-Trimethoxystyrene**
(previously known)

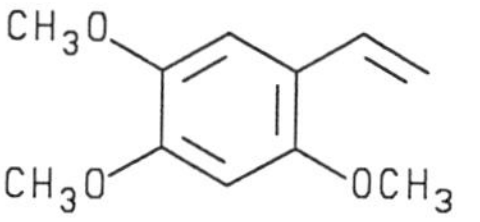

Mol. Wt.: 194
Bioactivity: Brine shrimp toxicity: LC_{50} 8 ppm
Weakly cytotoxic to 9KB and P-388
Spectral Data: UV, IR, PMR, Mass Spec.
Organism: *Duguetia panamensis* (Annonaceae)
Location: Panama
Reference: 1158, 1164

$C_{13}H_{10}O_4$ **Psychorubrin**

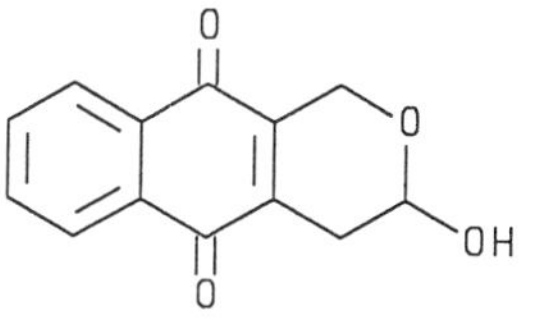

Mol. Wt.: 230
Bioactivity: KB: ED_{50} 3.0 μg/ml
Melting Point: 150-152°C
Spectral Data: UV, IR, PMR, Mass Spec.
Organism: *Psychotria rubra* (Rubiaceae)
Location: Taiwan
Reference: 407

$C_{13}H_{12}O_7$ **Tricrozarin B**

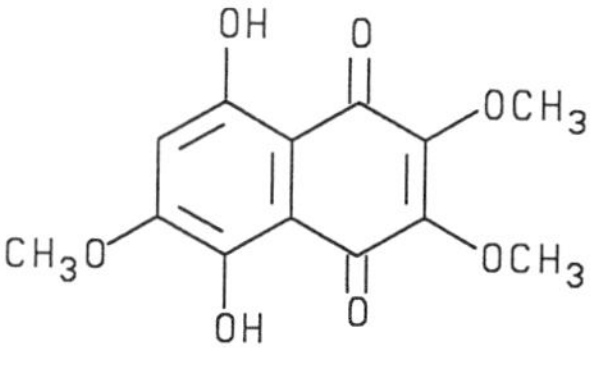

Mol. Wt.: 280
Bioactivity: Sarcoma 180 (ip): T/C 146%
(5.0 mg/kg/day for 10 days on days 1-10)
Hela S3: IC_{50} 0.007 μg/ml
Melting Point: 176-177°C
Spectral Data: UV, IR, CMR, PMR, Mass Spec.
Organism: *Tritonia crocosmaeflora* Lemoine (Iridaceae)
Location: Kagoshima, Japan
Reference: 706

$C_{17}H_{14}O_5$

Afromosin
(previously known)

Mol. Wt.: 298
Bioactivity: Inhibition of TPA-enhanced EBV-EA activation in Raji cells
Inhibition of TPA-stimulated ^{32}P incorporation into HeLa cell phospholipids
Organism: *Wisteria brachybotrys* (Leguminosae)
Location: Shikoku, Japan
Reference: 607, 1001, 1078

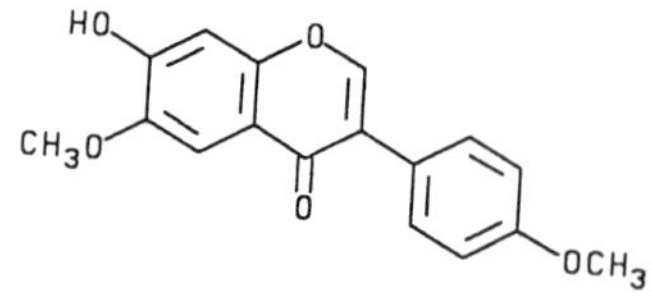

$C_{17}H_{22}O_2$

Cicutoxin
(previously known

Mol. Wt.: 258
Bioactivity: P-388: T/C 165 (1 mg/kg, 3 day dosing)
KB: ED_{50} 2.0 μg/ml
Central nervous system toxin
Melting Point: Syrup
$[\alpha]_D^{25}$: -11.8 Solvent: Alc
Spectral Data: IR, CMR, PMR
Organism: *Cicuta maculata* L. (Umbelliferae)
Location: North Carolina
Reference: 605

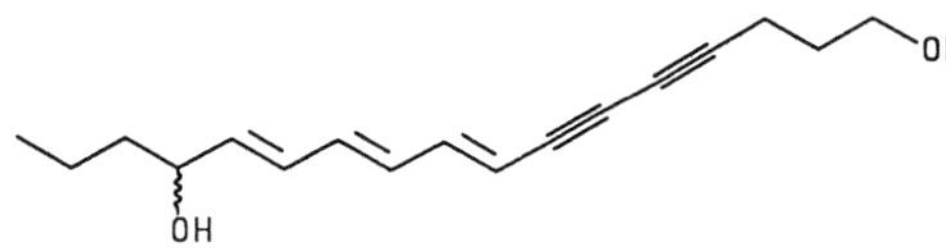

$C_{18}H_{20}O_6$

Combretastatin A-1

Mol. Wt.: 332
Bioactivity: P-388: T/C 129 (11 mg/kg)
ED_{50} 0.99 μg/ml
Inhibits microtubule assembly
Inhibits binding of colchicine to tubulin
Melting Point: 113-115°C
Spectral Data: UV, IR, CMR, PMR, Mass Spec., x-ray c.s.
Organism: *Combretum caffrum* (Eckl. and Zeyh) Kuntze (Combretaceae)
Location: South Africa
Reference: 893

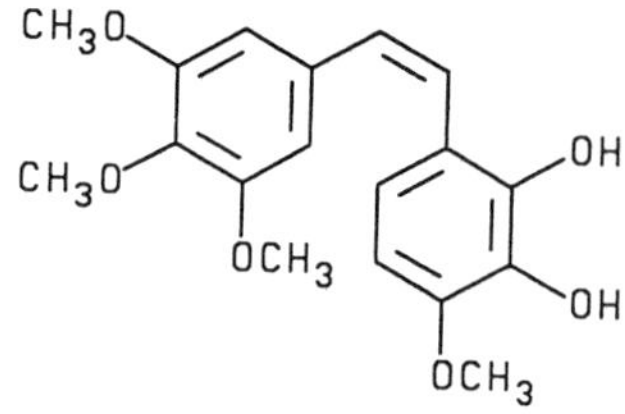

$C_{18}H_{22}O_6$ **Combretastatin B-1**

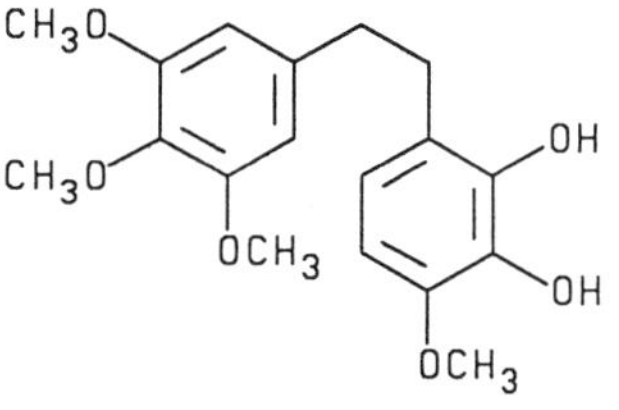

Mol. Wt.: 334
Bioactivity: P-388: ED_{50} 1.7 μg/ml
Inhibits microtubule assembly
Inhibits binding of colchicine to tubulin
Melting Point: Oil
Spectral Data: UV, IR, CMR, PMR, Mass Spec.
Organism: *Combretum caffrum* (Eckl. and Zeyh) Kuntze (Combretaceae)
Location: South Africa
Reference: 893

$C_{19}H_{12}O_7$ **Daphnoretin**
(previously known)

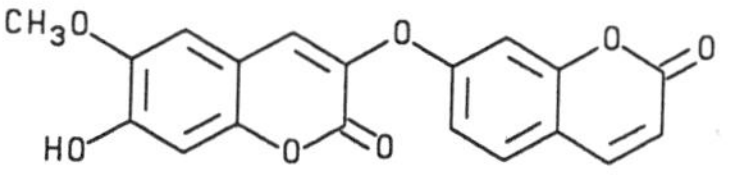

Mol. Wt.: 352
Bioactivity: P-388: ED_{50} 3.4 μg/ml
Melting Point: 245-247°C
Organism: *Wikstroemia elliptica* Merrill (Thymelaeaceae)
Location: Hawaii
Reference: 250, 392

$C_{19}H_{16}O_5$ **3',4'-Deoxypsorospermin**

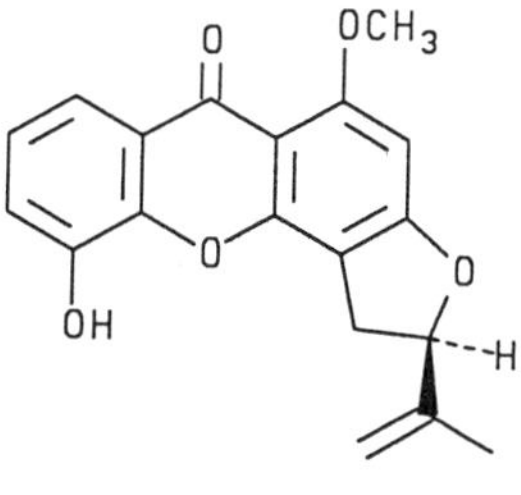

Mol. Wt.: 324
Bioactivity: 9KB: ED_{50} 0.8 μg/ml
Melting Point: 228-230°C
$[\alpha]_D^{20}$: -46 Solvent: Me
Spectral Data: UV, CD, IR, PMR, Mass Spec.
Organism: *Psorospermum febrifugum* Spach. (Guttiferae)
Location: Tanzania
Reference: 384

$C_{19}H_{17}O_6Cl$ **3′,4′-Deoxy-4′-chloropsorospermin-3′-ol**

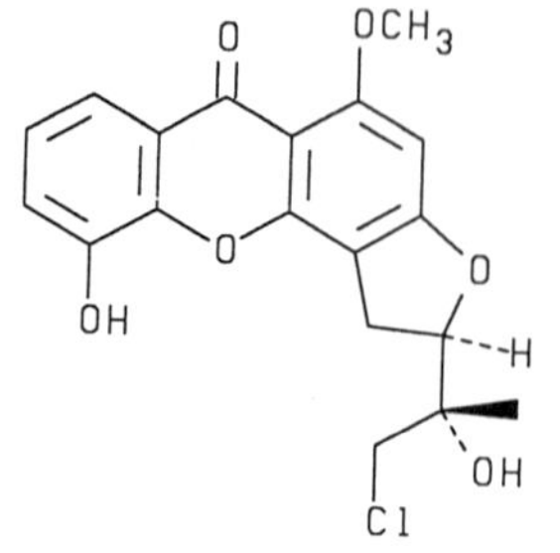

Mol. Wt.: 376
Bioactivity: P-388: T/C 135 (8 mg/kg)
9KB: ED_{50} 0.1 μg/ml
Melting Point: 269-270°C
$[\alpha]_D^{20}$: -114 Solvent: Me
Spectral Data: UV, CD, IR, PMR, Mass Spec.
Organism: *Psorospermum febrifugum* Spach. (Guttiferae)
Location: Tanzania
Reference: 384

$C_{19}H_{18}O_7$ **3′,4′-Deoxypsorospermin-3′,4′-diol**

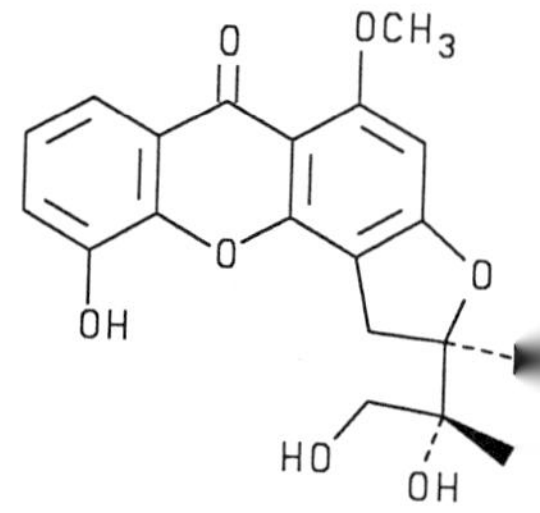

Mol. Wt.: 358
Bioactivity: 9KB: ED_{50} 7 μg/ml
Melting Point: 278-279°C
$[\alpha]_D^{20}$: -114 Solvent: Me
Spectral Data: UV, CD, IR, PMR, Mass Spec.
Organism: *Psorospermum febrifugum* Spach. (Guttiferae)
Location: Tanzania
Reference: 384

$C_{20}H_{24}O_7$ **10-(1′,2′,3′-Trihydroxy-3′-methylbutanyl)spatheliachromen**

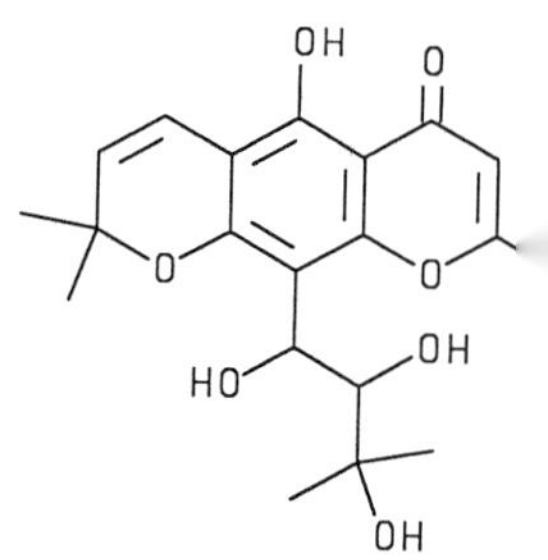

Mol. Wt.: 376
Bioactivity: 9PS: ED_{50} 0.5 μg/ml
Melting Point: 120-122°C
Spectral Data: UV, IR, PMR, Mass Spec.
Organism: *Spathelia sorbifolia* L. (Rutaceae)
Location: Jamaica
Reference: 1054

$C_{21}H_{20}O_6$ **Curcumin**
(previously known)

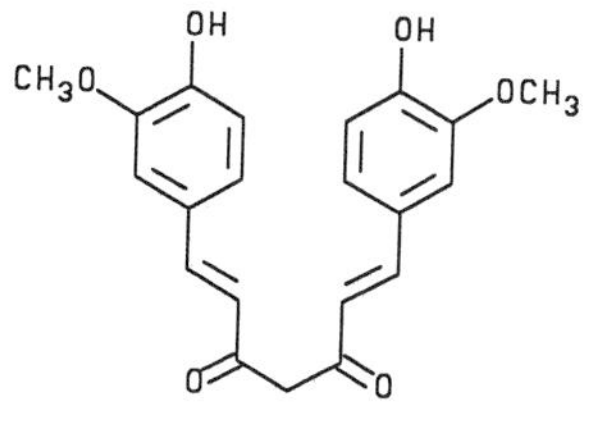

Mol. Wt.: 368
Bioactivity: Dalton's lymphoma: 100% at 4 μg/ml
Leukemic lymphocytes: 100% at 8 μg/ml
Normal lymphocytes: 100% at 8 μg/ml
Reduction in growth of tumor induced by Dalton's lymphoma at 1 mg/animal
Melting Point: 183°C
Organism: *Curcuma longa* L. (Zingiberaceae)
Reference: 630

$C_{21}H_{22}O_5$ **Vismione B**
(previously known)

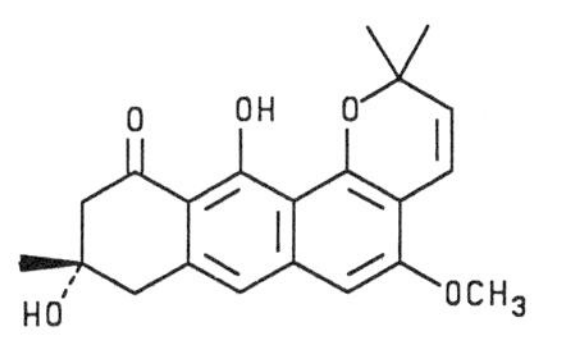

Mol. Wt.: 354
Bioactivity: P-388/S: ID_{50} 10 μg/ml
P-388/R: ID_{50} 3.0 μg/ml
9KB: ID_{50} 10.0 μg/ml
Melting Point: 200-202°C
$[\alpha]_D$: +24 Solvent: Chf
Spectral Data: UV, IR, PMR, Mass Spec.
Organism: *Vismia baccifera* var. *dealbata* (H.B.K.)
V. lindeniana
V. falcata
(Guttiferae)
Location: Venezuela
Reference: 158, 228, 229

$C_{21}H_{24}O_5$ **Desacetylvismione A**
(previously known)

Mol. Wt.: 356
Bioactivity: P-388/S: ID_{50} 0.4 μg/ml
P-388/R: ID_{50} 0.3 μg/ml
9KB: ID_{50} 0.7 μg/ml
Melting Point: 163-165°C (dec.)
$[\alpha]_D$: +7.0 Solvent: Chf
Organism: *Vismia lindeniana* Dcne.
V. macrophylla
V. falcata
(Guttiferae)
Location: Columbia; Venezuela
Reference: 158, 228

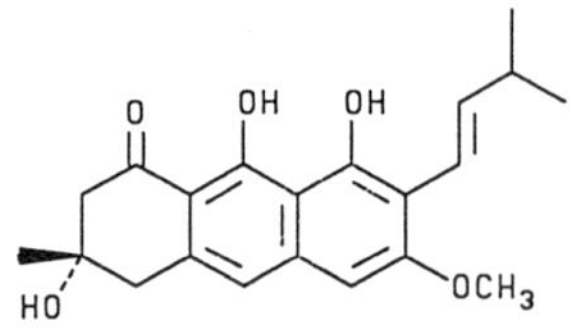

$C_{21}H_{24}O_5$ **5-O-Methylsorbifolin**
(previously known)

Mol. Wt.: 356
Bioactivity: 9PS: ED_{50} 0.3 μg/ml
Melting Point: 120-121°C
Spectral Data: PMR, Mass Spec.
Organism: *Spathelia sorbifolia* L.
(Rutaceae)
Location: Jamaica
Reference: 1054, 1085

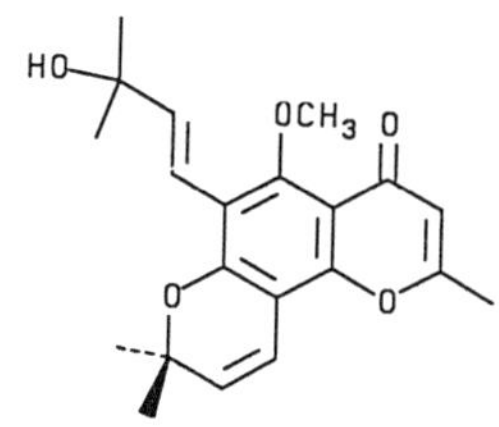

$C_{21}H_{34}O$ **Ginkgol**
(previously known)

Mol. Wt.: 302
Bioactivity: Sarcoma 180 antitumor activity
Melting Point: Oil
Spectral Data: UV, IR, CMR, PMR, Mass Spec.
Organism: *Ginkgo biloba* L.
(Ginkgoaceae)
Location: Japan
Reference: 481, 770

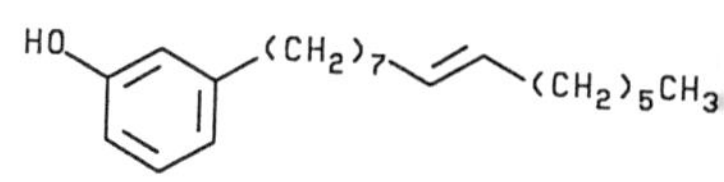

$C_{21}H_{34}O_2$ **Bilobol**
(previously known)

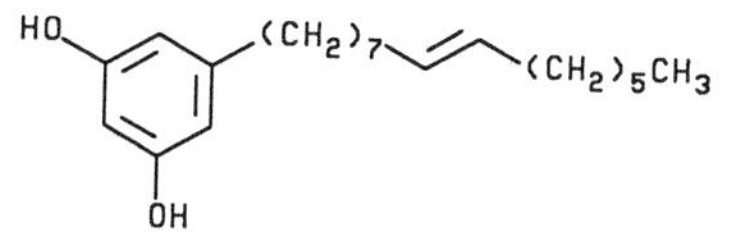

Mol. Wt.: 318
Bioactivity: Sarcoma 180 antitumor activity
Melting Point: 36°C
Spectral Data: UV, IR, CMR, PMR, Mass Spec.
Organism: *Ginkgo biloba* L. (Ginkgoaceae)
Location: Japan
Reference: 481, 770

$C_{22}H_{24}O_6$ **Vismione C**
(previously known)

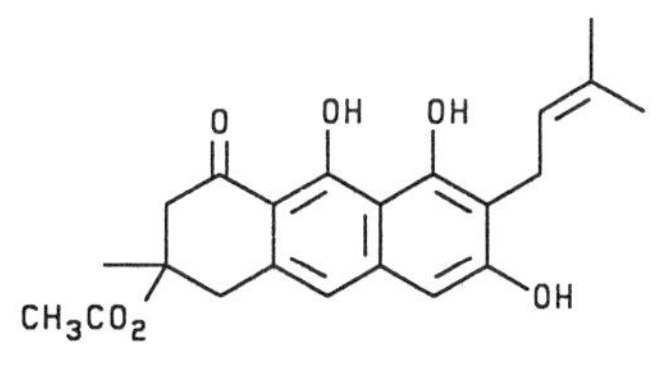

Mol. Wt.: 384
Bioactivity: 9KB: ID_{50} 2.1 μg/ml
Melting Point: 100-105°C
Spectral Data: UV, PMR, Mass Spec.
Organism: *Psorospermum febrifugum* Spach.
P. glaberrimum
(Guttiferae)
Location: Nigeria; Ivory Coast
Reference: 96, 158, 227

$C_{22}H_{34}O_3$ **Ginkgol acid**
(previously known)

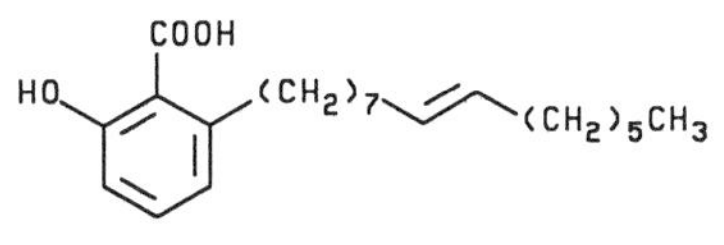

Mol. Wt.: 346
Bioactivity: Sarcoma 180 antitumor activity
Antimicrobial activity
Melting Point: 41-42°C
Spectral Data: UV, IR, CMR, PMR, Mass Spec.
Organism: *Ginkgo biloba* L. (Ginkgoaceae)
Location: Japan
Reference: 481, 770

$C_{23}H_{24}O_6$ **Acetylvismione B**
(previously known)

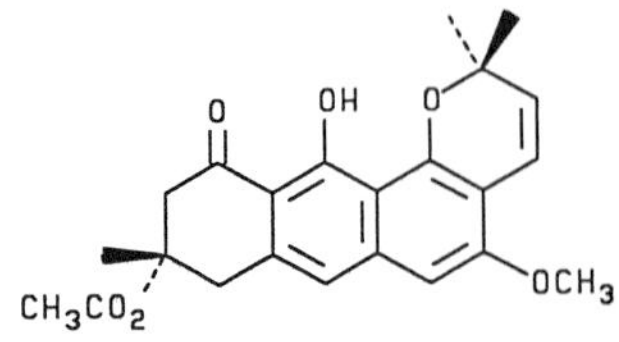

Mol. Wt.:	396
Bioactivity:	P-388/S: ID_{50} 5.0 μg/ml
	P-388/R: ID_{50} 2.0 μg/ml
Melting Point:	115-120°C (dec.)
Spectral Data:	UV, IR, PMR, Mass Spec.
Organism:	*Vismia japurensis* Reich (Guttiferae)
Location:	Brazil
Reference:	158, 776

$C_{23}H_{26}O_6$ **Vismione A**
(previously known)

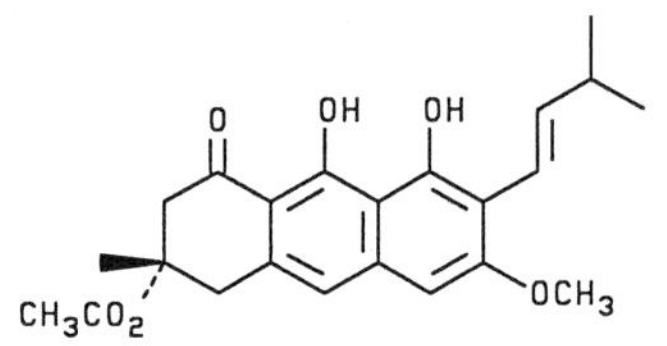

Mol. Wt.:	398
Bioactivity:	B16: T/C 148 (5mg/kg/5 days)
	M5076: T/C 145-147 (5mg/kg/9 days)
	P-388/S: ID_{50} 0.45 μg/ml
	P-388/R: ID_{50} 1.1 μg/ml
	9KB: ID_{50} 0.25 μg/ml
Melting Point:	140-141°C
$[\alpha]_D$:	+54 Solvent: Chf
Spectral Data:	UV, IR, PMR, Mass Spec., x-ray c.s.
Organism:	*Vismia baccifera* var. *dealbata* (H.B.K.)
	V. lindeniana
	V. falcata
	(Guttiferae)
Location:	Venezuela
Reference:	158, 228, 229

$C_{24}H_{28}O_9$ **Mallotochromanol**

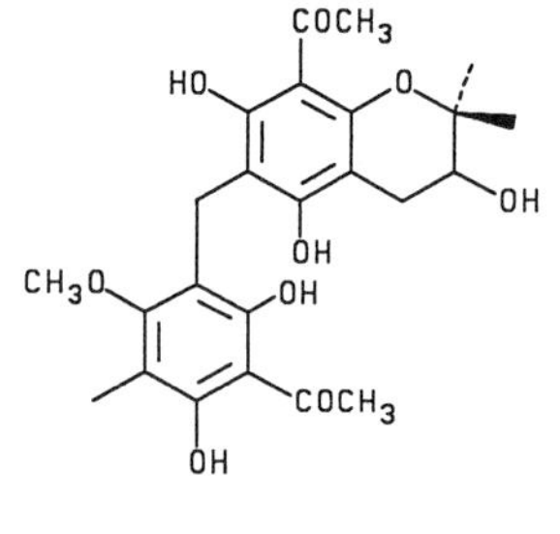

Mol. Wt.:	460
Bioactivity:	KB: ED_{50} 8.60 μg/ml (acetate)
	L-5178Y: ED_{50} 4.50 μg/ml (acetate)
Melting Point:	216-218°C
$[\alpha]_D^{23}$:	-0.74 Solvent: Chf
Spectral Data:	UV, CD of benzoate, IR, CMR, PMR, Mass Spec.
Organism:	*Mallotus japonicus* Muell. Arg. (Euphorbiaceae)
Location:	Japan
Reference:	36

$C_{25}H_{24}O_6$ **Cudraisoflavone-A**

Mol. Wt.: 420
Bioactivity: P-388: Cytotoxic at 1 μg/ml
Melting Point: 167-170°C
Spectral Data: UV, PMR, Mass Spec.
Organism: *Cudrania cochinchinensis* (Moraceae)
Location: Hong Kong
Reference: 1050

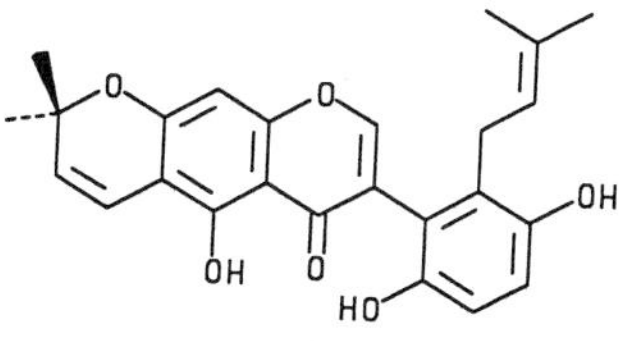

$C_{25}H_{30}O_5$ **Vismione F**
(previously known)

Mol. Wt.: 410
Bioactivity: P-388/S: ID_{50} 2.0 μg/ml
9KB: ID_{50} 2.8 μg/ml
Melting Point: 144-146°C
Spectral Data: UV, PMR, Mass Spec.
Organism: *Psorospermum corymbiferum* Hochr.
P. glaberrimum
(Guttiferae)
Location: Ivory Coast
Reference: 95, 158, 227

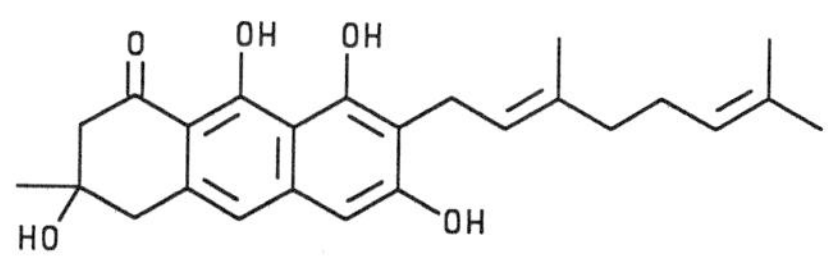

$C_{26}H_{30}O_8$ **Butyrylmallotochromene**

Mol. Wt.: 470
Bioactivity: KB: ED_{50} 3.3 μg/ml
Melting Point: 175-176°C
Spectral Data: UV, IR, CMR, PMR, Mass Spec.
Organism: *Mallotus japonicus* Muell. Arg.
(Euphorbiaceae)
Location: Japan
Reference: 315

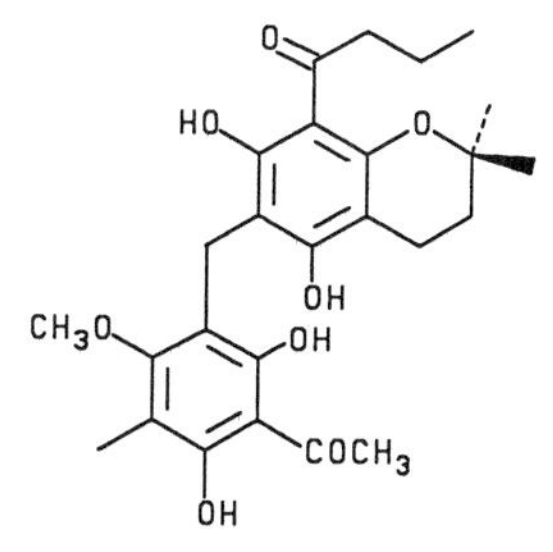

$C_{26}H_{30}O_8$ **Isobutyrylmallotochromene**

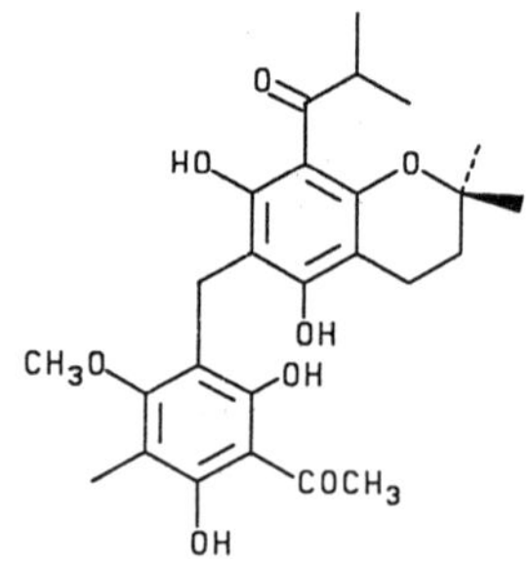

Mol. Wt.:	470
Bioactivity:	KB: ED_{50} 0.4 μg/ml
Melting Point:	180-181°C
Spectral Data:	UV, IR, CMR, PMR, Mass Spec.
Organism:	*Mallotus japonicus* Muell. Arg. (Euphorbiaceae)
Location:	Japan
Reference:	315

$C_{26}H_{32}O_9$ **Mallotolerin**

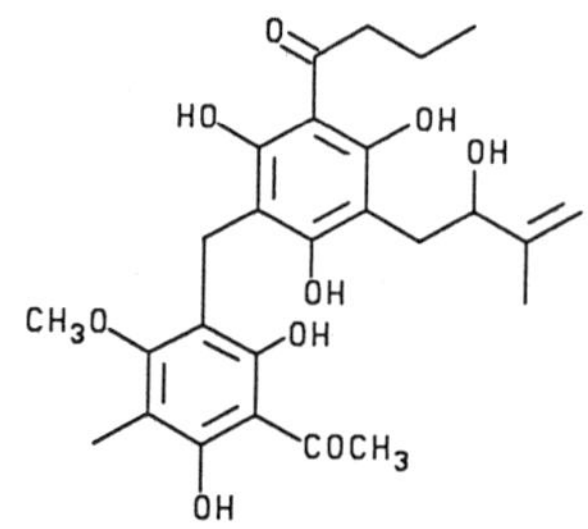

Mol. Wt.:	488
Bioactivity:	KB: ED_{50} 0.95 μg/ml L-5178Y: ED_{50} 0.82 μg/ml
Melting Point:	197-198°C
$[\alpha]_D^{23}$:	-0.30 Solvent: Chf
Spectral Data:	UV, IR, CMR, PMR, Mass Spec.
Organism:	*Mallotus japonicus* (Euphorbiaceae)
Location:	Japan
Reference:	36

$C_{27}H_{24}O_7$ **Larreantin**

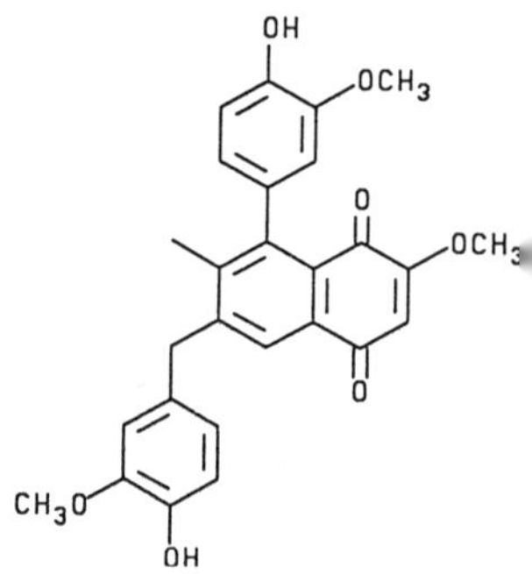

Mol. Wt.:	460
Bioactivity:	P-388: ED_{50} 0.38 μg/ml
Melting Point:	204-206°C
Spectral Data:	UV, IR, CMR, PMR, Mass Spec.
Organism:	*Larrea tridentata* (DC) Coville (Zygophyllaceae)
Location:	Arizona
Reference:	680

$C_{27}H_{32}O_6$

Acetylvismione D
(previously known)

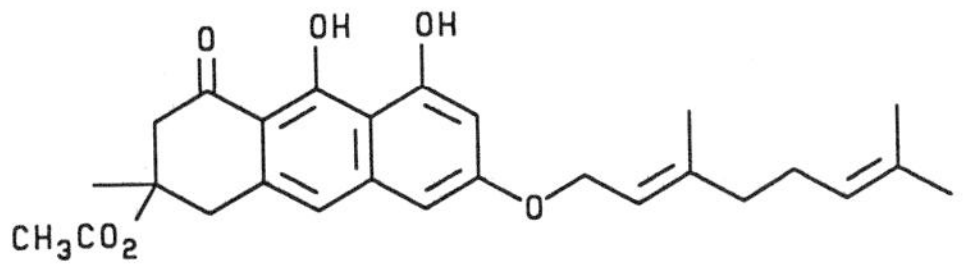

Mol. Wt.: 452
Bioactivity: P-388/S: ID_{50} 1.8 μg/ml
9KB: ID_{50} 5.0 μg/ml
Melting Point: 65-66°C
$[\alpha]_D^{22}$: +6.0 Solvent: Chf
Spectral Data: UV, IR, PMR, Mass Spec.
Organism: *Psorospermum febrifugum* Spach. (Guttiferae)
Location: Zaire
Reference: 94, 158

$C_{27}H_{32}O_6$

Acetylvismione F
(previously known)

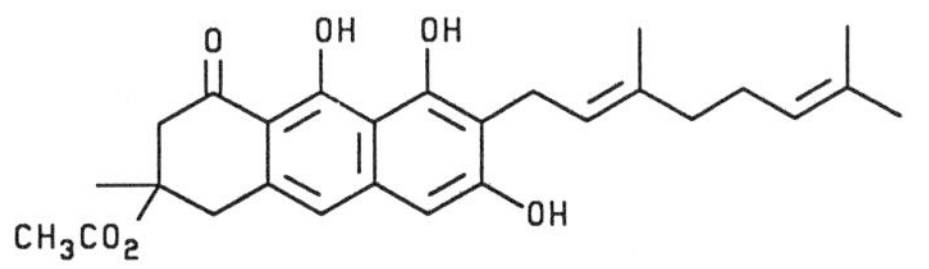

Mol. Wt.: 452
Bioactivity: P-388/S: ID_{50} 2.7 μg/ml
P-388/R: ID_{50} 3.0 μg/ml
9KB: ID_{50} 1.0 μg/ml
Melting Point: 119-121°C (dec.)
Spectral Data: UV, IR, PMR, Mass Spec.
Organism: *Psorospermum corymbiferum* Hochr. (Guttiferae)
Location: Ivory Coast
Reference: 158, 227

$C_{27}H_{32}O_6$

Vismione G
(previously known)

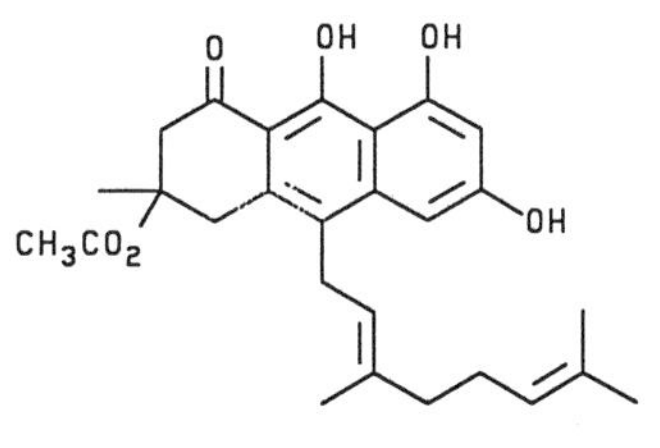

Mol. Wt.: 452
Bioactivity: 9KB: ID_{50} 3.2 μg/ml
Melting Point: 185-188°C (dec.)
Spectral Data: UV, IR, PMR, Mass Spec.
Organism: *Psorospermum glaberrimum* Hochr. (Guttiferae)
Location: Ivory Coast
Reference: 158, 227

$C_{28}H_{24}O_5$ **Marchantin A**

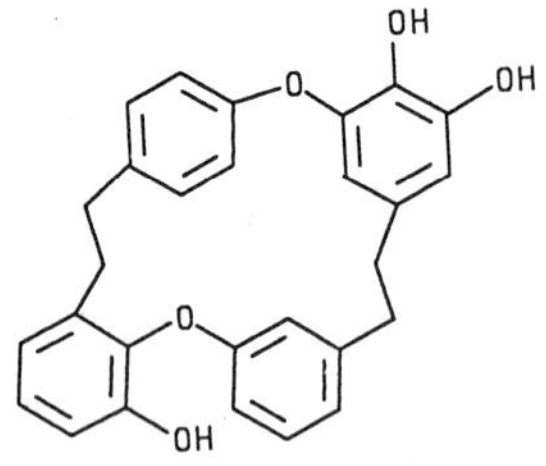

Mol. Wt.: 440
Bioactivity: KB: ED_{50} 8.4 μg/ml
P-388: T/C 117
Spectral Data: PMR, x-ray c.s. (of derivative)
Organism: *Marchantia polymorpha*
M. paleacea var. *diptera*
M. tosana
(Bryophyta)
Reference: 42, 591

$C_{44}H_{74}O_{18}$ **Glycoside 1a**

Mol. Wt.: 890
Bioactivity: Sarcoma 180: 71.9% tumor inhibition in mice at 10 mg/kg
Melting Point: 100-102°C
Spectral Data: IR, CMR, PMR, Mass Spec.
Organism: *Ipomoea bahiensis* Willd
(Convolvulaceae)
Reference: 69

NPF-86IA
Polyphenol

Mol. Wt.: 5620
Bioactivity: Inhibition of 5'-nucleotidase activity
Ehrlich ascites carcinoma: ILS: 100% at 20 mg/kg
Ehrlich ascites carcinoma strain E: 50% inhibition at 27 μg/ml
HeLa: 50% inhibition at 6.2 μg/ml
HL-60: 50% inhibition at 17 μg/ml
Toxicity (mice): LD_{50}: >150 mg/kg (ip); >500 mg/kg (po)
Melting Point: >300°C
Spectral Data: UV, IR
Organism: *Areca catechu* (Palmae)
Location: Southeast Asia
Reference: 490, 1116

NPF-86IB
Polyphenol

Mol. Wt.: 5000
Bioactivity: Inhibition of 5'-nucleotidase activity
Ehrlich ascites carcinoma: ILS: 100% at 20 mg/kg
Moderate cytotoxicity against Ehrlich ascites carcinoma, HeLa and HL-60 cells
Toxicity (mice): LD_{50}: >150 mg/kg (ip); >500 mg/kg (po)
Melting Point: >300°C
Spectral Data: UV, IR
Organism: *Areca catechu* (Palmae)
Location: Southeast Asia
Reference: 490, 1116

NPF-86IIA
Polyphenol

Mol. Wt.:	29,400
Bioactivity:	Inhibition of 5'-nucleotidase activity Antitumor activity against Ehrlich ascites carcinoma Moderate cytotoxicity against Ehrlich ascites carcinoma, HeLa and HL-60 cells Toxicity (mice): LD_{50}: >150 mg/kg (ip); >500 mg/kg (po)
Melting Point:	>300°C
Spectral Data:	UV, IR
Organism:	*Areca catechu* (Palmae)
Location:	Southeast Asia
Reference:	490, 1116

NPF-86IIB
Polyphenol

Mol. Wt.:	8610
Bioactivity:	Inhibition of 5'-nucleotidase activity Antitumor activity against Ehrlich ascites carcinoma Moderate cytotoxicity against Ehrlich ascites carcinoma, HeLa and HL-60 cells Toxicity (mice): LD_{50} >150 mg/kg (ip); >500 mg/kg (po)
Melting Point:	>300°C
Spectral Data:	UV, IR
Organism:	*Areca catechu* (Palmae)
Location:	Southeast Asia
Reference:	490, 1116

Semi-Syntheses or Synthetic Modifications

Compound	Activity	Reference
4-Acetamino-α,α-bis(7-hydroxy-5-isopropyltropon-2-yl)toluene	P388: T/C 171 (5 mg/kg) KB: ED_{50} <0.3 μg/ml	1201
7-O-Acetylafromosin	Inhibition of TPA-enhanced EBV-EA activation in Raji cells Inhibition of TPA-stimulated ^{32}P incorporation into HeLa cell phospholipids	607, 1001, 1078
7-O-Acetylformononetin	Inhibition of TPA-enhanced EBV-EA activation in Raji cells Inhibition of TPA-stimulated ^{32}P incorporation into HeLa cell phospholipids	607, 1001, 1078
Acetylhalleridone	P388: IC_{50} 0.5 μg/ml HeLa-S_3: IC_{50} 4.1 μg/ml	818
Benzoylhalleridone	P388: IC_{50} 0.5 μg/ml HeLa-S_3: IC_{50} 1.6 μg/ml	818
α,α-Bis(7-hydroxy-5-isopropyltropon-2-yl)-furan	P388: T/C 177 (5 mg/kg)	1201
α,α-Bis(7-hydroxy-5-isopropyltropon-2-yl)-4-hydroxytoluene	P388: T/C 195 (5 mg/kg) KB: ED_{50} <0.3 μg/ml	1201
α,α-Bis(7-hydroxy-5-isopropyltropon-2-yl)-4-methoxytoluene	P388: T/C 173 (5 mg/kg) KB: ED_{50} <0.3 μg/ml	1200, 1201, 1202
α,α-Bis(7-hydroxy-5-isopropyltropon-2-yl)-3,4-methylenedioxytoluene	P388: T/C 193 (10 mg/kg) KB: ED_{50} 0.5 μg/ml	1201

Compound	Activity	Reference
α,α-Bis(7-hydroxy-5-isopropyltropon-2-yl)-naphthalene	P388: T/C 180 (5 mg/kg) KB: ED_{50} 2.6 μg/ml	1201
α,α-Bis(7-hydroxy-5-isopropyltropon-2-yl)-thiophene	P388: T/C 178 (5 mg/kg) KB: ED_{50} 0.6 μg/ml	1201
α,α-Bis(7-hydroxy-5-iso-propyltropon-2-yl)toluene	P388: T/C 188 (5 mg/kg) KB: ED_{50} <0.3 μg/ml	1200, 1201, 1202
Butanoylhalleridone	P388: IC_{50} 0.6 μg/ml HeLa-S_3: IC_{50} 2.7 μg/ml	818
Butyrylmallotochromene tetraacetate	KB: ED_{50} 2.6 μg/ml	315
1'-Chlorobenzoyl-halleridone	P388: IC_{50} 0.4 μg/ml HeLa-S_3: IC_{50} 1.0 μg/ml	818
2'-Chlorobenzoyl-halleridone	P388: IC_{50} <0.1 μg/ml HeLa-S_3: IC_{50} 1.2 μg/ml	818
3'-Chlorobenzoyl-halleridone	P388: IC_{50} 0.7 μg/ml HeLa-S_3: IC_{50} 0.9 μg/ml	818
Demethyl-α-lapachone (cis/trans mixture)	KB: ED_{50} 0.4 μg/ml	407
Hexanoylhalleridone	P388: IC_{50} 0.3 μg/ml HeLa-S_3: IC_{50} 1.8 μg/ml	818
Isobutyrylmallotochromene tetraacetate	KB: ED_{50} 2.7 μg/ml	315
2-Methylnaphtho[1,2-b]-furan-4,5-dione	KB: ED_{50} 0.6 μg/ml	407

Compound	Activity	Reference
2-Methylnaphtho[2,3-b]-furan-4,9-dione	KB: ED_{50} 0.3 μg/ml	407
2H-Naphtho[2,3-b]pyran-5,10-dione	KB: ED_{50} 0.4 μg/ml	407
Octanoylhalleridone	P388: IC_{50} 0.3 μg/ml HeLa-S_3: IC_{50} 0.8 μg/ml	818

Chapter 8 HIGHER PLANT ALKALOIDS, AMIDES, AND PEPTIDES

$C_{14}H_{13}NO_6$ — **7-Deoxynarciclasine**
(syn. **Margetine**, **Lycoricidine**)
(previously known)

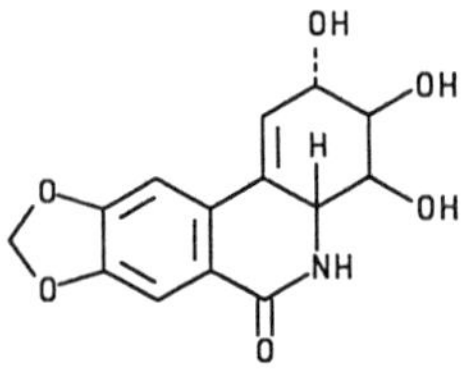

Mol. Wt.:	291
Bioactivity:	P-388: T/C 161 (12.5 mg/kg) P-388: ED_{50} 0.02 μg/ml
Melting Point:	251-252°C
$[\alpha]_D^{33}$:	+157.3 Solvent: DMSO
Spectral Data:	UV, IR, CMR, PMR, Mass Spec., x-ray c.s.
Organism:	*Pancratium littorale* Jacq. (Amaryllidaceae)
Location:	Hawaii
Reference:	761, 762, 843, 847, 882, 896

$C_{14}H_{15}NO_8$ — **Pancratistatin**

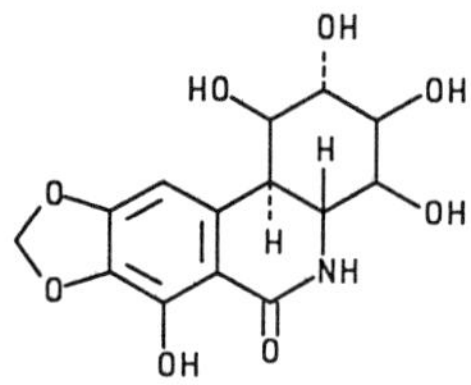

Mol. Wt.:	325
Bioactivity:	P-388: T/C 206 (12.5 mg/kg) P-388: ED_{50} 0.01 μg/ml M-5076: T/C 184 (3.0 mg/kg)
Melting Point:	322-324°C (dec.)
$[\alpha]_D^{34}$;	+48 Solvent: DMSO
Spectral Data:	UV, IR, CMR, PMR, Mass Spec., x-ray c.s.
Organism:	*Pancratium littorale* Jacq. (Amaryllidaceae)
Location:	Hawaii
Reference:	882

$C_{15}H_{10}N_2O_3$ — **1-Hydroxy-11-methoxycanthin-6-one**

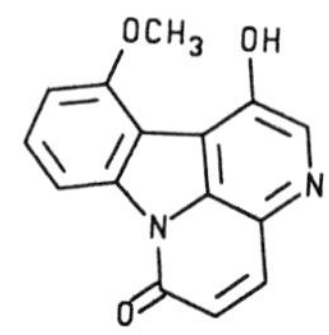

Mol. Wt.:	266
Bioactivity:	KB: ED_{50} 2.0 μg/ml
Melting Point:	220-223°C (dec.)
Spectral Data:	UV, IR, PMR, Mass Spec.
Organism:	*Brucea antidysenterica* (Simaroubaceae)
Location:	Ethiopia; Kenya
Reference:	320, 395

$C_{15}H_{10}N_2O_3$ **11-Hydroxy-1-methoxycanthin-6-one**

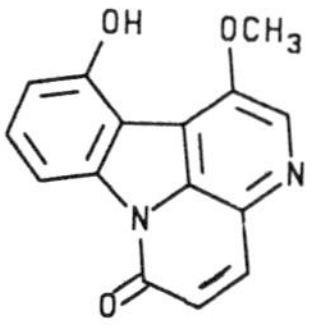

Mol. Wt.: 266
Bioactivity: KB: ED_{50} 2.0 μg/ml
Melting Point: 237-240°C (dec.)
Spectral Data: UV, IR, PMR, Mass Spec.
Organism: *Brucea antidysenterica* (Simaroubaceae)
Location: Ethiopia; Kenya
Reference. 320, 395

$C_{16}H_{11}NO_3$ **Aristolactam-AII**
(previously known)

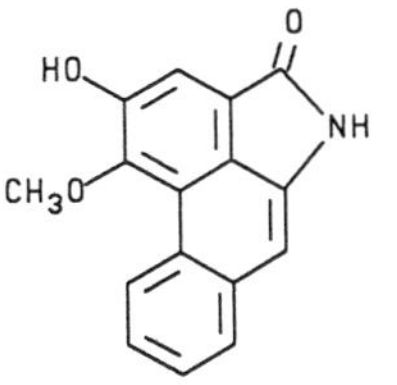

Mol. Wt.: 265
Bioactivity: PS: ED_{50} 3.2 μg/ml
KB: ED_{50} 2.1 μg/ml
Melting Point: 271°C
Spectral Data: Mass Spec.
Organism: *Pararistolochia flos-avis* (A.Cheval.) Hutch. and Dalz. (Aristolochiaceae)
Location: Ghana
Reference: 211, 1049

$C_{16}H_{12}N_2O_3$ **1,11-Dimethoxycanthin-6-one**

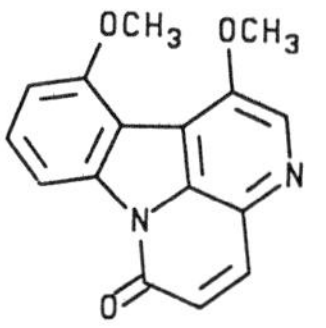

Mol. Wt.: 280
Bioactivity: KB: ED_{50} 1.0 μg/ml
P-388: T/C 122 (25 mg/kg)
Melting Point: 217-220°C (dec.)
Spectral Data: UV, IR, CMR, PMR, Mass Spec.
Organism: *Brucea antidysenterica* (Simaroubaceae)
Location: Ethiopia
Reference: 321

$C_{17}H_9O_3$ **Liriodenine**
(Oxoushinsunine)
(previously known)

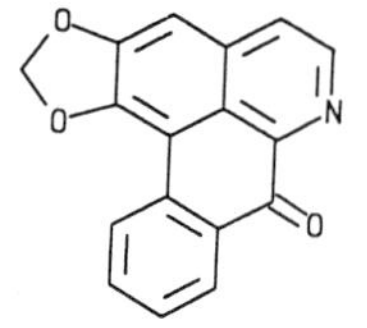

Mol. Wt.: 275
Bioactivity: KB: ED_{50} 1.00 $\mu g/ml$
A-549: ED_{50} 0.7 $\mu g/ml$
HCT-8: ED_{50} 0.7 $\mu g/ml$
P-388: ED_{50} 0.6 $\mu g/ml$
L1210: ED_{50} 2.3 $\mu g/ml$
Melting Point: 286-288°C
$[\alpha]_D^{24}$: ±0 Solvent: Me
Spectral Data: IR, PMR, Mass Spec.
Organism: *Thalictrum sessile*
(Ranunculaceae)
Paramichelia baillonii (Pierre) Hu
(Magnoliaceae)
Location: Taiwan; Thailand
Reference: 67, 68, 117, 953, 1193

$C_{18}H_{23}NO_5$ **Sinococuline**

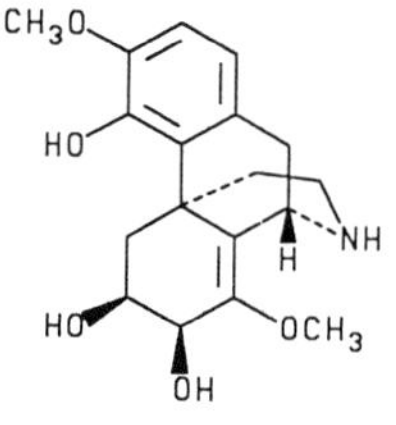

Mol. Wt.: 333
Bioactivity: P-388: T/C 200 (100 mg/kg/day
for 5 days)
Activity against Sarcoma 180 (ascites)
$[\alpha]_D^{26}$: -77 Solvent: Me
Spectral Data: UV, CD, CMR, PMR, Mass Spec.
Organism: *Cocculus trilobus*
(Menispermaceae)
Reference: 483

$C_{20}H_{16}N_2O_5$ **11-Hydroxy-(20S)-camptothecin**
(previously known)

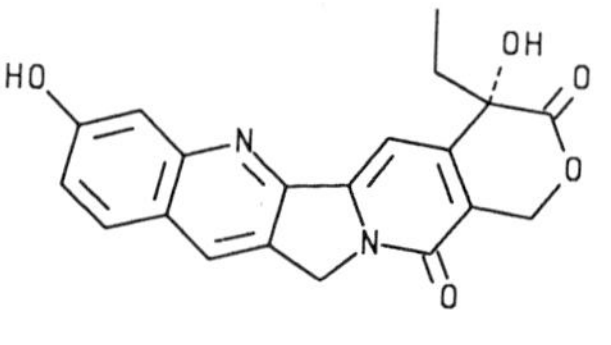

Mol. Wt.: 364
Bioactivity: L1210: T/C 357 (60 mg/kg x 4
for 2 days)
Tested as racemate
Melting Point: 320-324°C
$[\alpha]_D^{21}$: -30.7 Solvent: Py
Spectral Data: IR, PMR
Organism: *Camptotheca acuminata* Decsne.
(Nyssaceae)
Reference: 659, 1152

$C_{20}H_{24}N_2O_2$ **Akagerine**

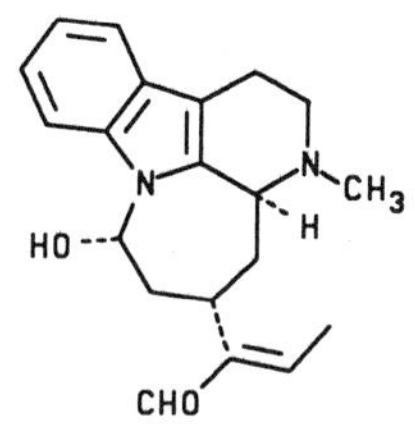

Mol. Wt.: 324
Bioactivity: 2002: 100% toxicity at 10 μg/ml
L1210: 100% toxicity at 10 μg/ml
B16, HeLa: lesser effect
Melting Point: 188°C
Spectral Data: UV, CD, IR, PMR, Mass Spec., x-ray c.s.
Organism: *Strychnos usambarensis* (Loganiaceae)
Location: Central Africa
Reference: 27, 640

$C_{21}H_{16}ClNO_5$ **Chelirubine chloride**
(previously known)

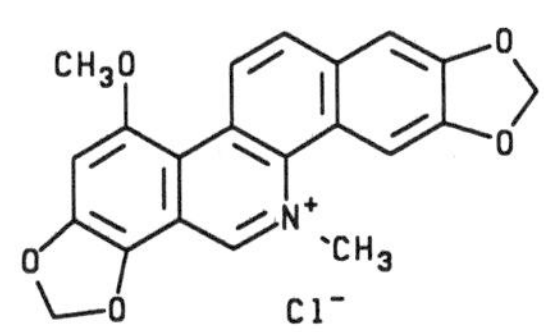

Mol. Wt.: 397
Bioactivity: Sarcoma 180: 93% inhibition at 10 mg/kg for 5 days
Toxic at 30 mg/kg for 5 days
Organism: *Chelidonium majus* (Papaveraceae)
Reference: 469, 1020, 1021

$C_{21}H_{18}ClNO_4$ **Nitidine chloride**
(previously known)

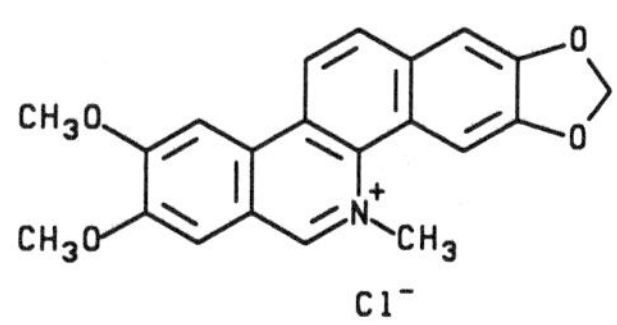

Mol. Wt.: 383
Bioactivity: 9KB: ED_{50} 0.1 μg/ml
P-388: T/C 240-260 (30-50 mg/kg)
Sarcoma 180: 96% inhibition at 30 mg/kg for 5 days
Melting Point: 281-282°C
Spectral Data: UV, IR, PMR, Mass Spec.
Organism: *Fagara macrophylla* (Rutaceae)
Location: Ghana
Reference: 41, 469, 470, 1153

$C_{21}H_{26}N_2O_2$ **Vincadifformine**
(previously known)

Mol. Wt.: 338
Bioactivity: in vitro Inhibition of leukemia P-388 cell growth and nucleic acid/protein synthesis
Melting Point: 124-125°C
$[\alpha]_D$: 0 Solvent: Me
Organism: *Vinca minor* L. (Apocynaceae)
Reference: 240, 1037

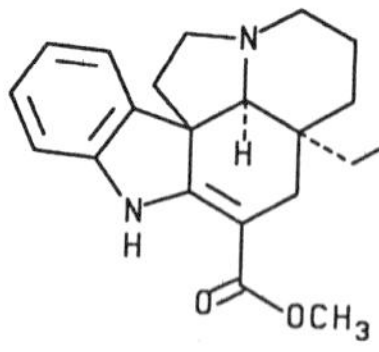

$C_{21}H_{33}NO_7$ **Lasiocarpine**

Mol. Wt.: 411
Bioactivity: Antitumor activity
Melting Point: 95-96°C
Spectral Data: IR, CMR, PMR, Mass Spec.
Organism: *Heliotropium marifolium* Retz
H. maris mortui
H. arbainense
(Boraginaceae)
Location: Gaipur, India; Israel
Reference: 494, 1217

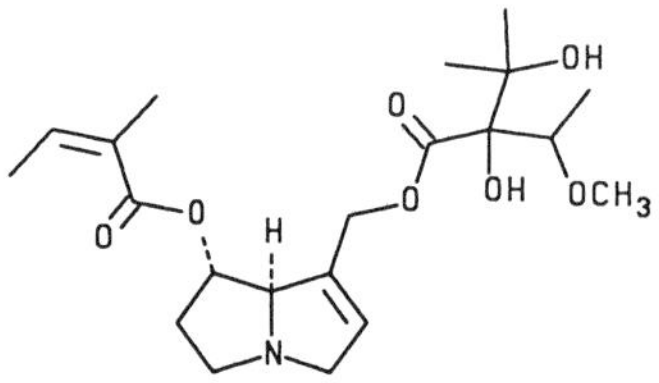

$C_{22}H_{21}NO_5$ **6-Methoxy-5,6-dihydronitidine**

Mol. Wt.: 379
Bioactivity: 9KB: ED_{50} 0.1 μg/ml
P-388: T/C 240-260 (30-50 mg/kg)
Melting Point: 270°C
Spectral Data: UV, IR, PMR, Mass Spec.
Organism: *Fagara macrophylla*
(artefact of isolation)
(Rutaceae)
Location: Ghana
Reference: 1153

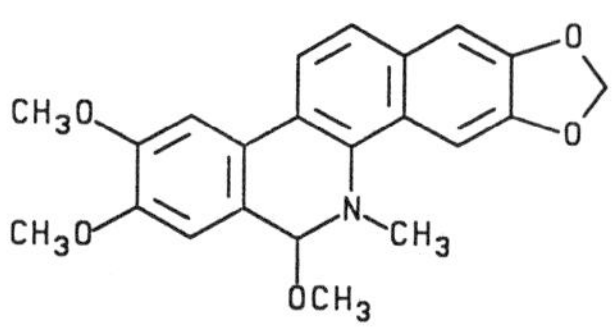

$C_{22}H_{30}N_2O_2$ **Vincaminoreine**
(previously known)

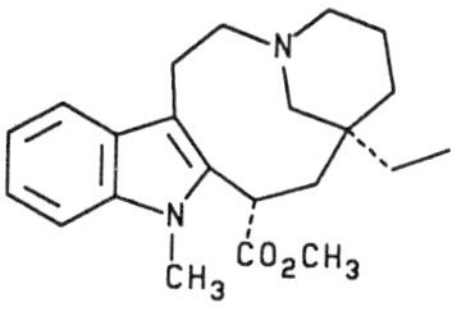

Mol. Wt.: 354
Bioactivity: in vitro Inhibition of leukemia P-388 cell growth and nucleic acid/protein synthesis
Melting Point: 138-139°C
$[\alpha]_D$: +26.5 Solvent: Chf
Organism: *Vinca minor* L. (Apocynaceae)
Reference: 751, 1037

$C_{22}H_{30}N_2O_2$ **Vincaminorine**
(previously known)

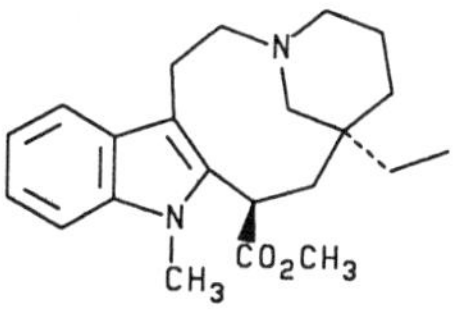

Mol. Wt.: 354
Bioactivity: in vitro Inhibition of leukemia P-388 cell growth and nucleic acid/protein synthesis
Melting Point: 130-131°C
Spectral Data: UV, IR
$[\alpha]_D^{21}$: +46 ±2 Solvent: Alc
Organism: *Vinca minor* L. (Apocynaceae)
Reference: 1037, 1107

$C_{29}H_{28}N_4$ **Usambarensine**

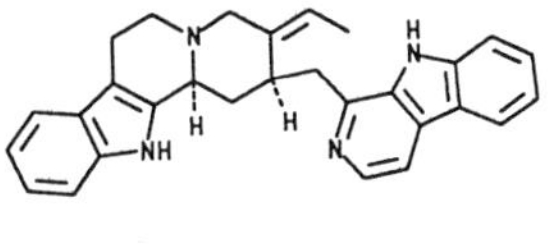

Mol. Wt.: 432
Bioactivity: Cytotoxicity: B16: 100% at 10 $\mu g/ml$
2002: 100% at 10 $\mu g/ml$
L1210: 100% at 10 $\mu g/ml$
HeLa: 100% at 10 $\mu g/ml$
Organism: *Strychnos sp.* (Loganiaceae)
Location: Central Africa
Reference: 640

$C_{29}H_{30}N_4$ **Dihydrousambarensine**

Mol. Wt.: 434
Bioactivity: Cytotoxicity: B16: 100% at 10 μg/ml
2002: 100% at 10 μg/ml
L1210: 100% at 1 μg/ml
HeLa: 100% at 10 μg/ml
Organism: *Strychnos sp.*
(Loganiaceae)
Location: Central Africa
Reference: 640

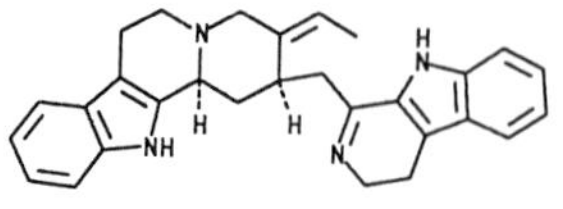

$C_{30}H_{34}N_4$ **Usambarine**

Mol. Wt.: 450
Bioactivity: Cytotoxicity: B16: 100% at 10 μg/ml
2002: 100% at 10 μg/ml
L1210: 100% at 10 μg/ml
HeLa: 100% at 10 μg/ml
Melting Point: 215°C
Spectral Data: UV, CD, IR, PMR, Mass Spec.
Organism: *Strychnos usambarensis*
(Loganiaceae)
Location: Central Africa
Reference: 26, 640

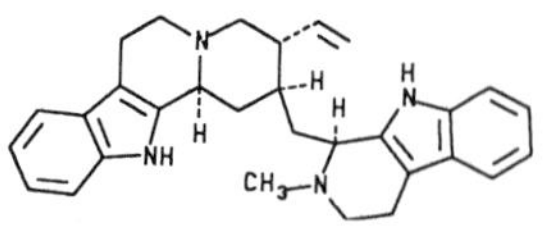

$C_{30}H_{34}N_4O$ **10-Hydroxyusambarine**

Mol. Wt.: 466
Bioactivity: Cytotoxicity: B16: 100% at 10 μg/ml
2002: 100% at 10 μg/ml
L1210: 100% at 10 μg/ml
HeLa: 100% at 10 μg/ml
Organism: *Strychnos sp.*
(Loganiaceae)
Reference: 640

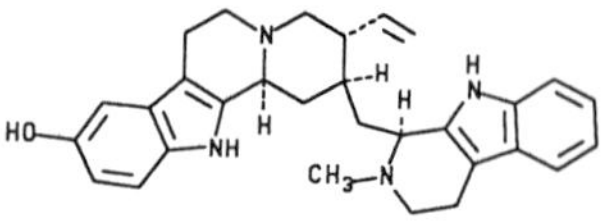

$C_{30}H_{34}N_4O$ **11-Hydroxyusambarine**

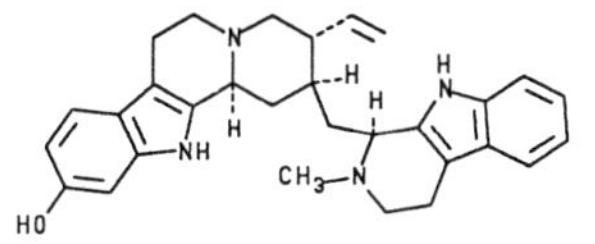

Mol. Wt.: 466
Bioactivity: Cytotoxicity: B16: 100% at 10 μg/ml
2002: 100% at 10 μg/ml
L1210: 100% at 10 μg/ml
HeLa: lesser effect
Organism: *Strychnos sp.*
(Loganiaceae)
Reference: 640

$C_{30}H_{36}N_4$ **Dihydrousambarine**

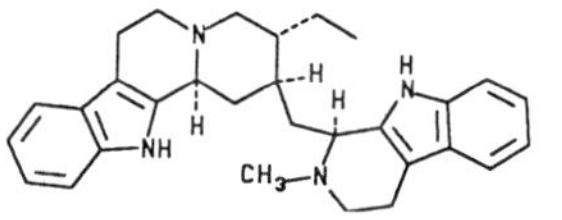

Mol. Wt.: 452
Bioactivity: Cytotoxicity: B16: 100% at 10 μg/ml
2002: 100% at 10 μg/ml
L1210: 100% at 1 μg/ml
HeLa: 100% at 10 μg/ml
Organism: *Strychnos usambarensis*
(Loganiaceae)
Location: Central Africa
Reference: 53, 640

$C_{30}H_{43}NO_6$ **(-)-Bisparthenolidine**

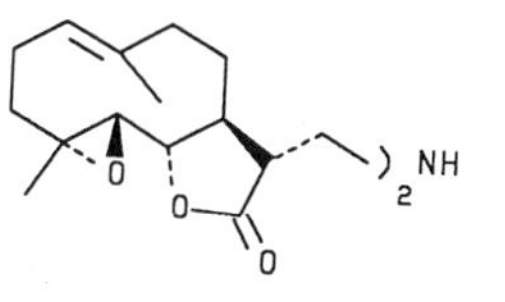

Mol. Wt.: 513
Bioactivity: 9KB: ED_{50} 0.6 μg/ml
Melting Point: 100-103°C
$[\alpha]_D^{20}$: -112 Solvent: Chf
Spectral Data: IR, CMR, PMR, Mass Spec.
Organism: *Paramichelia baillonii*
(Pierre) Hu
(syn. *Magnolia baillonii*,
Michelia baillonii, *Aromadendron*
baillonii, and *A. spongocarpum*)
(Magnoliaceae)
Location: Doi Suthep, Thailand
Reference: 953

$C_{31}H_{43}NO_7$ **Anopterine**
(previously known)

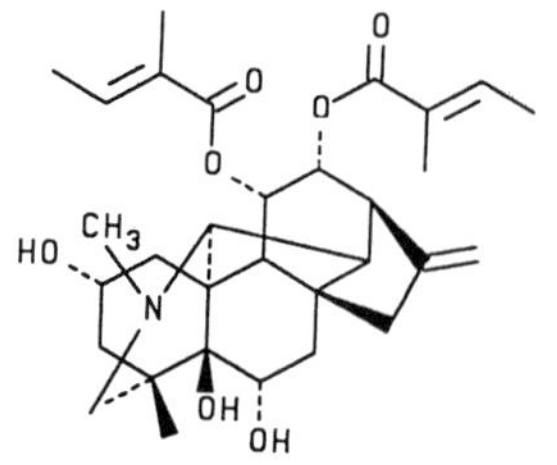

Mol. Wt.: 541
Bioactivity: KB: ED_{50} $5x10^{-2}$ μg/ml
P-388: T/C 122 (13 mg/kg)
Melting Point: 222-223°C
Spectral Data: CMR, PMR, Mass Spec.
Organism: *Anopterus glandulosus*
A. macleayanus
(Escalloniaceae)
Location: Tasmania; New South Wales
Reference: 397, 499, 1151

$C_{31}H_{43}NO_8$ **7β-Hydroxyanopterine**
(previously known)

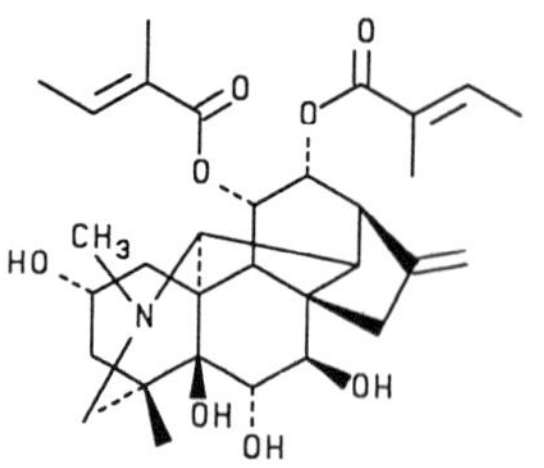

Mol. Wt.: 557
Bioactivity: KB: ED_{50} $1x10^{-3}$ μg/ml
P-388: T/C 140 (4.4 mg/kg)
Melting Point: 248-249°C
$[\alpha]_D$: -12 Solvent: Chf/Me
Spectral Data: CMR, PMR, Mass Spec.
Organism: *Anopterus glandulosus*
A. macleayanus
(Escalloniaceae)
Location: Tasmania; New South Wales
Reference: 398, 499, 1151

$C_{31}H_{43}NO_9$ **4',7β-Dihydroxyanopterine**
(previously known)

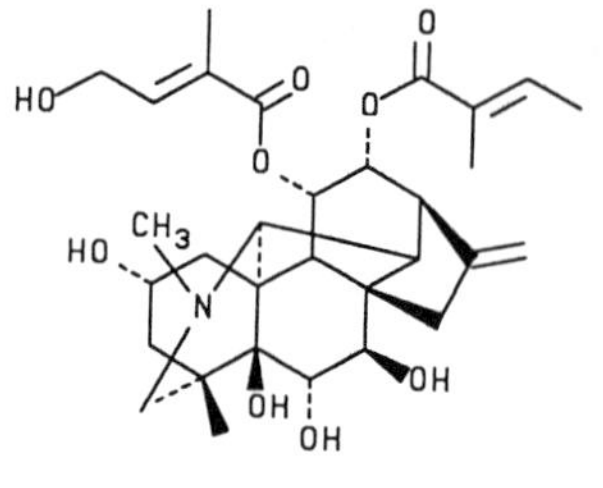

Mol. Wt.: 573
Bioactivity: KB: ED_{50} $5x10^{-2}$ μg/ml
P-388: T/C 120 (3.5 mg/kg)
Melting Point: 246-248°C
$[\alpha]_D^{25}$: -6.5 Solvent: Me
Spectral Data: CMR, PMR, Mass Spec.
Organism: *Anopterus glandulosus*
A. macleayanus
(Escalloniaceae)
Location: Tasmania; New South Wales
Reference: 398, 499, 1151

$C_{33}H_{41}NO_8$	**11α-Benzoyl-7β-hydroxy-11α-destigloylanopterine** (previously known)
Mol. Wt.:	579
Bioactivity:	KB: ED_{50} $1x10^{-3}$ μg/ml P-388: T/C 125 (1.5 mg/kg)
Melting Point:	268-269°C
$[\alpha]_D^{25}$:	-9.5 Solvent: Me
Spectral Data:	PMR, Mass Spec.
Organism:	*Anopterus glandulosus* *A. macleayanus* (Escalloniaceae)
Location:	Tasmania; New South Wales
Reference:	398, 499, 1151

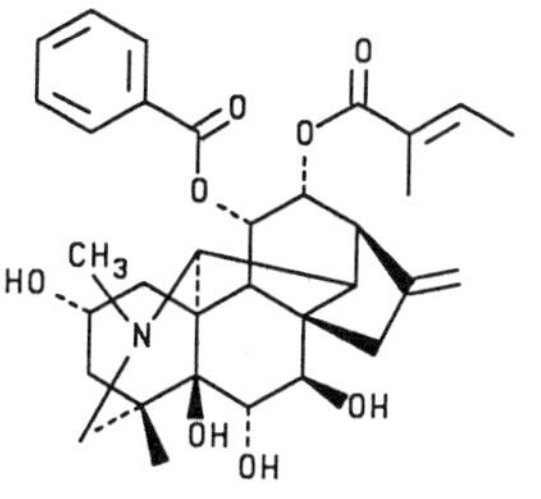

$C_{33}H_{45}ClN_2O_{10}$	**15-Methoxyansamitocin P-3**
Mol. Wt.:	664
Bioactivity:	Cytotoxicity
Spectral Data:	PMR, Mass Spec.
Organism:	*Isothecium subdiversiforme* *Thamnobryum sandei* (Bryophyta)
Location:	Japan
Reference:	961

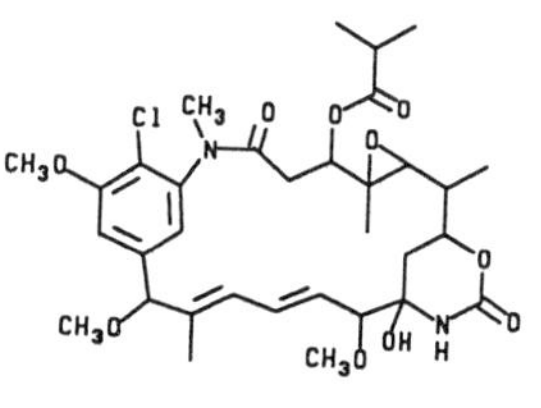

$C_{35}H_{43}N_5O$	**Strychnopentamine**
Mol. Wt.:	549
Bioactivity:	Cytotoxicity: B16: 100% at 10 μg/ml 2002: 100% at 10 μg/ml L1210: 100% at 1 μg/ml HeLa: 100% at 10 μg/ml
Organism:	*Strychnos usambarensis* (Loganiaceae)
Location:	Tanzania
Reference:	640, 1094

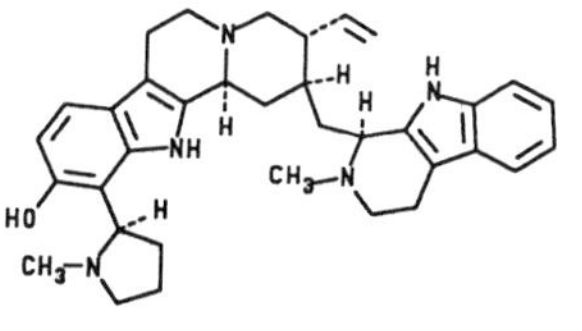

$C_{35}H_{43}N_5O_2$ **Strychnophylline**

Mol. Wt.: 565
Bioactivity: Cytotoxicity: B16: 100% at 10 μg/ml
2002: 100% at 10 μg/ml
L1210: 100 % at 10 μg/ml
HeLa: very little effect
Organism: *Strychnos sp.*
(Loganiaceae)
Reference: 640

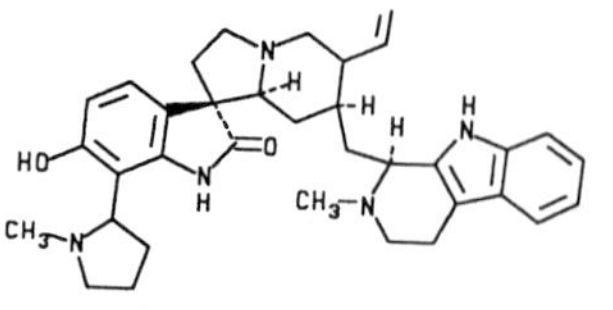

$C_{40}H_{46}N_2O_8$ **(+)-Thalifarazine**

Mol. Wt.: 682
Bioactivity: KB: ED_{50} 1.50 μg/ml
HCT-8: ED_{50} 4.3 μg/ml
A-549: ED_{50} 6.5 μg/ml
P-388: ED_{50} 3.8 μg/ml
L-1210: ED_{50} 5.7 μg/ml
$[\alpha]_D$: +72 Solvent: Me
Spectral Data: UV, CD, IR, PMR, Mass Spec.
Organism: *Thalictrum sessile*
T. cultratum
(Ranunculaceae)
Location: Taiwan; Pakistan
Reference: 447, 1193

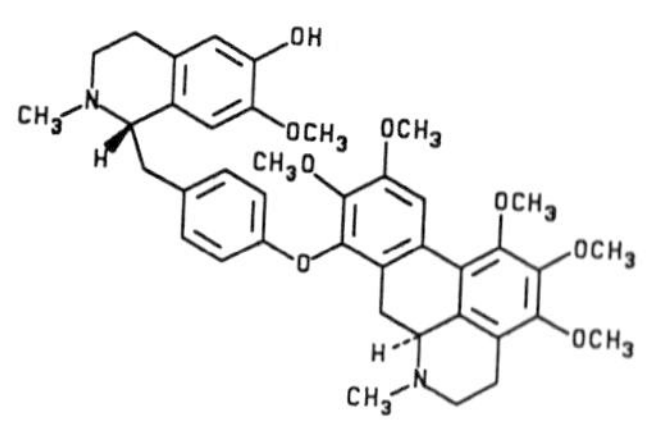

$C_{44}H_{50}N_8$ **Alkaloid B**

Mol. Wt.: 690
Activity: Cytotoxicity against cultured rat hepatoma cells (HTC line)
$[\alpha]_D^{20}$: +215 Solvent: Alc
-10 Solvent: Chf
Spectral Data: UV, IR, CMR, Mass Spec.
Organism: *Psychotria forsteriana* A. Gray
(Rubiaceae)
Location: Vanuatu, New Hebrides
Reference: 945

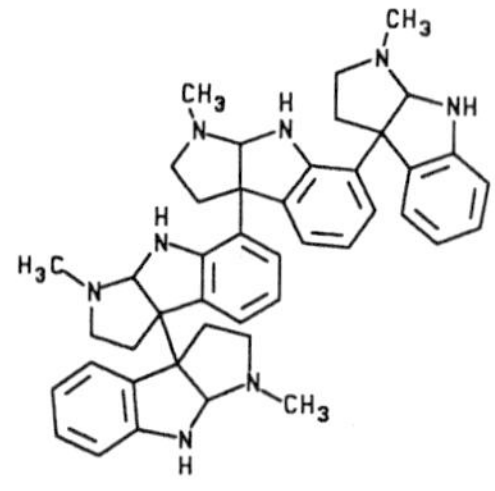

$C_{44}H_{50}N_8$ **Alkaloid C**

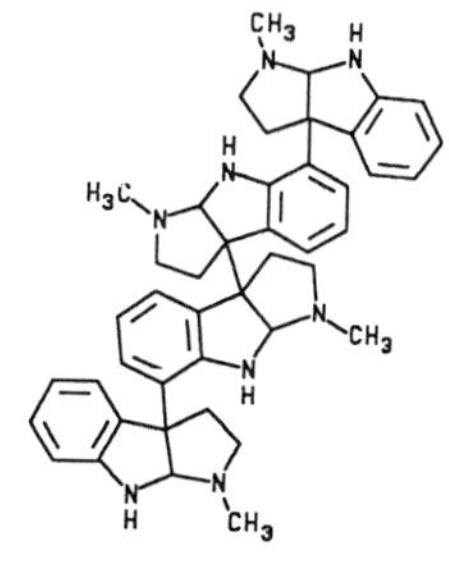

Mol. Wt.: 690
Bioactivity: Cytotoxicity against cultured rat hepatoma cells (HTC line)
$[\alpha]_D^{20}$: +32.5 Solvent: Alc
+116 Solvent: Chf
Spectral Data: UV, IR, CMR, Mass Spec.
Organism: *Psychotria forsteriana* A.Gray (Rubiaceae)
Location: Vanuatu, New Hebrides
Reference: 945

$C_{49}H_{75}N_7O_{15}$ **FR900359**

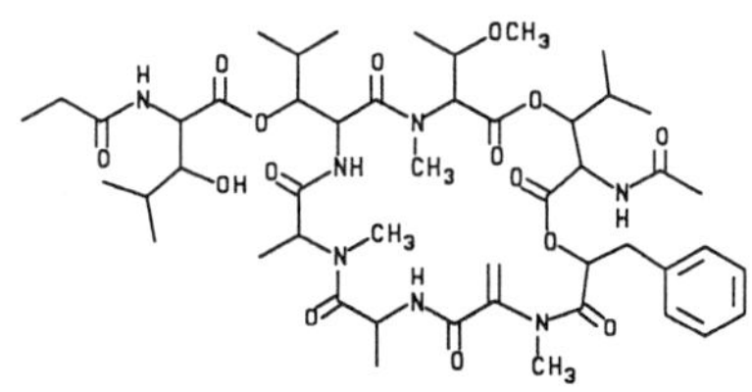

Mol. Wt.: 1002
Bioactivity: Cytotoxic to cultured rat fibroblasts and myelocytic leukemia cells
Inhibits platelet aggregation, decreases blood pressure and causes hypotension in rats
Spectral Data: IR, CMR, PMR, Mass Spec.
Organism: *Ardisia crenata sims* (gymnosperm)
Location: Japan
Reference: 313, 314

$C_{55}H_{62}N_{10}$ **Alkaloid D**

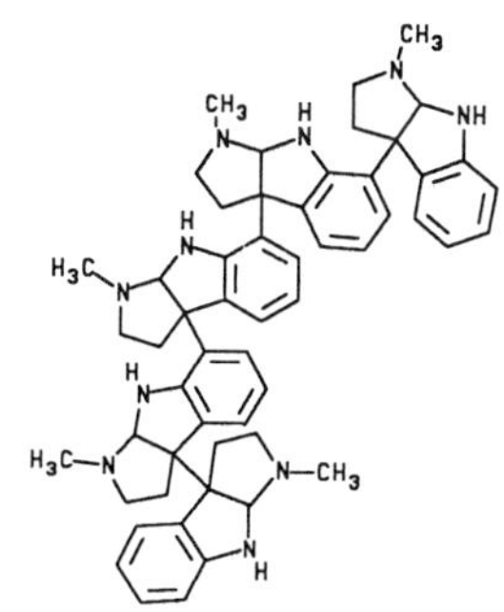

Mol. Wt.: 863
Bioactivity: Cytotoxicity against cultured rat hepatoma cells (HTC line)
$[\alpha]_D^{20}$: +183.3 Solvent: Alc
Spectral Data: UV, IR, CMR, Mass Spec.
Organism: *Psychotria forsteriana* A.Gray (Rubiaceae)
Location: Vanuatu, New Hebrides
Reference: 945, 946

$C_{55}H_{62}N_{10}$ **Alkaloid E**

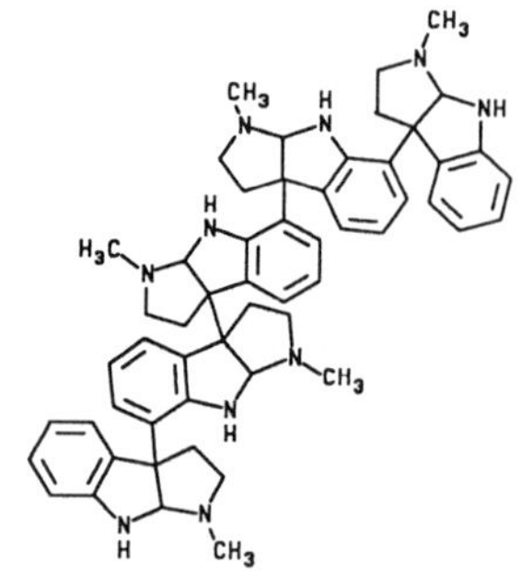

Mol. Wt.: 863
Bioactivity: Cytotoxicity against cultured rat hepatoma cells (HTC line)
$[\alpha]_D^{20}$: +153 Solvent: Alc
+49 Solvent: Chf
Spectral Data: UV, IR, CMR, Mass Spec.
Organism: *Psychotria forsteriana* A.Gray (Rubiaceae)
Location: Vanuatu, New Hebrides
Reference: 945

Ricin A

Mol. Wt.: ~62,000
Bioactivity: Sarcoma 180: ILS 62 ± 7%
Sarcoma 180: ED_{50} $1x10^{-10}$ g/ml; $1x10^{-4}$ μg/ml
LTK: ED_{50} $2.6x10^{-10}$ g/ml; $2.6x10^{-4}$ μg/ml
3T3: ED_{50} $7.8x10^{-10}$ g/ml; $7.8x10^{-4}$ μg/ml; LD_{50} 5 μg/kg (ip)
Organism: *Ricinus communis* L. (Euphorbiaceae)
Location: China
Reference: 658

A. Total Syntheses

Compound	Activity	Reference
Avicine chloride	Sarcoma 180 (ip): 62% inhibition at 100 mg/kg for 5 days	469, 470
20(S)-Camptothecin	KB: ED_{50} $4x10^{-2}$ μg/ml P388: ED_{50} $3x10^{-2}$ μg/ml L1210: T/C 250 (10 mg/kg)	1159
7-Methoxy-5-methyl-2,3;9,10-bis(methylenedioxy)benzo[c]phenanthridium chloride	Sarcoma 180: 91% inhibition at 10 mg/kg for 5 days Toxic at 30 mg/kg for 5 days	469
7-Methoxynitidine chloride	Sarcoma 180 (ip): 56% inhibition at 30 mg/kg for 5 days	469, 470
10-Methoxynitidine chloride	Sarcoma 180 (ip): 73% inhibition at 3 mg/kg for 5 days Toxic at 10 mg/kg for 5 days	469
9-[(2-Methyl-4-methylene-5-oxotetrahydrofuran-2-yl)-methyl]adenine	L1210: ED_{50} 0.3 μg/ml KB: ED_{50} 5.0 μg/ml	645
9-[(2-Methyl-4-methylene-5-oxotetrahydrofuran-2-yl)-methyl]guanine	L1210: ED_{50} 1.3 μg/ml	645
9-[(2-Methyl-4-methylene-5-oxotetrahydrofuran-2-yl)-methyl]hypoxanthine	L1210: ED_{50} 2.0 μg/ml	645
6-Methylnitidine chloride	Sarcoma 180 (ip): 83% inhibition at 100 mg/kg for 5 days	469

B. Semi-Syntheses or Synthetic Modifications

Compound	Reference
Ellipticine Glycosides	435

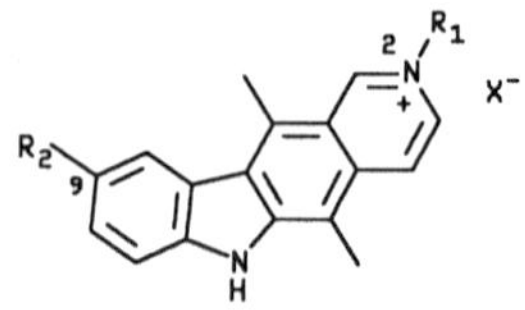

R_1	R_2	X	Activity	mg/kg	ILS%	Cures
β-D-Allopyranosyl	OH	Br	L1210 (ip-ip)	10	>254	1/6
α-L Arabinofuranosyl	OH	Br	L1210 (ip-ip)	10	>379	2/6
β-L-Arabinofuranosyl	OH	OAc	L1210 (ip-ip)	30	>269	1/6
β-D-Arabinofuranosyl	OH	OAc	L1210 (ip-ip)	30	>262	1/6
α-L-Arabinopyranosyl	OH	Br	L1210 (ip-ip)	30	>860	5/6
			L1210 (ip-iv)	30	>344	2/6
			P388 (ip-ip)	40	>789	6/6
			P388 (ip-iv)	20	>394	2/6
			EAC (ip-ip)	40	>518	5/6
			Sarcoma 180 (ip-ip)	80	>353	2/6
α-D-Arabinopyranosyl	OH	Br	L1210 (ip-ip)	20	>606	3/6
α-L-5'-Deoxyarabinofuranosyl	OH	Cl	L1210 (ip-ip)	30	>261	1/6
β-L-5'-Deoxyarabinofuranosyl	OH	OAc	L1210 (ip-ip)	30	>217	1/6
β-D-2'-Deoxyribofuranosyl	OH	Cl	L1210 (ip-ip)	10	>390	2/6
β-D-5'-Deoxyribofuranosyl	OH	Cl	L1210 (ip-ip)	30	>230	1/6
β-L-Fucopyranosyl	OH	Br	L1210 (ip-ip)	30	>583	3/6
β-D-Fucopyranosyl	OH	Br	L1210 (ip-ip)	30	124	0/6
β-D-Galactopyranosyl	OH	Br	L1210 (ip-ip)	20	>729	4/6
L-Lyxofuranosyl	OH	Cl	L1210 (ip-ip)	10	>552	3/6
D-Lyxofuranosyl	OH	Cl	L1210 (ip-ip)	30	>967	6/6
			P388 (ip-ip)	20	>510	4/6

R_1	R_2	X	Activity	mg/kg	ILS%	Cures
α-L-Lyxopyranosyl	OH	Cl	L1210 (ip-ip)	30	>786	5/6
			P388 (ip-ip)	20	>585	4/6
α-D-Lyxopyranosyl	OH	Cl	L1210 (ip-ip)	10	>651	4/6
α-L-Mannopyranosyl	OH	Br	L1210 (ip-ip)	5	>362	2/6
L-Rhamnopyranosyl	OH	Br	L1210 (ip-ip)	80	>1016	6/6
			P388 (ip-ip)	40	>789	6/6
	OH	OAc	L1210 (ip-ip)	30	>615	3/6
β-L-Ribofuranosyl	OH	Br	L1210 (ip-ip)	10	>391	2/6
β-L-Ribopyranosyl	OH	Br	L1210 (ip-ip)	30	>944	6/6
β-D-Ribopyranosyl	OH	Br	L1210 (i-ip)	30	112	0/6
α-D-Talopyranosyl	OH	Br	L1210 (ip-ip)	10	>212	1/6
β-L-Xylofuranosyl	OH	Cl	L1210 (ip-ip)	30	>387	2/6
β-D-Xylofuranosyl	OH	Cl	L1210 (ip-ip)	30	>682	4/6
			P388 (ip-ip)	20	>628	5/6
			P388 (ip-iv)	16	>417	2/6
			EAC (ip-ip)	40	>501	5/6
			Sarcoma 180 (ip-ip)	40	>335	2/6
L-Xylopyranosyl	OH	Br	L1210 (ip-ip)	10	>396	2/6
D-Xylopyranosyl	OH	Br	L1210 (ip-ip)	30	>857	5/6

Chapter 9 FUNGI AND OTHER LOWER PLANT BIOSYNTHETIC PRODUCTS

$C_7H_6O_4$ **BMY-28438**
(3,7-Dihydroxytropolone)

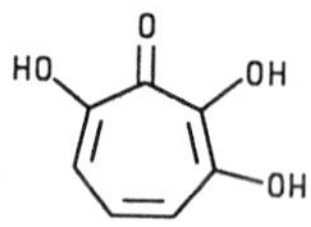

Mol. Wt.:	154
Bioactivity:	B16: IC_{50} 0.04 μg/ml B16: T/C 181 at 1.3 mg/kg/day Inhibition of macromolecule biosynthesis in L1210: DNA: IC_{50} 9.4 μg/ml RNA: IC_{50} 14 μg/ml Protein: IC_{50} 11 μg/ml Weak antibacterial activity Antifungal activity
Melting Point:	>166°C (sublimation)
Spectral Data:	UV, IR, CMR, PMR, Mass Spec.
Organism:	*Streptomyces tropolofaciens* sp. nov. K611-97 (Streptomycetaceae) Culture
Reference:	1040

$C_7H_9ClN_2O$ **Clazamycin**
(Epimers A and B)

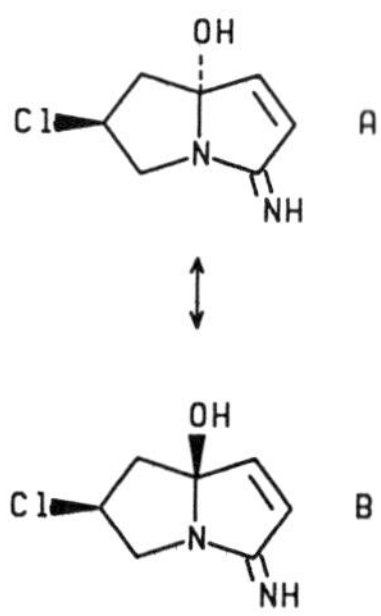

Mol. Wt.:	172
Bioactivity:	L1210: T/C >130 (12.5~100 μg/mouse) L1210: ID_{90} 1.6 μg/ml LD_{50} (iv) 50~100 mg/kg (A) and >100 mg/kg (B) LD_{50} (ip) 26 mg/kg Antiviral activity against HSV1 and HSV2 at 12 μg/ml Activity against *Pseudomonas* spp.
Melting Point:	110°C (dec.) (A) (HCl)
$[\alpha]_D^{25}$:	-56 (A) Solvent: Aq (HCl)
$[\alpha]_D^{24}$:	+96 (B) Solvent: Aq (HCl)
Spectral Data:	UV, IR, CMR, PMR, Mass Spec., x-ray c.s. of epimer A
Organism:	*Streptomyces* No. MF990-BF4; *S. puniceus* subsp. *doliceus* NRRL 11160 (Streptomycetaceae) Culture
Reference:	118, 241, 438, 799

$C_8H_{12}N_4O_5$ **LL-D05139β (Alanylazaserine)**

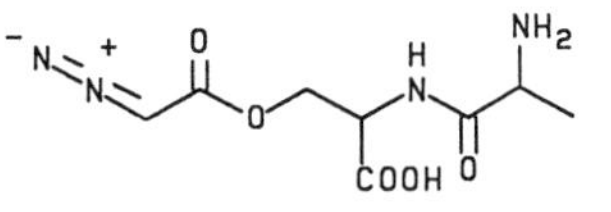

Mol. Wt.: 244
Bioactivity: Cytotoxic activity against human lung and colon tumor cells and against P-388 leukemia
Peak β-galactosidase induction at ~5 μg/ml
Antibacterial activity
$[\alpha]_D^{26}$: +57 ±5 Solvent: Aq
Spectral Data: UV, IR, CMR, PMR, Mass Spec.
Organism: *Glycomyces harbinensis* (NRRL 15337)
Culture of soil sample
Location: Harbin, China
Reference: 282, 646, 649

$C_9H_9NO_3$ **Erbstatin**

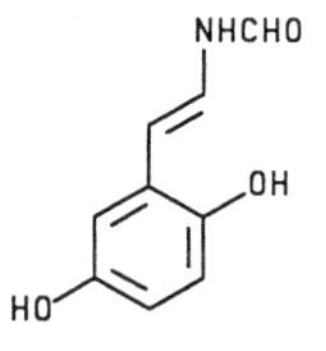

Mol. Wt.: 179
Bioactivity: Human epidermoid carcinoma cells (A-431): IC_{50} 3.6 μg/ml
IMC-carcinoma cells: IC_{50} 3.0 μg/ml
LD_{50} (ip) >200 mg/kg
Inhibition of tyrosine kinase: IC_{50} 0.55 μg/ml
Weak antibacterial activity against
Staphylococcus aureus
Pseudomonas aeruginosa
Micrococcus lysodeikticus
Proteus mirabilis
Melting Point: 150.5-152.0°C
$[\alpha]_D^{25}$: 0 Solvent: Me
Spectral Data: UV, IR, CMR, PMR, x-ray c.s.
Organism: Stain no. MH435-hF3 (closely related to *Streptomyces viridosporus*)
Culture
Reference: 393, 798, 1126

$C_{10}H_{14}O_5$	**Acetomycin** (previously known)
Mol. Wt.:	214
Bioactivity:	L1210: IC_{50} 2.2 μg/ml HCT-8: IC_{50} 1.5 μg/ml Active in the HCT-8 resting cell agar diffusion assay at 25 μg/ml Activity in human stem cell assay Antimicrobial activity
Melting Point:	115-116°C
$[\alpha]_D$:	-167 Solvent: Alc
Organism:	Actinomycete culture WP-2661
Reference:	275, 694

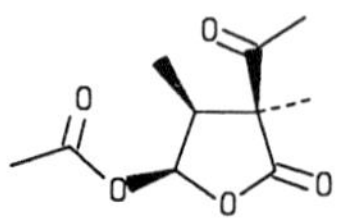

$C_{11}H_{16}O_4$	**Methylenolactocin**
Mol. Wt.:	212
Bioactivity:	Ehrlich carcinoma: T/C 166 at 0.2 mg/mouse Antimicrobial activity
Melting Point:	82.5-83.5°C
$[\alpha]_D^{26}$:	-2.37 Solvent: Me
Spectral Data:	UV, IR, CMR, PMR, Mass Spec.
Organism:	*Penicillium* sp. Strain No. 24-4 Culture of soil isolate (Moniliaceae)
Location:	Osaka, Japan
Reference:	863

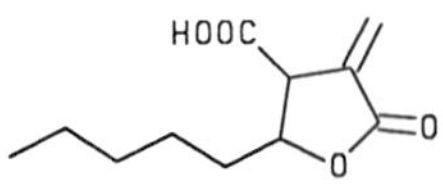

$C_{14}H_{15}N_3O_6$ **FR-900482**

Mol. Wt.: 321

Bioactivity: P-388: MIC 0.4 μg/ml
B16: MIC 0.4 μg/ml
EL4: MIC 0.4 μg/ml
FM3A: MIC 0.4 μg/ml
L1210: MIC 0.8 μg/ml
BHK-21: MIC 0.8 μg/ml
Acute toxicity: LD_{50} 32 mg/kg
Antitumor activity:
P-388: T/C 305 at 10.0 mg/kg
L1210: T/C 190 at 10.0 mg/kg
B16: T/C 350 at 10.0 mg/kg
MM46: T/C >300 at 3.2 mg/kg
Ehrlich: T/C >270 at 3.2 mg/kg
EL4: T/C 169 at 10 mg/kg
AH130: T/C >429 at 1.0 mg/kg
AMC60: T/C >333 at 3.2 mg/kg
Tumor growth inhibition:
LX-1: 97% at 18.0 mg/kg
MX-1: 100% at 18.0 mg/kg
SC-6: 100% at 18.0 mg/kg
LC-6: 100% at 18.0 mg/kg
Antitumor activity towards drug resistant P-388 leukemia
Antimicrobial activity vs *Bacillus stearothermophilus* var. *calidolactis* C953 at 0.03 μg/ml

Melting Point: 175°C (dec.)

$[\alpha]_D^{23}$: +8.0 Solvent: Aq

Spectral Data: UV, IR, CMR, PMR, Mass Spec., x-ray c.s. of derivative

Organism: *Streptomyces sandaensis* No. 6897 (Streptomycetaceae) Culture

Reference: 422, 489, 571, 1006

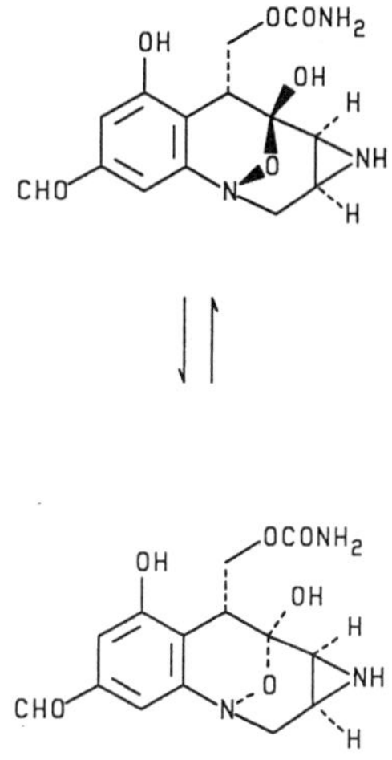

$C_{15}H_{22}O_3$ **FS-1**

Mol. Wt.: 250

Bioactivity: Cytotoxic

Melting Point: Oil

Spectral Data: UV, CD, IR, CMR, PMR, Mass Spec.

Organism: *Fusarium sporotrichioides* MC-72083 (Tuberculariaceae) Culture

Reference: 201

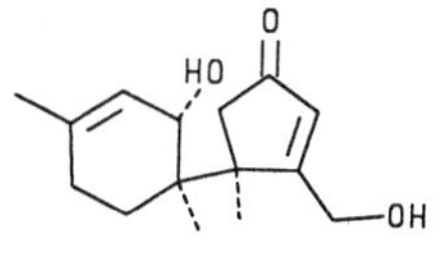

$C_{15}H_{22}O_3$ **8β-Hydroxytrichothecene**

Mol. Wt.: 250
Bioactivity: Cytotoxic
Melting Point: Oil
Spectral Data: IR, CMR, PMR, Mass Spec.
Organism: *Fusarium sporotrichioides* MC-72083 (Tuberculariaceae) Culture
Reference: 201

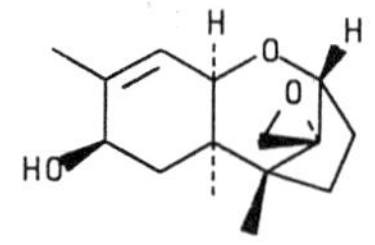

$C_{16}H_{12}N_2O_6$ **PD 116,152 (Methyl 6-formyl-4,7,9-trihydroxy-8-methyl-1-phenazinecarboxylate)**

Mol. Wt.: 328
Bioactivity: P-388 (ip): T/C 149 (12.5 mg/kg/day for 9 days)
L1210: IC_{50} $5.2x10^{-7}M$
HCT-8: IC_{50} $7.1x10^{-7}M$
Antimicrobial activity: broad spectrum
Weak
Melting Point: 255°C
Spectral Data: UV, IR, CMR, PMR, Mass Spec., x-ray c.s.
Organism: *Streptomyces* sp. (NRRL 15783) (Streptomycetaceae) Culture
Reference: 1024

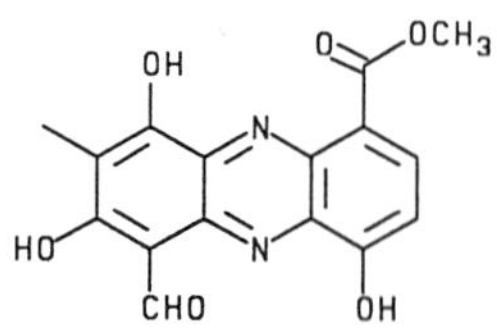

$C_{17}H_{14}N_2O_5$ **DC-86-M**

Mol. Wt.: 326
Bioactivity: Sarcoma 180 (sc-ip): T/C 277 (20 mg/kg)
LD_{50}: <25 mg/kg
Antimicrobial activity
Melting Point: 185-187°C
$[\alpha]_D$: -43.8 Solvent: Chf
Spectral Data: UV, IR, PMR, Mass Spec.
Organism: *Streptomyces luteogriseus* DO-86 (Streptomycetaceae) Culture of soil sample
Location: Japan
Reference: 43, 1072

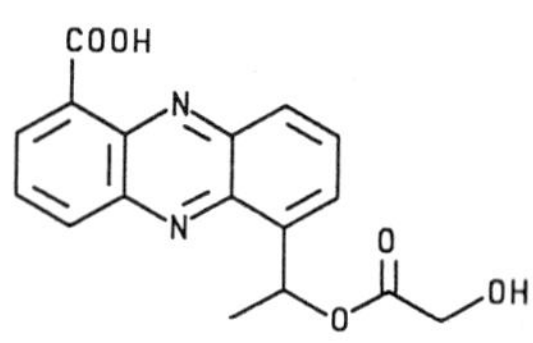

$C_{18}H_{32}N_4O_6$ **Bisucaberin**

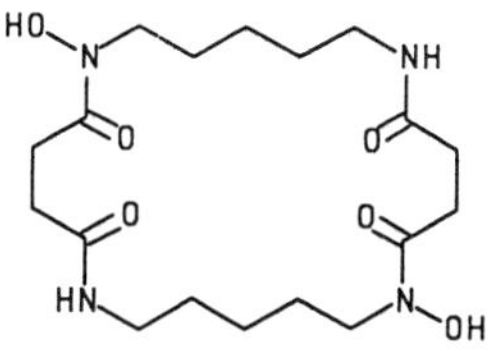

Mol. Wt.: 400
Bioactivity: L1210: 85% inhibition at 18 μg/ml
IC_{50} 3.9 μg/ml
IMC carcinoma: 85% inhibition at 18 μg/ml
IC_{50} 5.1 μg/ml
Fibrosarcoma 1023: 85% inhibition at 18 μg/ml (>98% viable)
Macrophage-mediated cytolysis
Inhibition of macromolecular synthesis
Melting Point: 180°C (dec.)
Spectral Data: UV, IR, CMR, PMR, Mass Spec., x-ray c.s.
Organism: *Alteromonas haloplanktis* strain SB-1123 (Pseudomonadaceae)
Location: Japan
Reference: 507, 1070

$C_{19}H_{14}O_6$ **PD 116,779 (2-Hydroxytetrangomycin)**

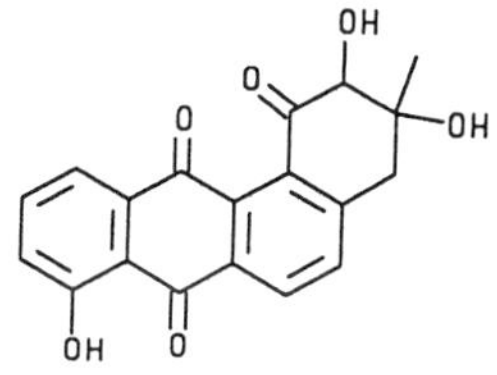

Mol. Wt.: 338
Bioactivity: L1210: IC_{50} $3.55x10^{-7}M$
HCT-8: IC_{50} $4.08x10^{-7}M$
Melting Point: 205°C
Spectral Data: UV, IR, PMR, Mass Spec.
Organism: Actinomycete isolate (WP 3688) (unidentified)
Reference: 545

$C_{19}H_{16}N_2O_2$ **Neihumicin**

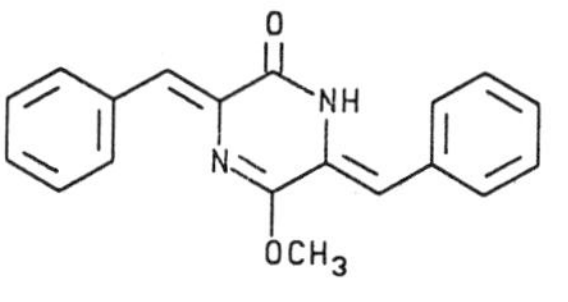

Mol. Wt.: 304
Bioactivity: KB: ED_{50} 0.94 μg/ml
Antimicrobial activity towards *Saccharomyces cerevisiae* and *Penicillium italicum*
Melting Point: 175~176°C
Spectral Data: UV, IR, PMR, Mass Spec., x-ray c.s.
Organism: *Micromonospora neihuensis* sp.nov. (Micromonosporaceae)
Culture of soil isolate
Location: Taiwan
Reference: 1192, 1204, 1210

$C_{20}H_{28}O_6$ **Terpentecin**

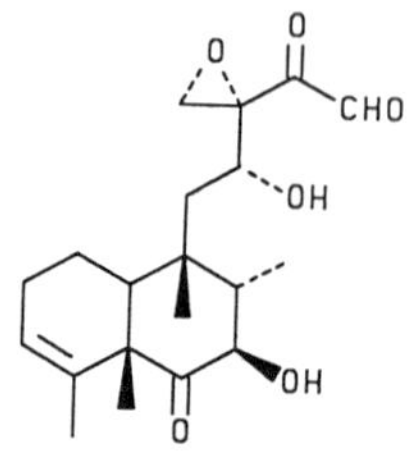

Mol. Wt.: 364
Bioactivity: P-388 (ip): T/C >175 (62.5 μg/mouse/day for 10 days)
L1210 (ip): T/C 200 (15.6 μg/mouse/day for 10 days)
Ehrlich ascites carcinoma: T/C >369 (15.6 μg/mouse/day for 10 days)
LD_{50} (ip): 100 mg/kg
Antibacterial activity (against both gram-positive + gram-negative)
Melting Point: 115-119°C
$[\alpha]_D^{26}$: -28.5 Solvent: Chf
Spectral Data: UV, IR, CMR, PMR, Mass Spec.
Organism: *Kitasatosporia* sp. strain MF730-N6, (Actinomycete)
Soil sample
Location: Japan
Reference: 476, 1077

$C_{23}H_{33}NO_6$ **Aranorosin**

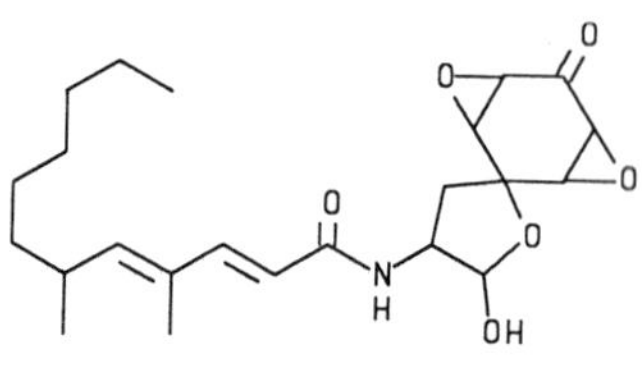

Mol. Wt.: 419
Bioactivity: Toxicity (ip): LD_{50} 5 mg/kg
Antitumor activity
Active against fungi and gram-positive bacteria
Melting Point: 150°C (dec.)
$[\alpha]_D^{20}$: -2.42 Solvent: Chf
Spectral Data: UV, IR, CMR, PMR, Mass Spec.
Organism: *Pseudoarachniotus roseus* (Gymnoascaceae)
Culture of soil sample
Location: Maharashtra, India
Reference: 291, 292, 952

$C_{24}H_{20}N_4O_8$ **10'-<u>O</u>-Demethylstreptonigrin**

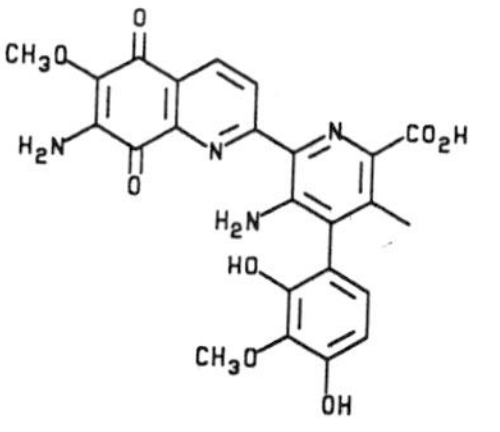

Mol. Wt.: 492
Bioactivity: P-388: IC_{50} 0.58 μg/ml
P-388 resistant to adriamycin: IC_{50} 0.41 μg/ml
Weak antibacterial activity
Melting Point: 177-181°C (dec.)
Spectral Data: UV, IR, CMR, PMR
Organism: *Streptomyces albus*
MG883-12F2
(Streptomycetaceae)
Culture
Reference: 475

$C_{24}H_{30}N_2O_{11}$ **Quinocarmycin citrate**
(KW 2152; DC 52 citrate)

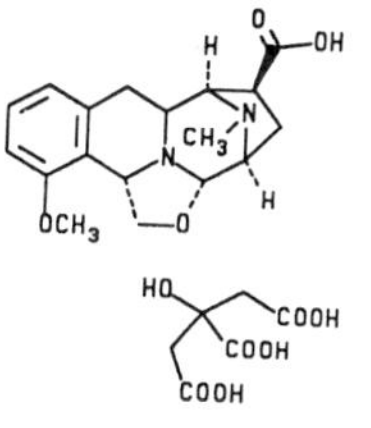

Mol. Wt.: 522
Bioactivity: P-388: T/C 215 (6.1 mg/kg/day for 7 days)
P-388/MMC: T/C 168 (5.4 mg/kg/day for 7 days)
P-388/ADM: T/C 168 (3.6 mg/kg/day for 7 days)
Active against MX-1 human mammary carcinoma
Inhibition of RNA but not of DNA synthesis
<u>In vitro</u>: P-388: IC_{50} $1.1x10^{-7}$M
L1210: IC_{50} $7.2x10^{-7}$ M
B16: IC_{50} $7.3x10^{-7}$M
Sarcoma 180: IC_{50} $3.4x10^{-6}$M
HeLa S_3: IC_{50} $1.6x10^{-7}$M
KB: IC_{50} $1.0x10^{-7}$M
SK-MEL-28: IC_{50} $1.0x10^{-7}$M
Organism: *Streptomyces melanovinaceus*
(Streptomycetaceae)
Reference: 312

$C_{25}H_{36}O_9$ **4-Propanoyl HT-2**

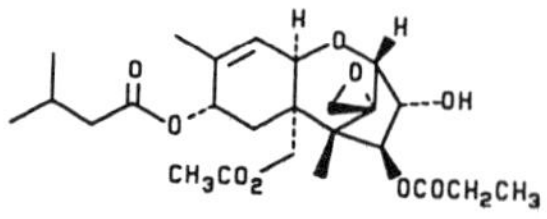

Mol. Wt.: 480
Bioactivity: Cytotoxic
Melting Point: 141-142°C
Spectral Data: IR, CMR, PMR, Mass Spec.
Organism: *Fusarium sporotrichioides*
MC-72083
(Tuberculariaceae)
Culture
Reference: 201

$C_{26}H_{26}ClN_3O_8$ **DC89-A1**

Mol. Wt.: 543
Bioactivity: P-388: T/C 144 at 0.50 mg/kg
Sarcoma 180: T/C 0.17% at 8 mg/kg
Toxicity (mice) (iv): LD_{50} 14 mg/kg
Antibacterial activity
$[\alpha]_D^{20}$: -126 Solvent: Me
Spectral Data: UV, IR, CMR, PMR, Mass Spec.
Organism: *Streptomyces* sp. (FERM BP988)
(Streptomycetaceae)
Culture from soil sample
Location; Japan
Reference: 450

$C_{27}H_{21}Cl_2N_3O_7$ **Rebeccamycin**
(previously known)

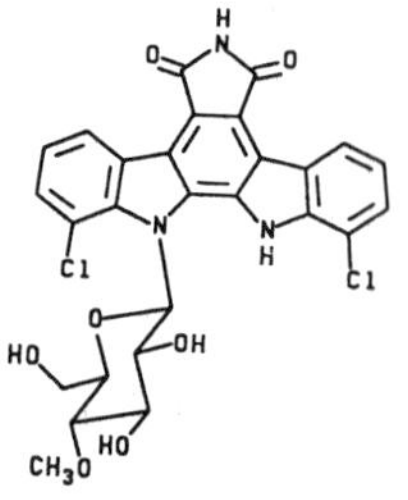

Mol. Wt.: 570
Bioactivity: P-388: T/C 168 (128 mg/kg for 5 days)
L1210: T/C 175 (256 mg/kg for 9 days)
B16: T/C 150 (128 mg/kg for 9 days)
Inhibition of human lung
adenocarcinoma cells: IC_{50} 6.0 μg/ml
Inhibition of DNA synthesis: 43%
at 100 μg/ml
Antimicrobial activity against
Staphylococcus aureus and
Streptococcus faecalis
Melting Point: 326-330°C (dec.)
$[\alpha]_D$: +131 Solvent: THF
Organism: *Nocardia aerocolonigenes*
(Nocardiaceae)
(syn. *Saccharothrix aerocolonigenes*)
Strain C-38,383
Culture of Panamanian soil sample
Reference: 122, 809

$C_{28}H_{19}NO_9$ **4181-B**

Mol. Wt.: 513
Bioactivity: KB: ED_{50} 0.005 μg/ml
P-388: activity at 0.625 - 5 mg/kg/day
Antimicrobial activity
Melting Point: >260°C
Spectral Data: UV, IR, PMR, Mass Spec.
Organism: *Streptomyces griseus* (Streptomycetaceae)
Culture of soil isolate
Location: China
Reference: 858

$C_{28}H_{24}ClNO_{10}$ **Actinoplanone B**

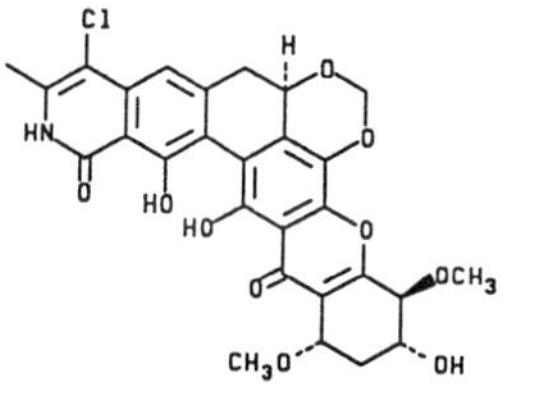

Mol. Wt.: 569
Bioactivity: HeLa: IC_{50} $5x10^{-3}$ μg/ml
Antifungal and antibacterial (gram-positive) activity
Melting Point: 240-243°C
$[\alpha]_D^{25}$: -649.4 Solvent: Chf
Spectral Data: UV, CD, IR, CMR, PMR, Mass Spec.
Organism: *Actinoplanes* sp. R-304 (Actinoplanaceae)
Culture of soil isolate
Location: Okinawa, Japan
Reference: 585, 586

$C_{28}H_{25}ClN_2O_{10}$ **Actinoplanone A**

Mol. Wt.: 584
Bioactivity: HeLa: IC_{50} $4x10^{-5}$ $\mu g/ml$
P-388: IC_{50} $8x10^{-5}$ $\mu g/ml$
YAC-1: IC_{50} $1.6x10^{-4}$ $\mu g/ml$
Raji: IC_{50} $9x10^{-6}$ $\mu g/ml$
L-929(1): IC_{50} $5.4x10^{-4}$ $\mu g/ml$
CHO: IC_{50} $4x10^{-4}$ $\mu g/ml$
VERO: IC_{50} $9x10^{-5}$ $\mu g/ml$
KB: IC_{50} $1.3x10^{-3}$ $\mu g/ml$
HLC: IC_{50} $4x10^{-4}$ $\mu g/ml$
PLC: IC_{50} $1x10^{-4}$ $\mu g/ml$
KN: IC_{50} $4x10^{-4}$ $\mu g/ml$
Antifungal and antibacterial activity
Inhibition of DNA synthesis
Melting Point: 276-278°C (dec.)
$[\alpha]_D^{25}$: -619.8 Solvent: Chf
Spectral Data: UV, CD, IR, CMR, PMR, Mass Spec.
Organism: *Actinoplanes* sp. R-304 (Actinoplanaceae)
Culture of soil isolate
Location: Okinawa, Japan
Reference: 585, 586

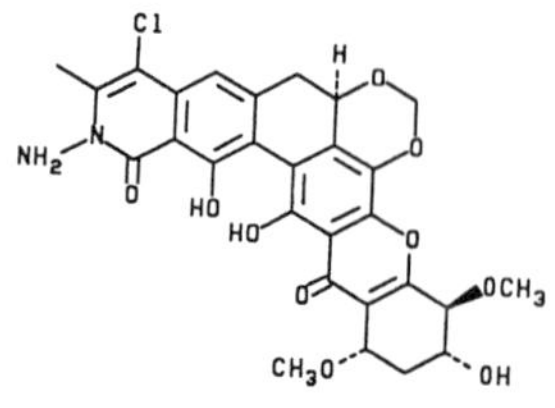

$C_{28}H_{25}NO_{10}$ **Actinoplanone D**

Mol. Wt.: 535
Bioactivity: HeLa: IC_{50} $1.1x10^{-2}$ $\mu g/ml$
Antifungal activity
Melting Point: 222-224°C (dec.)
$[\alpha]_D^{25}$: -624.1 Solvent: Chf
Spectral Data: UV, IR, CMR, PMR, Mass Spec.
Organism; *Actinoplanes* sp. R-304 (Actinoplanaceae)
Culture of soil isolate
Location: Okinawa, Japan
Reference: 586

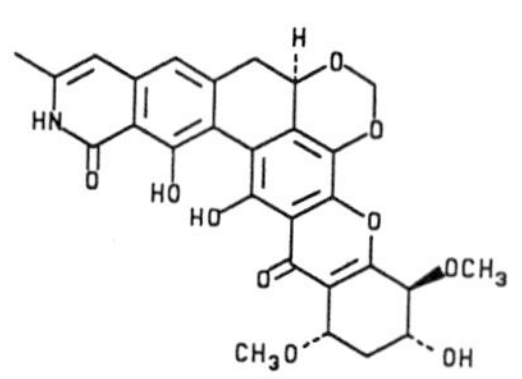

$C_{28}H_{26}N_2O_{10}$ **Actinoplanone C**

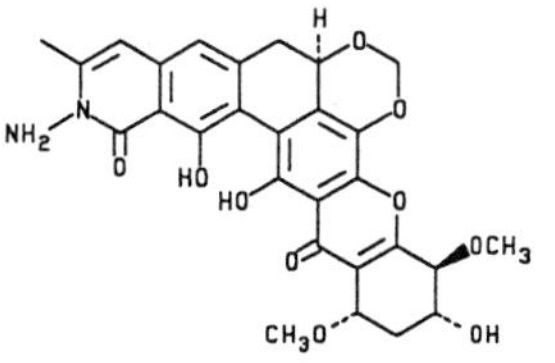

Mol. Wt.: 550
Bioactivity; HeLa: IC_{50} <4x10^{-5} μg/ml
Antifungal activity
Melting Point: 278-280°C (dec.)
$[\alpha]_D^{25}$: -646.1 Solvent: Chf
Spectral Data: UV, IR, CMR, PMR, Mass Spec.
Organism: *Actinoplanes* sp. R-304
(Actinoplanaceae)
Culture of soil isolate
Location: Okinawa, Japan
Reference: 586

$C_{28}H_{38}N_2O_8$ **Herbimycin B**
(previously known)

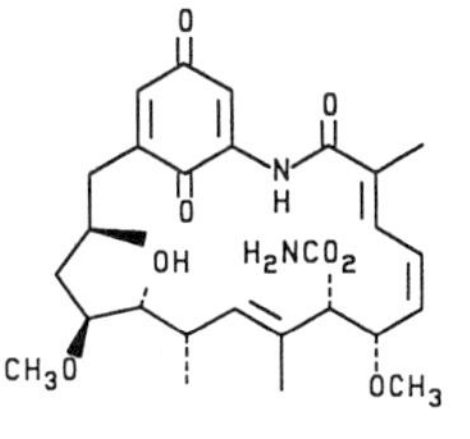

Mol. Wt.: 530
Bioactivity: HeLa: IC_{50} 3.2 μg/ml
Ehrlich: IC_{50} 0.8 μg/ml
herbicidal and anti-tobacco-mosaic virus activity
Spectral Data: CMR
Organism: *Streptomyces hygroscopicus*
AM-3672
(Streptomycetaceae)
Reference: 487, 999

$C_{29}H_{21}NO_9$ **4181-A**

Mol. Wt.: 527
Bioactivity: KB: ED_{50} 0.003 μg/ml
P-388: activity at 5-40 mg/kg/day
Antimicrobial activity
Melting Point: >300°C
Spectral Data: UV, IR, PMR, Mass Spec.
Organism: *Streptomyces griseus*
(Streptomycetaceae)
Culture of soil isolate
Location: Sichuan, China
Reference: 858

$C_{29}H_{32}O_{11}$ **Roritoxin D**

Mol. Wt.: 556
Bioactivity: L1210: ID_{50} 0.0021 μg/ml
Melting Point: 294-297°C (dec.)
$[\alpha]_D^{25}$: +30.0 Solvent: Chf
Spectral Data: UV, CD, IR, CMR of the acetate, PMR, Mass Spec.
Organism: *Myrothecium roridum* CL-514 (ATCC 20605) (Tuberculariaceae) Rice culture
Reference: 496

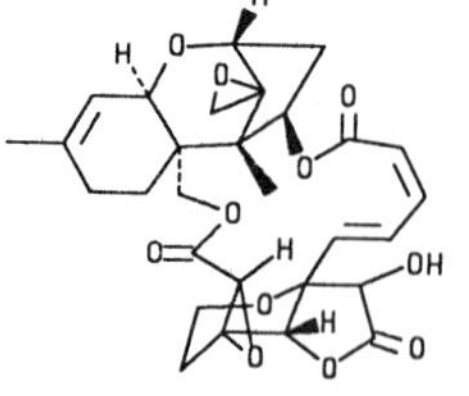

$C_{29}H_{32}O_{12}$ **Roritoxin C**

Mol. Wt.: 572
Bioactivity: L1210: ID_{50} 0.0042 μg/ml
Melting Point: 288-290°C (dec.)
$[\alpha]_D^{25}$: +8.9 Solvent: Chf
Spectral Data: UV, CD, IR, CMR of the acetate, PMR, Mass Spec.
Organism: *Myrothecium roridum* CL-514 (ATCC 20605) (Tuberculariaceae) Rice culture
Reference: 496

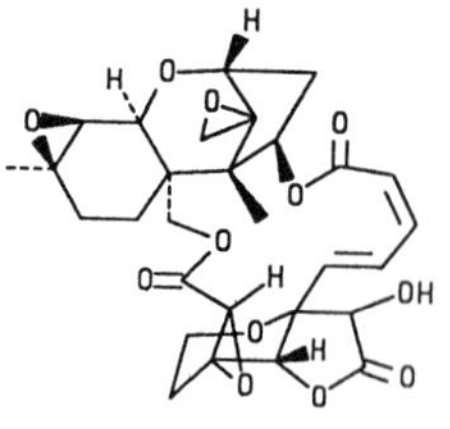

$C_{29}H_{34}O_{10}$ **Roritoxin A**

Mol. Wt.: 542
Bioactivity: L1210: ID_{50} 0.0011 μg/ml
Melting Point: 220-225°C
$[\alpha]_D^{25}$: +16 Solvent: Chf
Spectral Data: UV, CD, IR, CMR, PMR, Mass Spec.
Organism: *Myrothecium roridum* CL-514(ATCC 20605) (Tuberculariaceae) Rice culture
Reference: 496

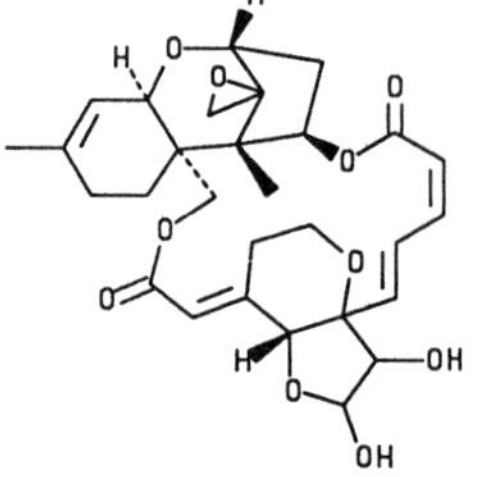

$C_{29}H_{34}O_{11}$ **Roritoxin B**

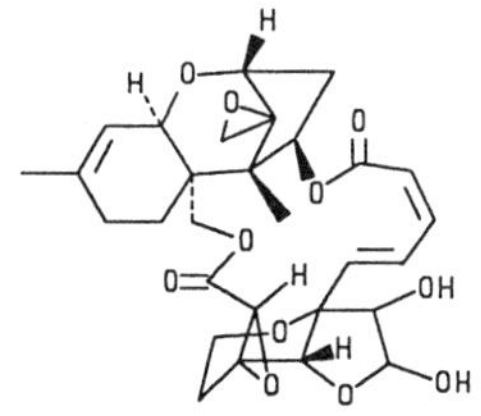

Mol. Wt.: 558
Bioactivity: P-388: toxic at 80 μg/kg
L1210: ID_{50} 0.0017 μg/ml
Melting Point: 262-265°C (dec.)
$[\alpha]_D^{25}$: +2.6 Solvent: Chf
Spectral Data: UV, CD, IR, CMR, PMR, Mass Spec.
Organism: *Myrothecium roridum*
CL-514(ATCC 20605)
(Tuberculariaceae)
Rice culture
Reference: 496

$C_{29}H_{38}N_4O_8$ **Saframycin Mx 2**

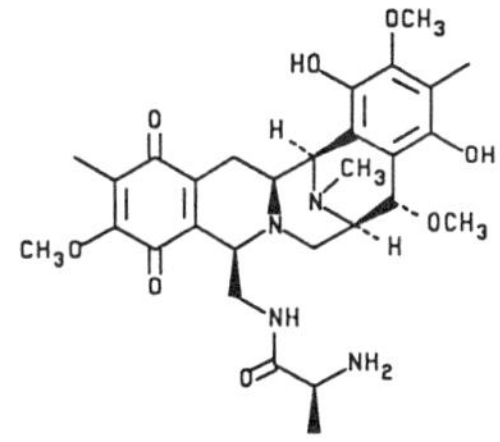

Mol. Wt.: 570
Bioactivity: Antitumor active antibiotic
$[\alpha]_D^{20}$: -119.8 Solvent: Me
Spectral Data: UV, IR, CMR, PMR, Mass Spec.
Organism: *Myxococcus xanthus*
Strain Mx x48
(Myxococcaceae)
Culture of soil sample
Location: Tunisia
Reference: 1108

$C_{29}H_{38}N_4O_9$ **Saframycin Mx 1**

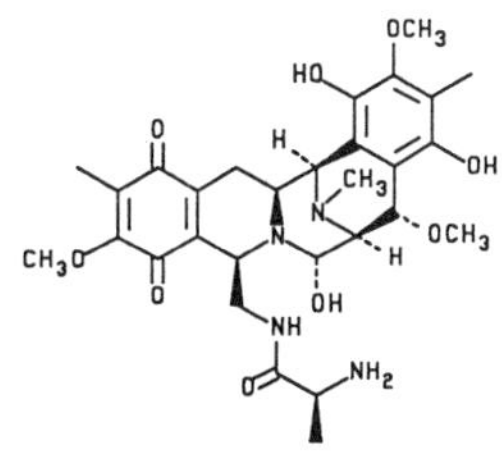

Mol. Wt.: 586
Bioactivity: Antitumor activity
Inhibition of DNA, RNA and protein syntheses in *Staphylococcus aureus* at 0.5 μg/ml
Inhibition of RNA synthesis in *Escherichia coli*
Antibacterial activity
$[\alpha]_D^{20}$: -70.7 Solvent: Me
Spectral Data: UV, IR, CMR, PMR, Mass Spec.
Organism: *Myxococcus xanthus*
Strain Mx x48
(Myxococcaceae)
Culture of soil sample
Location: Tunisia
Reference: 463, 1108

$C_{29}H_{40}N_2O_9$ **Herbimycin C**
(syn. **TAN-420-D**)

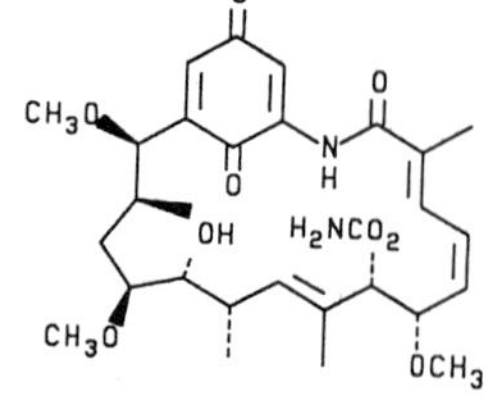

Mol. Wt.:	560
Bioactivity:	P-388: ED_{50} 0.17 μg/ml KB: ED_{50} 0.12 μg/ml HeLa: IC_{50} 7.3 μg/ml Ehrlich: IC_{50} 1.2 μg/ml Herbicidal and anti-tobacco-mosaic virus activity
Melting Point:	203°C (dec.)
$[\alpha]_D^{23}$:	+210 Solvent: Chf
Spectral Data:	UV, IR, CMR, PMR, Mass Spec.
Organism:	*Streptomyces hygroscopicus* AM-3672 and AM-3675 (Streptomycetaceae) Culture
Reference:	660, 999, 1081

$C_{29}H_{42}N_2O_9$ **Dihydro-herbimycin C**
(syn. **TAN-420-C**)
(previously known)

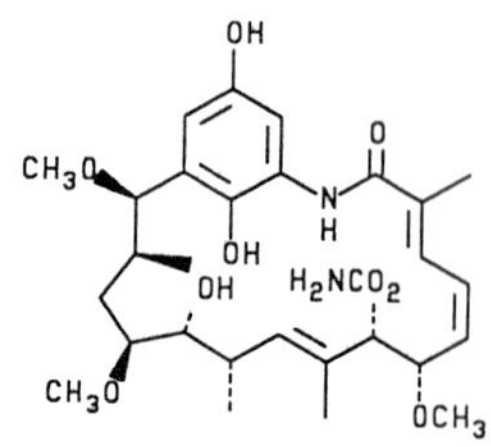

Mol. Wt.:	562
Bioactivity:	P-388: ED_{50} 0.34 μg/ml KB: ED_{50} 3.49 μg/ml
Melting Point:	155-157°C
Spectral Data:	UV, IR, PMR
Organism:	*Streptomyces hygroscopicus* AM-3675 (Streptomycetaceae) Culture
Reference:	660, 1081

$C_{30}H_{21}NO_9$	**Fredericamycin A**	
Mol. Wt.:	539	
Bioactivity:	KB: ED_{50} $7x10^{-1}$ $\mu g/ml$ P-388: ED_{50} $5x10^{-4}$ $\mu g/ml$ L1210: ED_{50} $2x10^{-4}$ $\mu g/ml$ Transplantable CD8F tumor: T/C 7 (median tumor weight) at 1.25 mg/kg P-388: T/C 200 (0.5 mg/kg) Ehrlich: T/C 295 Meth-A-fibrosarcoma: T/C 242	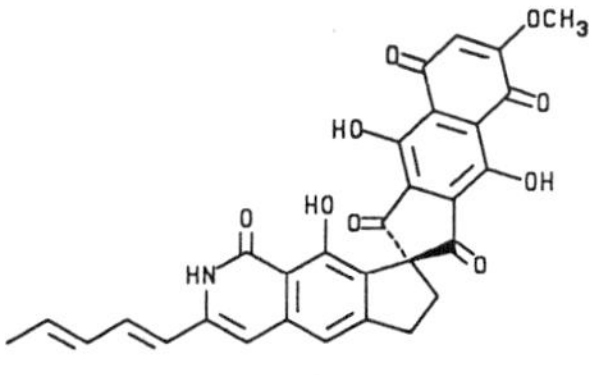
Spectral Data:	UV, CD, IR, CMR, PMR, Mass Spec., x-ray c.s.	
Organism:	*Streptomyces griseus* FCRC-48 (Streptomycetaceae)	
Reference:	541, 542, 745	

$C_{30}H_{33}N_3O_{10}$	**Azinomycin A**	
Mol Wt.:	595	
Bioactivity:	P-388: T/C 176 (16 $\mu g/kg/day$ for 10 days) B16: T/C 175 (16 $\mu g/kg/day$ for 10 days) Ehrlich carcinoma: T/C 256 (8 $\mu g/kg/day$ for 10 days) L5178Y: IC_{50} 0.07 $\mu g/ml$ Antimicrobial activity against gram positive and gram negative	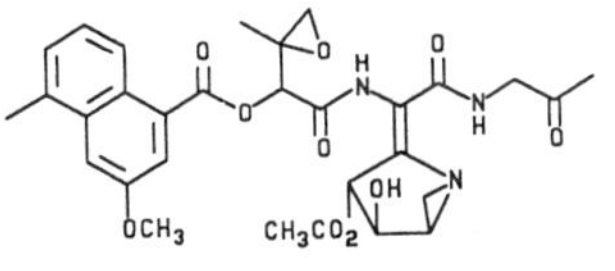
Melting Point:	140°C (dec.)	
Spectral Data:	UV, IR, CMR, PMR, Mass Spec.	
Organism:	*Streptomyces griseofuscus* S42227 (FERM P-8443) (Streptomycetaceae)	
Location:	Gunma, Japan	
Reference:	473, 789, 1209	

$C_{30}H_{42}N_2O_9$ **Herbimycin A**
(syn. **TAN-420-F**)
(previously known)

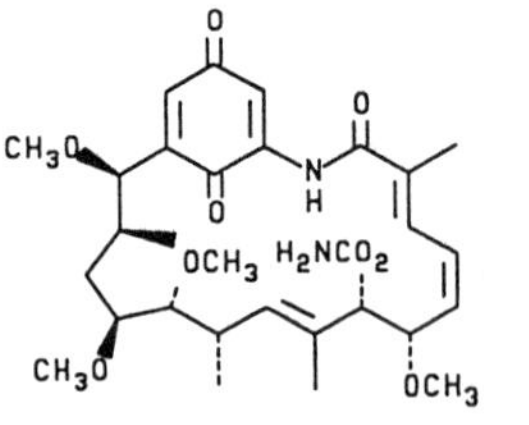

Mol. Wt.: 574
Bioactivity: P-388: ED_{50} 0.0051 μg/ml
KB: ED_{50} 0.12 μg/ml
HeLa: IC_{50} 3.5 μg/ml
Ehrlich: IC_{50} 0.4 μg/ml
Herbicidal and anti-tobacco-mosaic virus activity
Melting Point: 230°C
Spectral Data: CMR, PMR, x-ray c.s.
Organism: *Streptomyces hygroscopicus* AM-3672 and AM-3675 (Streptomycetaceae) Culture
Reference: 329, 660, 855, 856, 999, 1081

$C_{30}H_{44}N_2O_9$ **Dihydro-herbimycin A**
(syn. **TAN-420-E**)
(previously known)

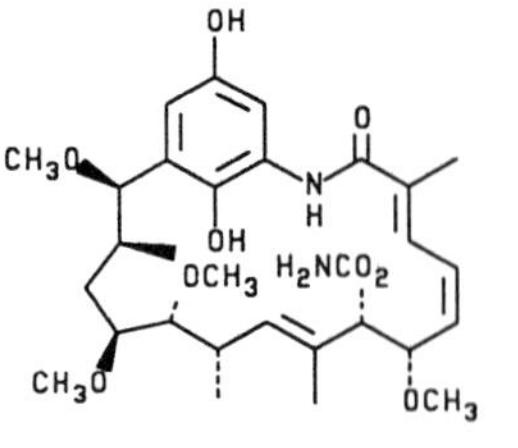

Mol. Wt.: 576
Bioactivity: P-388: ED_{50} 0.022 μg/ml
KB: ED_{50} 0.30 μg/ml
Melting Point: 163-165°C
Spectral Data: UV, IR, PMR
Organism: *Streptomyces hygroscopicus* AM-3675 (Streptomycetaceae) Culture
Reference: 660, 1081

$C_{30}H_{46}O_7$ **Saponaceolide A**

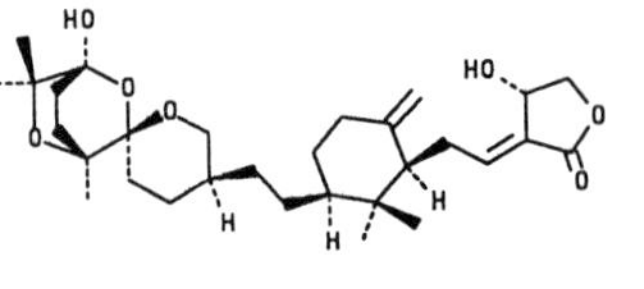

Mol. Wt.: 518
Bioactivity: Human colon adenocarcinoma: ID_{50} 450 ±112 ng/ml
Melting Point: 145-146°C
$[\alpha]_D^{20}$: +78.14 Solvent: Chf
Spectral Data: IR, CMR, PMR, Mass Spec., x-ray c.s.
Organism: *Tricholoma saponaceum* (Fr.) Kummer (Tricholomataceae)
Location: Northern Italy
Reference: 224

$C_{31}H_{29}ClN_2O_{10}$	**Actinoplanone E**
Mol. Wt.:	624
Bioactivity:	HeLa: IC_{50} $1.3x10^{-4}$ $\mu g/ml$ Antifungal activity
Melting Point:	190-193°C
$[\alpha]_D^{25}$:	-516.7 Solvent: Chf
Spectral Data:	UV, IR, CMR, PMR, Mass Spec.
Organism:	*Actinoplanes* sp. R-304 (Actinoplanaceae) Culture of soil isolate
Location:	Okinawa, Japan
Reference:	586

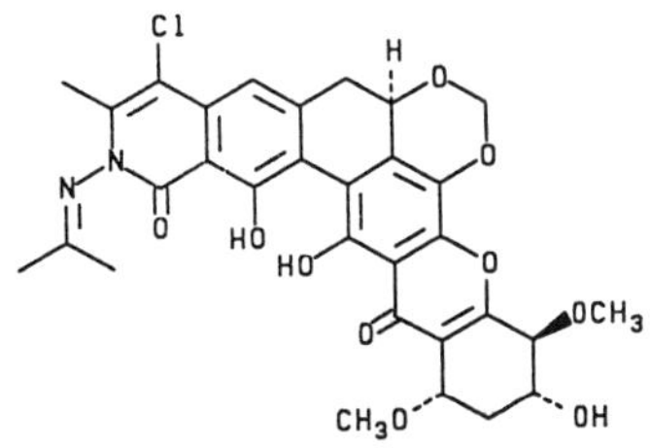

$C_{31}H_{33}N_3O_{11}$	**Azinomycin B**
Mol. Wt.:	623
Bioactivity:	P-388: T/C 293 (16 $\mu g/kg/day$ for 10 days) B16: T/C 164 (8 $\mu g/kg/day$ for 10 days) Ehrlich carcinoma: T/C 261 (32 $\mu g/kg/day$ for 10 days) L5178Y: IC_{50} 0.11 $\mu g/ml$ Antimicrobial activity against gram positive + negative bacteria
Melting Point:	190°C (dec.)
$[\alpha]_D^{20}$:	+48 Solvent: Chf
Spectral Data:	UV, IR, CMR, PMR, Mass Spec.
Organism:	*Streptomyces griseofuscus* S42227 (Streptomycetaceae)
Location:	Gunma, Japan
Reference:	473, 789, 1209

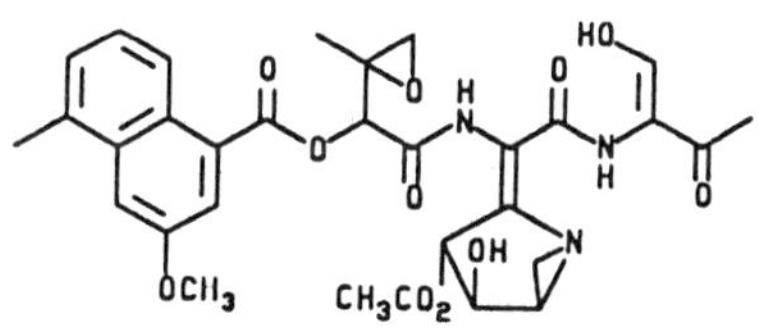

$C_{31}H_{44}N_4O_6$ **WF-3161**
(previously known)

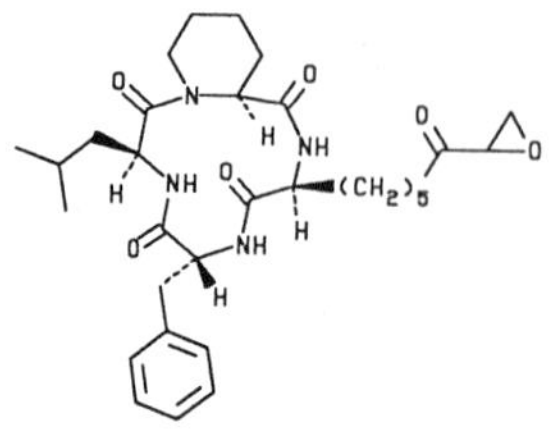

Mol. Wt.: 568
Bioactivity: P-388: T/C 175 (100 mg/kg/day for 4 days)
P-388: LD_{50} 200 mg/kg
Antimicrobial activity against *Trichophyton asteroides*
Melting Point: 181-183°C
$[\alpha]_D^{25}$: -120 Solvent: Chf
Spectral Data: CMR, PMR
Organism: *Petriella guttulata* (Microascaceae)
Reference: 532, 1125

$C_{31}H_{44}O_6$ **Anguinomycin A**

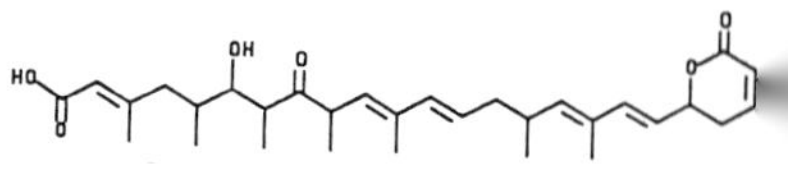

Mol. Wt.: 512
Bioactivity: P-388: T/C 147 (50 μg/kg/day)
Lewis lung carcinoma: T/C 159 (31.3 μg/kg/day)
Melting Point: Oil
$[\alpha]_D^{27}$: -139 Solvent: Me
Spectral Data: UV, IR, CMR, PMR, Mass Spec.
Organism: *Streptomyces* sp. R2827 (Streptomycetaceae)
Culture
Reference: 405

$C_{32}H_{29}ClN_2O_{11}$ **Actinoplanone F**

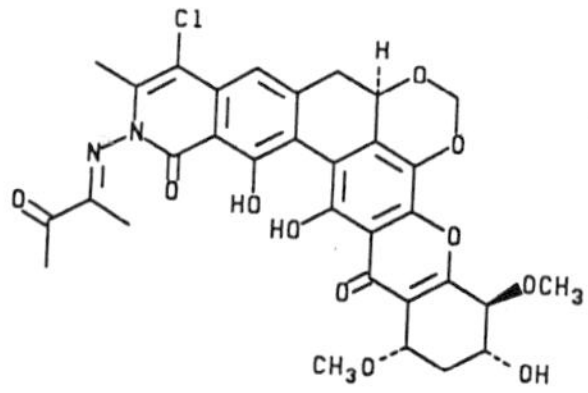

Mol. Wt.: 652
Bioactivity: HeLa: IC_{50} $2x10^{-3}$ μg/ml
Antifungal and antibacterial (gram-positive) activity
Melting Point: 281-282°C (dec.)
$[\alpha]_D$: -569.1 Solvent: Chf
Spectral Data: UV, IR, CMR, PMR, Mass Spec.
Organism: *Actinoplanes* sp. R-304 (Actinoplanaceae)
Culture of soil isolate
Location: Okinawa, Japan
Reference: 586

$C_{32}H_{30}N_2O_{11}$ **Actinoplanone G**

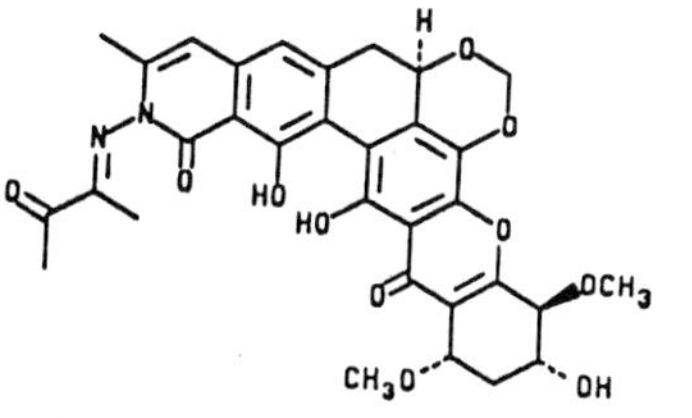

Mol. Wt.: 618
Bioactivity: HeLa: IC_{50} <4x10^{-5} μg/ml
Antifungal activity
Melting Point: 173-176°C
$[\alpha]_D^{25}$: -582.3 Solvent: Chf
Spectral Data: UV, IR, CMR, PMR, Mass Spec.
Organism: *Actinoplanes* sp. R-304
(Actinoplanaceae)
Culture of soil isolate
Location: Okinawa, Japan
Reference: 586

$C_{32}H_{46}O_6$ **Anguinomycin B**

Mol. Wt.: 526
Bioactivity: P-388: T/C 140 (50 μg/kg/day)
Lewis lung carcinoma:
T/C 201 (15.6 μg/kg/day)
(5/6 mice cured at 31.3 μg/kg/day)
Melting Point: Oil
$[\alpha]_D^{27}$: -130 Solvent: Me
Spectral Data: UV, IR, CMR, PMR, Mass Spec.
Organism: *Streptomyces* sp. R2827
(Streptomycetaceae)
Culture
Reference: 405

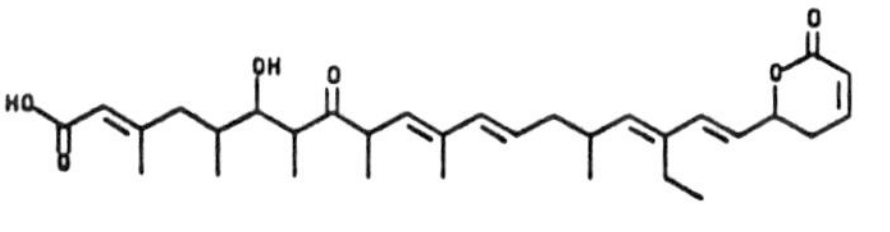

$C_{32}H_{46}O_6$ **Leptomycin A**

Mol. Wt.: 526
Bioactivity: Cytotoxic to SV-40 transformed C3H-2K cells
Antimicrobial activity
Melting Point: Oil
$[\alpha]_D$: -31.8 Solvent: Me
Spectral Data: UV, IR, CMR, PMR, Mass Spec.
Organism: *Streptomyces* sp. ATS1287 (Streptomycetaceae)
Culture of soil sample
Location: Japan
Reference: 327, 389, 390

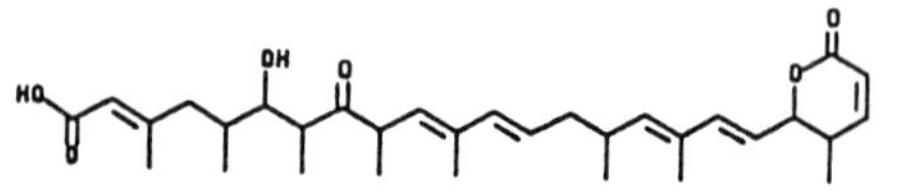

$C_{32}H_{46}O_7$ **Kazusamycin B**

Mol. Wt.: 542
Bioactivity: P-388: IC_{100} 1.6x10^{-3} μg/ml
L1210: IC_{50} 1.8x10^{-3} μg/ml
Antimicrobial activity
Melting Point: 53-55°C
$[\alpha]_D^{20}$: -152.0 Solvent: Chf
Spectral Data: UV, IR, CMR, PMR, Mass Spec.
Organism: *Streptomyces* sp. No. 81-484 (Streptomycetaceae)
Culture
Reference: 327

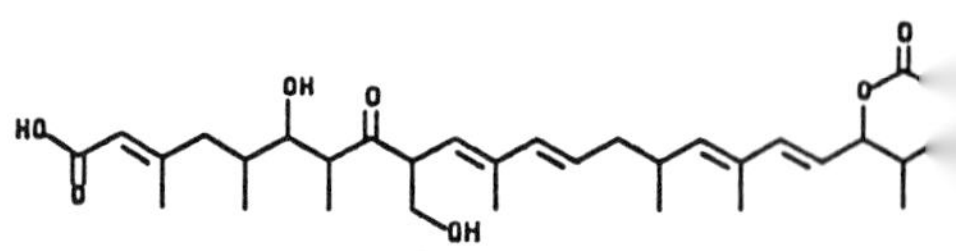

$C_{32}H_{46}O_7$ **PD 124,895**

Mol. Wt.:	542
Bioactivity:	P-388: T/C 153 (100 μg/kg/day for 5 days) L1210: IC_{50} $1.1x10^{-3}$ μg/ml HCT-8: IC_{50} $1.0x10^{-3}$ μg/ml
Melting Point:	40-50°C
$[\alpha]_D$:	+158 Solvent: Chf
Spectral Data:	UV, IR, CMR, PMR, Mass Spec.
Organism:	*Streptomyces* sp. (Streptomycetaceae)
Reference:	446

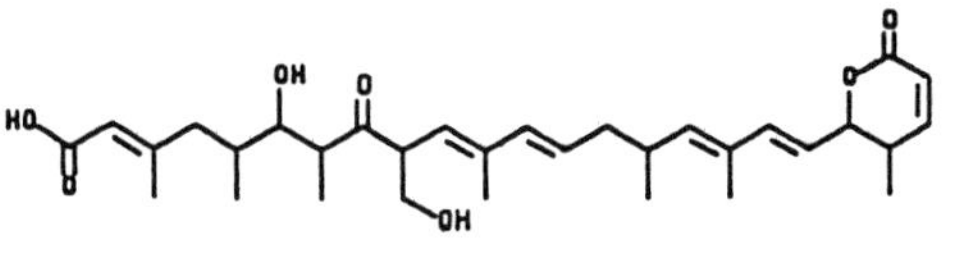

$C_{33}H_{35}NO_{13}$ **Elsamicin A**

Mol. Wt.:	653
Bioactivity:	P-388: T/C 239 (1 mg/kg/day for 9 days) L1210: T/C 150 (3 mg/kg/day for 9 days) B16: T/C 296 (3 mg/kg/day for 9 days) Acute toxicity: LD_{50} 38 mg/kg Antibacterial activity against gram positive bacteria and anaerobes
Melting Point:	225-226°C
$[\alpha]_D{}^{26}$:	+124 Solvent: Py
Spectral Data:	UV, IR, CMR, PMR, Mass Spec., x-ray c.s.
Organismn:	Actinomycete Strain No. J907-21 (ATCC 39417) (unidentified) Soil sample
Location;	El Salvador
Reference:	602, 1041

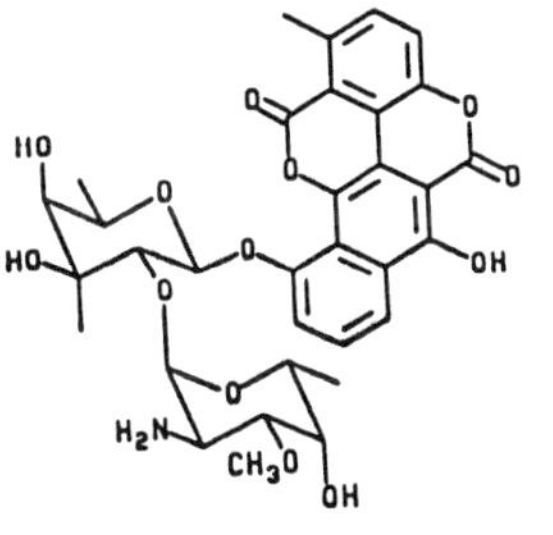

$C_{33}H_{39}NO_{13}$ **Barminomycin I**

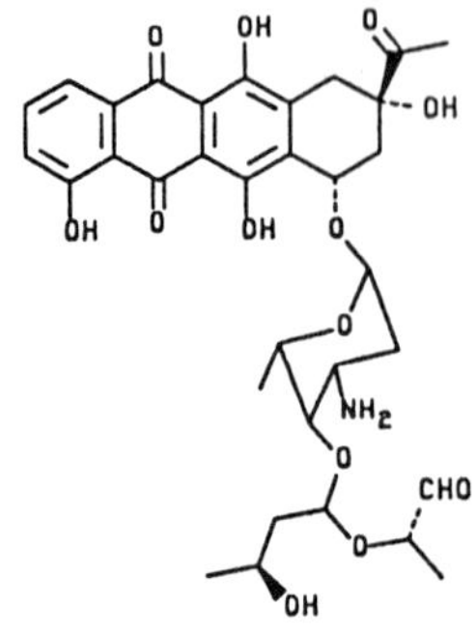

Mol. Wt.: 657
Bioactivity: P-388: IC_{50}~10^{-5} μg/ml
L1210: T/C 140~500
(0.39~1.5 μg/kg/day)
Antimicrobial activity
Spectral Data: UV, IR, CMR of derivative, PMR, Mass Spec.
Organism: *Actinomadura roseoviolacea* or *A. carminata*
Strain MG463-yF4
(Thermomonosporaceae)
Culture of soil isolate
Location: Kochi, Japan
Reference: 1115

$C_{33}H_{39}NO_{13}$ **Barminomycin II**

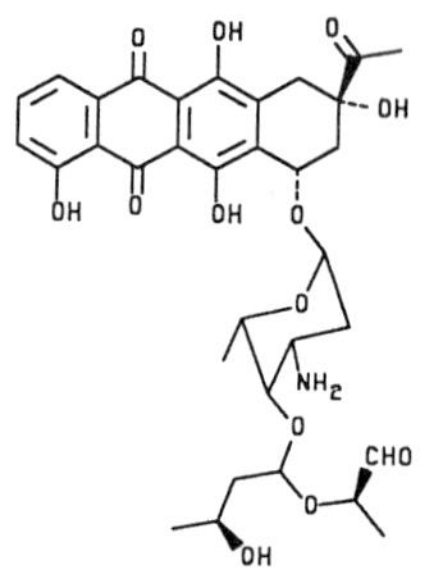

Mol. Wt.: 657
Bioactivity: P-388: IC_{50}~$2x10^{-5}$ μg/ml
L1210: T/C 140~500
(0.39~1.5 μg/kg/day)
Spectral Data: UV, IR, CMR of derivative, PMR, Mass Spec.
Organism: *Actinomadura roseoviolacea* or *A. carminata*
Strain MG463-yF4
(Thermomonosporaceae)
Culture of soil isolate
Location: Kochi, Japan
Reference: 1115

$C_{33}H_{48}O_6$

Cl-940
(PD 114,720)
(Elactocin)

Mol. Wt.: 540
Bioactivity: P-388 (ip-ip): T/C 153 (1.0 mg/kg)
L1210 (ip-ip): T/C 128 (0.25 mg/kg)
B16 (ip-ip): T/C 201 (0.225 mg/kg)
B16 (sc-ip): T/C 135 (1.8 mg/kg)
Mammary adenocarcinoma 16/C (ip-ip): T/C 163 (1.875 mg/kg)
Mammary adenocarcinoma 16/C (sc-ip): T/C 4.0 (4.8 mg/kg)
M5076 (ip-ip): T/C 217 (3.2 mg/kg)
LC12 (sc-iv): T/C 32 (8.0 mg/kg)
ROS (sc-iv): T/C 6.0 (3.0 mg/kg)
L1210: IC_{50} 0.22 nM
Lewis lung carcinoma: IC_{50} 0.37 nM
Pancreatic carcinoma 02: IC_{50} 2.8 nM
Mammary adenocarcinoma 16/C': IC_{50} 0.61 nM
HCT-8 human colon: IC_{50} 0.37 nM
A549 human lung: IC_{50} 0.45 nM
MCF-7 human mammary carcinoma: IC_{50} 0.19 nM
P388: IC_{50} 0.463 nM
P-388/ADR: IC_{50} 0.704 nM
P-388/AMSA: IC_{50} 0.352 nM
P-388/MITOX: IC_{50} 0.463 nM
$[\alpha]_D^{23}$: -105.4 Solvent: Me
Organism: Unidentified actinomycete (ATCC 39366) soil sample
Location: Pennsylvania
Reference: 939, 978

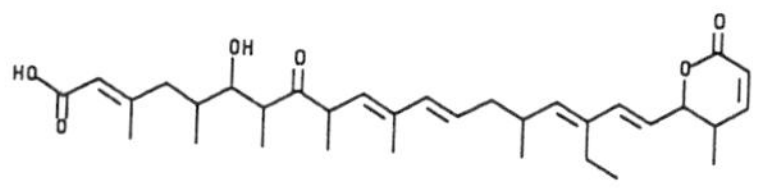

$C_{33}H_{48}O_6$

Leptomycin B

Mol. Wt.: 540
Bioactivity: Cytotoxic to SV-40 transformed C3H-2K cells; Antimicrobial activity
Melting Point: Oil
$[\alpha]_D$: -24.5 Solvent: Me
Spectral Data: UV, IR, CMR, PMR, Mass Spec.
Organism: *Streptomyces* sp. ATS1287 (Streptomycetaceae)
Culture of soil sample
Location: Japan
Reference: 327, 389, 390

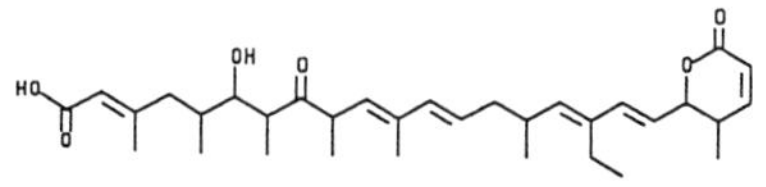

$C_{33}H_{48}O_7$ **PD 114,721**
(Kazusamycin A)

Mol. Wt.: 556

Bioactivity:
P388 (ip-ip): T/C 161 (0.225 mg/kg)
L1210 (ip-ip): T/C 142 (0.25 mg/kg)
B16 (ip-ip): T/C 184 (0.056 mg/kg)
B16 (sc-ip): T/C 130 (0.45 mg/kg)
Mammary adenocarcinoma 16/C (ip-ip): T/C 161 (0.936 mg/kg)
Mammary adenocarcinoma 16/C (sc-ip): T/C 3.7 (4.8 mg/kg)
M5076 (ip-ip): T/C 217 (3.2 mg/kg)
ROS (sc-iv): T/C 15 (1.5 mg/kg)
Ehrlich carcinoma (ip-ip): T/C 242 (0.04 mg/kg)
Sarcoma 180 (ip-ip): T/C 319 (0.08 mg/kg)
IMC carcinoma (ip-ip): T/C 363 (0.02 mg/kg)
IMC solid tumor (sc-ip): 63% inhibition (0.04 mg/kg)
Meth A fibrosarcoma (ip-ip): T/C 195 (0.04 mg/kg)
Lewis lung carcinoma (ip-ip): T/C 151 (0.04 mg/kg)
HeLa: 99.4% inhibition (21 μg/ml)
L1210: IC_{50} 0.33 nM
Lewis lung carcinoma: IC_{50} 1.6 nM
Pancreatic carcinoma: IC_{50} 8.0 nM
HCT-8: IC_{50} 1.7 nM
A549: IC_{50} 1.2 nM
MCF-7: IC_{50} 0.66 nM
Antimicrobial activity

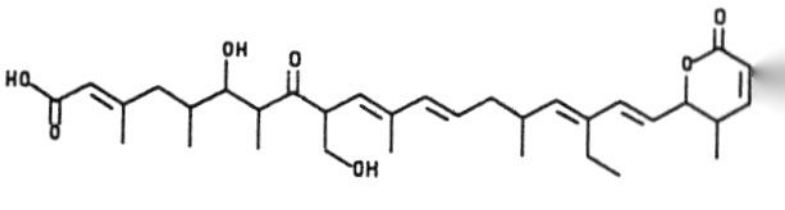

$[\alpha]_D^{20}$: -83.5 Solvent: Me

Spectral Data: UV, IR, CMR, PMR, Mass Spec.

Organism: *Streptomyces* sp. No. 81-484 (Streptomycetaceae)
Unidentified actinomycete (ATCC 39366)
Culture

Reference: 327, 599, 600, 939, 978, 1127

$C_{34}H_{45}NO_7$ **WF-1360C**

Mol. Wt.: 579

Bioactivity: P-388: IC_{50} 0.0015 μg/ml
Inhibition of tubulin polymerization: IC_{50} 7μM
Antimicrobial, antifungal activity

$[\alpha]_D^{23}$: +197 Solvnet: Chf

Spectral Data: UV, IR, CMR, PMR, Mass Spec.

Organism: *Rhizopus chinensis* Rh-2
Rhizopus sp. No. F-1360
(Mucoraceae)
Culture

Reference: 570, 1073

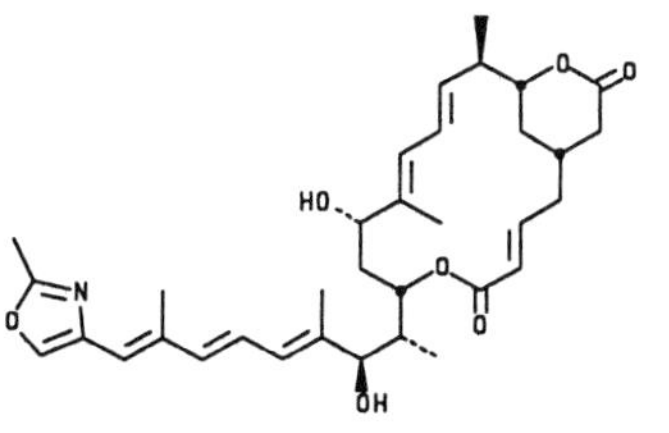

$C_{34}H_{45}NO_8$ **WF-1360B**

Mol. Wt.: 595

Bioactivity: P-388: IC_{50} 0.0008 μg/ml
Inhibition of tubulin polymerization: IC_{50} 7 μM
Antimicrobial, antifungal activity

$[\alpha]_D^{23}$: +110 Solvent: Chf

Spectral Data: UV, IR, CMR, PMR, Mass Spec.

Organism: *Rhizopus chinensis* Rh-2
Rhizopus sp. No. F-1360
(Mucoraceae)
Culture

Reference: 570, 1073

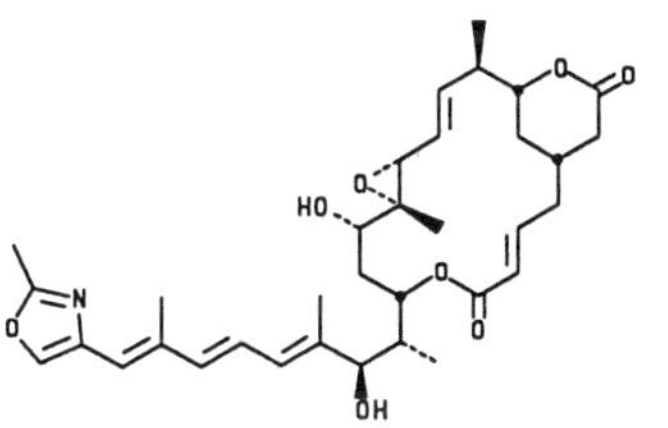

$C_{34}H_{45}NO_8$ **WF-1360D**

Mol. Wt.: 595

Bioactivity: P-388: IC_{50} 0.12 μg/ml
Antimicrobial (weak) and antifungal activity

$[\alpha]_D^{23}$: +57 Solvent: Chf

Spectral Data: IR, Mass Spec.

Organism: *Rhizopus* sp. No. F-1360
(Mucoraceae)

Reference: 570

$C_{34}H_{45}NO_9$

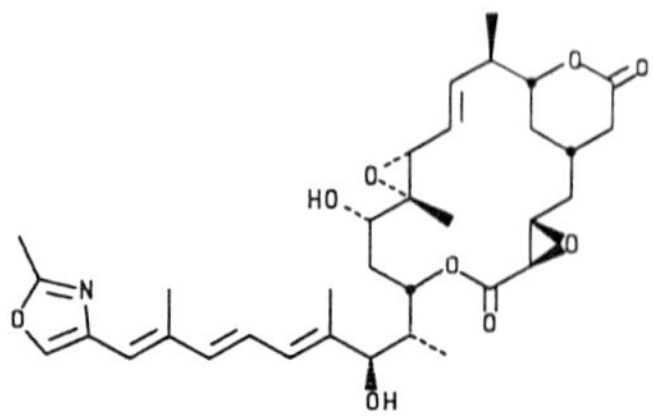

Mol. Wt.: 611
Bioactivity: Inhibition of tubulin polymerization: IC_{50} 7 μm
Organism: *Rhizopus chinensis* Rh-2 (Mucoraceae) Culture
Reference: 1073

$C_{35}H_{33}NO_{12}$ **Neocarzinostatin chromophore (NCS-chr)**

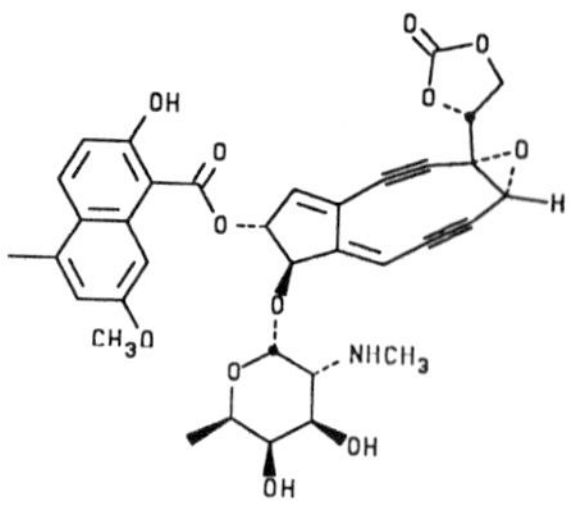

Mol. Wt.: 659
Bioactivity: Yoshida sarcoma: minimum effective dose 0.1 mg/kg [in combination with apo-NCS protein: MED 0.005 mg/kg]
Toxicity (iv): LD_{50} 1.8 mg/kg; (ip): >10 mg/kg
Significant antimicrobial activity
Inhibition of DNA synthesis
Induction of DNA strand breakage
Melting Point: 125°C (dec.) (hydrochloride)
$[\alpha]_D^{20}$: -171 Solvent: Me (1%)
Spectral Data: UV, IR, CMR, PMR, Mass Spec.
Organism: *Streptomyces carzinostaticus* var. F-41 (Streptomycetaceae) Culture
Reference: 257, 258, 595, 786

$C_{35}H_{47}NO_7$

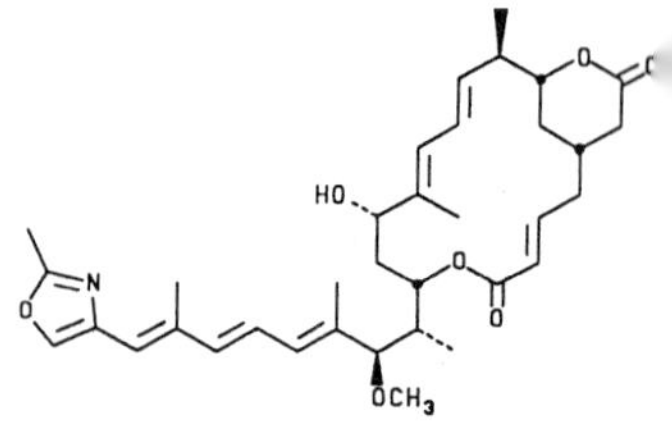

Mol. Wt.: 593
Bioactivity: Inhibition of tubulin polymerization: IC_{50} 7 μM
Organism: *Rhizopus chinensis* Rh-2 (Mucoraceae) Culture
Reference: 1073

$C_{35}H_{47}NO_8$ **WF-1360F**

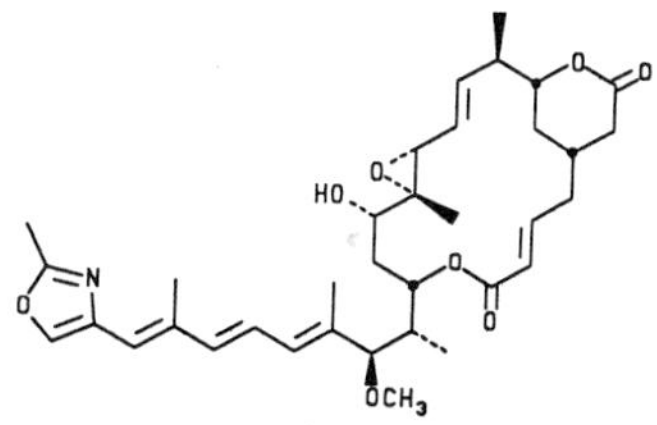

Mol. Wt.: 609
Bioactivity: P-388: IC_{50} 0.0002 μg/ml
Inhibition of tubulin polymerization: IC_{50} 5 μM
Antimicrobial and antifungal activity
$[\alpha]_D^{23}$: +97 Solvent: Chf
Spectral Data: UV, IR, CMR, PMR, Mass Spec.
Organism: *Rhizopus chinensis* Rh-2
Rhizopus sp. No. F-1360
(Mucoraceae)
Culture
Reference: 570, 1073

$C_{35}H_{47}NO_9$ **Rhizoxin (WF-1360) (FR-900216)**
(previously known)

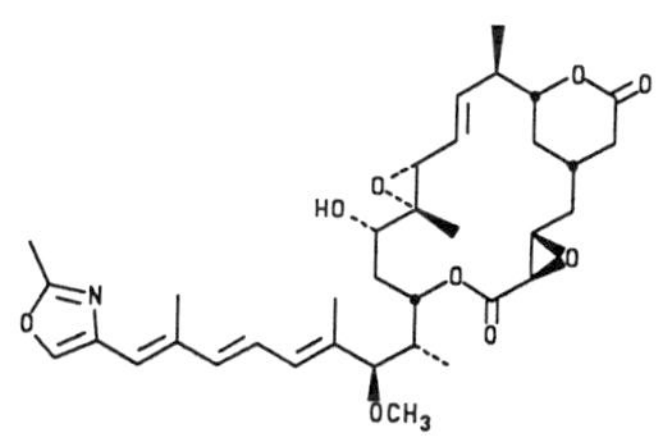

Mol. Wt.: 625
Bioactivity: P-388: IC_{50} 0.0001 μg/ml
L1210: T/C 151 (1.0 mg/kg/day)
B16: T/C 153 (0.5 mg/kg/day)
LD_{50}: 2.5 mg/kg
Inhibition of fusion of male and female sea urchin pronuclei at $1.6x10^{-8}$M
Inhibition of cilia formation at $16x10^{-8}$M
50% Inhibition of DNA synthesis at ~$1.6x10^{-5}$M
Inhibition of tubulin polymerization: IC_{50} $5x10^{-6}$M
Antimicrobial activity
$[\alpha]_D^{20}$: +140 Solvent: Chf
Spectral Data: UV, IR, CMR, PMR, Mass Spec.
Organism: *Rhizopus chinensis* Rh-2
Rhizopus sp. No. F-1360
(Mucoraceae)
Culture
Reference: 491, 570, 574, 1073

$C_{37}H_{53}NO_9$ **WF-1360E**

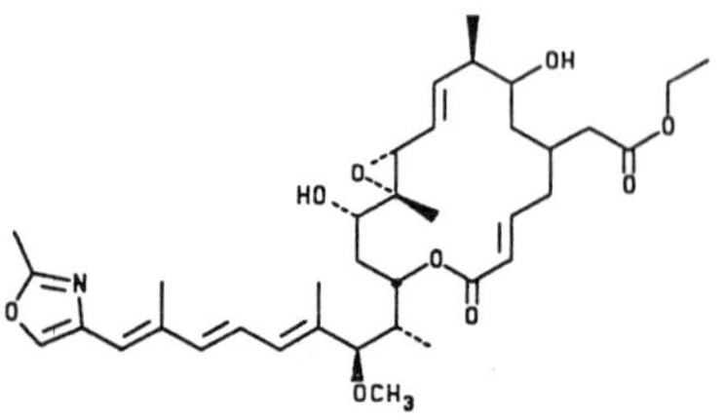

Mol. Wt.: 655
Bioactivity: P-388: IC_{50} 0.0016 μg/ml
Antimicrobial (weak) and antifungal activity
$[\alpha]_D^{23}$: +58 Solvent: Chf
Spectral Data: UV, IR, CMR, PMR, Mass Spec.
Organism; *Rhizopus* sp. No. F-1360 (Mucoraceae)
Reference: 570

$C_{40}H_{46}ClNO_9$ **Naphthomycin**
(previously known)

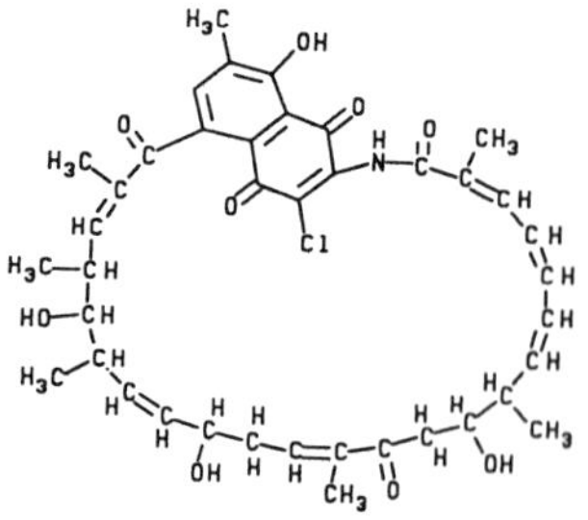

Mol. Wt.: 719
Bioactivity: Ehrlich carcinoma (ip):
T/C >269 (8mg/kg/day)
IMC carcinoma (ip):
T/C 228 (8 mg/kg/day)
P-388: IC_{50} 0.44 μg/ml
L5178Y: IC_{50} 0.83 μg/ml
L1210: IC_{50} 1.31 μg/ml
Melting Point: ~200°C
$[\alpha]_D$: +432 Solvent: Chf
Organism: *Streptomyces* sp. (Streptomycetaceae)
Soil sample
Location: Iwo Jima, Japan
Reference: 49, 846, 1185

$C_{42}H_{52}N_2O_{12}$ **DC92-B**

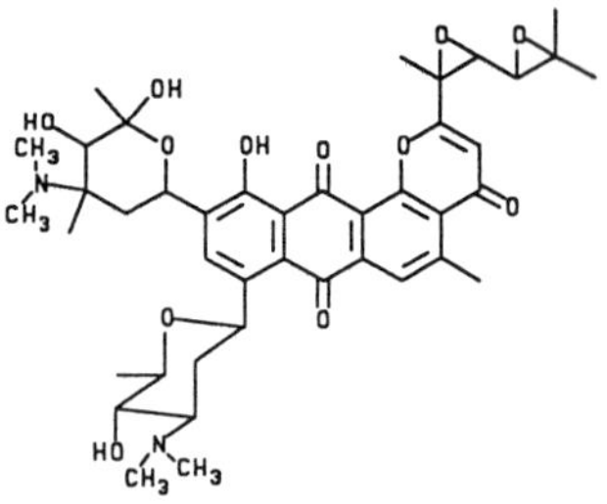

Mol. Wt.: 776
Bioactivity: P-388 (ip-ip): T/C 143 (0.10 mg/kg)
Sarcoma 180 (sc-iv): T/C 34 (0.10 mg/kg/day for 5 days)
Toxicity: LD_{50} 0.145 mg/kg in mice
Antimicrobial activity
Spectral Data: UV, IR, CMR, PMR, Mass Spec.
Organism: *Actinomadura* sp. (Thermomonosporaceae)
Culture of soil isolate
Location: Tokyo, Japan
Reference: 1071

$C_{45}H_{72}O_{12}$ **Oligomycin B**
(previously known)

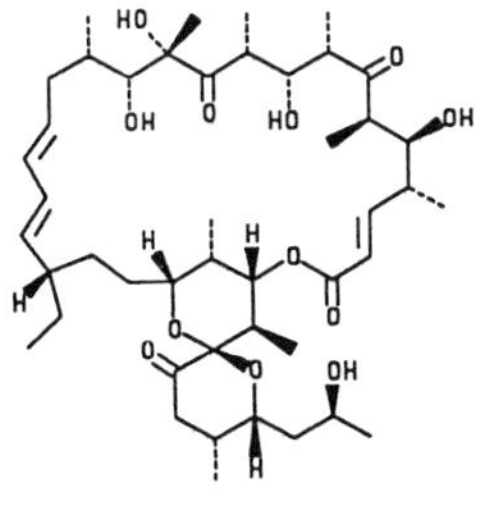

Mol. Wt.: 805
Bioactivity: HeLa: IC_{50} $1.5x10^{-2}$ μg/ml
Antifungal activity
Melting Point: 160-161°C
$[\alpha]_D$: -46.4 Solvent: Di
Spectral Data: UV, IR, CMR, x-ray c.s.
Organism: *Streptomyces diastatochromogenes*
Streptomyces sp. MCI-2225
(Streptomycetaceae)
Culture
Reference: 152, 587, 1144

$C_{45}H_{72}O_{13}$ **Oligomycin E**

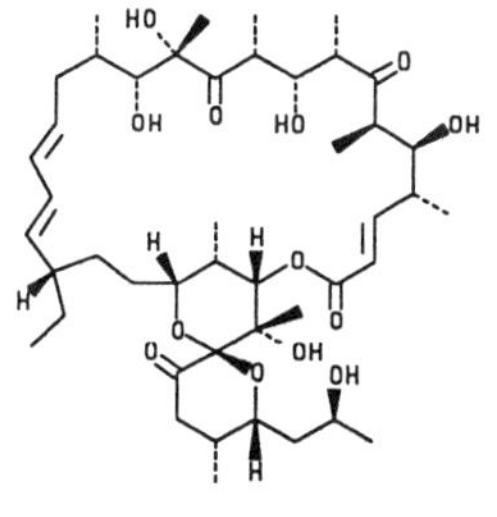

Mol. Wt.: 821
Bioactivity: HeLa: IC_{50} $1.4x10^{-2}$ μg/ml
Antibacterial (gram-positive)
activity
Melting Point: 120.5-121.5°C
$[\alpha]_D$: -49.1 Solvent: Di
Spectral Data: UV, IR, CMR, PMR, Mass Spec.
Organism: *Streptomyces* sp. MC1-2225
(Streptomycetaceae)
Culture of soil isolate
Location: Tasmania
Reference: 587

$C_{45}H_{74}O_{10}$ **Oligomycin C**
(previously known)

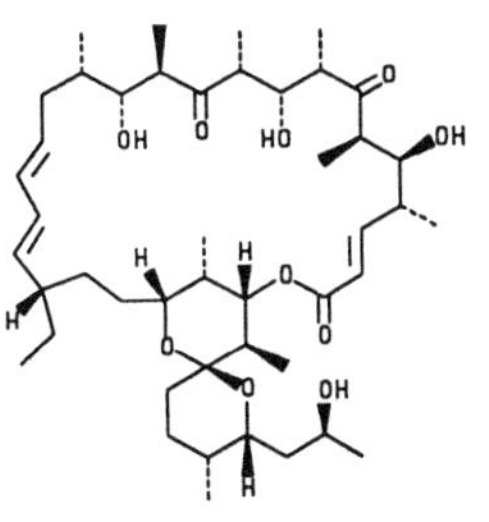

Mol. Wt.: 775
Bioactivity: HeLa: IC_{50} $10.6x10^{-2}$ μg/ml
Antifungal activity
Melting Point: 198-200°C
$[\alpha]_D$: -80.7 Solvent: Di
Spectral Data: UV, IR, CMR, PMR, Mass Spec.
Organism: *Streptomyces diastatochromogenes*
(Streptomycetaceae)
Culture
Reference: 152, 587

$C_{45}H_{74}O_{11}$ **Oligomycin A**
(previously known)

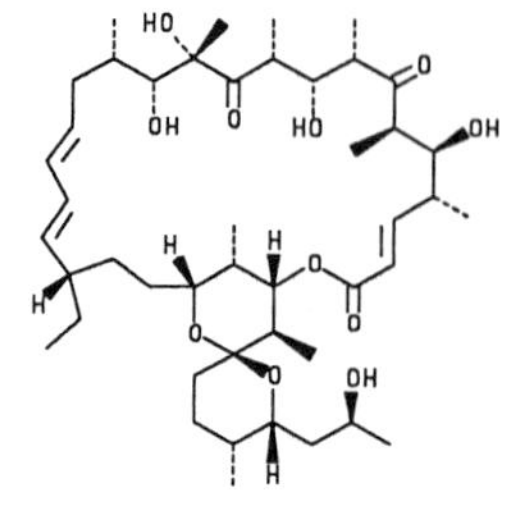

Mol. Wt.: 791
Bioactivity: HeLa: IC_{50} $8x10^{-3}$ $\mu g/ml$
Antifungal activity
Melting Point: 150-151°C
$[\alpha]_D$: -54.5 Solvent: Di
Spectral Data: UV, IR, CMR, PMR, Mass Spec.
Organism: *Streptomyces diastatochromogenes* sp. MC1-225
Streptomyces sp.
(Streptomycetaceae)
Culture
Reference: 152, 587

$C_{47}H_{76}N_8O_{14}$ **A83586C**

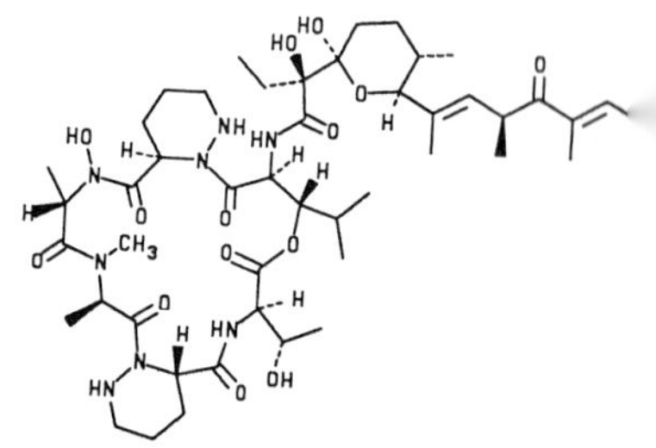

Mol. Wt.: 978
Bioactivity: CCRF-CEM: IC_{50} 0.0135 $\mu g/ml$
Antimicrobial activity
Melting Point: 189-191°C
$[\alpha]_D^{25}$: +116.1 Solvent: Chf
Spectral Data: UV, IR, CMR, PMR, Mass Spec.
x-ray c.s.
Organism: *Streptomyces karnatakensis*
(Streptomycetaceae)
Culture of soil sample
Location: Guam
Reference: 1025

$C_{49}H_{60}N_4O_{14}$ **Chromoxymycin**

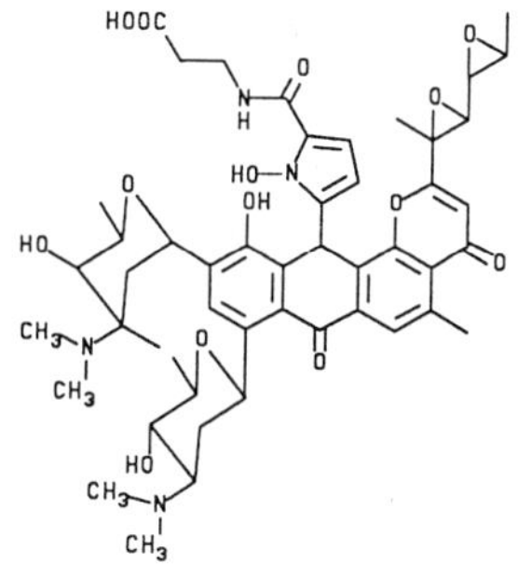

Mol. Wt.: 929
Bioactivity: P-388: T/C 193 (200 mg/kg/day for 4 days)
B16: T/C 184 (50 mg/kg/day for 4 days)
LD_{50} 1,000 mg/kg
Antimicrobial activity against *Staphylococcus aureus* and *Bacillus subtilis*
Melting Point: 85°C (dec.)
$[\alpha]_D^{23}$: +291 Solvent: Aq
Spectral Data: UV, IR, CMR, PMR, Mass Spec.
Organism: *Streptomyces libani* subsp. *rubropurpureus* No. 6362 (Streptomycetaceae)
Culture of soil sample
Location: Osaka, Japan
Reference: 437, 488, 533

$C_{55}H_{74}IN_3O_{21}S_4$ **Calicheamicin γ_1'**

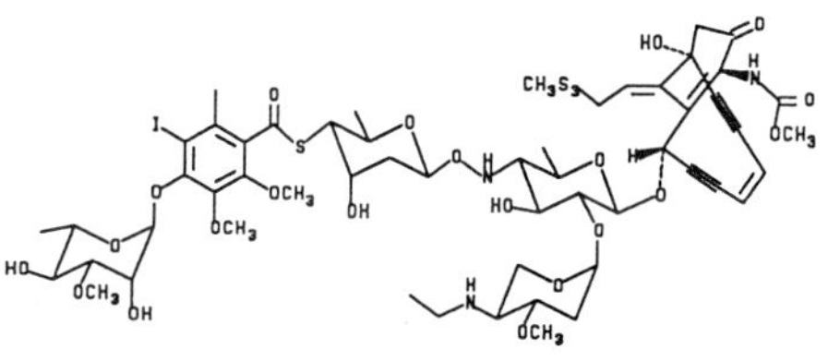

Mol. Wt.: 1369
Bioactivity: Antitumor activity against murine tumors at 0.5-1.5 μg/kg
$[\alpha]_D^{26}$: -124 Solvent: Alc
Spectral Data: CD, CMR, PMR, Mass Spec., x-ray c.s.
Organism: *Micromonospora echinospora* ssp. *calichensis* (Micromonosporaceae)
Reference: 217, 543, 647, 648

$C_{58}H_{78}N_4O_{22}S_4$ **Esperamicin A_{1b}**

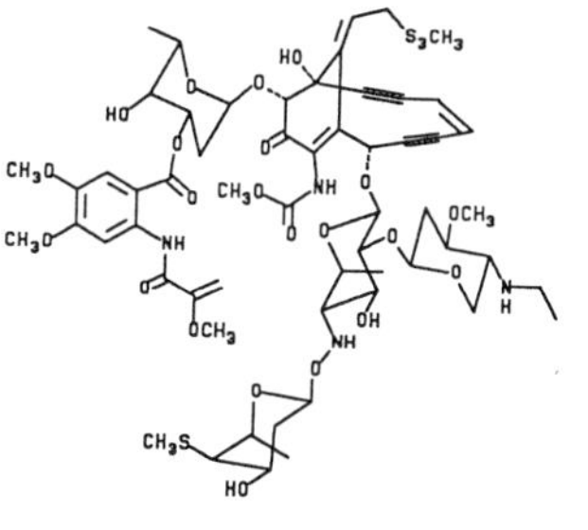

Mol. Wt.: 1312
Bioactivity: DNA - damaging antitumor activity
Antibiotic activity
Spectral Data: CMR, PMR, Mass Spec. (degradation products)
Organism: *Actinomadura verrucosospora* (Thermomonosporaceae)
Location: Argentina
Reference: 217, 353, 690

$C_{59}H_{80}N_4O_{22}S_4$ **Esperamicin A_1**

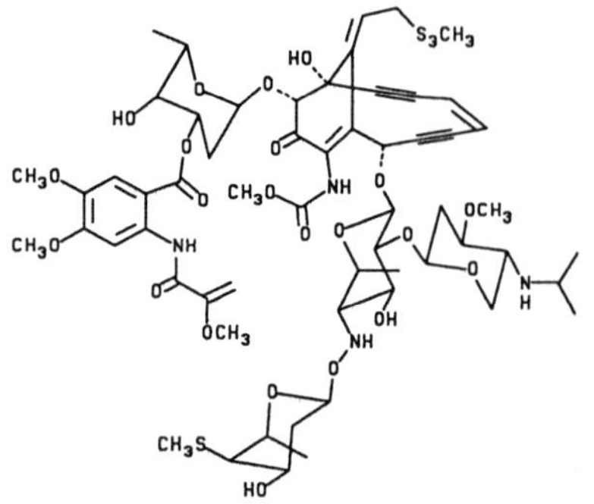

Mol. Wt.: 1326
Bioactivity: DNA - damaging antitumor activity
Antibiotic activity
Melting Point: 156-158°C (dec.)
$[\alpha]_D^{27}$: -191 Solvent: Chf
Spectral Data: CMR, PMR, Mass Spec. (degradation products)
Organism: *Actinomadura verrucosospora* (Thermomonosporaceae)
Location: Argentina
Reference: 217, 353, 690

$C_{59}H_{80}N_4O_{22}S_4$ **Esperamicin A_2**

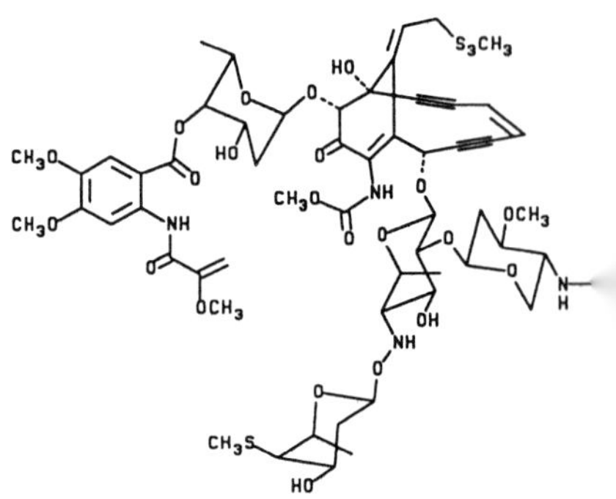

Mol. Wt.: 1326
Bioactivity: DNA - damaging antitumor activity
Antibiotic activity
Melting Point: 147-149°C
$[\alpha]_D$: -179.4 Solvent: Chf
Spectral Data: CMR, PMR, Mass Spec. (degradation products)
Organism: *Actinomadura verrucosospora* (Thermomonosporaceae)
Location: Argentina
Reference: 217, 353

$C_{80}H_{112}N_2O_{37}$ **Arugomycin (AGM)**

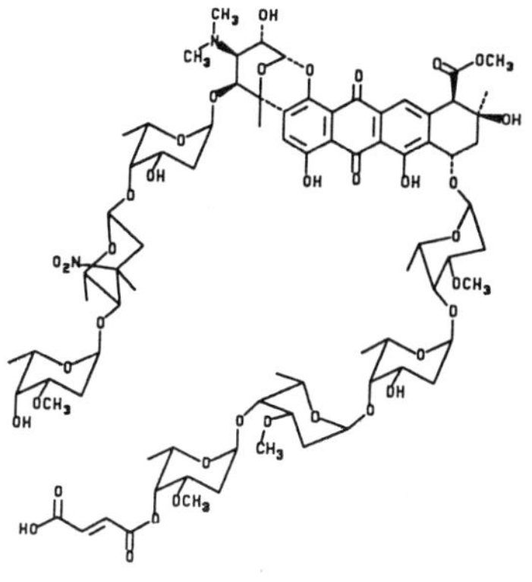

Mol. Wt.: 1694
Bioactivity: Sarcoma 180: T/C >464 (1 mg/kg)
Ehrlich ascites: T/C 189 (0.50 mg/kg)
LD_{50} 1.75 mg/kg (ip)
Antimicrobial activity
Growth inhibition and induction of phagocytic activity of M1 cells
Induction of differentiation of Friend erythroleukemia cells 75.4% at 0.125 μg/ml
Inhibition of RNA synthesis in L-5178Y cells: IC_{50} 0.4 μg/ml
Inhibition of DNA synthesis in L-5178Y cells: IC_{50} 1.8 μg/ml
Melting Point: 208~212°C
$[\alpha]_D^{25}$: +112 Solvent: Chf:Me (9:1)
Spectral Data: UV, IR, CMR, PMR, Mass Spec.
Organism: *Streptomyces violaceochromogenes* Strain No. 1098-AV_2 (Streptomycetaceae) Culture of soil sample
Location: Japan
Reference: 530, 531, 1008

β-D-Glucans

Mol. Wt.: 9,000-200,000
Bioactivity: Inhibition of solid S-180 ascites: 99% at 1 m/kg
Spectral Data: CMR
Organism: *Phytophthora parasitica* (Pythiaceae)
Reference: 116

Glycoprotein (SAGP)

Mol. Wt.: 46,000
Bioactivity: Tumor growth inhibition
Organism: *Streptococcus pyogenes* Su cloned in *E. coli* (Streptococcaceae)
Reference: 508

Schizophyllan
(β-1,3-D-Glucan)

Mol. Wt.: $>5.0x10^4$
Bioactivity: Antitumor activity against Sarcoma 180
Organism: *Schizophyllum commune* (Agaricaceae) Culture
Reference: 596

AS-1
(β-1,3-Glucan)

Mol. Wt.: $\sim 1.2x10^6$
Bioactivity: S-180: Tumor growth inhibition ratio 49.7% (0.5 mg/kg/day for 9 days)
Spectral Data: CMR
Organism: *Cochliobolus miyabeanus* (Pyrenophoraceae) Culture
Reference: 803

TS-CAGIII
(β-1,3-Glucan)

Mol. Wt.: $>2.0x10^6$
Bioactivity: Sarcoma 180 (ip): 98% inhibition at 100 μg/mouse (4/10 regressions); Sarcoma 180 (il): 90% inhibition (20 μg/mouse)
$[\alpha]_D$: +18 Solvent: 0.4N NaOH
Spectral Data: CMR
Organism: *Sclerotinia sclerotiorum* IFO 9395 (Sclerotiniaceae) Culture
Reference: 1011

Polysaccharide H_{11}
(1,3)-(1,6)-β-D-Glucan
(PCME-H_{11})

Mol. Wt.:	~$5.0x10^6$
Bioactivity:	Sarcoma 180 (sc): 96% inhibition (8 mg/kg/day) Sarcoma 180 (ip): T/C 136 (100 mg/kg/day- impure fraction) Ehrlich carcinoma (sc): 78% inhibition (30 mg/kg/day- impure fraction) IMC carcinoma (ip): T/C 191 (50 mg/kg/day- impure fraction)
Melting Point:	>300°C
$[\alpha]_D^{26}$:	-28.2 Solvent: Aq
Spectral Data:	UV, IR, CMR
Organism:	*Poria cocos* (Schw.)Wolf (Polyporaceae)
Reference:	509, 510, 511

SSG
(β-1,3-Glucan)

Mol. Wt.:	>$5.0x10^6$
Bioactivity:	Sarcoma 180 (sc): 93% inhibition (100 μg/day for 5 days)
$[\alpha]_D$:	-2.0 Solvent: 8M urea-0.2N NaOH
Spectral Data:	CMR
Organism:	*Sclerotinia sclerotiorum* IFO 9395 (Sclerotiniaceae)
Reference:	841, 842

Melanocidin A
(polysaccharide)

Mol. Wt.:	>1,000,000
Bioactivity:	Inhibition of 5'-nucleotidase activity from snake venom Antitumor activity against B16 melanoma
Melting Point:	>300°C
$[\alpha]_D^{20}$:	+40 Solvent: Aq
Spectral Data:	UV, IR, CMR
Organism:	*Nocardioides* sp. Strain 1681J (Nocardiaceae) Culture
Reference:	837, 1118

Nucleoticidin
(polysaccharide)

Mol. Wt.:	>1,000,000
Bioactivity:	Inhibition of 5'-nucleotidase activity from snake venom and rat liver membrane Antitumor activity against Sarcoma 180
Melting Point:	>300°C
$[\alpha]_D^{20}$:	-140 Solvent: 0.1N NaOH
Spectral Data:	UV, IR
Organism:	*Pseudomonas* sp. Strain YM-3229G (Pseudomonadaceae) Culture
Reference:	836, 1117

CA-II
[(1→3)-β-D-Glucan]

Bioactivity:	Sarcoma 180 (ip): 59.6% inhibition (10 mg/kg/day for 10 days)
Spectral Data:	IR
Organism:	*Ganoderma lucidum* (Polyporaceae) Culture
Reference:	1027

HW-II
[(1→3)-β-D-Glucan]

Bioactivity:	Sarcoma 180 (ip): 97.9% inhibition (10 mg/kg/day for 10 days)
Spectral Data:	IR
Organism:	*Ganoderma lucidum* (Polyporaceae) Culture
Reference:	1027

MY-1 (DNA/RNA fraction)
Nucleic acid

Bioactivity:	Inhibition of tumor growth: IMC: 100% inhibition at 300 μg x6 (10/10 regression) Meth A: 100% inhibition at 300 μg x6 (9/10 regression) B16: 99% inhibition at 300 μg x6 (8/11 regression) S1509a: 100% inhibition at 100 μg x6 (8/8 regression) MM46: 100% inhibition at 300 μg x6 (11/11 regression)
Organism:	*Mycobacterium bovis* BCG (Mycobacteriaceae)
Reference:	1003

PVG
(β-1,3-Glucan)

Bioactivity:	Sarcoma 180: 98% inhibition (75 μg/day for 10 days)
$[\alpha]_D$:	+28 Solvent: Aq
Spectral Data:	CMR
Organism:	*Peziza vesiculosa* (Pezizaceae)
Reference:	735

A. Total Syntheses

Compound	Activity	Reference
Acivicin	Antitumor activity	787
1-Amino-20-guanidino-10-hydroxy-4,8,11-triazaeicosane-9,12-dione	L1210: T/C >429 (3.13 mg/kg/day)	1123
1-Amino-21-guanidino-11-hydroxy-4,9,12-triazauneicosane-10,13-dione	L1210: T/C >416 (0.78 mg/kg/day)	1124
3-Benzylidene-6-(m-chlorobenzylidene)-2-methoxy-3,6-dihydropyrazin-5-one	KB: ED_{50} 0.29 μg/ml	1210
(S_c,R_s)-Chlorosparsomycin	L1210: ID_{50} 0.29 μM	1137
(+)-9-O-α-L-Daunosaminyl-4-demethoxydaunorubicin	P388: IC_{50} $3x10^{-6}$ mM T/C 163 (5 mg/kg)	558
(-)-15-Deoxy-11-O-methylspergualin	L1210: T/C 400 (12.5 mg/kg) Toxic at 50 mg/kg/day	1122
15-Deoxyspergualin	L1210 (ip): T/C 382 (3.1 mg/kg/day) L1210 (po): T/C >705 (100 mg/kg/day)	474, 1122, 1124
3,6-Di-(2,4,5-trimethoxybenzylidene)-piperazine-2,5-dione	KB: ED_{50} 0.27 μg/ml	1210
3,6-Di-(m-chlorobenzylidene)-2-methoxy-3,6-dihydropyrazin-5-one	KB: ED_{50} 0.40 μg/ml	1210

Compound	Activity	Reference
3,6-Dibenzylidene-2-ethoxy-3,6-dihydro-pyrazin-5-one	KB: ED_{50} 0.08 μg/ml	1210
Guanine 7-oxide	P388, L1210 activity	823
Islandic acid I aldehyde, methyl ester	L1210: 100% inhibition (10 μg/ml)	1004
Islandic acid I methyl ester	L1210: 100% inhibition (10 μg/ml)	1004
($\underline{S}_c$,$\underline{S}_s$)-2-[β-(6-Methyl-5-uracilyl)acrylamido]-3-[n-decylsulfinyl]propanol	L1210: ID_{50} 0.14 μM	1137
Phenylsparsomycin	L1210: ID_{50} 0.11 μM	1137
Rosellisin aldehyde	L1210: 96% inhibition (10 μg/ml)	1004
U-71,184	P388 and L1210 curative Active against B-16, M5076 and mammary carcinoma 16/C at 50-200 μg/kg (iv)	1161, 1162

B. Semi-Syntheses or Synthetic Modifications

Compound	Activity	Reference
AG2	P388: T/C 159 (30 mg/kg) L-5178Y: inhibition of RNA synthesis: IC_{50} 0.7 μg/ml	530, 531, 1008

Compound	Activity	Reference
AG3	P388: T/C 158 (16 mg/kg) L-5178Y: inhibition of RNA synthesis: IC_{50} 2.0 μg/ml	530, 531, 1008
AG4	L5178Y: inhibition of RNA synthesis: IC_{50} 2.5 μg/ml	530, 531, 1008
AG6	P388: T/C 158 (8.0 μg/ml)	530, 531, 1008
AG7	Differentiation of Friend erythroleukemia: 59.7% at 0.10 μg/ml L-5178Y: inhibition of RNA synthesis: IC_{50} 1.1 μg/ml Ehrlich ascites: T/C 270 (2.0 mg/kg)	1008
1-Allylelymoclavine	L5178Y: ED_{50} 4.0 μM	259
19-Bromoherbimycin A	Ehrlich ascites: T/C 190 (50 mg/kg for 5 days)	1000
6-Butyl-6-noragroclavine	L5178Y: ED_{50} 2.9 μM	260
1-Butylagroclavine	L5178Y: ED_{50} 1.0 μM	260, 261
6-Chloro-6-demethoxy-herbimycin A	Ehrlich ascites: T/C 200 (25 mg/kg for 5 days)	1000

Compound	Degree of substitution	Sarcoma 180 inhibition	Reference
CM-Curdlan	0.21	99.9% (100 μg/day for 5 days)	840, 975
	0.08	99.1% (500 μg/day for 5 days)	
	0.28	98.5% (100 μg/day for 5 days)	
	0.38	99.9% (20 μg/day for 5 days)	
CM-SSG	0.04	99.2% (100 μg/day for 5 days)	840
	0.09	99.1% (500 μg/day for 5 days)	
	0.14	93.2% (500 μg/day for 5 days)	

Compound	Activity	Reference
7-Decarbamoyl-7,8-O-carbonyl-8,9-dihydro-8-hydroxyherbimycin A	Ehrlich ascites: T/C 150 (50 mg/kg for 5 days)	1000
7-Decarbamoyl-19-chloroherbimycin A	Ehrlich ascites: T/C 129 (50 mg/kg for 5 days)	1000
7-Decarbamoyl-8,9-epoxyherbimycin A	Ehrlich ascites: T/C 146 (25 mg/kg for 5 days)	1000
7-Decarbamoyl-herbimycin A	Ehrlich ascites: T/C 200 (50 mg/kg for 5 days)	1000
9,19-Dibromo-7-decarbamoyl-7,8-O-carbonyl-8,9-dihydro-8-hydroxyherbimycin A	Ehrlich ascites: T/C 134 (25 mg/kg for 5 days)	1000
4,5-Dichloro-4,5-dihydro-7-decarbamoyloxy-6-demethoxy-6-enoherbimycin A	Ehrlich ascites: T/C 215 (50 mg/kg for 5 days)	1000
1-(3',3'-Dimethylbutyl)-agroclavine	L5178Y: ED_{50} 3.0 μM	260
1,O-Dimethyllysergol	L5178Y: ED_{50} 3.6 μM	259
1,O-Dipropylelymoclavine	L5178Y: ED_{50} 5.7 μM	259
8,9-Epoxy-19-bromo-herbimycin A	Ehrlich ascites: T/C 144 (50 mg/kg for 5 days)	1000
6-Ethyl-6-noragroclavine	L5178Y: ED_{50} 7.1 μM	260
1-Ethylagroclavine	L5178Y: ED_{50} 2.4 μM	260, 261

Compound	Activity	Reference
FK973	P-388: IC_{50} 0.012 μM L1210: IC_{50} 0.044 μM B16: IC_{50} 0.28 μM LLC: IC_{50} 2.5 μM Colon 38: IC_{50} 1.2 μM CCRF-CEM: IC_{50} 0.023 μM PC10: IC_{50} 0.7 μM MKN45: IC_{50} 0.4 μM Antitumor activity (ip-ip): P-388: T/C ≥243 at 3.2 mg/kg L1210: T/C 163 at 5.6 mg/kg B16: T/C >375 at 1.0 mg/kg M5076: T/C >286 at 10 mg/kg Colon 56: T/C ≥249 at 10 mg/kg Ehrlich: T/C >333 at 0.32 mg/kg MH134: T/C 229 at 5.6 mg/kg P-388/MMC: T/C 145 at 3.2 mg/kg P-388/CPM: T/C 176 at 10 mg/kg P-388/VCR: T/C 200 at 10 mg/kg P-388/ADR: T/C 145 at 10 mg/kg (sc-iv): M5076: 1-T/C 85 at 10 mg/kg Colon 38: 1-T/C 100 at 10 mg/kg B16: 1-T/C 100 at 10 mg/kg LLC: 1-T/C 66 at 10 mg/kg LX-1: 1-T/C 90 at 5.6 mg/kg MX-1: 1-T/C 99 at 3.2 mg/kg SC-6: 1-T/C 84 at 5.6 mg/kg Weak hematoxicity	707, 1007
6-Heptyl-6-noragroclavine	L5178Y: ED_{50} 3.9 μM	260
1-Heptylagroclavine	L5178Y: ED_{50} 4.4 μM	260
6-Hexyl-6-noragroclavine	L5178Y: ED_{50} 3.4 μM	260
1-Hexylagroclavine	L5178Y: ED_{50} 1.6 μM	260
6-Methyl-8β-(2′-hydroxycyclohexylidene-methyl)ergoline-1	L5178Y: ED_{50} 5.2 μM	259

Compound	Activity	Reference
6-Methyl-8β-(2'-oxocyclohexylidene-methyl)ergoline-1	L5178Y: ED_{50} 4.0 μM	259
1-Methylagroclavine	L5178Y: ED_{50} 5.2 μM	260
1-(2'-Methylpropyl)-agroclavine	L5178Y: ED_{50} 3.2 μM	260, 261
MX	P388 (iv): ILS 111 (6.67 mg/kg)	598
MX2	P388 (iv): ILS 140 (3.33 mg/kg) L1210 (iv): ILS 89 (3 mg/kg)	598
MY5	P388: ILS 142 (60 mg/kg)	598
1-Pentyl-6-cyano-6-noragroclavine	L5178Y: ED_{50} 4.5 μM	260
1-Pentyl-6-noragroclavine	L5178Y: ED_{50} 1.4 μM	260
6-Pentyl-6-noragroclavine	L5178Y: ED_{50} 5.1 μM	260
1-Pentyl-6-propyl-6-noragroclavine	L5178Y: ED_{50} 1.3 μM	260
1-Pentylagroclavine	L5178Y: ED_{50} 0.87 μM	260
6-Propyl-6-noragroclavine	L5178Y: ED_{50} 5.3 μM	260
1-Propylagroclavine	L5178Y: ED_{50} 1.3 μM	260, 261
1-Propylelymoclavine	L5178Y: ED_{50} 2.2 μM Inhibition of DNA synthesis	259

Compound	Activity	Reference
1-Propylelymoclavine-O-butyrate	L5178Y: ED_{50} 2.7 μM	259
2,3,4,5-Tetrahydro-herbimycin A	Ehrlich ascites: T/C 193 (25 mg/kg for 5 days)	1000

Chapter 10 MARINE ALGAE BIOSYNTHETIC PRODUCTS

$C_{11}H_{14}N_4O_4$ **Tubercidin**
(previously known)

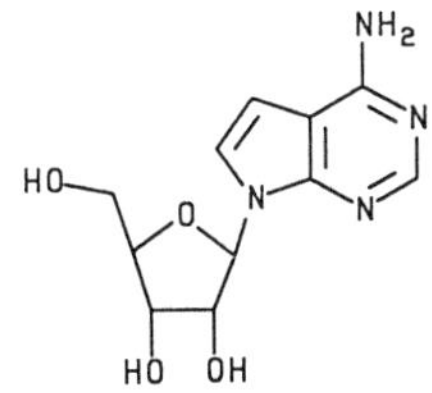

Mol. Wt.: 266
Bioactivity: KB: MIC 70 ng/ml
Induction of HL-60 cell adhesion
NIH/3T3: cytotoxic activity at 70 ppb
Antimicrobial activities
Spectral Data: UV, CD, CMR, PMR
Organism: *Tolypothrix distorta*
T. byssoidea (Berk) Kirchner
Plectonema radiosum
Saytonema saleyeriense var. *indica*
(Cyanophyta)
Cultures of isolates
Location: Oahu, Hawaii; Fiji and South Africa
Reference: 31, 50, 1034, 1062

$C_{12}H_{13}N_5O_4$ **Toyocamycin**
(previously known)

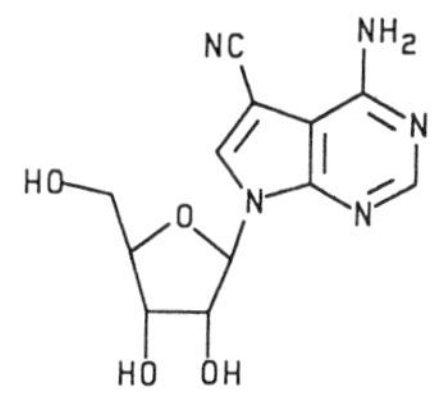

Mol. Wt.: 291
Bioactivity: KB: MIC 60 ng/ml
Antifugal activity
Spectral Data: CMR, PMR
Organism: *Tolypothrix tenuis*
(Cyanophyta)
Culture of isolate
Location: Oahu, Hawaii
Reference: 816, 1034

$C_{17}H_{24}N_4O_9$ **Tubercidin 5'-α-D-glucopyranose**

Mol. Wt.: 428
Bioactivity: KB: MIC 560 ng/ml
Induction of HL-60 cell adhesion
Antimycotic activity
$[\alpha]_D^{25}$: +10 Solvent: Aq
Spectral Data: UV, IR, CMR, PMR, Mass spec.
Organism: *Tolypothrix distorta*
Plectonema radiosum
Cultures of isolates
(Cyanophyta)
Location: Oahu, Hawaii and Fiji
Reference: 1034

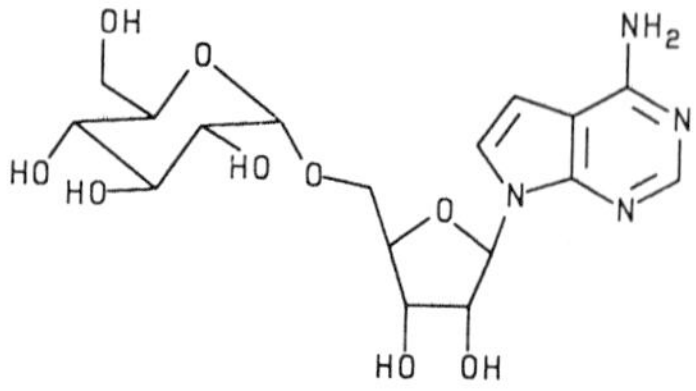

$C_{18}H_{23}N_5O_9$ **Toyocamycin 5'-α-D-glucopyranose**

Mol. Wt.: 453
Bioactivity: KB: MIC 300 ng/ml
Induction of HL-60 cell adhesion
Fungicidal activity
$[\alpha]_D^{25}$: +2.1 Solvent: Aq
Spectral Data: UV, IR, CMR, PMR, Mass Spec.
Organism: *Tolypothrix tenuis*
(Cyanophyta)
Culture of isolate
Reference: 1034

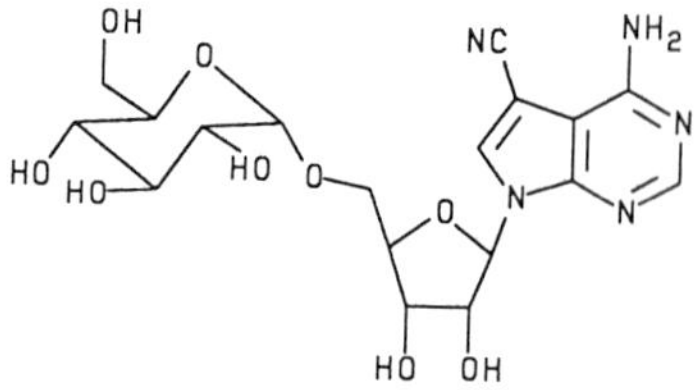

$C_{19}H_{28}O_3$ **Nordictyotalide**

Mol. Wt.: 304
Bioactivity: B16: IC_{50} 1.58 μg/ml
$[\alpha]_D$: −31 Solvent: Chf
Spectral Data: IR, CMR, PMR, Mass Spec.
Organism: *Dictyota dichotoma*
(Phaeophyta)
Location: Okinawa, Japan
Reference: 471

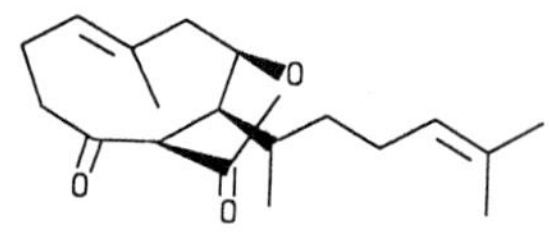

$C_{20}H_{30}O_3$ **Dictyotalide A**

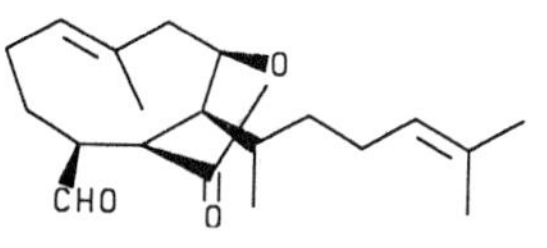

Mol. Wt.: 318
Bioactivity: B16: IC_{50} 2.57 μg/ml
Melting Point: −102 Solvent: Chf
Spectral Data: IR, CMR, PMR, Mass Spec.
Organism: *Dictyota dichotoma* (Phaeophyta)
Location: Okinawa, Japan
Reference: 471

$C_{21}H_{20}O_8$ **Hormothamnione**

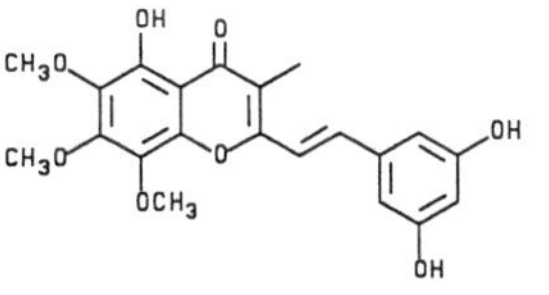

Mol. Wt.: 400
Bioactivity: P388: ID_{50} 4.6 ng/ml
HL−60: ID_{50} 0.1 ng/ml
Melting Point: 270°C
Spectral Data: UV, IR, PMR, Mass spec., x−ray c.s. (triacetate)
Organism: *Hormothamnion enteromorphoides* Grunow (Cyanophyta)
Location: Puerto Rico
Reference: 348

$C_{22}H_{32}O_4$ **4-Acetoxydictyolactone**

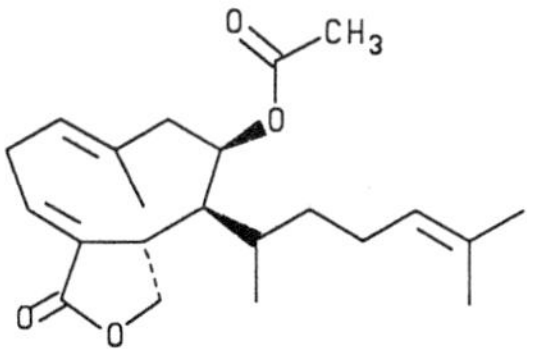

Mol. Wt.: 360
Bioactivity: B16: IC_{50} 1.6 μg/ml
$[\alpha]_D$: −224 Solvent: Chf
Spectral Data: UV, IR, CMR, PMR, Mass. Spec.
Organism: *Dictyota dichotoma* (Phaeophyta)
Location: Okinawa, Japan
Reference: 471

$C_{22}H_{32}O_4$ **Dictyotalide B**

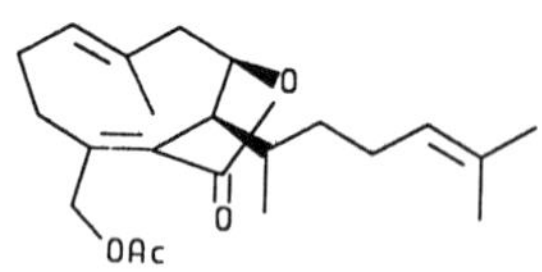

Mol. Wt.: 360
Bioactivity: B16: IC_{50} 0.58 μg/ml
$[\alpha]_D$: +50.3 Solvent: Chf
Spectral Data: UV, IR, CMR, PMR, Mass Spec.
Organism: *Dictyota dichotoma* (Phaeophyta)
Location: Okinawa, Japan
Reference: 471

$C_{26}H_{37}BrO_7$ **Isoparguerol 7,16-diacetate**

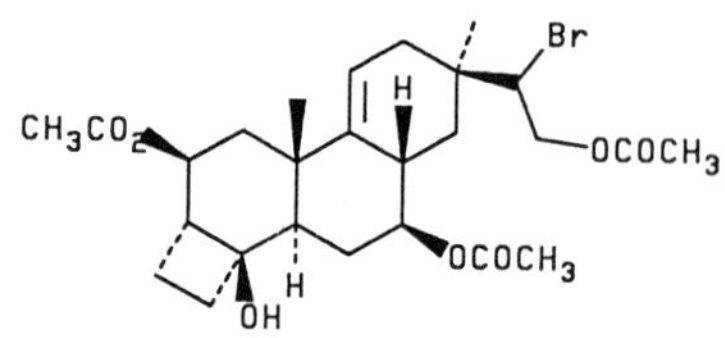

Mol. Wt.: 541
Bioactivity: P388: IC_{50} 9.9 μg/ml
Hela: IC_{50} 6.3 μg/ml
Melting Point: 176–178°C
$[\alpha]_D$: +8.9
Spectral Data: IR, PMR
Organism: *Laurencia obtusa* (Rhodophyta)
Location: Japan
Reference: 1064

$C_{26}H_{37}BrO_7$ **Parguerol 16,19-diacetate**

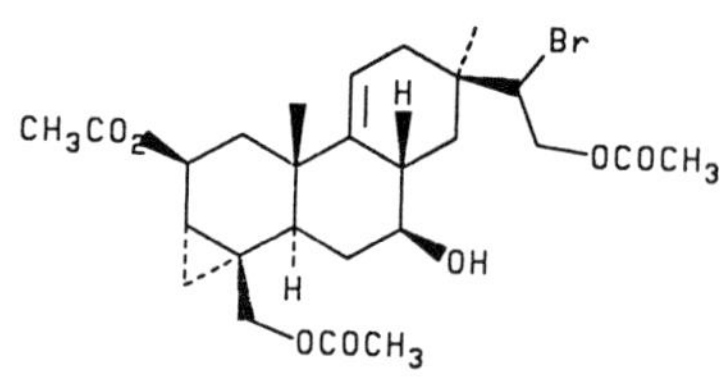

Mol. Wt.: 541
Bioactivity: P388: IC_{50} 3.5 μg/ml
Hela: IC_{50} 3.1 μg/ml
$[\alpha]_D$: -37.8
Spectral Data: IR, PMR
Organism: *Laurencia obtusa* (Rhodophyta)
Location: Japan
Reference: 1064

$C_{28}H_{39}BrO_8$ **Parguerol triacetate**

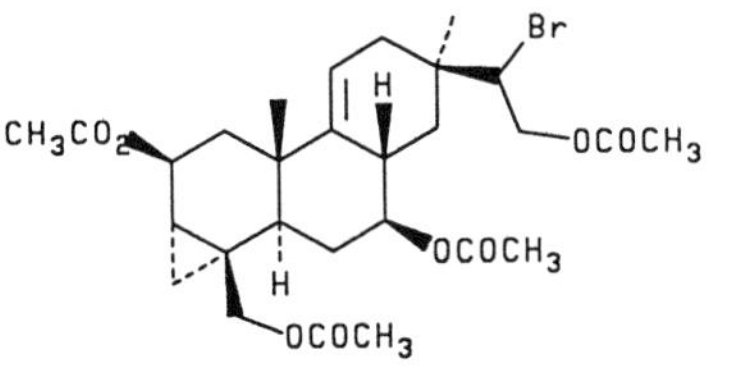

Mol. Wt.: 583
Bioactivity: P388: IC_{50} 8.5 μg/ml
Hela: IC_{50} 6.3 μg/ml
$[\alpha]_D$: −24
Spectral Data: IR, PMR
Organism: *Laurencia obtusa* (Rhodophyta)
Location: Japan
Reference: 1064

$C_{30}H_{51}BrO_5$

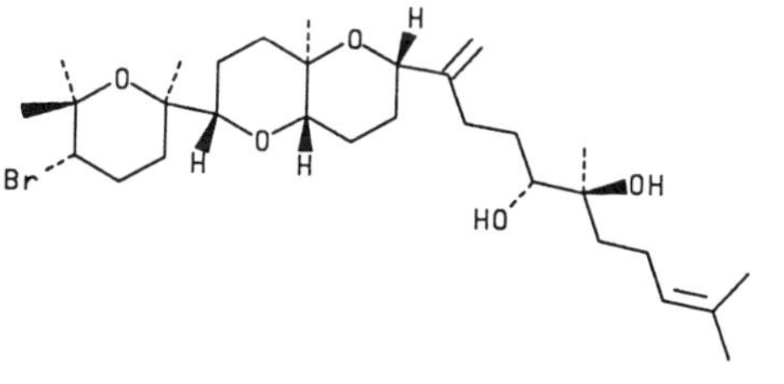

Mol. Wt.: 571
Bioactivity: P388: ED_{50} 30 ng/ml
Melting Point: 64.5–66°C
$[\alpha]_D$: +7.8
Spectral Data: IR, CMR, PMR
Organism: *Laurencia obtusa* (Hud) Lamouroux (Rhodophyta)
Location: Japan
Reference: 1065

$C_{30}H_{51}BrO_5$

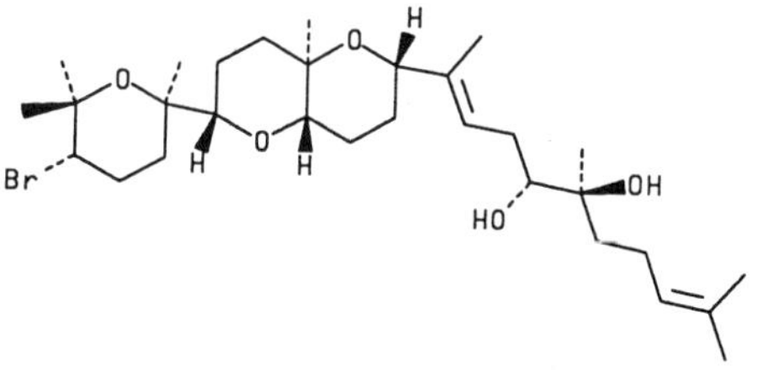

Mol. Wt.: 571
Bioactivity: P388: ED_{50} 30 ng/ml
Melting Point: 69–70°C
$[\alpha]_D$: +6.4
Spectral Data: IR, CMR, PMR
Organism: *Laurencia obtusa* (Hud) Lamouroux (Rhodophyta)
Location: Japan
Reference: 1065

$C_{30}H_{53}BrO_6$

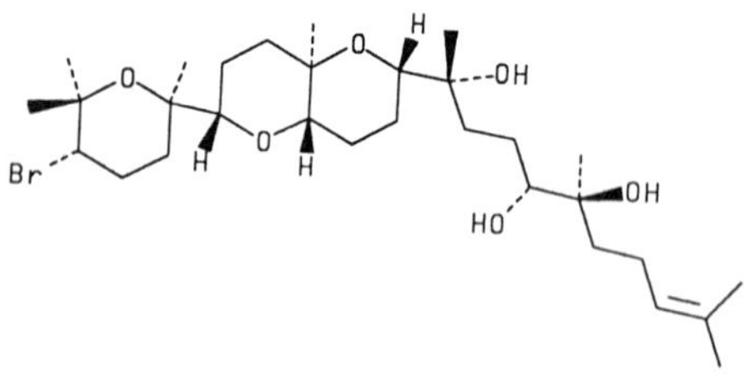

Mol. Wt.: 589
Bioactivity: P388: ED_{50} 30 ng/ml
Melting Point: 98.5–100°C
$[\alpha]_D$: 0
Spectral Data: IR, CMR, PMR, Mass Spec.
Organism: *Laurencia obtusa* (Hud) Lamouroux (Rhodophyta)
Location: Japan
Reference: 1065

$C_{31}H_{46}O_7$ **Amphidinolide A**

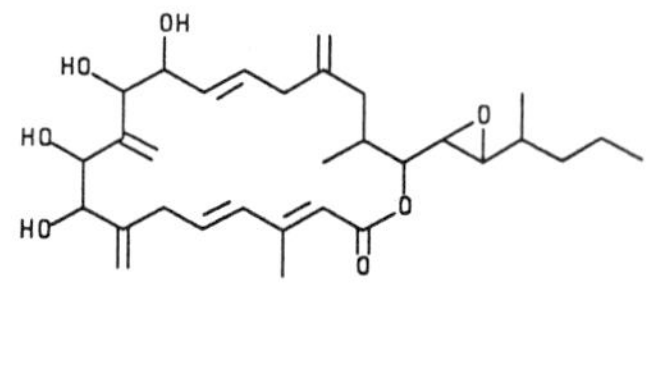

Mol. Wt.: 530
Bioactivity: L1210: IC_{50} 2.4 μg/ml
L5178Y: IC_{50} 3.9 μg/ml
Melting Point: 130–133°C
$[\alpha]_D^{24}$: +46 Solvent: Chf
Spectral Data: UV, IR, CMR, PMR, Mass Spec.
Organism: *Amphidinium sp.* (Pyrrophyta) Culture of flatworm isolate
Location: Okinawa, Japan
Reference: 579, 580

$C_{32}H_{50}O_8$ **Amphidinolide B**

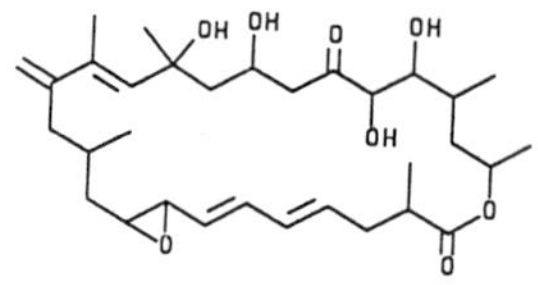

Mol. Wt.: 562
Bioactivity: L1210: IC_{50} 0.14 ng/ml
$[\alpha]_D^{25}$: −45 Solvent: Chf
Spectral Data: UV, IR, CMR, PMR, Mass Spec.
Organism: *Amphidinium sp.* (Pyrrophyta) Culture of flatworm isolate
Location: Okinawa, Japan
Reference: 466, 579

$C_{34}H_{55}BrO_8$

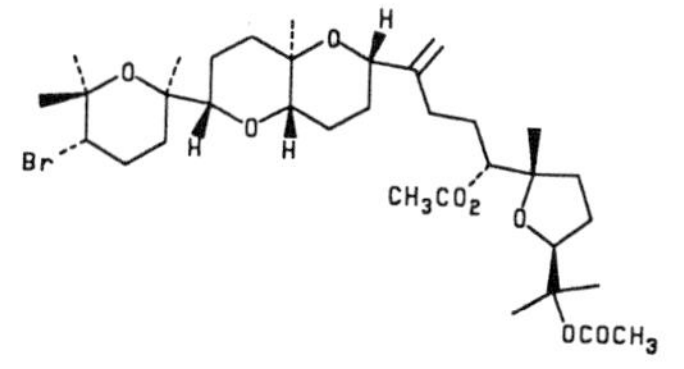

Mol. Wt.: 671
Bioactivity: P388: ED_{50} 50 ng/ml
Melting Point: 94–95°C
$[\alpha]_D$: +8.8
Spectral Data: IR, CMR, PMR
Organism: *Laurencia obtusa* (Hud) Lamouroux (Rhodophyta)
Location: Japan
Reference: 1065

$C_{34}H_{55}BrO_8$

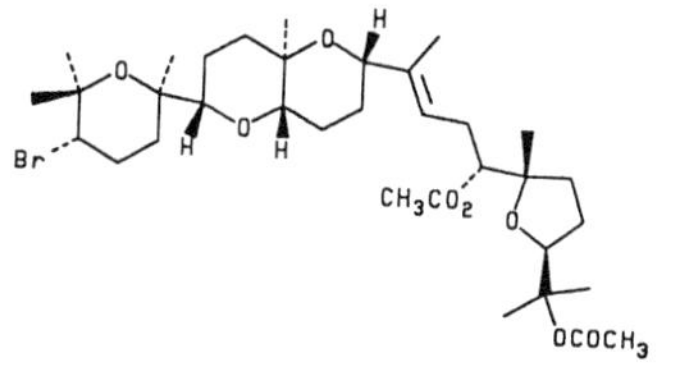

Mol. Wt.: 671
Bioactivity: P388: ED_{50} 100 ng/ml
Melting Point: 163–164°C
$[\alpha]_D$: +12.9
Spectral Data: IR, CMR, PMR
Organism: *Laurencia obtusa* (Hud) Lamouroux (Rhodophyta)
Location: Japan
Reference: 1065

$C_{41}H_{62}O_{10}$ **Amphidinolide C**

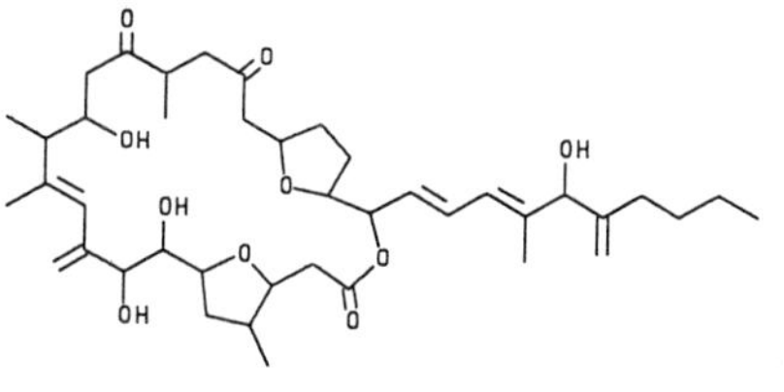

Mol. Wt.: 714
Bioactivity: L1210: IC_{50} 5.8 ng/ml
$[\alpha]_D^{26}$: −106 Solvent: Chf
Spectral Data: UV, IR, CMR, PMR, Mass. Spec.
Organism: *Amphidinium sp.* (Pyrrophyta) Culture of flat worm isolate
Location: Okinawa, Japan
Reference: 579, 581

$C_{45}H_{73}NO_{12}$ **Scytophycin B**

Mol. Wt.: 820
Bioactivity: Toxic to KB and NIH/3T3 mouse fibroblast cells
P388: T/C 136 (3.25 μg/ml mouse for 6 days)
Lewis lung carcinoma: T/C 129 (4 μg/ml/mouse for 9 days)
$[\alpha]_D$: −24 Solvent: Me
Spectral Data: UV, CD, IR, CMR, PMR, Mass Spec.
Organism: *Scytonema pseudohofmanni* Bharadwaja (Cyanophyta)
Culture of soil isolate
Location: Hawaii
Ref: 464, 764, 765

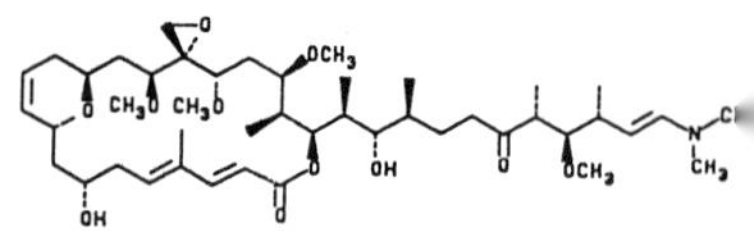

$C_{45}H_{75}NO_{11}$ **Scytophycin C**

Mol. Wt.: 806
Bioactivity: Cytotoxic and antifungal activity
$[\alpha]_D$: −23 Solvent: Me
Spectral Data: UV, CD, IR, CMR, PMR, Mass. Spec., x-ray c.s. (of derivative)
Organism: *Scytonema pseudohofmanni* Bharadwaja (Cyanophyta)
Culture of soil isolate
Location: Hawaii
Reference: 464, 764

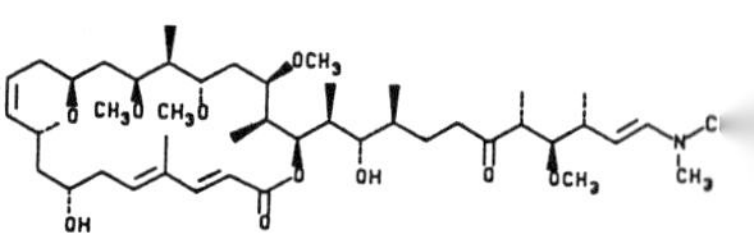

$C_{45}H_{75}NO_{12}$ **Scytophycin A**

Mol. Wt.: 822
Bioactivity: Toxic to KB and NIH/3T3 mouse fibroblast cells
P388: T/C 125 (1 μg/mouse for 8 days)
$[\alpha]_D$: −35 Solvent: Me
Spectral Data: UV, CD, IR, CMR, PMR, Mass Spec.
Organism: *Scytonema pseudohofmanni* Bharadwaja (Cyanophyta)
Culture of soil isolate
Location: Hawaii
Reference: 464, 764, 765

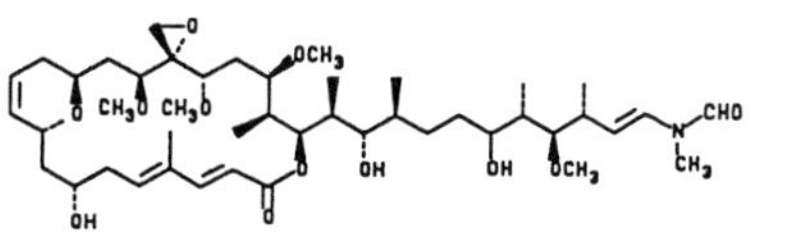

$C_{45}H_{75}NO_{12}$ **Scytophycin D**

Mol. Wt.: 822
Bioactivity: Cytotoxic and antifungal activity
$[\alpha]_D$: −32 Solvent: Me
Spectral Data: UV, IR, CD, CMR, PMR, Mass Spec.
Organism: *Scytonema pseudohofmanni* Bharadwaja (Cyanophyta)
Culture of soil isolate
Location: Hawaii
Reference: 464, 764

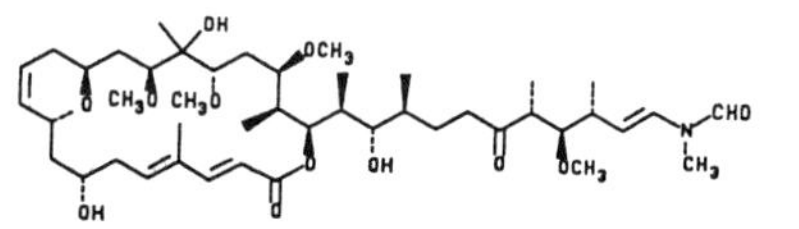

$C_{45}H_{75}NO_{12}$ **Scytophycin E**

Mol. Wt.: 822
Bioactivity: Cytotoxic and antifungal activity
$[\alpha]_D$: −38 Solvent: Me
Spectral Data: UV, CD, IR, CMR, PMR, Mass Spec.
Organism: *Scytonema pseudohofmanni* Bharadwaja (Cyanophyta)
Culture of soil isolate
Location: Hawaii
Reference: 464, 764

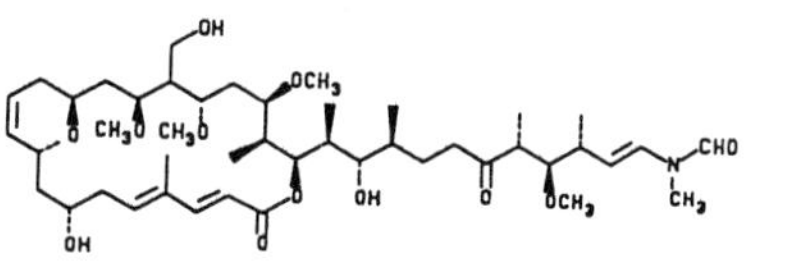

$C_{56}H_{85}NO_{13}$	**Prorocentrolide**
Mol. Wt.:	981
Bioactivity:	L1210: IC_{50} 20 μg/ml Lethal to mice at 0.4 mg/kg Antimicrobial activity
$[\alpha]_D^{23}$:	+136.5 Solvent: Me
Spectral Data:	UV, IR, CMR, PMR, Mass Spec.
Organism:	*Prorocentrum lima* (Pyrrophyta)
Location:	Okinawa, Japan
Reference:	1100

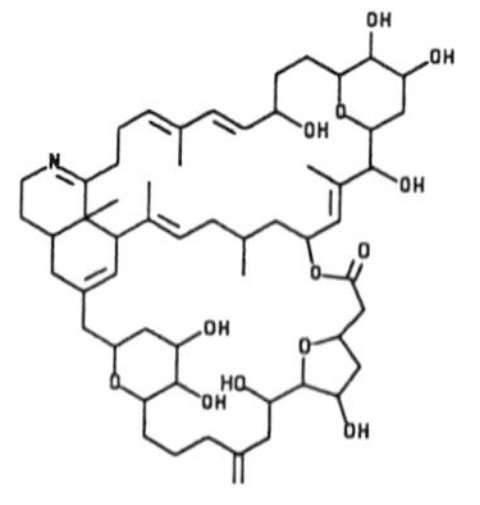

A. Total Syntheses

Compound	Activity	Reference
Unit of stypoldione	P388: 96% inhibition at $1x10^{-4}$M	298

B. Semi-Syntheses or Synthetic Modifications

Compound	Activity	Reference
Glycoprotein hydrolysate	L1210: IC_{50} 5 μg/ml Sarcoma 180 activity	711

Chapter 11 MARINE INVERTEBRATE AND OTHER LOWER ANIMAL BIOSYNTHETIC PRODUCTS

$C_{10}H_{15}BrCl_2O$ **Aplysiapyranoid C**

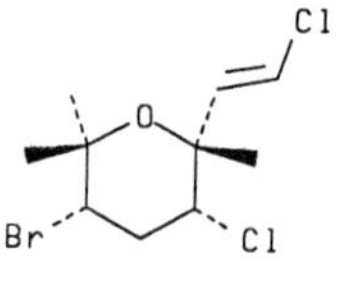

Mol. Wt.	302
Bioactivity:	Moderate cytotoxicity against Vero, MDCK and B16 cells: IC_{50} 19–96 μg/ml
Melting Point:	Oil
$[\alpha]_D$:	+52 Solvent: Chf
Spectral Data:	IR, CMR, PMR, Mass Spec.
Organism:	*Aplysia kurodai* Baba (Mollusca)
Location:	Nabeta Bay, Japan
Reference:	629

$C_{10}H_{15}BrCl_2O$ **Aplysiapyranoid D**

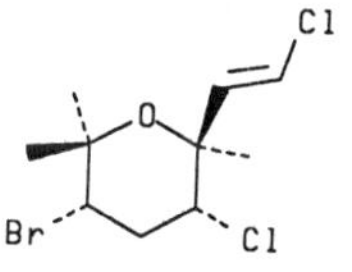

Mol. Wt.:	302
Bioactivity:	Moderate cytotoxicity against Vero, MDCK, B16 cells: IC_{50} 19–96 μg/ml Moser cells: IC_{50} 14 μg/ml
Melting Point:	Oil
$[\alpha]_D$:	+3.4 Solvent: Chf
Spectral Data:	IR, CMR, PMR, Mass Spec.
Organism:	*Aplysia kurodai* Baba (Mollusca)
Location:	Nabeta Bay, Japan
Reference:	629

$C_{10}H_{15}Br_2ClO$ **Aplysiapyranoid A**

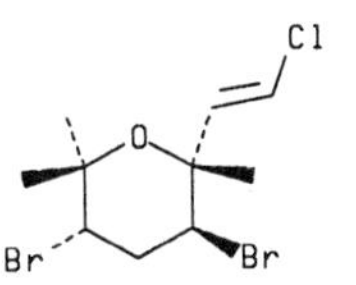

Mol. Wt.:	346
Bioactivity:	Moderate cytotoxicity against Vero, MDCK and B16 cells: IC_{50} 19–96 μg/ml
Melting Point:	Oil
$[\alpha]_D$:	+4.4 Solvent: Chf
Spectral Data:	IR, CMR, PMR, Mass Spec.
Organism:	*Aplysia kurodai* Baba (Mollusca)
Location:	Nabeta Bay, Japan
Reference:	629

$C_{10}H_{15}Br_2ClO$ **Aplysiapyranoid B**

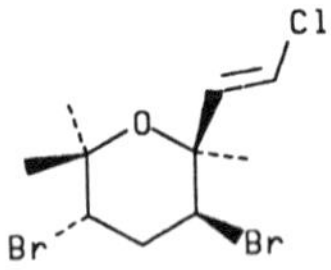

Mol. Wt.: 346
Bioactivity: Moderate cytotoxicity against Vero, MDCK and B16 cells: IC_{50} 19–96 μg/ml
Melting Point: 46–49°C
$[\alpha]_D$: −27 Solvent: Chf
Spectral Data: IR, CMR, PMR, Mass Spec., x-ray c.s.
Organism: *Aplysia kurodai* Baba (Mollusca)
Location: Nabeta Bay, Japan
Reference: 457, 629

$C_{12}H_8N_2O_2$ **Demethyl(oxy)aaptamine**

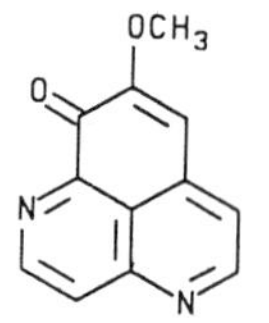

Mol. Wt.: 212
Bioactivity HeLa cells: ED_{50} 0.87 μg/ml
Antimicrobial activity against gram-positive and gram-negative bacteria (*Staphylococcus aureus*, *Bacillus subtilis*, *Proteus vulgaris*)
Melting Point: 198–200°C (dec.)
Spectral Data: UV, IR, CMR, PMR, Mass Spec.
Organism: *Aaptos aaptos* (Porifera)
Location: Okinawa, Japan
Reference: 801

$C_{12}H_{10}N_2O_2$ **Demethylaaptamine**

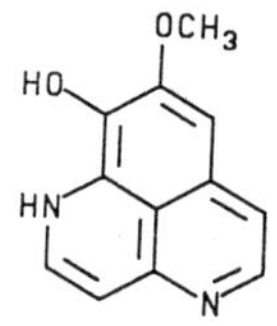

Mol. Wt.: 214
Bioactivity: HeLa cells: ED_{50} ~ 1.7 μg/ml
Antimicrobial activity against gram-positive and gram-negative bacteria (*Staphylococcus aureus*, *Bacillus subtilis*, *Proteus vulgaris*)
Melting Point: 248–251°C (dec.) (HCl)
Spectral Data: UV, IR, CMR, PMR, Mass Spec. (HCl)
Organism: *Aaptos aaptos* (Porifera)
Location: Okinawa, Japan
Reference: 801

$C_{12}H_{11}NO_4$ **Renierol**

Mol. Wt.: 233
Bioactivity: L1210: IC_{50} 3.0 μg/ml
Antibacterial activity against *Staphylococcus aureus*
Spectral Data: UV, IR, CMR, PMR, Mass Spec.
Organism: *Xestospongia caycedoi* Zea and van Soest
(Porifera)
Location: Sand Island, Fiji
Reference: 723

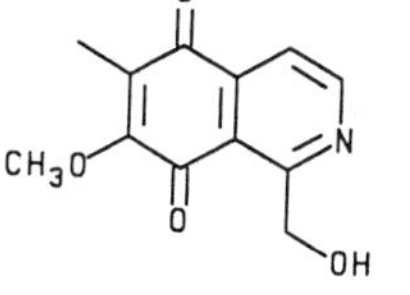

$C_{12}H_{18}O_2$ **Clavularin A**
(previously known)

Mol. Wt.: 194
Bioactivity: Cytotoxicity against PV_4 cultured cells transformed with polyoma virus
Spectral Data: CD, PMR
Organism: *Clavularia koellikeri*
(Coelenterata)
Location: Okinawa, Japan
Reference: 270, 271, 272

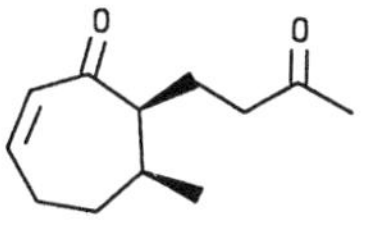

$C_{12}H_{18}O_2$ **Clavularin B**
(previously known)

Mol. Wt.: 194
Bioactivity: Cytotoxicity against PV_4 cultured cells transformed with polyoma virus
Spectral Data: CD, PMR
Organism: *Clavularia koellikeri*
(Coelenterata)
Location: Okinawa, Japan
Reference: 270, 271, 272

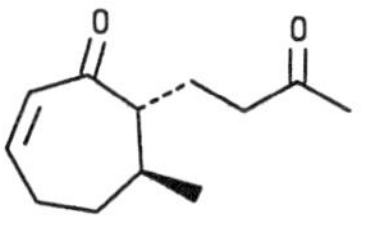

$C_{15}H_{22}O$ **(S)-(+)-Curcuphenol**

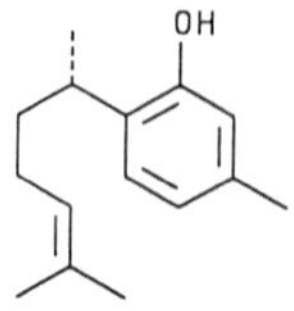

Mol. Wt.: 218

Bioactivity A-549 (lung): minimum inhibitory concentration 10 μg/ml
HCT-8 (colon): minimum inhibitory concentration 0.1 μg/ml
MDAMB (mammary): minimum inhibitory concentration 0.1 μg/ml
P388: IC_{50} 7 μg/ml
Inhibition of gastric H,K-ATPase: IC_{50} 8.3 x 10^{-6}M
Antifungal activity against *Candida albicans*

$[\alpha]_D$: +29.1 Solvent: Chf

Spectral Data: UV, IR, CMR, PMR, Mass Spec.

Organism: *Didiscus flavus* van Soest
Epipolasis sp.
(Porifera)

Location: Bahamas, Belize; Izu Archipelago

Reference: 334, 1189

$C_{15}H_{26}O_3$ **Nephtheoxydiol**

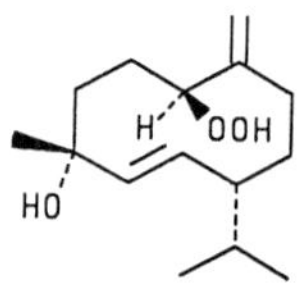

Mol. Wt.: 254

Bioactivity: B16: IC_{50} 0.1 μg/ml

$[\alpha]_D^{21}$: +14 Solvent: Chf

Spectral Data: CD, IR, CMR, PMR, Mass Spec.

Organism: *Nephthea* sp.
(Coelenterata)

Location: Okinawa, Japan

Reference: 563

$C_{15}H_{27}N$ **(6R,7S)-7-Amino-7,8-dihydro-α-bisabolene (Aminobisabolene)**

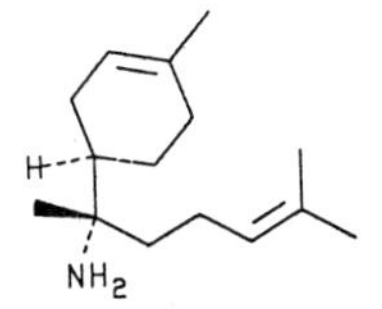

Mol. Wt.: 221
Bioactivity: Cytotoxicity: CCRF-CEM: IC_{50} 3.1 μg/ml
Antimicrobial activity
Melting Point: Oil
$[\alpha]_D^{20}$: +59.9 Solvent: Chf
$[\alpha]_D^{16}$: +59.0 Solvent: Me
Spectral Data: IR, CMR, PMR, Mass Spec.; x-ray c.s. of derivatives
Organism: *Halichondria* sp.
Theonella sp.
(Porifera)
Location: Ponape, Marshall Islands; Okinawa, Japan
Reference: 565, 569, 1045

$C_{16}H_{25}N$

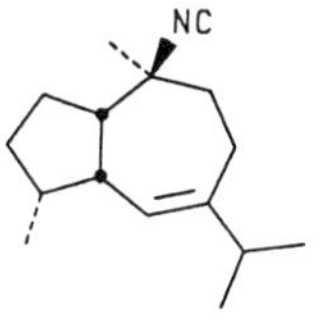

Mol. Wt.: 231
Bioactivity: L1210: ED_{50} 0.19 μg/ml
HeLa: ED_{50} 0.27 μg/ml
Melting Point: 57–59°C
$[\alpha]_D$: −60.1 Solvent: Chf
Spectral Data: IR, CMR, PMR, Mass Spec., x-ray c.s.
Organism: Unidentified sp.
(Porifera)
Location: Wakayama, Japan
Reference: 1068

$C_{17}H_{20}O_3$ **15-Acetoxytubipofuran**

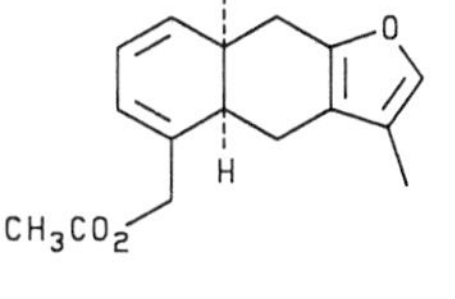

Mol. Wt.: 272
Bioactivity: B-16: IC_{50} 33 μg/ml
Ichthyotoxic at 20 μg/ml
Melting Point: Oil
$[\alpha]_D$: +10.7 Solvent: Chf
Spectral Data: UV, CD, IR, CMR, PMR, Mass Spec.
Organism: *Tubipora musica*
(Coelenterata)
Location: Okinawa, Japan
Reference: 453

$C_{18}H_{11}ClN_2O$ **Fascaplysin**

Mol. Wt.: 306
Bioactivity: L1210: IC_{50} 0.2 μg/ml
Antimicrobial activity
Melting Point: 232–235°C
Spectral Data: UV, IR, CMR, PMR, Mass Spec., x-ray c.s.
Organism: *Fascaplysinopsis* sp. Bergquist (Porifera)
Location: Fiji
Reference: 943

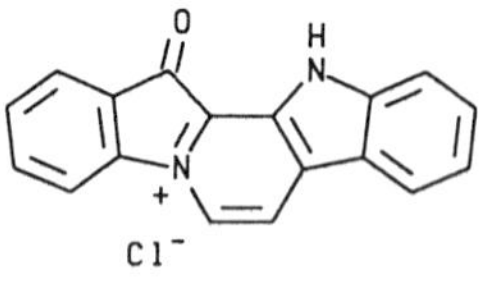

$C_{18}H_{12}BrN_3O_2S$ **Discorhabdin B**

Mol. Wt.: 414
Bioactivity: P388: ED_{50} 0.1 μg/ml
P388: T/C 117 at 0.25 mg/kg
Antimicrobial activity
Melting Point: >360°C (hydrochloride)
$[\alpha]_D$: +400 Solvent: Me
Spectral Data: UV, IR, CMR, PMR, Mass Spec. (hydrochloride)
Organism: *Latrunculia* sp. (Porifera)
Location: New Zealand
Reference: 875

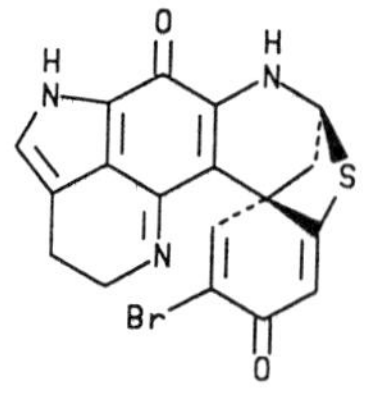

$C_{18}H_{12}BrN_3O_2S$ **Prianosin B**

Mol. Wt.: 414
Bioactivity: L1210: IC_{50} 2.0 μg/ml
L5178Y: IC_{50} 1.8 μg/ml
Melting Point: 250–251°C (dec.)
$[\alpha]_D^{30}$ +360 Solvent: Chf
Spectral Data: UV, CD, IR, CMR, PMR, Mass Spec.
Organism: *Prianos melanos* (Porifera)
Location: Okinawa, Japan
Reference: 170

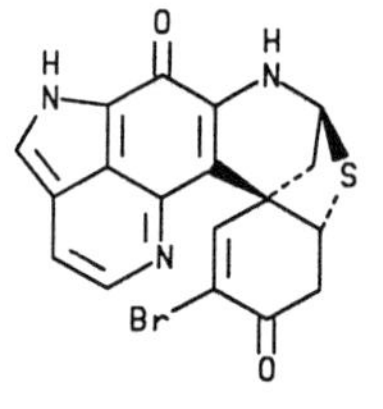

$C_{18}H_{13}Br_2N_3O_2$ **Discorhabdin C**

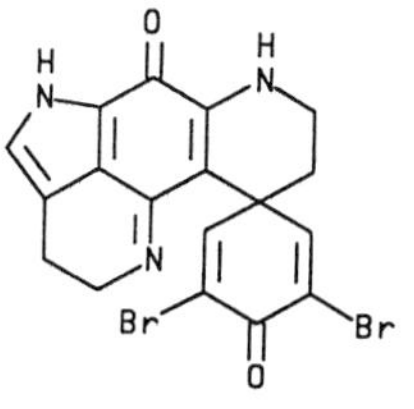

Mol. Wt.: 463
Bioactivity: L1210: ED_{50} < 100 ng/ml
P388: ED_{50} 0.03 μg/ml
Toxic to mice at 2 mg/kg
Antimicrobial activity
Melting Point: >360°C (HCl)
$[\alpha]_D$: 0° (HCl) Solvent: Not given
Spectral Data: UV, IR, (hydrochloride); CMR, PMR, Mass spec., x-ray c.s.
Organism: *Latrunculia* sp.
(Porifera)
Location: New Zealand
Reference: 874, 875

$C_{18}H_{13}N_3O_2S$ **Discorhabdin D**

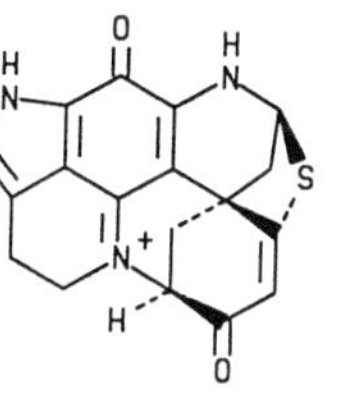

Mol. Wt.: 335
Bioactivity: P388: IC_{50} 6 μg/ml
P388: T/C 132 (20 mg/kg)
Antimicrobial activity
Melting Point: >360°C (HCl)
$[\alpha]_D$: 0 Solvent: Me
$[\alpha]_{578}$: -45 Solvent: Me
Spectral Data: UV, IR, CMR, PMR, Mass Spec. (hydrochloride)
Organism: *Latrunculia brevis*
Prianos sp.
(Porifera)
Location: New Zealand; Okinawa, Japan
Reference: 876

$C_{18}H_{14}BrN_3O_2S$ **Discorhabdin A**
(syn. **Prianosin A**)

Mol. Wt.: 416

Bioactivity:
P388: ED_{50} 0.05 μg/ml
L1210: IC_{50} 37 ng/ml
L5178Y: IC_{50} 14 ng/ml
KB: IC_{50} 73 ng/ml
Induction of Ca^{2+} release from sarcoplasmic reticulum
Toxic to mice at 2 mg/kg
Antimicrobial activity

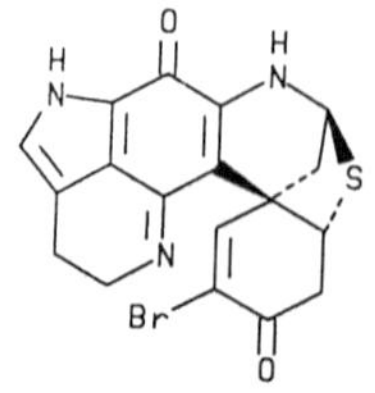

Melting Point: >300°C

$[\alpha]_D^{24}$: +248 Solvent: Chf

Spectral Data: UV, CD, IR, CMR, PMR, Mass Spec., x-ray c.s.

Organism: *Latrunculia brevis*
Prianos melanos
(Porifera)

Location: New Zealand; Okinawa, Japan

Reference: 170, 575, 875

$C_{18}H_{15}N_3O_2S$ **Prianosin D**

Mol. Wt.: 337

Bioactivity:
L1210: IC_{50} 0.18 μg/ml
L5178Y: IC_{50} 0.048 μg/ml
KB: IC_{50} 0.46 μg/ml
Induction of Ca^{2+} release from sarcoplasmic reticulum

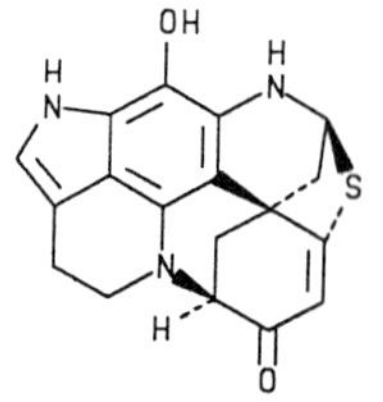

Melting Point: >300°C

$[\alpha]_D^{26}$: +344 Solvent: Me

Spectral Data: UV, CD, IR, CMR, PMR, Mass Spec. (acetate)

Organism: *Prianos melanos*
(Porifera)

Location: Okinawa, Japan

Reference: 170

$C_{18}H_{15}N_3O_3S$	**Prianosin C**
Mol. Wt.:	353
Bioactivity:	L1210: IC_{50} 0.15 μg/ml L5178Y: IC_{50} 0.024 μg/ml KB: IC_{50} 0.57 μg/ml
Melting Point:	>300°C
$[\alpha]_D^{22}$:	+358 Solvent: Me
Spectral Data:	UV, CD, IR, CMR, PMR, Mass Spec. (acetate)
Organism:	*Prianos melanos* (Porifera)
Location:	Okinawa, Japan
Reference:	170

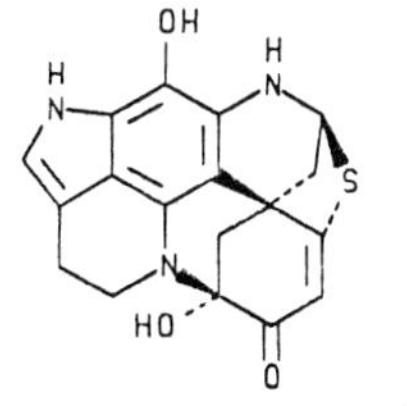

$C_{18}H_{39}NO$	**2-Aminooctadecan-3-ol**
Mol. Wt.:	285
Bioactivity:	Cytotoxicity against PV_4 cultured cells transformed with polyoma virus at 10 μg/ml
Organism:	*Lemnalia* sp. (Coelenterata)
Location:	Queensland, Australia
Reference:	270

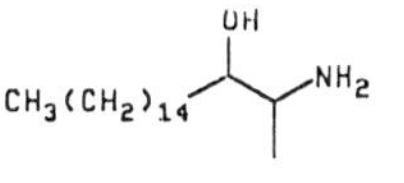

$C_{19}H_{33}NO_2$	**Dysidazirine**
Mol. Wt.:	307
Bioactivity:	Cytotoxic to L1210 cells at 0.27 μg/ml Inhibits growth of *Pseudomonas aeruginosa*, *Candida albicans*, and *Saccharomyces cerevisiae*
$[\alpha]_D$:	−165 Solvent: Me
Spectral Data:	UV, CD of derivative, IR, CMR, PMR, Mass Spec.
Organism:	*Dysidea fragilis* (Porifera)
Location:	Fiji
Reference:	759

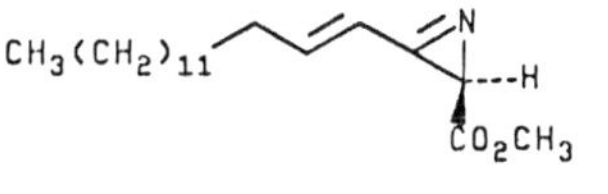

$C_{20}H_{12}O_5$

Halenaquinone
(previously known)

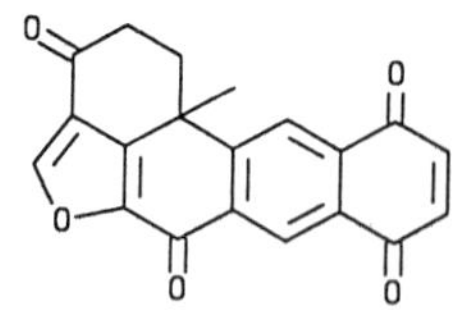

Mol. Wt.: 332
Bioactivity: P388: ED_{50} 2.9 μg/ml
Melting Point: >250° (dec.)
$[\alpha]_D$: +22.2 Solvent: Dcm
Organism: *Adocia* sp. (Porifera)
Location: Truk
Reference: 944, 982

$C_{20}H_{13}BrN_4O_2$

Bromotopsentin
(syn. **Topsentin-B2**)

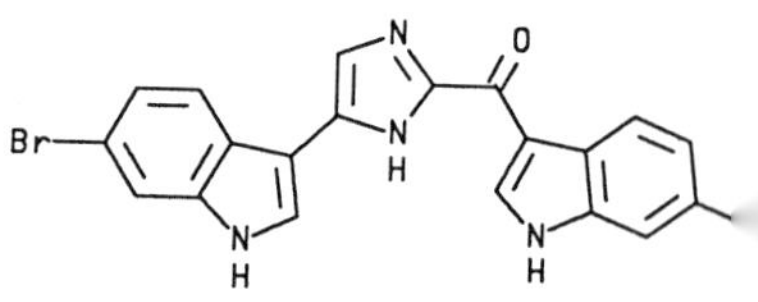

Mol. Wt.: 421
Bioactivity: P388: IC_{50} 7.0 μg/ml
P388: T/C 126 at 75 mg/kg
Antiviral activity towards HSV-1, *Vesicular stomatitis* virus and corona virus A-59
Weak ichthyotoxicity
Melting Point: 296-297°C
Spectral Data: UV, IR, CMR, PMR, Mass Spec.
Organism: *Spongosorites* spp. 1 and 3; *S. ruetzleri*
Topsentia genitrix
(Porifera)
Location: Bahamas; Mediterranean
Reference: 52, 1110

$C_{20}H_{14}N_4O$

Deoxytopsentin
(syn. **Topsentin-A**)

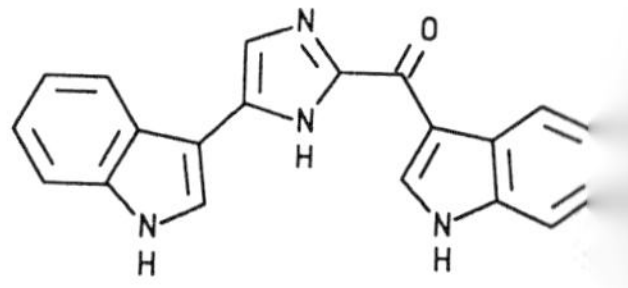

Mol. Wt.: 326
Bioactivity: P388: IC_{50} 12.0 μg/ml
Antiviral activity towards corona virus A-59
Weak ichthyotoxicity
Melting Point: 290-292°C
Spectral Data: UV, IR, CMR, PMR, Mass Spec.
Organism: *Topsentia genitrix* (Porifera)
Location: Mediterranean
Reference: 52, 1110

$C_{20}H_{14}N_4O_2$ | **Topsentin** (syn. **Topsentin-B1**)

Mol. Wt.: 342
Bioactivity: P388: IC_{50} 2.0 μg/ml
HCT-8: IC_{50} 20μg/ml
A-549: IC_{50} 20 μg/ml
T47D: IC_{50} 20 μg/ml
P388: T/C 137 at 150 mg/kg
B16: T/C 144 at 37.5 mg/kg
Antiviral activity towards HSV-1, *Vesicular stomatitis* virus and corona virus A-59
Weak ichthyotoxicity
Melting Point: 270°C
Spectral Data: UV, IR, CMR, PMR, Mass Spec.
Organism: *Spongosorites* spp. 1 and 3
S. ruetzleri
Topsentia genitrix
(Porifera)
Location: Bahamas; Mediterranean
Reference: 52, 1110

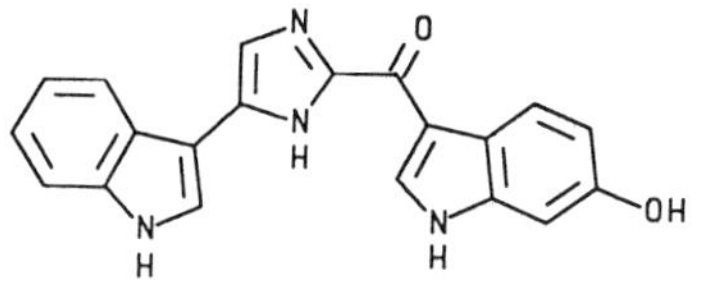

$C_{20}H_{15}BrN_4O$ | **4,5-Dihydro-6"-deoxybromotopsentin**

Mol. Wt.: 407
Bioactivity: P388: IC_{50} 4.0 μg/ml
Antiviral activity towards corona virus A-59
$[\alpha]_D^{24}$: +198 Solvent: Me
Spectral Data: UV, IR, CMR, PMR, Mass Spec.
Organism: *Spongosorites* sp. 3
(Porifera)
Location: Bahamas
Reference: 1110

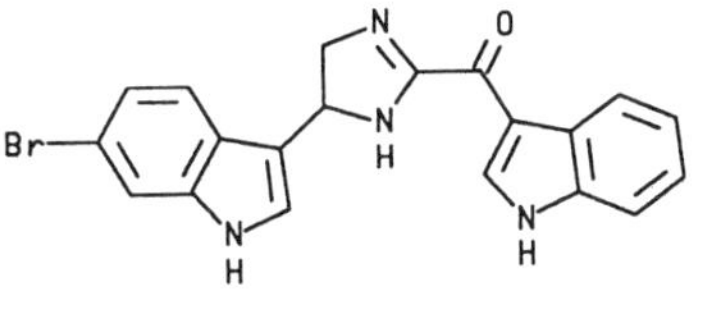

$C_{20}H_{28}O_4$

Kericembrenolide E

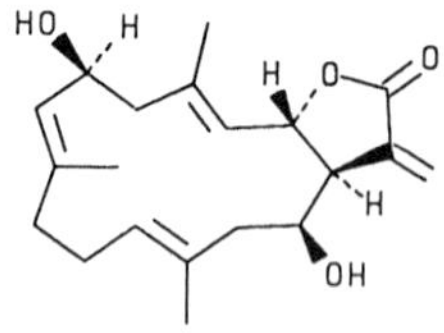

Mol. Wt.: 332
Bioactivity: B-16: IC_{50} 1.8 μg/ml
Melting Point: Oil
$[\alpha]_D^{21}$: -53 Solvent: Chf
Spectral Data: CMR
Organism: *Clavularia koellikeri* (Coelenterata)
Location: Okinawa, Japan
Reference: 590

$C_{20}H_{32}O_3$

Asperdiol

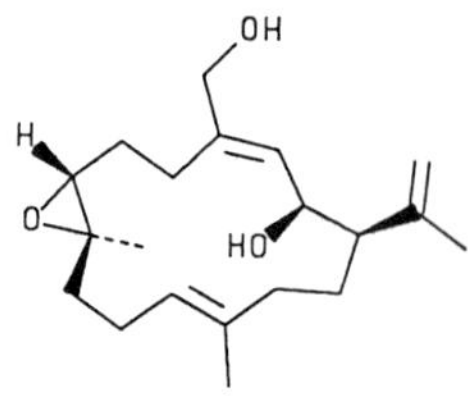

Mol. Wt.: 320
Bioactivity: KB: ED_{50} 24 μg/ml
P388: ED_{50} 6 μg/ml
LE: ED_{50} 6 μg/ml
Melting Point: 109–110°C (natural isolate)
119–120°C (synthetic racemate)
$[\alpha]_D^{20}$: -87 Solvent: Chf
Spectral Data: IR, CMR, PMR, Mass Spec.
Organism: *Eunicea asperula*
E. tourneforti
(Coelenterata)
Location: Caribbean
Reference: 522, 1095, 1166

$C_{20}H_{32}O_3$

Sclerophytin A

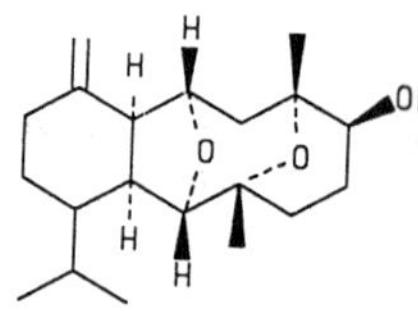

Mol. Wt.: 320
Bioactivity: L1210: cytotoxic at 0.001 μg/ml
Melting Point: 187°C
Spectral Data: IR, CMR, PMR, Mass Spec.
Organism: *Sclerophytum capitalis* (Coelenterata)
Location: Enewetak, Micronesia
Reference: 998

$C_{20}H_{32}O_4$ **Stolonidiol**

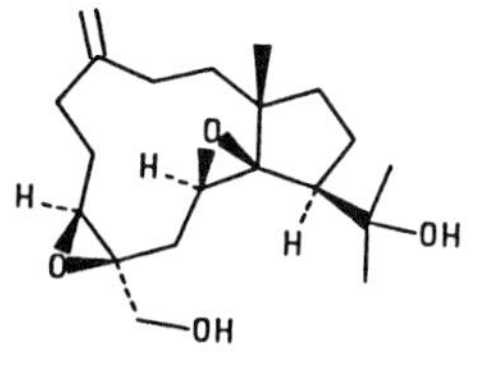

Mol. Wt.: 336
Bioactivity: P388 IC_{50} 0.015 μg/ml
Ichthyotoxicity: minimum lethal concentration (towards *Oryzias latipes*) 10 μg/ml
Melting Point: Oil
$[\alpha]_D$: −31 Solvent: Chf
Spectral Data: CD, IR, CMR, PMR, Mass Spec. x-ray c.s. (derivative)
Organism: *Clavularia* sp. (Coelenterata)
Location: Okinawa, Japan
Reference: 768, 769

$C_{20}H_{32}O_5$ **Methyl (3S*,6S*,14E,16E)-3,6-epidioxy-6-methoxy-octadeca-4,14,16-trienoate**

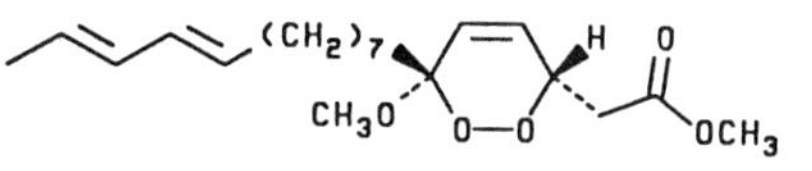

Mol. Wt.: 352
Bioactivity: P388: IC_{50} 0.05–0.1 μg/ml
Melting Point: 38–39°C
$[\alpha]_D^{20}$: +40.8 Solvent: Chf
Spectral Data: IR, CMR, PMR, Mass Spec.
Organism: *Plakortis lita* de Laubenfels (Porifera)
Location: Okinawa, Japan
Reference: 971

$C_{20}H_{34}O_5$ **Methyl (3S*,6S*,16E)-3,6-epidioxy-6-methoxy-octadeca-4,16-dienoate**

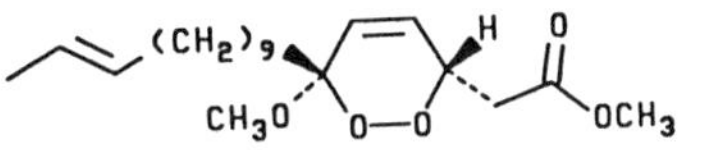

Mol. Wt.: 354
Bioactivity: P388: IC_{50} 0.05–0.1 μg/ml
Melting Point: 37.5°C
$[\alpha]_D^{20}$: +41.4 Solvent: Me
Spectral Data: IR, CMR, PMR, Mass Spec.
Organism: *Plakortis lita* de Laubenfels (Porifera)
Location: Okinawa, Japan
Reference: 971

$C_{20}H_{36}O_5$ **Methyl (3S*,6S*)-3,6-epidioxy-6-methoxyoctadec-4-enoate**

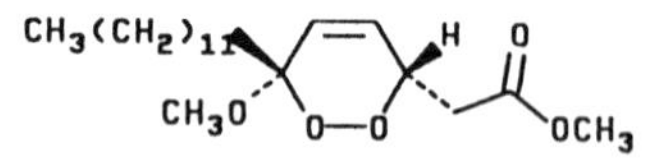

Mol. Wt.: 356
Bioactivity: P388: IC_{50} 0.05–0.1 μg/ml
Melting Point: 49°C
$[\alpha]_D^{20}$: +38.1 Solvent: Me
Spectral Data: IR, PMR, Mass Spec.
Organism: *Plakortis lita* de Laubenfels (Porifera)
Location: Okinawa, Japan
Reference: 971

$C_{21}H_{19}Br_3N_4O$ **Dragmacidin**

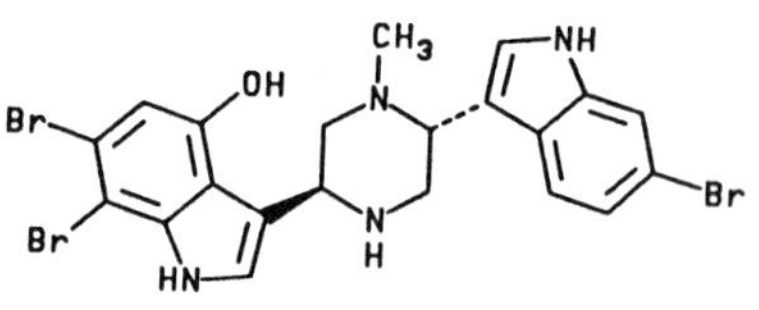

Mol. Wt.: 583
Bioactivity: P388: IC_{50} 15 μg/ml
A-549, HCT-8, and MDAMB: IC_{50} 1–10 μg/ml
$[\alpha]_D^{20}$: -3.0 Solvent: An
Spectral Data: UV, IR, CMR, PMR, Mass Spec.
Organism: *Dragmacidon* sp. Hallman (Porifera)
Location: Bahamas
Reference: 592

$C_{21}H_{20}N_4S$ **Dercitin**

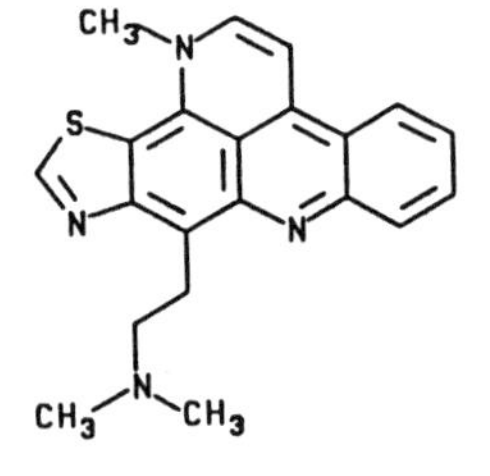

Mol. Wt.: 360
Bioactivity: P388: IC_{50} 0.05 μg/ml
A-549, T47D, and HCT-8: IC_{50} 1.0 μg/ml
P388: T/C 170 (5 mg/kg)
Activity against HSV-1
Complete inhibition of A-59 murine corona virus at 1 μg/well
Melting Point: 168°
Spectral Data: UV, CMR, PMR, Mass Spec.
Organism: *Dercitus* sp. (Porifera)
Location: Bahamas
Reference: 379

$C_{21}H_{29}BrO_4$ **Bromovulone 1**

Mol. Wt.: 425
Bioactivity: HL-60: IC_{50} 0.025 μg/ml
Melting Point Oil
Spectral Data: UV, CD, IR, PMR, Mass Spec.
Organism: *Clavularia viridis* (Coelenterata)
Location: Okinawa, Japan
Reference: 452

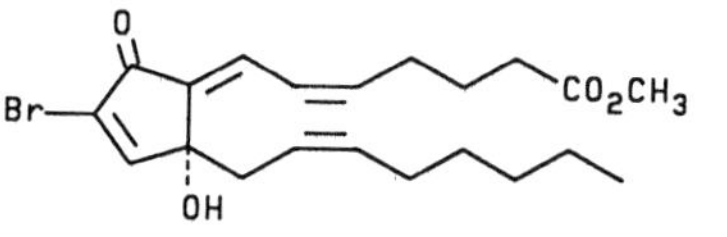

$C_{21}H_{29}ClO_5$

Mol. Wt.: 396
Bioactivity: HL-60: IC_{50} 0.04. μg/ml
Melting Point: Oil
$[\alpha]_D$: -24.1 Solvent: Chf
Spectral Data: UV, IR, PMR, Mass Spec.
Organism: *Clavularia viridis* (Coelenterata)
Location: Okinawa, Japan
Reference: 451

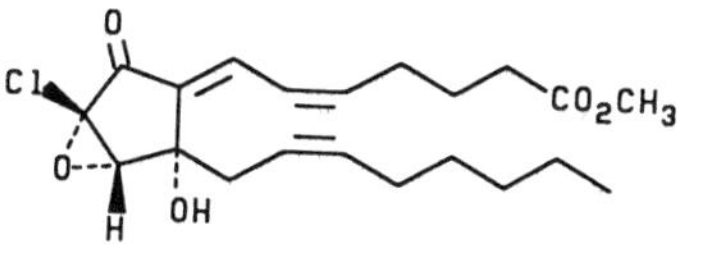

$C_{21}H_{29}IO_4$ **Iodovulone 1**

Mol. Wt.: 472
Bioactivity: HL-60: IC_{50} 0.03 μg/ml
Melting Point: Oil
Spectral Data: UV, IR, PMR, Mass Spec.
Organism: *Clavularia viridis* (Coelenterata)
Location: Okinawa, Japan
Reference: 452

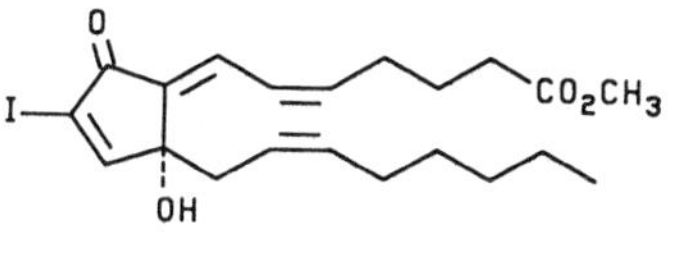

$C_{21}H_{29}NO_3$ **Smenospongine**

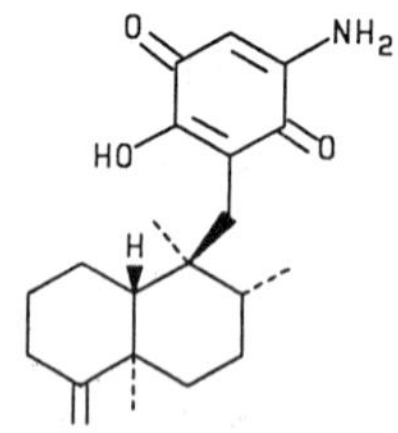

Mol. Wt: 343
Bioactivity: L1210: LD_{50} 1 μg/ml
Antibacterial activity
Melting Point: 153–155°C
Spectral Data: UV, CD, IR, CMR, PMR, Mass Spec.
Organism: *Smenospongia* sp. (Porifera)
Location: Red Sea
Reference: 601

$C_{21}H_{32}O_3$

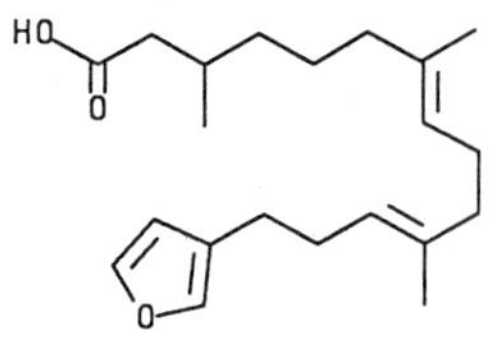

Mol. Wt.: 332
Bioactivity: Cytotoxicity
Melting Point: Oil
Spectral Data: IR, CMR, PMR, Mass Spec.
Organism: *Sarcotragus* sp. (Porifera)
Location: New Zealand
Reference: 51

$C_{22}H_{17}NO_6S$ **Adociaquinone B**

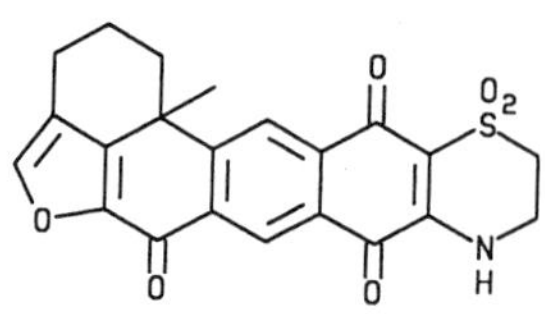

Mol. Wt.: 423
Bioactivity: P388: ED_{50} 2.4 μg/ml
Melting Point: >300°C (dec.)
$[\alpha]_D$: +22
Spectral Data: UV, IR, CMR, PMR, Mass Spec.
Organism: *Adocia* sp. (Porifera)
Location: Truk
Reference: 982

$C_{22}H_{24}Br_2N_4O_6S_2$ **Psammaplin A**

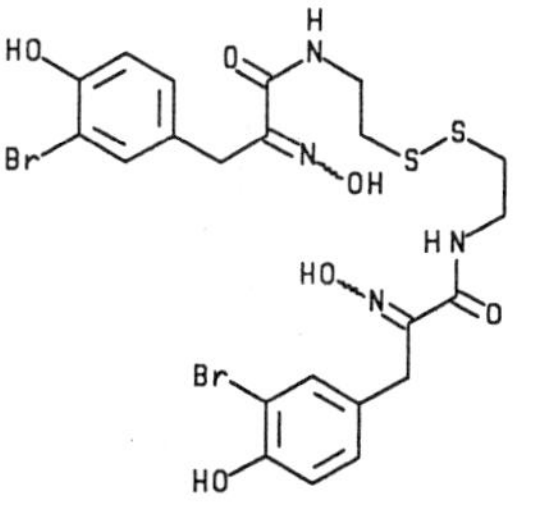

Mol. Wt.: 664
Bioactivity: P388: IC_{50} 0.3 μg/ml
Antimicrobial activity
Melting Point: 67–75°C
Spectral Data: UV, IR, CMR, PMR, Mass Spec.
Organism: *Thorectopsamma xana*
Psammaplysilla sp.
(Porifera)
Location: Guam; Tonga
Reference: 907, 940

$C_{22}H_{30}O_4$ **Isospongiaquinone**
(previously known)

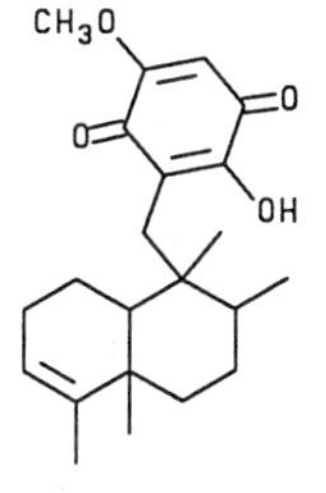

Mol. Wt.: 358
Bioactivity: P388: T/C 125 (10 mg/kg/dose)
L1210: IC_{50} 0.88 μg/ml
Coronary vasodilating activity
Cytotoxicity against PV_4 cells transformed w/polyoma virus at 10 μg/ml
Melting Point: 135.5–136°C
Organism: *Thorecta* sp.
(Porifera)
Location: New South Wales, Australia
Reference: 270, 465, 536

$C_{22}H_{30}O_4$ **Kericembrenolide A**

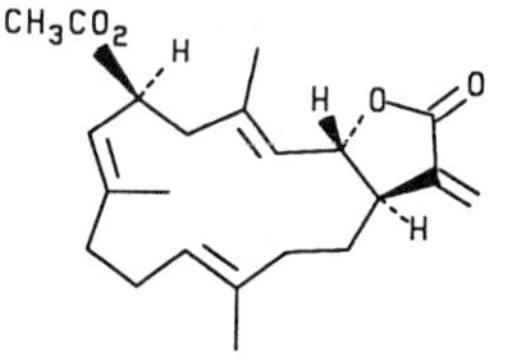

Mol. Wt.: 358
Bioactivity: B-16: IC_{50} 3.8 μg/ml
Melting Point: Oil
$[\alpha]_D^{22}$: −88 Solvent: Chf
Spectral Data: CMR; CD, PMR of derivative
Organism: *Clavularia koellikeri*
(Coelenterata)
Location: Okinawa, Japan
Reference: 590

$C_{22}H_{30}O_4$ **Kericembrenolide B**

Mol. Wt.: 358
Bioactivity: B-16: IC_{50} 2.5 μg/ml
Melting Point: Oil
$[\alpha]_D^{22}$: +97 Solvent: Chf
Spectral Data: CMR
Organism: *Clavularia koellikeri* (Coelenterata)
Location: Okinawa, Japan
Reference: 590

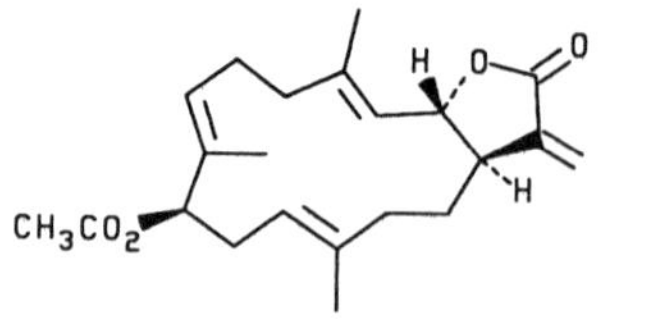

$C_{22}H_{30}O_4$ **Metachromin A**

Mol. Wt.: 358
Bioactivity: L1210: IC_{50} 2.40 μg/ml
Inhibition of coronary artery contraction in rabbit: IC_{50} $3x10^{-6}M$
Melting Point: 80–82°C
$[\alpha]_D^{27}$: -11 Solvent: Chf
Spectral Data: UV, IR, CMR, PMR, Mass Spec.
Organism: *Hippospongia* cf. *metachromia* (Porifera)
Location: Okinawa, Japan
Reference: 465

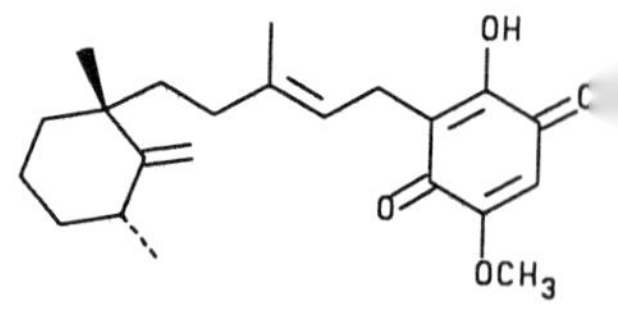

$C_{22}H_{30}O_5$ **Kericembrenolide D**

Mol. Wt.: 374
Bioactivity: B-16: IC_{50} 1.2 μg/ml
Melting Point: Oil
$[\alpha]_D^{22}$: -71 Solvent: Chf
Spectral Data: IR, CMR, PMR; CD of derivative
Organism: *Clavularia koellikeri* (Coelenterata)
Location: Okinawa, Japan
Reference: 590

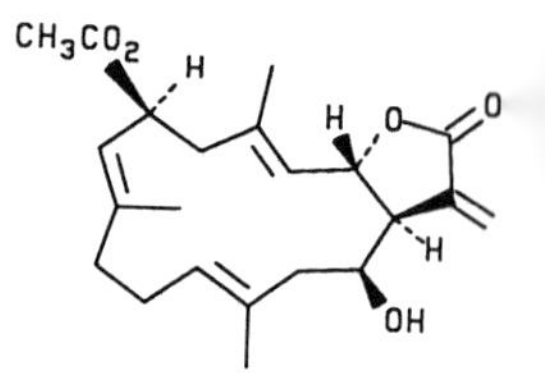

$C_{22}H_{31}NO_5S$

Latrunculin A
(previously known)

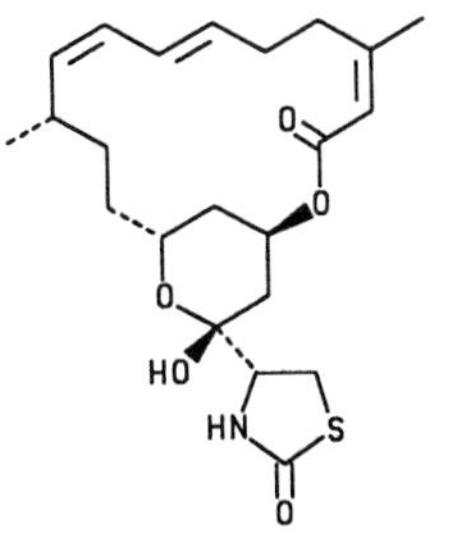

Mol. Wt.: 421
Bioactivity: KB: IC_{50} 150 ng/ml
HEP-2: toxic at 0.07 μg/ml
MA-104: toxic at 0.2 μg/ml
Organism: *Spongia mycofijiensis*
Hyattella sp.
(Porifera)
Chromodoris lochi
C. elizabethina
C. willani
Chromodoris sp.
(Mollusca)
Location: Indonesia; Fiji
Reference: 199, 506, 520

$C_{22}H_{34}O_5$

Stolonidiol monoacetate

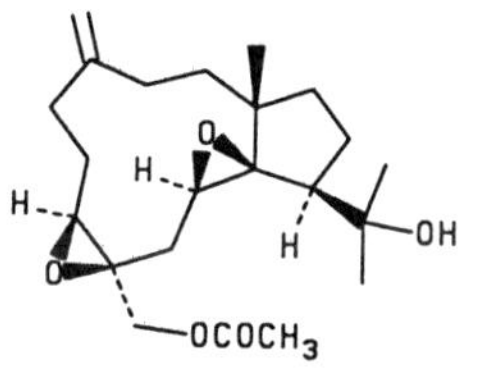

Mol. Wt.: 378
Bioactivity: P388: IC_{50} 0.015 μg/ml
Ichthyotoxicity: minimum lethal dose 17 μg/ml (towards *Oryzias latipes*)
Melting Point: Oil
$[\alpha]_D$: -26.8 Solvent: Chf
Spectral Data: CD of derivative, IR, PMR, Mass Spec.
Organism: *Clavularia* sp.
(Coelenterata)
Location: Okinawa, Japan
Reference: 768, 769

$C_{22}H_{36}N_2O$

Niphatyne A

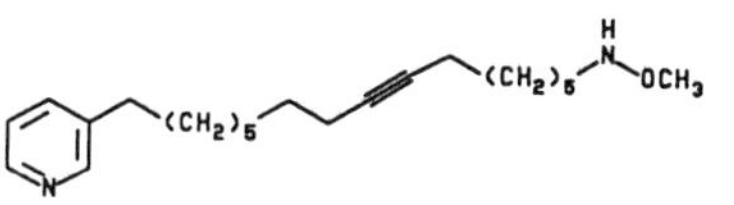

Mol. Wt.: 344
Bioactivity: P388: IC_{50} 0.5 μg/ml
Spectral Data: UV, IR, CMR, PMR, Mass Spec.
Organism: *Niphates* sp.
(Porifera)
Location: Viti Levu, Fiji
Reference: 906

$C_{22}H_{36}O_5$

Methyl (3S*,6S*,16E,18E)-3,6-epidioxy-6-methoxyeicosa-4,16,18-trienoate

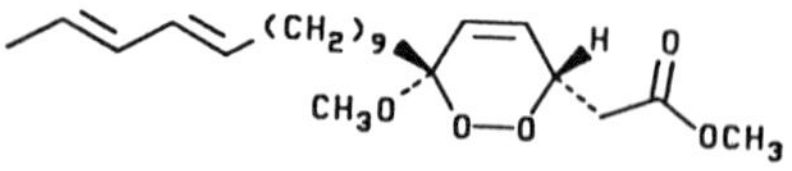

Mol. Wt.: 380
Bioactivity: P388: IC_{50} 0.05–0.1 μg/ml
Melting Point: 47.5°C
$[\alpha]_D^{20}$: +36.4 Solvent: Me
Spectral Data: IR, CMR, PMR, Mass Spec.
Organism: *Plakortis lita* de Laubenfels (Porifera)
Location: Okinawa, Japan
Reference: 971

$C_{23}H_{29}N_3$

Manzamine C

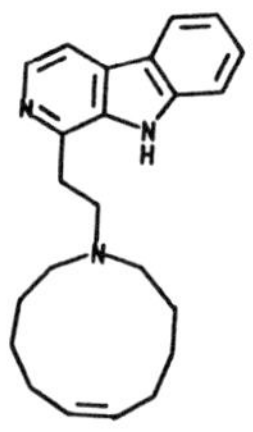

Mol. Wt.: 347
Bioactivity: P388: IC_{50} 3.0 μg/ml
Melting Point: 77–82°C
Spectral Data: UV, IR, CMR, PMR, x-ray c.s.
Organism: *Haliclona* sp. (Porifera)
Location: Okinawa, Japan
Reference: 965

$C_{23}H_{32}O_4$

Metachromin B

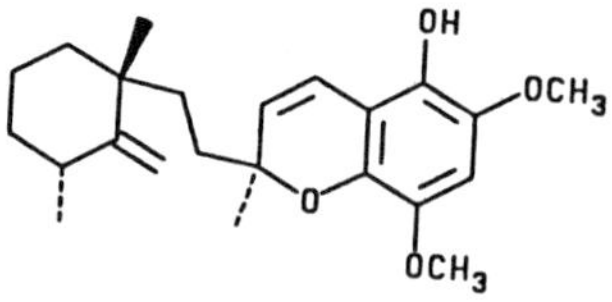

Mol. Wt.: 372
Bioactivity: L1210: IC_{50} 1.62 μg/ml
Inhibition of coronary artery contraction in rabbit: IC_{50} $3x10^{-6}M$
Melting Point: Oil
$[\alpha]_D^{24}$: +8.0 Solvent: Chf
Spectral Data: UV, IR, CMR, PMR, Mass Spec.
Organism: *Hippospongia* cf. *metachromia* (Porifera)
Location: Okinawa, Japan
Reference: 465

$C_{24}H_{26}N_4O_7S$ **Imbricatine**

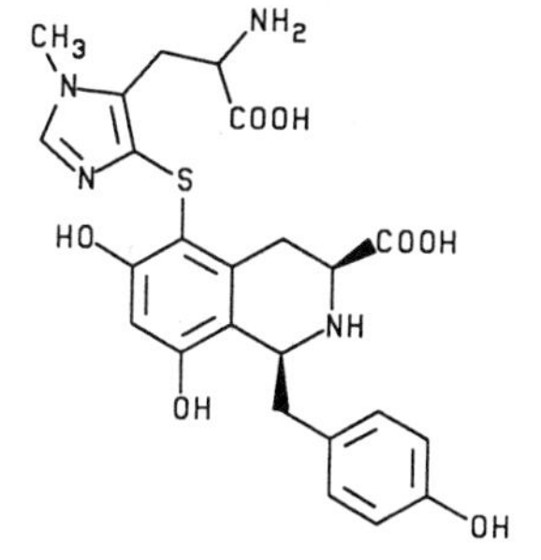

Mol. Wt.: 514
Bioactivity: P388: T/C 139 (0.5 mg/kg)
L1210: ED_{50} < 1 μg/ml
Induces *Stomphia coccinea* (sea anemone) swimming behavior
Spectral Data: CMR, PMR, Mass Spec.
Organism: *Dermasterias imbricata* (Echinodermata)
Location: Northeastern Pacific
Reference: 865

$C_{24}H_{32}O_6$ **Kericembrenolide C**

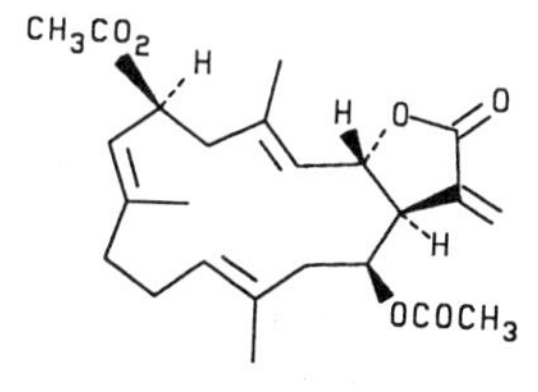

Mol. Wt.: 416
Bioactivity: B-16: IC_{50} 1.3 μg/ml
Melting Point: Oil
$[\alpha]_D^{22}$: -56 Solvent: Chf
Spectral Data: CMR
Organism: *Clavularia koellikeri* (Coelenterata)
Location: Okinawa, Japan
Reference: 590

$C_{24}H_{41}NO_{10}$ **Mycalamide A**

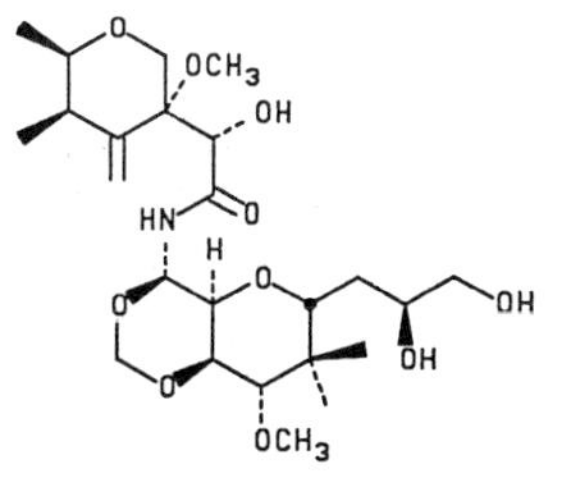

Mol. Wt.: 503
Bioactivity: Antiviral activity towards *Herpes simplex* Type 1 and Polio Type 1 viruses
Melting Point: Oil
$[\alpha]_{365}$: +110 Solvent: Chf
Spectral Data: IR, CMR, PMR, Mass Spec.
Organism: *Mycale* sp. (Porifera)
Location: Otago, New Zealand
Reference: 877

$C_{24}H_{44}O_5$ **Chondrillin**
(previously known)

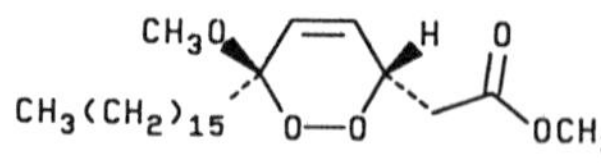

Mol. Wt.:	412
Bioactivity:	P388: IC_{50} 5 μg/ml
Melting Point:	31.5°
$[\alpha]_D^{20}$:	+40 Solvent: Me
Spectral Data:	IR, CMR, PMR, Mass Spec.
Organism:	*Plakortis lita* de Laubenfels (Porifera)
Location:	Okinawa, Japan
Reference:	971, 1171

$C_{25}H_{32}O_5$ **Tridachiapyrone-B**

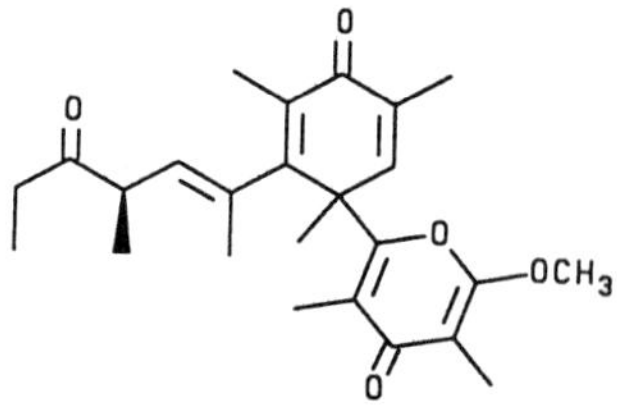

Mol. Wt.:	412
Bioactivity:	P388: ED_{50} 6 μg/ml
Melting Point:	Oil
Spectral Data:	UV, IR, CMR, PMR, Mass Spec.
Organism:	*Tridachia crispata* (Mollusca)
Location:	Jamaica
Reference:	613

$C_{25}H_{34}O_4$ **Tridachiapyrone-A**

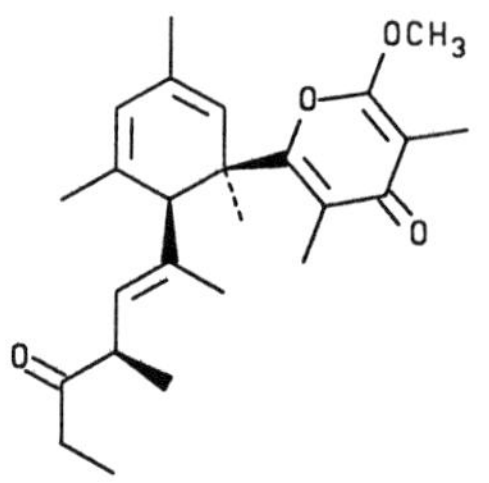

Mol. Wt.:	398
Bioactivity:	P388: ED_{50} 5 μg/ml
Melting Point:	Oil
Spectral Data:	UV, IR, PMR, Mass Spec.
Organism:	*Tridachia crispata* (Mollusca)
Location:	Jamaica
Reference:	613

$C_{25}H_{34}O_6$ **Tridachiapyrone-D**

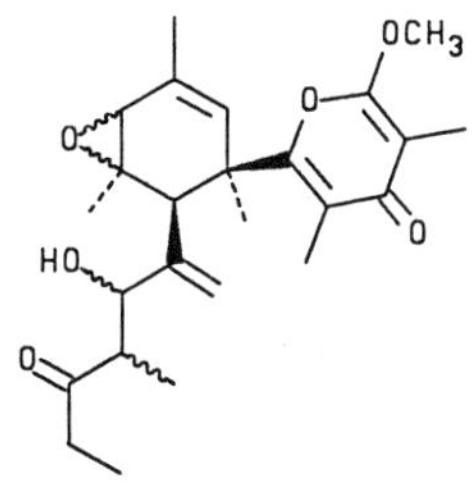

Mol. Wt.:	430
Bioactivity:	P388: ED_{50} 3.1 μg/ml
Melting Point:	Oil
Spectral Data:	UV, IR, PMR, Mass Spec.
Organism:	*Tridachia crispata* (Mollusca)
Location:	Jamaica
Reference:	613

$C_{26}H_{33}ClO_{10}$ **Brianthein Z**
(previously known)

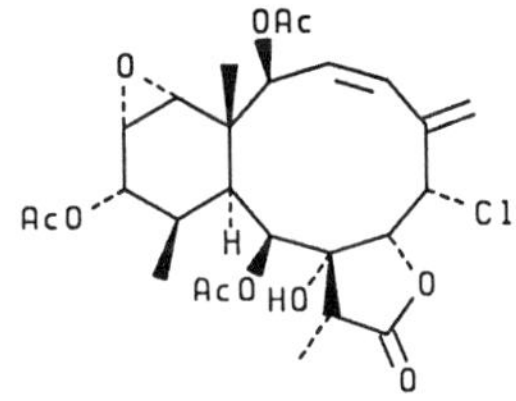

Mol. Wt.;	540
Bioactivity:	Cytotoxic to P388 at 10 μg/ml Active against mouse corona virus and HSV-1 at 80 μg/ml
Organism:	*Briareum asbestinum* (Coelenterata)
Location:	Bahamas
Reference:	204, 363

$C_{26}H_{44}O_5$ **Xestin A**

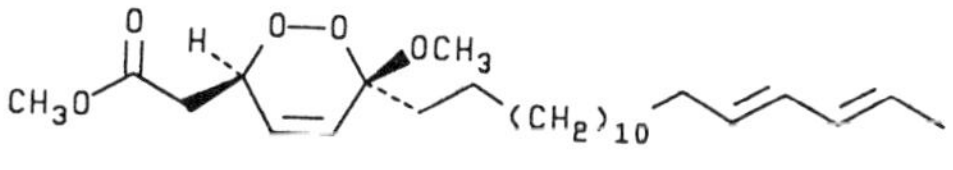

Mol. Wt.:	436
Bioactivity:	P388: IC_{50} 0.3 μg/ml A549 (lung), HCT-8, MD-AMB (mammary): <u>in vitro</u> activity at 5 μg/ml
Melting Point:	55–56°C
$[\alpha]_D^{20}$:	+26.5 Solvent: Dcm
Spectral Data:	UV, IR, CMR, PMR, Mass Spec.
Organism:	*Xestospongia* sp. (Porifera)
Location:	Viti Levu, Fiji
Reference:	910

$C_{26}H_{44}O_5$

Xestin B

Mol. Wt.: 436
Bioactivity: P388: IC_{50} 3 μg/ml
Melting Point: Oil
$[\alpha]_D^{20}$: +19.61 Solvent: Dcm
Spectral Data: UV, IR, CMR, PMR, Mass Spec.
Organism: *Xestospongia* sp. (Porifera)
Location: Viti Levu, Fiji
Reference: 910

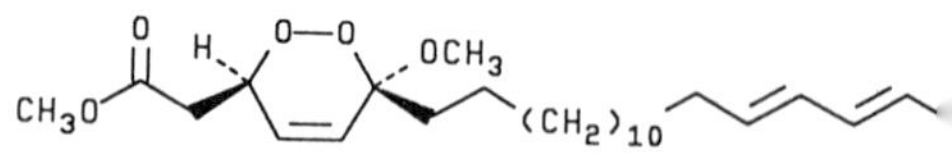

$C_{26}H_{48}O_3$

Ficulinic acid A

Mol. Wt.: 408
Bioactivity: L1210: ID_{50} 10 μg/ml
Melting Point: 33–35°C
Spectral Data: UV, IR, PMR, Mass Spec.
Organism: *Ficulina ficus* Gray (Porifera)
Location: Roscoff, France
Reference: 382

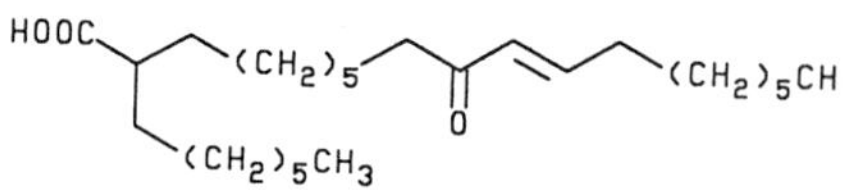

$C_{27}H_{43}N_5O$

Agelasimine-A

Mol. Wt.: 453
Bioactivity: L1210: ED_{50} 2–4 μg/ml
Inhibition of nucleoside transport: IC_{50} 6–14 μM
Smooth muscle relaxing effect: ED_{50} 3–10 μM
Ca^{2+} – Channel antagonism
α_1 Adrenergic blocking
Melting Point: Oil
$[\alpha]_D^{25}$: +2.3 Solvent: Me
Spectral Data: UV, IR, CMR, PMR, Mass Spec.
Organism: *Agelas mauritiana* (Porifera)
Location: Marshall Islands
Reference: 285

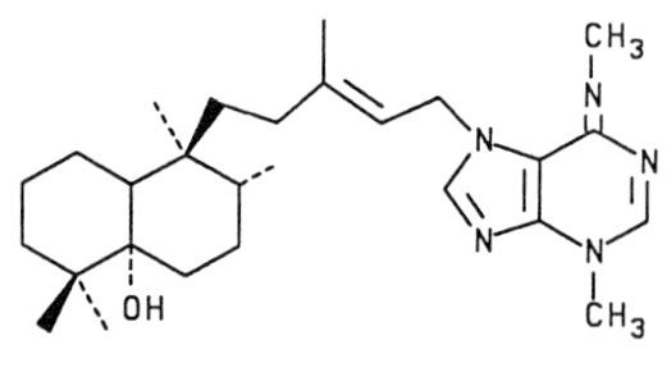

$C_{27}H_{45}N_5O$ **Agelasimine-B**

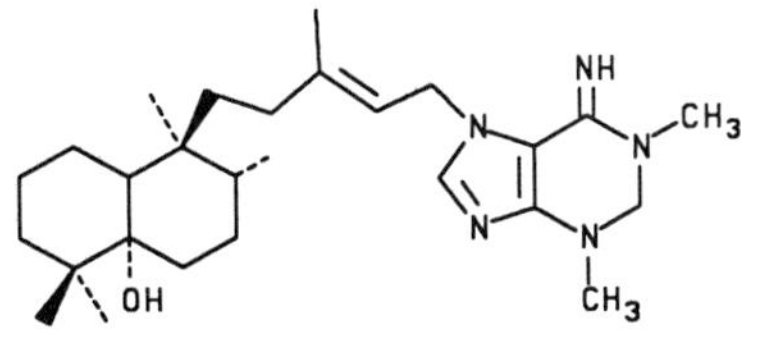

Mol. Wt.: 455
Bioactivity: L1210: ED_{50} 2–4 $\mu g/ml$
Inhibition of nucleoside transport: IC_{50} 6–14 μM
Ca^{2+} – Channel antagonism
α_1 Adrenergic blocking;
Smooth muscle relaxing effect: ED_{50} 3–10 μM
Melting Point: Oil
$[\alpha]_D^{25}$: +2.46 Solvent: Me
Spectral Data: UV, IR, CMR, PMR, Mass Spec.
Organism: *Agelas mauritiana* (Porifera)
Location: Marshall Islands
Reference: 285

$C_{27}H_{46}Na_2O_{10}S_2$ **5β-Cholestane-3α,4α,11β, 21-tetrol 3,21-disulfate**

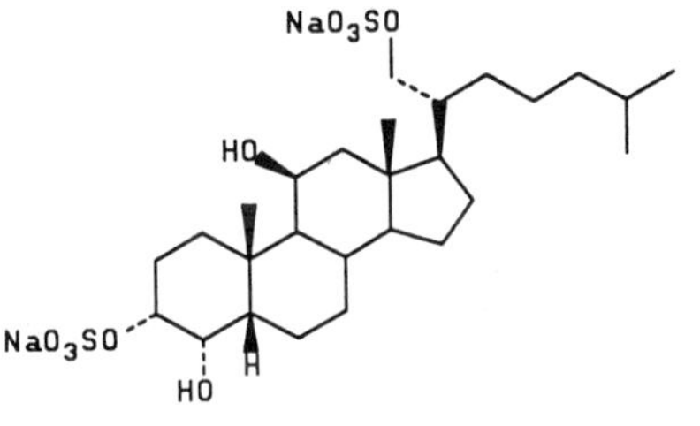

Mol. Wt.: 640
Bioactivity: Activity against mouse T-cells
Melting Point: 195–196°C
$[\alpha]_D$: +41.3 Solvent: Me
Spectral Data: CMR, PMR, Mass Spec.
Organism: *Ophiocoma dentata*
Ophiarthrum elegans
Ophiarachna incrassata
(Echinodermata)
Location: New Caledonia
Reference: 221

$C_{28}H_{52}O_3$ **Ficulinic acid B**

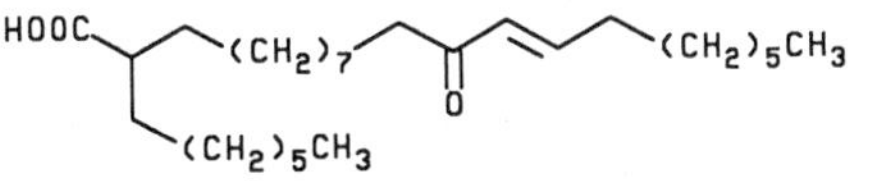

Mol. Wt.: 436
Bioactivity: L1210: ID_{50} 12 $\mu g/ml$
Melting Point: 31–32°C
Spectral Data: UV, IR, PMR, Mass Spec.
Organism: *Ficulina ficus* Gray (Porifera)
Location: Roscoff, France
Reference: 382

$C_{30}H_{41}ClO_{10}$ **Brianthein V**

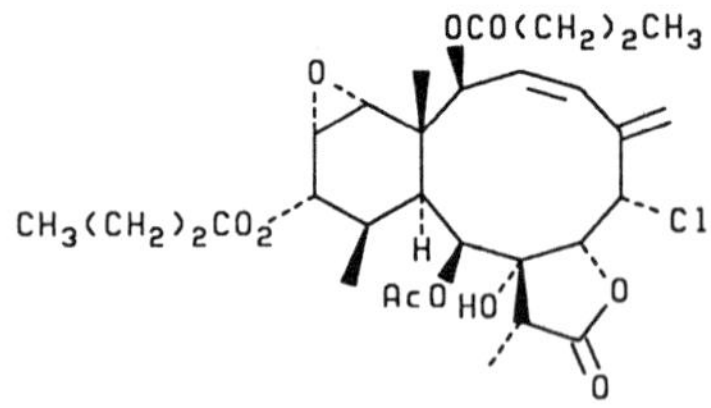

Mol. Wt.: 596
Bioactivity: Cytotoxic to P388 at 13 μg/ml
Antiviral to mouse corona virus at 50 μg/ml
Melting Point: 222°C
$[\alpha]_D^{20}$: -57 Solvent: Chf
Spectral Data: IR, CMR, PMR, Mass Spec., x-ray c.s.
Organism: *Briareum asbestinum* (Coelenterata)
Location: Bahamas
Reference: 204

$C_{30}H_{42}O_7$ **Fijianolide A**

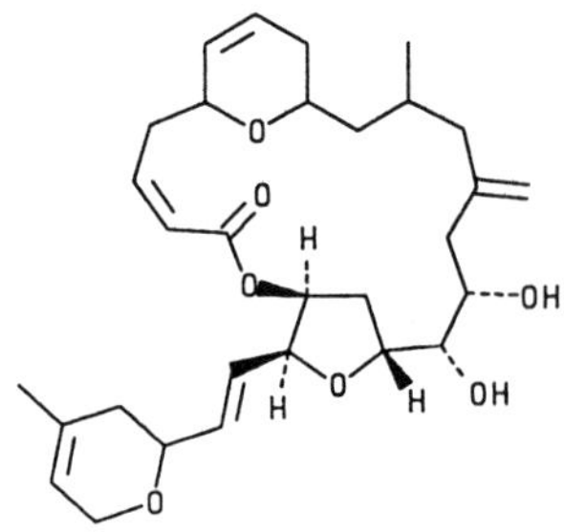

Mol. Wt.: 514
Bioactivity: P388: IC_{50} 9 μg/ml
HT-29: IC_{50} 11 μg/ml
A549: IC_{50} 12 μg/ml
HL-60: IC_{50} 14 μg/ml
Melting Point: Oil
$[\alpha]_D^{20}$: -8.0 Solvent: Chf
Spectral Data: UV, IR, CMR, PMR, Mass Spec.
Organism: *Spongia mycofijiensis* (Porifera)
Location: Vanuatu
Reference: 909

$C_{30}H_{42}O_7$ **Fijianolide B**

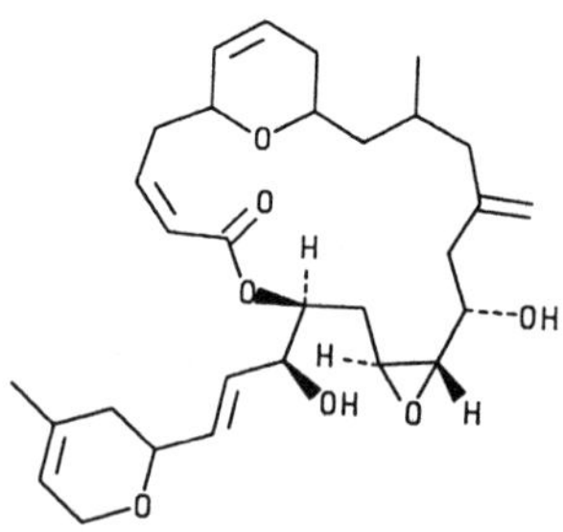

Mol. Wt.: 514
Bioactivity: P388: IC_{50} 6 μg/ml
HT-29: IC_{50} 0.5 μg/ml
A549: IC_{50} 2 μg/ml
HL-60: IC_{50} 5 μg/ml
(tested as the acetate)
Melting Point: Oil
$[\alpha]_D^{20}$: -8.0 (acetate) Solvent: Chf
Spectral Data: UV, IR, CMR, PMR, Mass Spec.
Organism: *Spongia mycofijiensis* (Porifera)
Location: Vanuatu
Reference: 909

$C_{30}H_{42}O_7$

Laulimalide

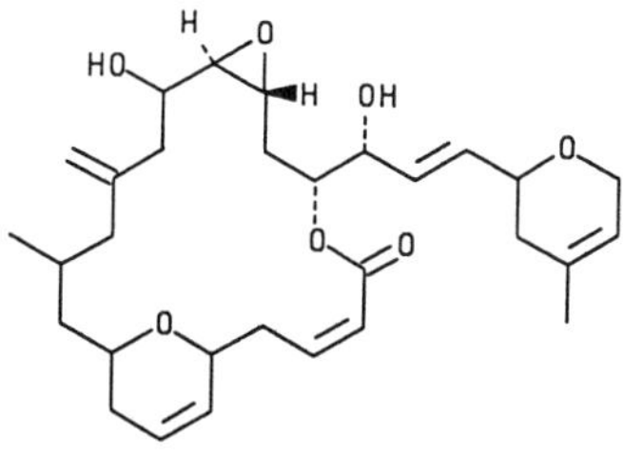

Mol. Wt.: 514
Bioactivity: KB: IC_{50} 15 ng/ml
Spectral Data: UV, IR, CMR, PMR, Mass Spec.
Organism: *Hyattella* sp.
(Porifera)
Chromodoris lochi
(Mollusca)
Location: Indonesia
Reference: 199

$C_{30}H_{48}O_2$

Duryne

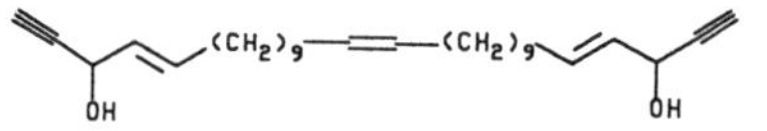

Mol. Wt.: 440
Bioactivity: P388: IC_{50} 0.07 μg/ml
HCT-8 (colon): MIC 0.1 μg/ml
A549 (lung): MIC 0.1 μg/ml
MCF7 (mammary): MIC 0.1 μg/ml
Melting Point: 44–45°C
$[\alpha]_D$: +29 Solvent: Chf
Spectral Data: UV, IR, CMR, PMR, Mass Spec.
Organism: *Cribrochalina dura* Wilson
(Porifera)
Location: Bahamas
Reference: 1188

$C_{31}H_{50}O_9$

5α-Cholest-7-ene-2α,3β,5α,6β,-9α,11α,19-heptol 11,19-diacetate

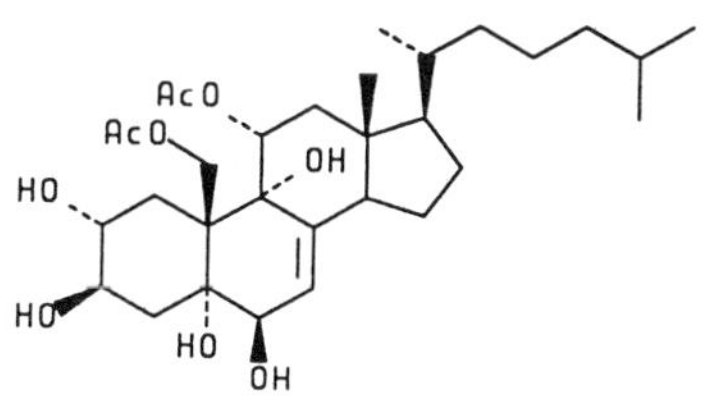

Mol. Wt.: 566
Bioactivity: KB: ED_{50} 4.7 μg/ml
Ichthyotoxicity: LD_{50} 18 μg/ml
Moderate microbial activity
Melting Point: 164°C
$[\alpha]_D^{25}$: -51.1 Solvent: Alc
Spectral Data: CMR, PMR, Mass Spec.
Organism: *Dysidea etheria*
(Porifera)
Location: Bermuda
Reference: 1173

$C_{32}H_{50}O_{11}$ **Tedanolide**

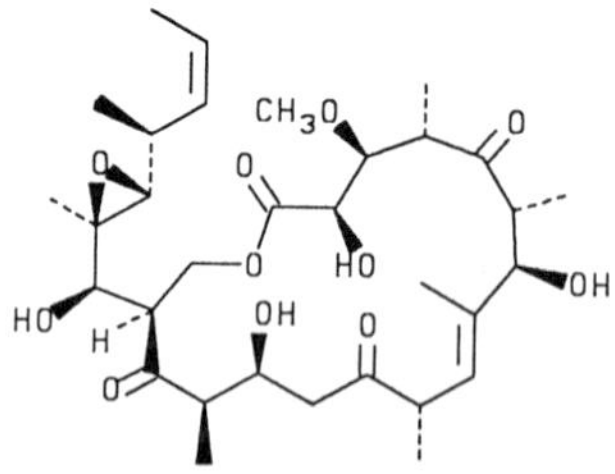

Mol. Wt.: 610
Bioactivity: PS: ED_{50} $1.6x10^{-5}$ $\mu g/ml$
KB: ED_{50} $2.5x10^{-4}$ $\mu g/ml$
Melting Point: 193–194°C
$[\alpha]_D$: +18.7 Solvent: Chf
Spectral Data: IR, CMR, PMR, x-ray c.s.
Organism: *Tedania ignis*
(Porifera)
Location: Summerland Key, Florida
Reference: 984

$C_{36}H_{44}N_4O$ **Keramamine-A**
(syn. **Manzamine A)**

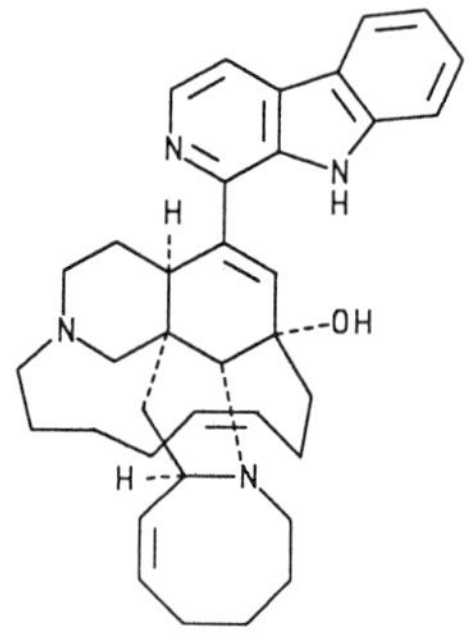

Mol. Wt.: 548
Bioactivity: Antimicrobial activity against *Staphylococcus aureus*
P388: IC_{50} 0.07 $\mu g/ml$
Melting Point: >240°C (dec.) (HCl)
$[\alpha]_D^{20}$: +50 Solvent: Chf
Spectral Data: UV, IR, CMR, PMR, Mass Spec., x-ray c.s.
Organism: *Pellina* sp.
Haliclona sp.
(Porifera)
Location: Okinawa, Japan
Reference: 797, 963

$C_{36}H_{44}N_4O_2$ **Manzamine E**

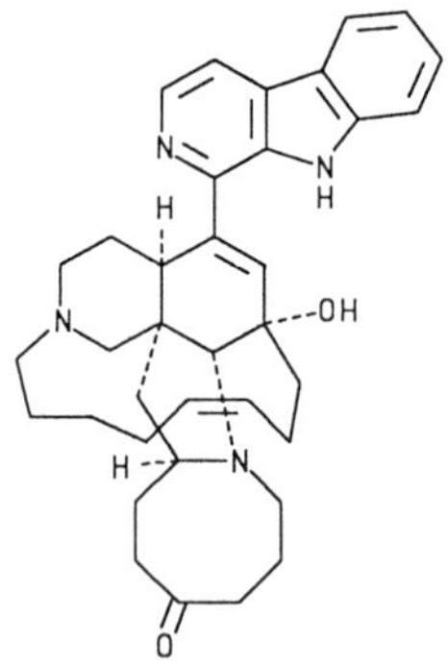

Mol. Wt.: 564
Bioactivity: P388: IC_{50} 5 $\mu g/ml$
Melting Point: 174–176°C
$[\alpha]_D$: +63.7 Solvent: Chf
Spectral Data: UV, IR, CMR, PMR, Mass Spec.
Organism: *Xestospongia* sp.
(Porifera)
Location: Okinawa, Japan
Reference: 449

$C_{36}H_{44}N_4O_3$ **Keramamine B**
(syn. **Manzamine F**)

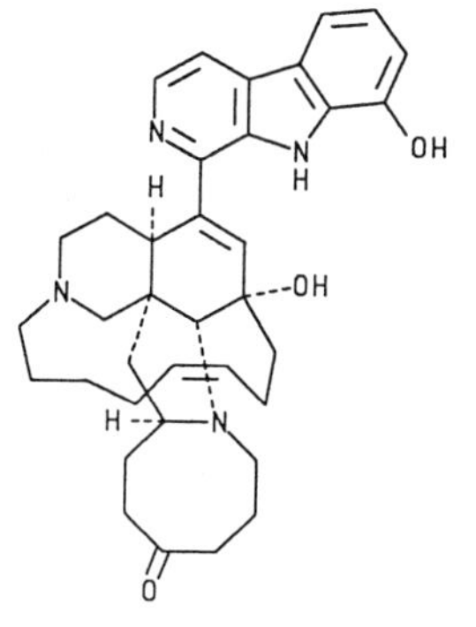

Mol. Wt.: 580
Bioactivity: P388: IC_{50} 5 μg/ml
Antimicrobial activity
Melting Point: >200°C (dec.)
$[\alpha]_D$: +59.9 Solvent: Chf
Spectral Data: UV, IR, CMR, PMR, Mass Spec.
Organism: *Xestospongia* sp.
Pellina sp.
(Porifera)
Location: Okinawa, Japan
Reference: 449, 797

$C_{36}H_{45}BrN_4O_6$ **Jaspamide**
[(+)-Jasplakinolide]

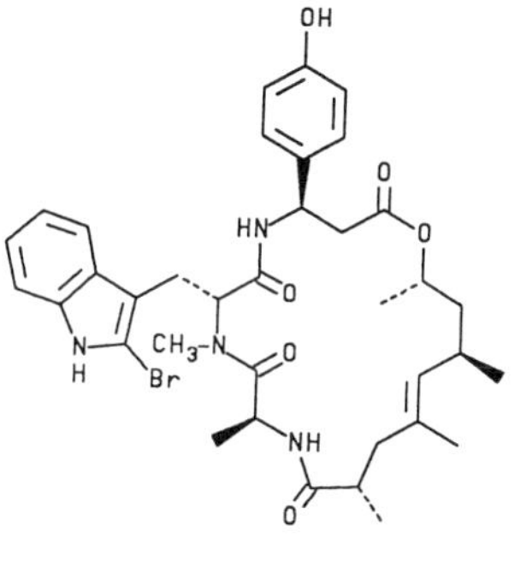

Mol. Wt.: 709
Bioactivity: Cytotoxicity to larynx epithelial carcinoma at 0.32 μg/ml and to human embryonic lung at 0.01 μg/ml
Antihelminthic activity against *Nippostrongylus braziliensis*: ED_{50} <1 μg/ml
Insecticidal activity against *Heliothis virescens*: LC_{50} 4 ppm
Antimicrobial activity towards *Candida albicans*
Ichthyotoxic activity
Melting Point: Oil
$[\alpha]_D$: +65.8 Solvent: Dcm
Spectral Data: UV, IR, CMR, PMR, Mass Spec., x-ray c.s.
Organism: *Jaspis* sp.
J. johnstoni
(syn. *Zapethea digonoxea*)
(Porifera)
Location: Fiji; Palau; Papua, New Guinea
Reference: 108, 210, 362, 1215

$C_{36}H_{46}N_4O$ **Manzamine B**

Mol. Wt.: 550
Bioactivity: P388: IC_{50} 6 μg/ml
Melting Point: 198–203°C
$[\alpha]_D^{20}$: +89 Solvent: Chf
Spectral Data: UV, IR, CMR, PMR, x-ray c.s.
Organism: *Haliclona* sp.
(Porifera)
Location: Okinawa, Japan
Reference: 965

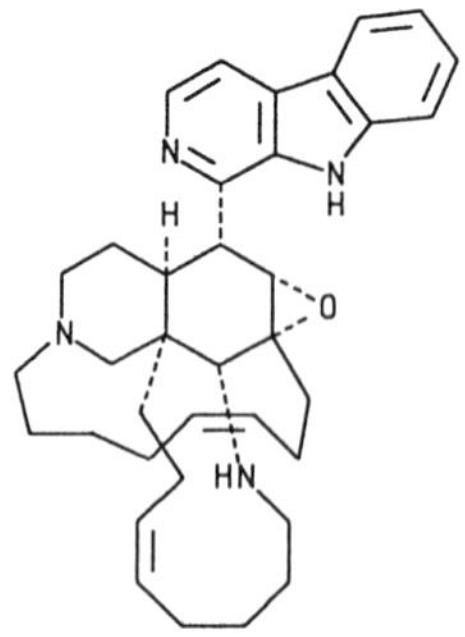

$C_{39}H_{58}O_{15}$ **Bryostatin 11**

Mol. Wt.: 766
Bioactivity: P388: ED_{50} $1.8x10^{-5}$ μg/ml
P388: T/C 164 at 92.5 μg/kg
Melting Point: 171–173°C
$[\alpha]_D^{27}$: +42.5 Solvent: Me
Spectral Data: UV, IR, PMR, Mass Spec.
Organism: *Bugula neritina*
(Bryozoa)
Location: Gulfs of California and Mexico
Reference: 887

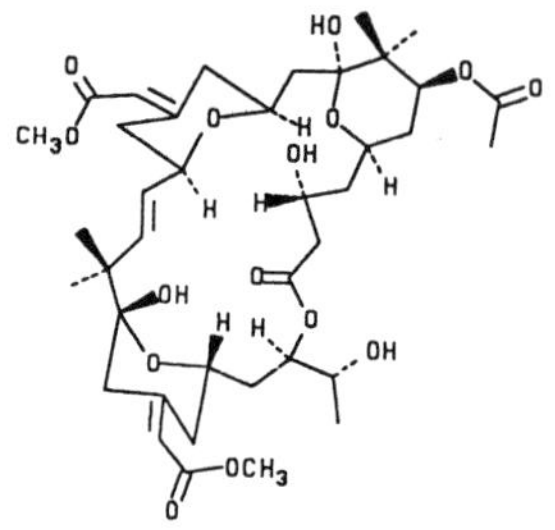

$C_{39}H_{63}N_5O_{12}$ **Onnamide A**

Mol. Wt.: 794
Bioactivity: Antiviral activity against *Herpes simplex* virus type-1, *Vesicular stomatitis* virus and Coronavirus A-59
$[\alpha]_D^{20}$: +99.1 Solvent: Me
Spectral Data: UV, IR, CMR, PMR, Mass Spec.
Organism: *Theonella* sp.
(Porifera)
Location: Okinawa, Japan
Reference: 972

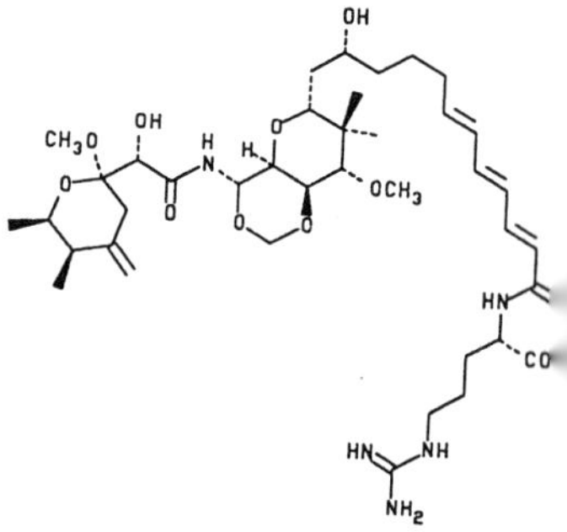

$C_{41}H_{62}O_{15}$ **Bryostatin 13**

Mol. Wt.: 794
Bioactivity: P388: ED_{50} 0.0054 μg/ml
Spectral Data: UV, IR, PMR, Mass Spec.
Organism: *Bugula neritina* (Bryozoa)
Location: California
Reference: 890

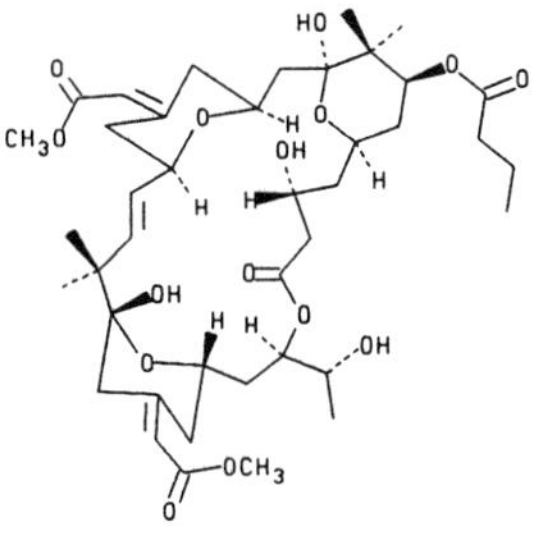

$C_{42}H_{64}O_{15}$ **Bryostatin 10**

Mol. Wt.: 808
Bioactivity: P388: ED_{50} 7.6x10^{-4} μg/ml
Melting Point: 161–164°C
$[\alpha]_D^{27}$: +99.8 Solvent: Me
Spectral Data: UV, IR, CMR, PMR, Mass Spec.
Organism: *Bugula neritina* (Bryozoa)
Location: Gulfs of California and Mexico
Reference: 887

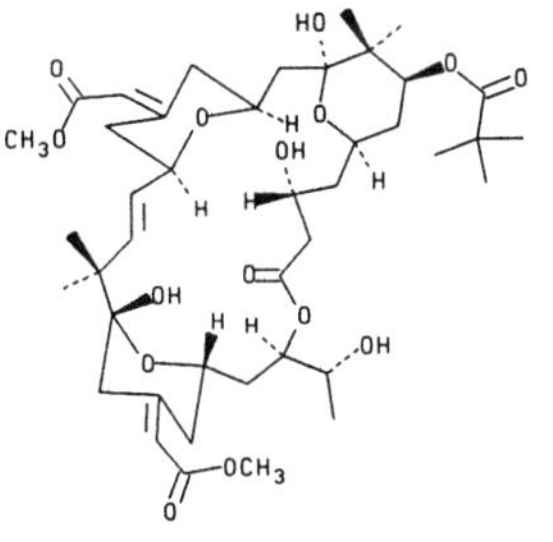

$C_{42}H_{66}O_{13}$ **Pouoside A**

Mol. Wt.: 779
Bioactivity: P388: ED_{50} 1.5 μg/ml
Melting Point: Oil
Spectral Data: IR, CMR, PMR, Mass Spec.
Organism: *Asteropus* sp. (Porifera)
Location Truk
Reference: 618

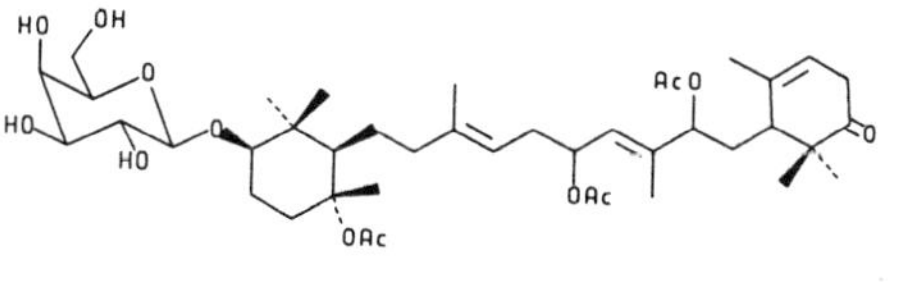

$C_{42}H_{68}N_6O_6S$ **Dolastatin 10**

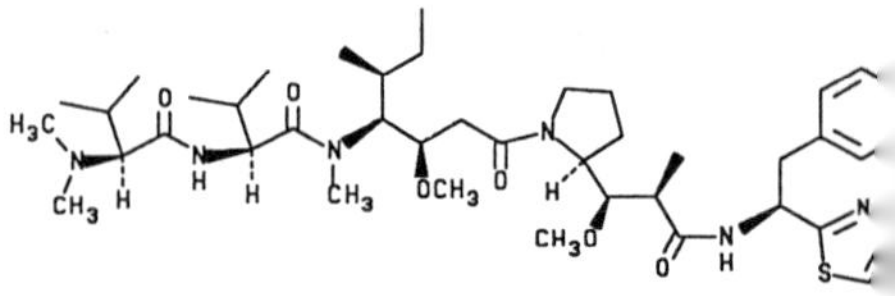

Mol. Wt.: 785
Bioactivity: NCI human melanoma xenograph (nude mouse): curative response 17-67% (3.25-26 μg/kg)
B16: T/C 238 (11.1 μg/kg)
P388: T/C 202 (4 μg/kg)
P388: ED_{50} 4.6 x 10^{-5} μg/ml
Melting Point: 107-112°C
$[\alpha]_D^{29}$: -68 Solvent: Me
Spectral Data: UV, CMR, PMR, Mass Spec.
Organism: *Dolabella auricularia* (Mollusca)
Location: Indian Ocean
Reference: 889, 892

$C_{43}H_{64}O_{17}$ **Bryostatin 9**

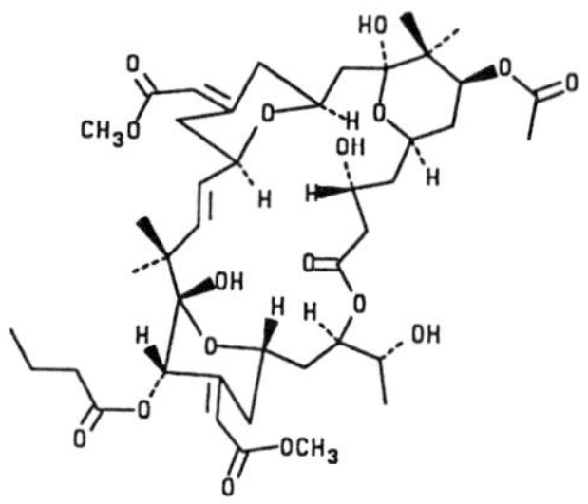

Mol. Wt.: 853
Bioactivity: P388: ED_{50} 1.2x10^{-3} μg/ml
P388: T/C 140 at 80 μg/kg
Melting Point: 159-162°C
$[\alpha]_D^{28}$: +87.31 Solvent: Me
Spectral Data: UV, IR, PMR, Mass Spec.
Organism: *Bugula neritina* (Bryozoa)
Location: California and Gulf of Mexico
Reference: 886, 890

$C_{44}H_{66}O_{16}$ **Bryostatin A**

Mol. Wt.: 851
Bioactivity: P388: ED_{50} 7.0x10^{-2} μg/ml
P388: T/C 148-163 at 0.63-0.25 mg/kg
Melting Point: 142-145°C
$[\alpha]_D^{27}$: +74.85 Solvent: Me
Spectral Data: UV, IR, PMR, Mass Spec.
Organism: *Lissodendoryx isodictyalis* (Porifera) cum *Bugula neritina* (Bryozoa)
Location: Gulf of California
Reference: 888

$C_{46}H_{64}N_4O_{13}$ **Ulapualide A**

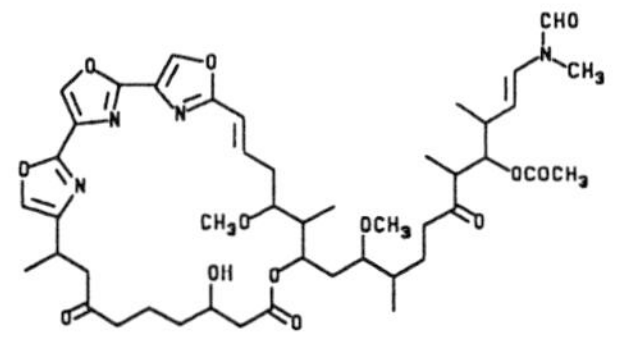

Mol. Wt.: 882
Bioactivity: L1210: IC_{50} 0.01–0.03 μg/ml
Growth inhibition of *Candida albicans*
Melting Point: Oil
$[\alpha]_D^{25}$: −42.9 Solvent: Me
Spectral Data: UV, CMR, PMR, Mass Spec.
Organism: *Hexabranchus sanguineus* (Mollusca)
Location: Oahu, Hawaii
Reference: 941

$C_{46}H_{70}O_{16}$ **Bryostatin B**

Mol. Wt.: 880
Bioactivity: P388: ED_{50} $6.9x10^{-3}$ μg/ml
P388: T/C 148–168 at 0.03–0.25 mg/kg
Melting Point: 137–140°C
$[\alpha]_D^{27}$: +71.30 Solvent: Me
Spectral Data: UV, IR, PMR, Mass Spec.
Organism: *Lissodendoryx isodictyalis* (Porifera)
cum *Bugula neritina* (Bryozoa)
Location: Gulf of California
Reference: 888

$C_{49}H_{72}O_{17}$ **Bryostatin 12**

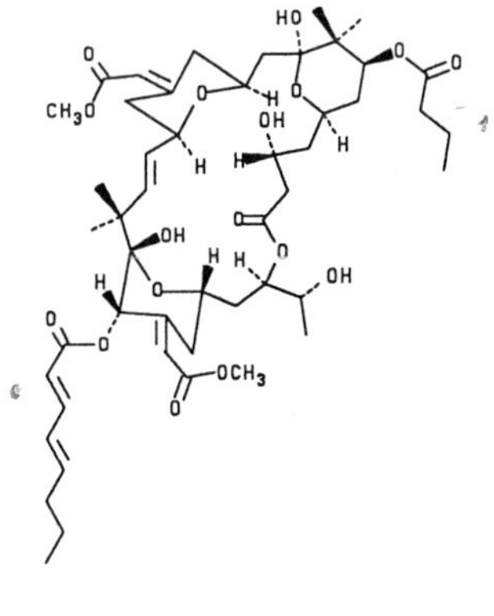

Mol. Wt.: 934
Bioactivity: P388: ED_{50} 0.014 μg/ml
P388: T/C 147–168 at 30–50 μg/kg
$[\alpha]_D^{27}$: +39 Solvent: Me
Spectral Data: UV, IR, CMR, PMR, Mass Spec.
Organism: *Bugula neritina* (Bryozoa)
Location: California
Reference: 890

$C_{50}H_{81}N_4O_{15}P$

Calyculin A

Mol. Wt.: 1010
Bioactivity: L1210: IC_{50} $7.4x10^{-4}$ μg/ml
P388: T/C 144 at 15 μg/kg
Ehrlich carcinoma: T/C 245.8 (15 μg/kg)
Starfish egg assay: IC_{50} $2x10^{-2}$ μg/ml
Sea urchin egg assay: IC_{50} $1x10^{-2}$ μg/ml
Melting Point: 247–249°C
$[\alpha]_D$: -60 Solvent: Alc
Spectral Data: UV, IR, CMR, PMR, ^{31}P NMR, Mass Spec., x-ray c.s.
Organism: *Discodermia calyx* (Porifera)
Location: Gulf of Sagami, Japan
Reference: 525, 526, 527

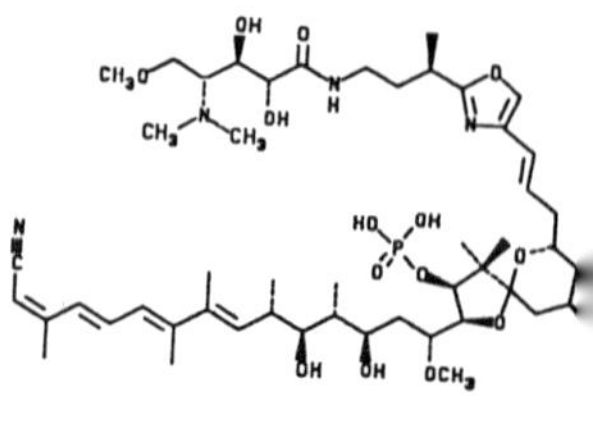

$C_{50}H_{81}N_4O_{15}P$

Calyculin B

Mol. Wt.: 1010
Bioactivity: L1210: IC_{50} $8.8x10^{-4}$ μg/ml
Starfish egg assay: IC_{50} $2x10^{-2}$ μg/ml
Sea urchin egg assay: IC_{50} $1x10^{-2}$ μg/ml
$[\alpha]_D^{24}$: -61 Solvent: Alc
Spectral Data: UV, IR, CMR, PMR, Mass Spec.
Organism: *Discodermia calyx* (Porifera)
Location: Gulf of Sagami, Japan
Reference: 526, 527

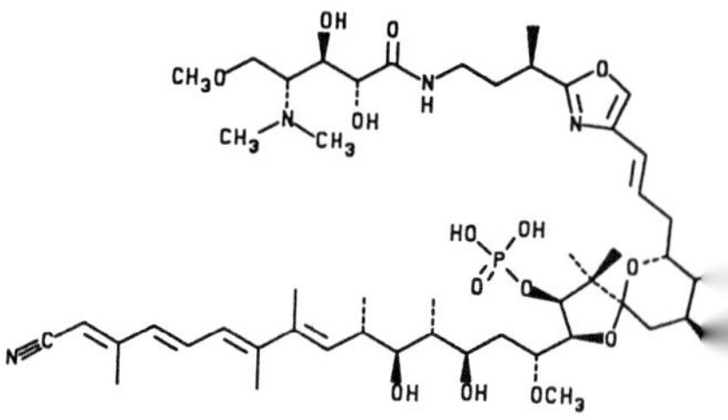

$C_{51}H_{74}N_4O_{16}$

Ulapualide B

Mol. Wt. 1000
Bioactivity: L1210: IC_{50} 0.01–0.03 μg/ml
Growth inhibition of *Candida albicans*
Melting Point: Oil
$[\alpha]_D^{25}$: -21.7 Solvent: Me
Spectral Data: UV, CMR, PMR, Mass Spec.
Organism: *Hexabranchus sanguineus* (Mollusca)
Location: Oahu, Hawaii
Reference: 941

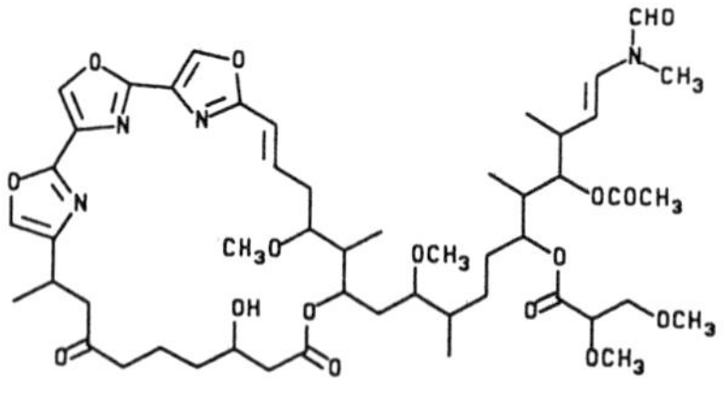

$C_{51}H_{83}N_4O_{15}P$ **Calyculin C**

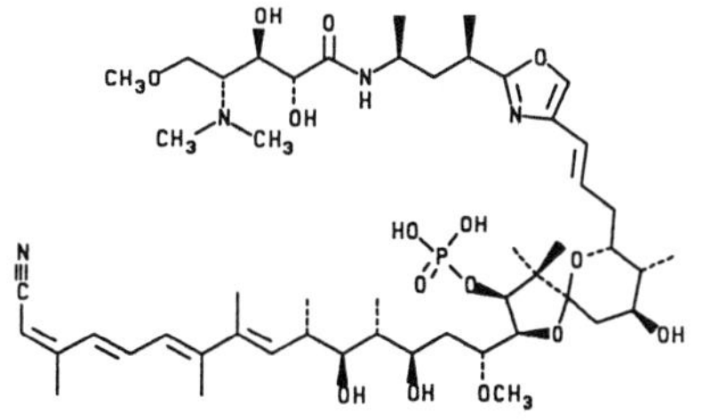

Mol. Wt.: 1024
Bioactivity: L1210: IC_{50} $8.6x10^{-4}$ μg/ml
Starfish egg assay: IC_{50} $2x10^{-2}$ μg/ml
Sea urchin egg assay: IC_{50} $5x10^{-3}$ μg/ml
$[\alpha]_D$: -65 Solvent: Alc
Spectral Data: UV, IR, CMR, PMR, Mass Spec.
Organism: *Discodermia calyx* (Porifera)
Location: Gulf of Sagami, Japan
Reference: 526, 527

$C_{51}H_{83}N_4O_{15}P$ **Calyculin D**

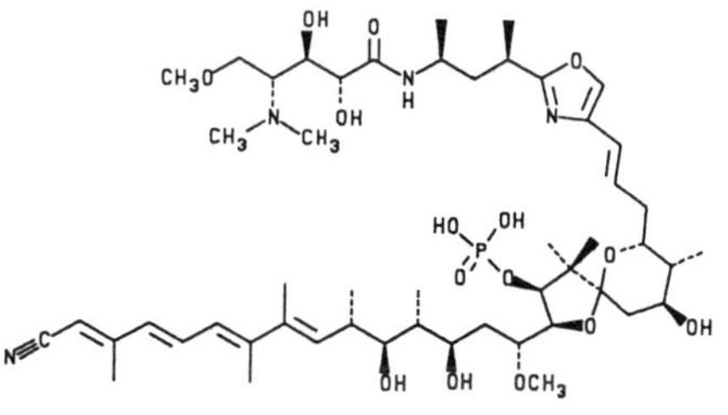

Mol. Wt.: 1024
Bioactivity: L1210: IC_{50} $1.5x10^{-3}$ μg/ml
Starfish egg assay: IC_{50} $5x10^{-2}$ μg/ml
Sea urchin egg assay: IC_{50} $5x10^{-3}$ μg/ml
$[\alpha]_D^{24}$: -41 Solvent: Alc
Spectral Data: UV, IR, CMR, PMR, Mass Spec.
Organism: *Discodermia calyx* (Porifera)
Location: Gulf of Sagami, Japan
Reference: 526, 527

$C_{57}H_{93}NaO_{28}S$ **Pectinioside A**

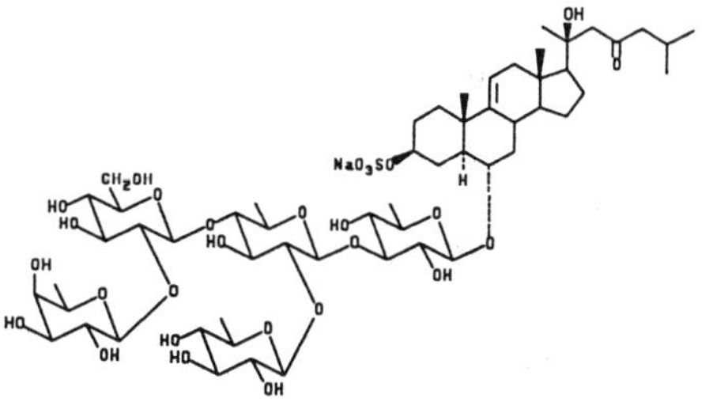

Mol. Wt.: 1282
Bioactivity: L1210: IC_{50} 10 μg/ml
KB: IC_{50} 10 μg/ml
Melting Point: >300°C (dec.)
$[\alpha]_D$: -6.59 Solvent: Py
Spectral Data: IR, CMR, Mass Spec.
Organism: *Asterina pectinifera* Muller et Troschel (Echinodermata)
Location: Fukuoka, Japan
Reference: 247, 822

$C_{59}H_{82}O_{21}$ **Norhalichondrin A**

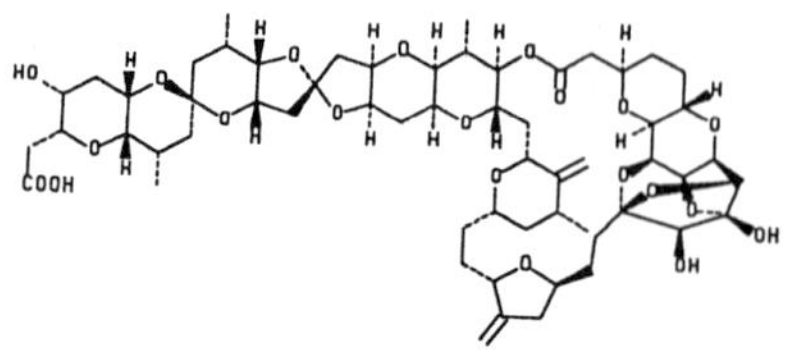

Mol. Wt.: 1128
Bioactivity: B16: IC_{50} 5.2 ng/ml
$[\alpha]_D$: -47.8 Solvent: Me
Spectral Data: IR, CMR, PMR, Mass Spec., CD, x-ray c.s. of derivatives
Organism: *Halichondria okadai* (Porifera)
Location: Japan
Reference: 423, 1121

$C_{60}H_{86}O_{19}$ **Halichondrin B**

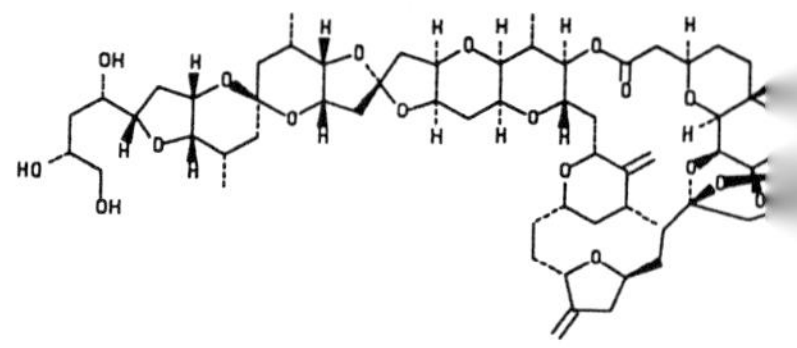

Mol. Wt.: 1112
Bioactivity: L1210: T/C >375 (100 μg/kg)
P388: T/C 323 (10.0 μg/kg)
B16: T/C 244 (5.0 μg/kg)
B16: IC_{50} 0.093 ng/ml
Melting Point: 164–166°C
$[\alpha]_D$: -58.9 Solvent: Me
Spectral Data: CMR, PMR, Mass Spec., IR of acetate
Organism: *Halichondria okadai* (Porifera)
Location: Japan
Reference: 423

$C_{60}H_{86}O_{20}$ **Halichondrin C**

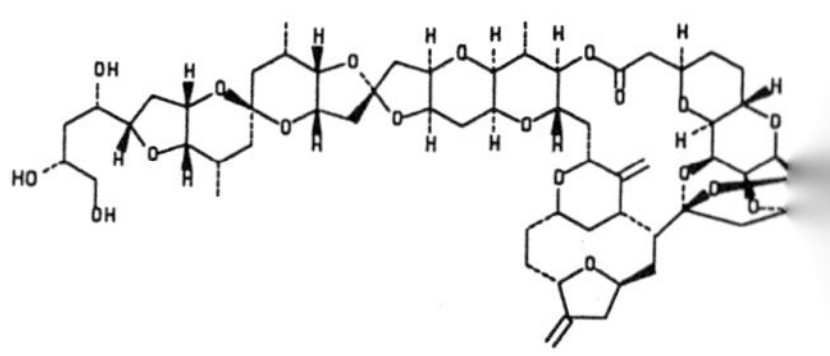

Mol. Wt.: 1128
Bioactivity: B16: IC_{50} 0.35 ng/ml
Melting Point: 169–172°C
$[\alpha]_D$: -41.6 Solvent: Me
Spectral Data: CMR, PMR, Mass Spec.
Organism: *Halichondria okadai* (Porifera)
Location: Japan
Reference: 423

$C_{61}H_{86}O_{19}$ **Homohalichondrin B**

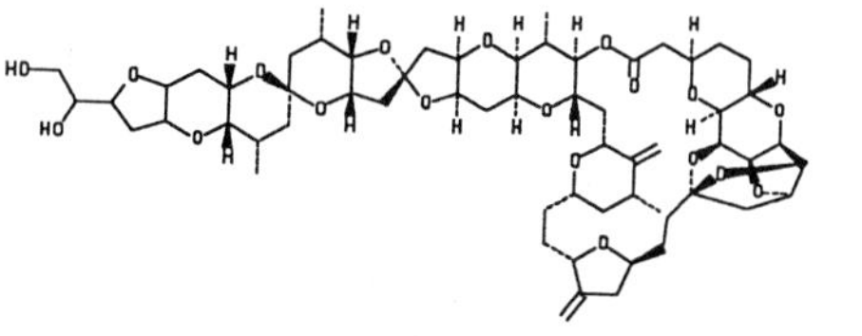

Mol. Wt.: 1124
Bioactivity: B16: IC_{50} 0.1 ng/ml
Spectral Data: PMR, Mass Spec.
Organism: *Halichondria okadai* (Porifera)
Location: Japan
Reference: 423

$C_{61}H_{86}O_{21}$ **Homohalichondrin A**

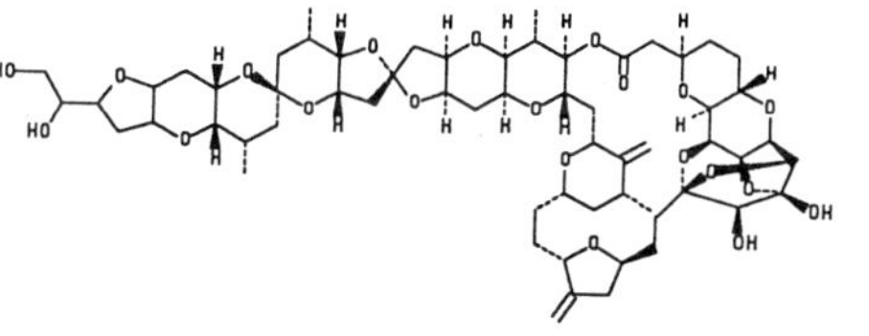

Mol. Wt.: 1156
Bioactivity: B16: IC_{50} 0.26 ng/ml
$[\alpha]_D$: -97.1 Solvent: Me
Spectral Data: CMR, PMR, Mass Spec.
Organism: *Halichondria okadai* (Porifera)
Location: Japan
Reference: 423

$C_{62}H_{100}N_2O_{26}$ **Sarasinoside A_1**

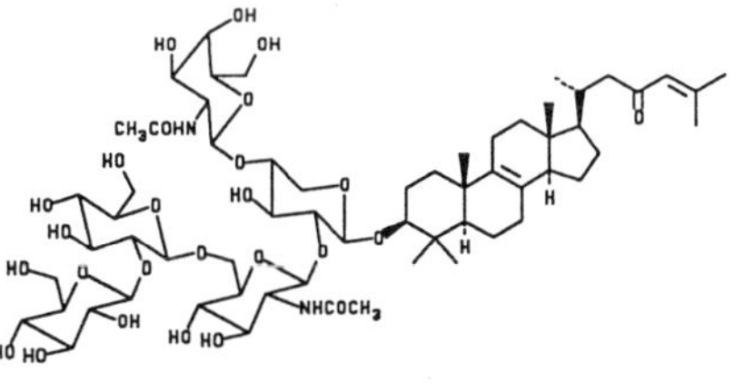

Mol. Wt.: 1290
Bioactivity: P388: ED_{50} 2.8 μg/ml
Ichthyotoxic to *Poecilia reticulata:* LD_{50} 0.39 μg/ml
Starfish egg assay: LD_{50} 10 μg/ml
Melting Point: 208–212°C
$[\alpha]_D$: –14 Solvent: Me
Spectral Data: UV, IR, CMR, PMR, Mass Spec., x-ray c.s. of the aglycone
Organism: *Asteropus sarasinosum*
Asteropus sp.
(Porifera)
Location: Guam, Truk, Palau
Reference: 567, 568, 985

$C_{62}H_{101}NaO_{32}S$ **Pectinioside E**

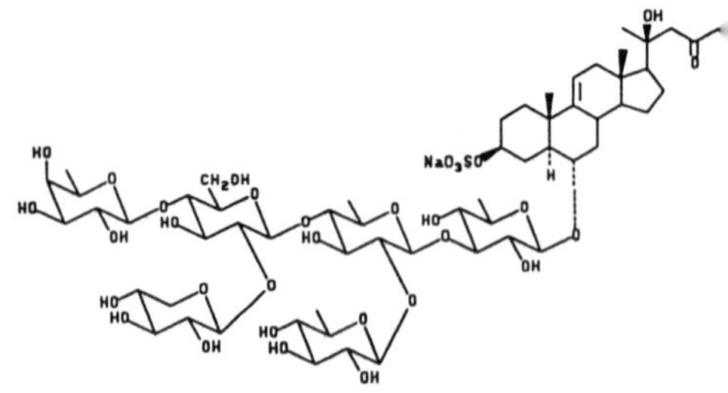

Mol. Wt.: 1414
Bioactivity: L1210: IC_{50} 8.8 μg/ml
KB: IC_{50} 11.5 μg/ml
Melting Point: 225–230°C
$[\alpha]_D^{25}$: -13 Solvent: Aq
Spectral Data: IR, CMR, PMR, Mass Spec.
Organism: *Asterina pectinifera* Muller et Troschel (Echinodermata)
Location: Fukuoka, Japan
Reference: 247

$C_{64}H_{105}NaO_{32}S$ **Pectinioside C**

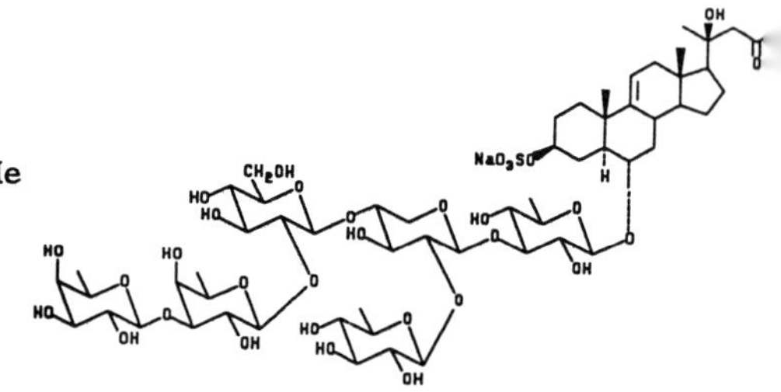

Mol. Wt.: 1442
Bioactivity: L1210: IC_{50} 11.0 μg/ml
KB: IC_{50} 10.8 μg/ml
Melting Point: 230–235°C (dec.)
$[\alpha]_D$: +5.38 Solvent: Me
Spectral Data: CD, IR, CMR, Mass Spec.
Organism: *Asterina pectinifera* (Echinodermata)
Location: Fukuoka, Japan
Reference: 247, 248

$C_{74}H_{128}O_{20}$ **Bistheonellide A** (syn. **Misakinolide A**)

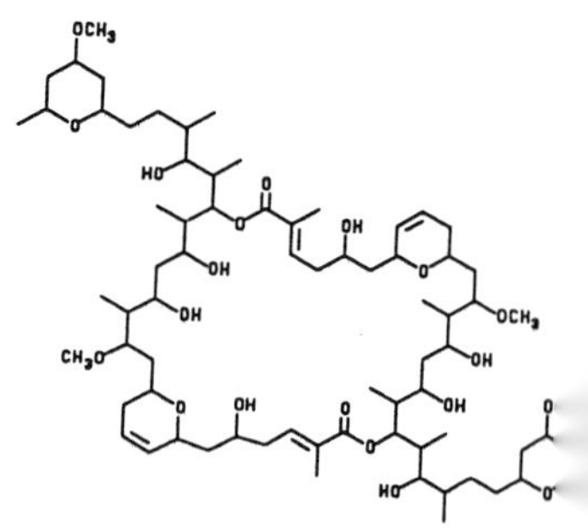

Mol. Wt.: 1338
Bioactivity: P388: IC_{50} 0.01 μg/ml
HCT, A549, and MD-AMB-231: IC_{50} 0.0005–0.005 μg/ml
L1210: IC_{50} 0.035 μg/ml
P388 (ip): T/C 140 (0.31 mg/kg)
Fertilized starfish egg assay: inhibition at 0.1 μg/ml
Antifungal activity
Melting Point: Oil
$[\alpha]_D^{20}$: -30 Solvent: Alc
Spectral Data: UV, IR, CMR, PMR, Mass Spec.
Organism: *Theonella* sp. (Porifera)
Location: Japan
Reference: 528, 529, 964

Kentin

Mol. Wt.:	18,000
Bioactivity:	Cytolytic activity
Organism:	*Stoichactis kenti* (Coelenterata)
Location:	Indo-Pacific
Reference:	64

Total Syntheses

Compound	Activity	Reference
Hydroxytopsentin	P388: IC_{50} 0.3 μg/ml	1110
Isotopsentin	P388: IC_{50} 4.0 μg/ml Antiviral activity	1110
Naphthoquinone hypotaurine derivative	P388: ED_{50} 2.9 μg/ml	982
Neoisotopsentin	P388: IC_{50} 1.8 μg/ml	1110
Neotopsentin	P388: IC_{50} 2.5 μg/ml	1110

Chapter 12 MARINE CHORDATA AND OTHER HIGHER ANIMAL BIOSYNTHETIC PRODUCTS

$C_8H_7BrO_4$ **(4S,5R,6R)-4-Acetoxy-2-bromo-5,6-epoxycyclohex-2-enone**

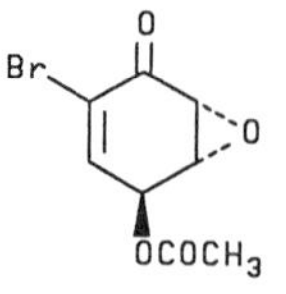

Mol. Wt.:	247
Bioactivity:	P388: IC_{50} 10 ng/ml
Melting Point:	93–94°C
$[\alpha]_D^{19}$:	+265 Solvent: Chf
Spectral Data:	IR, PMR, Mass Spec., x-ray c.s.
Organism:	*Ptychodera* sp (Chordata/Hemichordata)
Location:	Maui, Hawaii
Reference:	418

$C_8H_8Br_2O_4$ **(4S,5R,6S)-4-Acetoxy-2,6-dibromo-5-hydroxycyclohex-2-enone**

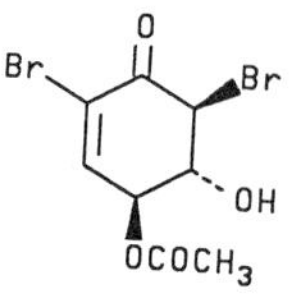

Mol. Wt.:	328
Bioactivity:	Antifeedant P388 cytotoxicity
Melting Point:	136–138°C
$[\alpha]_D^{25}$:	+109.7 Solvent: Chf
Spectral Data:	UV, IR, CMR, PMR, Mass Spec., x-ray c.s.
Organism:	*Ptychodera* sp. (Chordata/Hemichordata)
Location:	Maui, Hawaii
Reference:	418

$C_8H_{10}Br_2O_4$ **(1R,4S,5R,6S)-4-Acetoxy-2,6-dibromo-1,5-dihydroxycyclohexene**

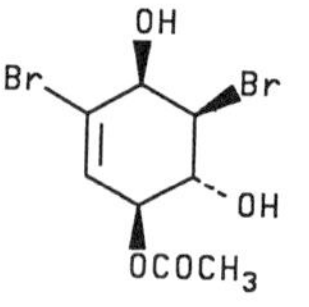

Mol Wt.:	330
Bioactivity:	P388 cytotoxicity
Melting Point:	150.5–151.5°C
Spectral Data:	IR, PMR, Mass Spec., x-ray c.s.
Organism:	*Ptychodera* sp. (Chordata/Hemichordata)
Location:	Maui, Hawaii
Reference:	418

$C_{11}H_{14}O_4$ **Didemnenone C**

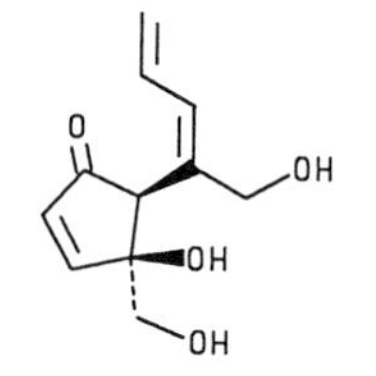

Mol. Wt.: 210
Bioactivity: L1210: IC_{50} 5.6 μg/ml
$[\alpha]_D$: −25.3 Solvent: Me
Spectral Data: UV, IR, CMR, PMR, Mass Spec.
Organism: *Didemnum voeltzkowi* (Chordata/Tunicata)
Location: Fiji
Reference: 661

$C_{11}H_{14}O_4$ **Didemnenone D**

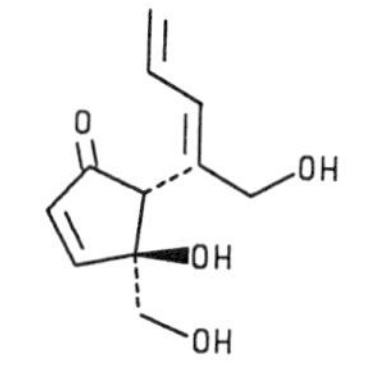

Mol. Wt.: 210
Bioactivity: L1210: IC_{50} 5.6 μg/ml
$[\alpha]_D$: −12.6 Solvent: Me
Spectral Data: UV, IR, CMR, PMR, Mass Spec.
Organism: *Didemnum voeltzkowi* (Chordata/Tunicata)
Location: Fiji
Reference: 661

$C_{14}H_{16}BrN_3O_2S$ **Eudistomin K sulfoxide**

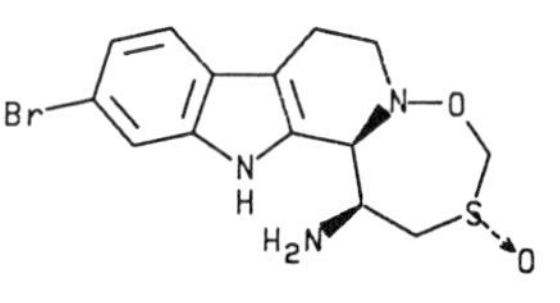

Mol. Wt.: 370
Bioactivity: Antiviral activity towards *Herpes simplex* Type 1 and Polio Type 1
Melting Point: Oil
$[\alpha]_D^{25}$: −3.3 Solvent: Me
Spectral Data: UV, IR, CMR, PMR; UV, CMR, PMR, Mass Spec. of acetate
Organism: *Ritterella sigillinoides* (Chordata/Tunicata)
Location: New Zealand
Reference: 631

$C_{16}H_{22}O_2$ **Cordiachromene A**
(CCA)

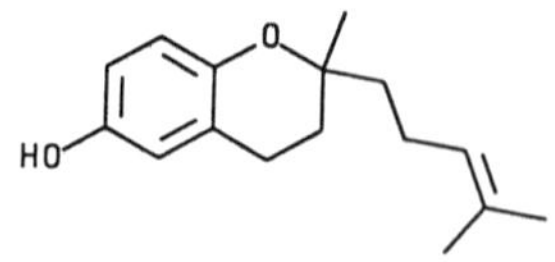

Mol. Wt. 246
Bioactivity: KB: IC_{50} 36 μg/ml
P388: IC_{50} 0.5 μg/ml
Antibacterial activity
(gram positive)
Organism: *Aplidium antillense* Gravier
A. constellatum
(Chordata/Tunicata)
Location: Guadeloupe; Georgia
Reference: 60, 1083

$C_{16}H_{22}O_2$ **Geranyl hydroquinone**
(GHQ)

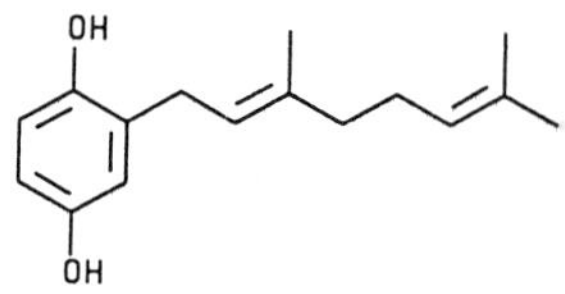

Mol. Wt.: 246
Bioactivity: KB: IC_{50} 4.3 μg/ml
P388: IC_{50} 0.034 μg/ml
Antibacterial activity
(gram positive)
Organism: *Aplidium antillense* Gravier
(Chordata/Tunicata)
Location: Guadeloupe
Reference: 60

$C_{18}H_8BrN_3O$ **2-Bromoleptoclinidinone**

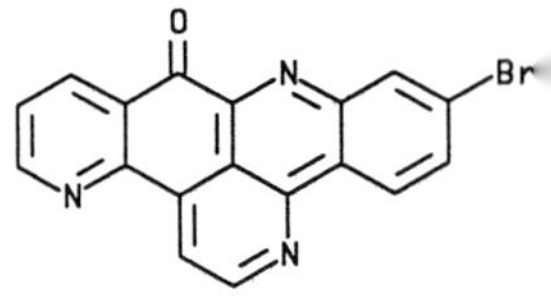

Mol. Wt.: 362
Bioactivity: P388: ED_{50} 0.4 μg/ml
Melting Point: >300°C
Spectral Data: UV, IR, CMR, PMR, Mass Spec.
Organism: *Leptoclinides* sp. (tentative)
(Chordata/Tunicata)
Location: Truk
Reference: 79

$C_{18}H_9N_3O$ **Ascididemin**

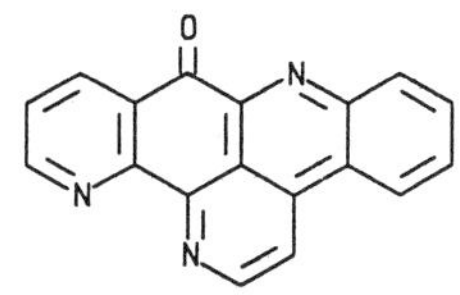

Mol. Wt.:	283
Bioactivity:	L1210: IC_{50} 0.39 μg/ml Ca- releasing activity
Melting Point:	>300°C
Spectral Data:	UV, IR, CMR, PMR, Mass Spec.
Organism:	*Didemnum* sp. (Chordata/Tunicata)
Location:	Okinawa, Japan
Reference:	576

$C_{18}H_{34}N_2O$ **Pseudodistomin A**

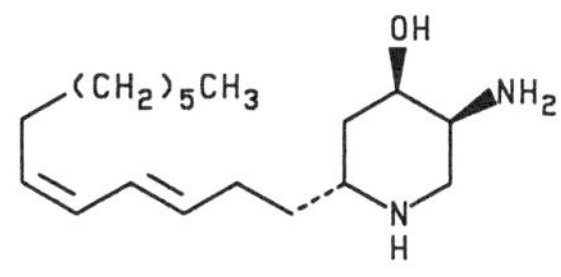

Mol. Wt.:	294
Bioactivity:	L1210: IC_{50} 2.5 μg/ml L5178Y: IC_{50} 2.4 μg/ml Calmodulin antagonist
Melting Point:	Oil (acetate)
$[\alpha]_D^{24}$:	+36 Solvent: Me (acetate)
Spectral Data:	UV, IR, CMR, PMR, Mass Spec. (acetate)
Organism:	*Pseudodistoma kanoko* Tokioka et Nishikawa (Chordata/Tunicata)
Location:	Okinawa, Japan
Reference:	467

$C_{18}H_{34}N_2O$ **Pseudodistomin B**

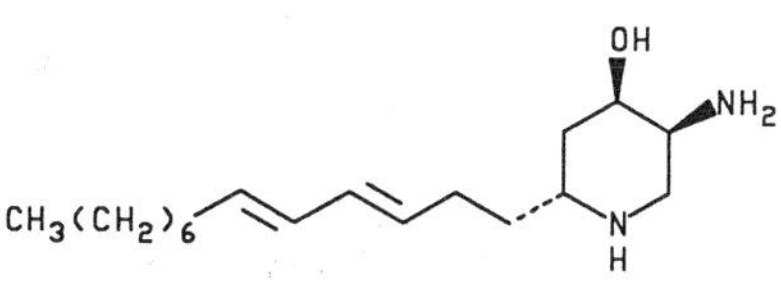

Mol. Wt.:	294
Bioactivity:	L1210: IC_{50} 0.4 μg/ml L5178Y: IC_{50} 0.7 μg/ml Calmodulin antagonist
Melting Point:	Oil (acetate)
$[\alpha]_D^{24}$:	+35 Solvent: Me (acetate)
Spectral Data:	UV, IR, CMR, PMR, Mass Spec. (acetate)
Organism:	*Pseudodistoma kanoko* Tokioka et Nishikawa (Chordata/Tunicata)
Location:	Okinawa, Japan
Reference:	467

$C_{22}H_{19}N_3O_2$ **Cystodytins A and B (mixture)**

Mol. Wt.: 357
Bioactivity: L1210: IC_{50} 0.22 μg/ml
Ca- releasing activity
Melting Point: 181–183°C
Spectral Data: UV, IR, Mass Spec.; CMR, PMR (A); CMR, PMR (B)
Organism: *Cystodytes dellechiajei* (Chordata/Tunicata)
Location: Okinawa, Japan
Reference: 578

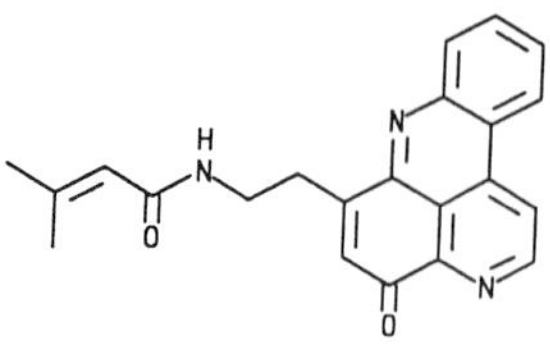

A

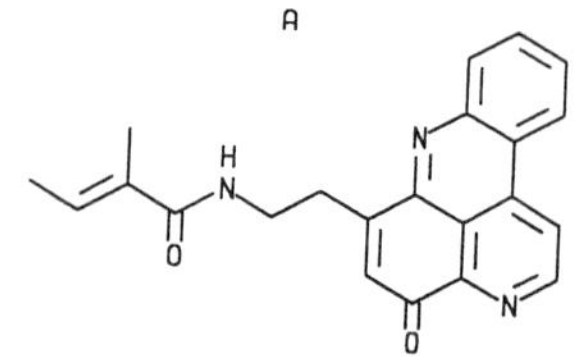

B

$C_{22}H_{21}N_3O_3$ **Cystodytin C**

Mol. Wt.: 375
Bioactivity: L1210: IC_{50} 0.24 μg/ml
Ca- releasing activity
Melting Point: 257–259°C
Spectral Data: UV, IR, CMR, PMR, Mass Spec.
Organism: *Cystodytes dellechiajei* (Chordata/Tunicata)
Location: Okinawa, Japan
Reference: 578

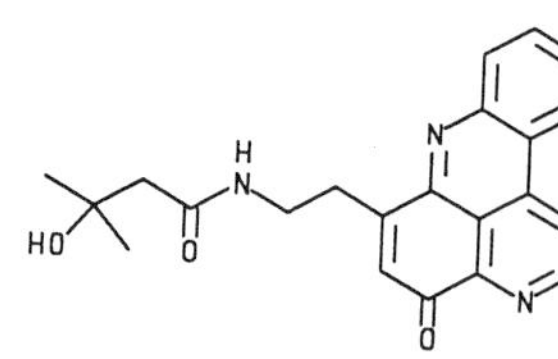

$C_{36}H_{52}N_8O_6S_2$ **Ascidiacyclamide (previously known)**

Mol. Wt.: 756
Bioactivity: Cytotoxic
Spectral Data: x-ray c.s.
Organism: *Ascidian* sp. (Chordata/Tunicata)
Reference: 468

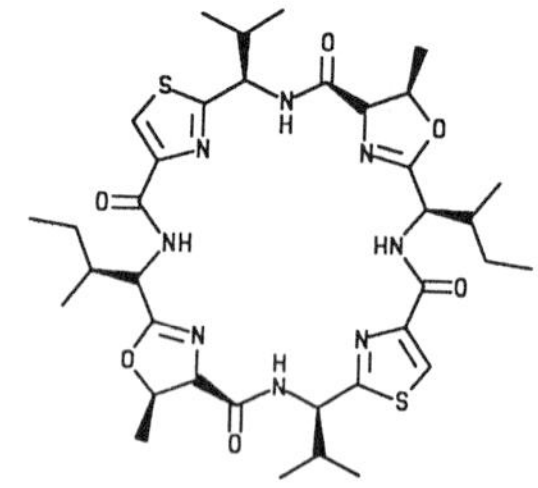

$C_{40}H_{58}N_2O_7$ **Iejimalide A**

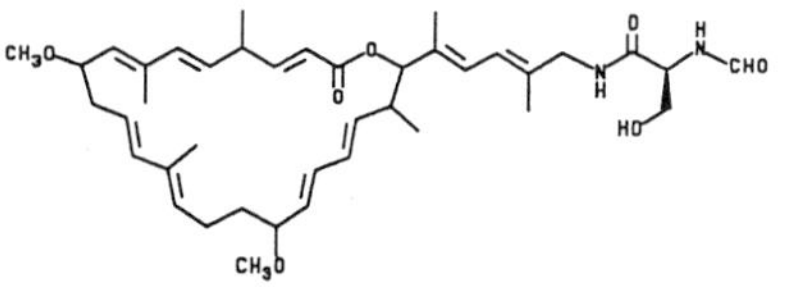

Mol. Wt.: 678
Bioactivity: L1210: IC_{50} 62 ng/ml
L5178Y: IC_{50} 22 ng/ml
Melting Point: 71–73°C
$[\alpha]_D^{23}$: −36.4 Solvent: Chf
Spectral Data: UV, IR, CMR, PMR, Mass Spec.
Organism: *Eudistoma* cf. *rigida*
(Chordata/Tunicata)
Location: Okinawa, Japan
Reference: 577

$C_{40}H_{68}N_2O_8$ **Bistramide A**

Mol. Wt.: 705
Bioactivity: Cytotoxicity
Neurotoxicity
Spectral Data: CMR, PMR, Mass Spec.
Organism: *Lissoclinum bistratum* Sluiter
(Chordata/Tunicata)
Location: New Caledonia
Reference: 355

$C_{41}H_{60}N_2O_7$ **Iejimalide B**

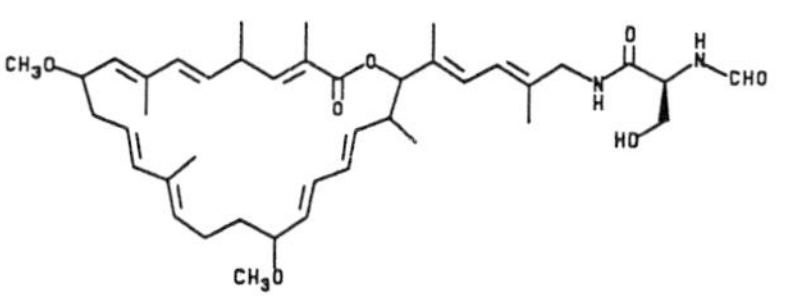

Mol. Wt.: 692
Bioactivity: L1210: IC_{50} 32 ng/ml
L5178Y: IC_{50} 1.0 ng/ml
Melting Point: 69–71°C
$[\alpha]_D^{23}$: −17.6 Solvent: Chf
Spectral Data: UV, IR, CMR, PMR, Mass Spec.
Organism: *Eudistoma* cf. *rigida*
(Chordata/Tunicata)
Location: Okinawa, Japan
Reference: 577

$C_{49}H_{77}NO_{11}S$ **Patellazole A**

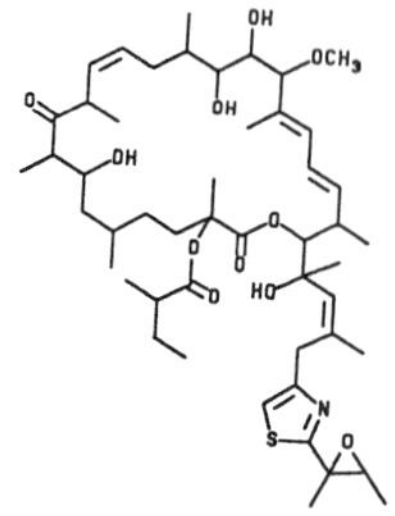

Mol. Wt.: 889
Bioactivity: Cytotoxicity: Human cell lines: IC_{50} 10^{-3}–10^{-6} μg/ml
Antifungal activity towards *Candida albicans*
Organism: *Lissoclinum patella* (Chordata/Tunicata)
Location: Fiji
Reference: 1216

$C_{49}H_{77}NO_{12}S$ **Patellazole B**

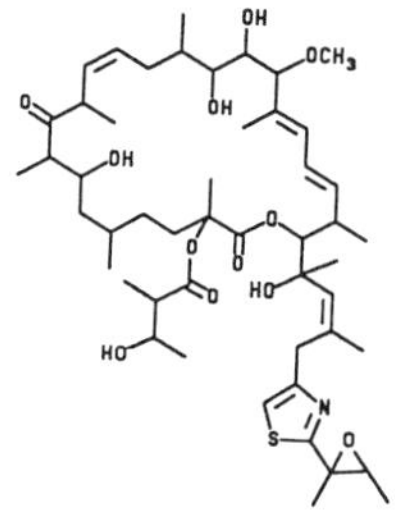

Mol. Wt.: 905
Bioactivity: KB: IC_{50} 300 pg/ml
Human cell lines: IC_{50} 10^{-3}–10^{-6} μg/ml
Antifungal activity towards *Candida albicans*
Spectral Data: UV, IR, CMR, PMR, Mass Spec.
Organism: *Lissoclinum patella* (Chordata/Tunicata)
Location: Guam, Fiji
Reference: 200, 1216

$C_{49}H_{77}NO_{13}S$ **Patellazole C**

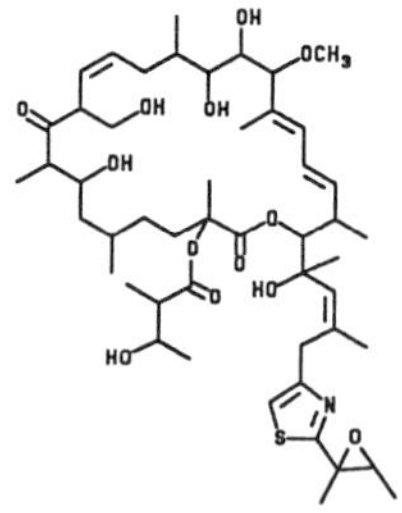

Mol. Wt.: 921
Bioactivity: Human cell lines: IC_{50} 10^{-3}–10^{-6} μg/ml
Antifungal activity towards *Candida albicans*
$[\alpha]_D$: −100° Solvent: Dcm
Spectral Data: UV, IR, CMR, PMR, Mass Spec.
Organism: *Lissoclinum patella* (Chordata/Tunicata)
Location: Fiji
Reference: 1216

$C_{54}H_{74}N_2O_{10}$ **Cephalostatin 1**

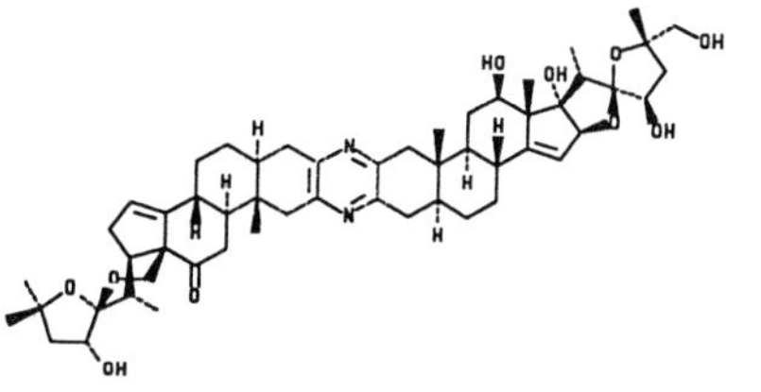

Mol. Wt.: 912
Bioactivity: P388: ED_{50} 10^{-7}–10^{-9} μg/ml
Melting Point: 326°C (dec.)
$[\alpha]_D$: +102 Solvent: Me
Spectral Data: UV, IR, CMR, PMR, Mass Spec., x-ray c.s.
Organism: *Cephalodiscus gilchristi* (Chordata/Hemichordata)
Location: Indian Ocean
Reference: 885

$C_{54}H_{74}N_2O_{11}$ **Cephalostatin 2**

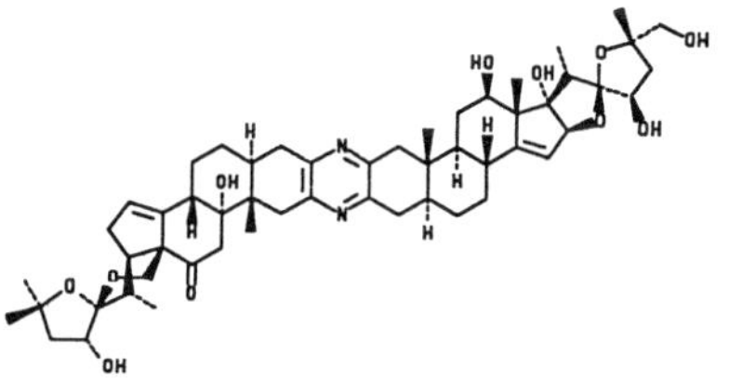

Mol. Wt.: 928
Bioactivity: P388: ED_{50} 10^{-7}–10^{-9} μg/ml
Melting Point: >350°C
$[\alpha]_D$: +111 Solvent: Me
Spectral Data: UV, IR, CMR, PMR, Mass Spec.
Organism: *Cephalodiscus gilchristi* (Chordata/Hemichordata)
Location: Indian Ocean
Reference: 884

$C_{54}H_{74}N_2O_{12}$ **Cephalostatin 4**

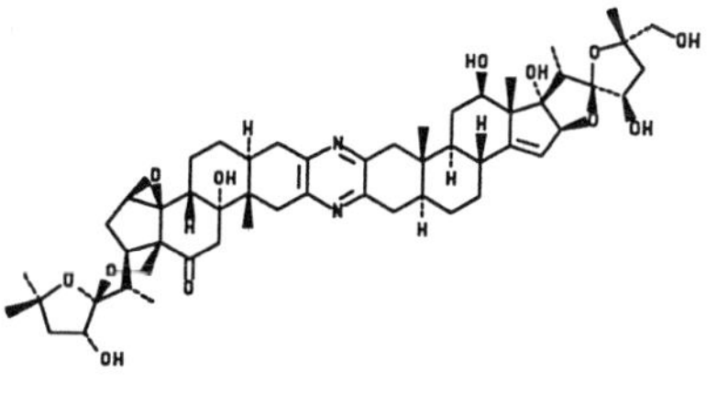

Mol. Wt.: 944
Bioactivity: P388: ED_{50} 10^{-7}–10^{-9} μg/ml
Melting Point: >350°C
$[\alpha]_D$: +89 Solvent: Me
Spectral Data: UV, IR, CMR, PMR, Mass Spec.
Organism: *Cephalodiscus gilchristi* (Chordata/Hemichordata)
Location: Indian Ocean
Reference: 884

$C_{55}H_{76}N_2O_{11}$ **Cephalostatin 3**

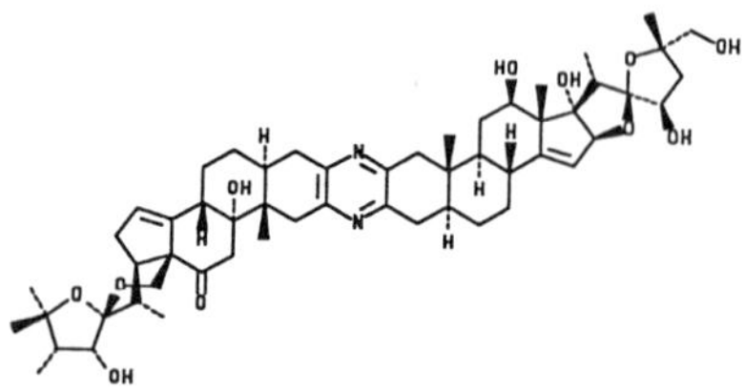

Mol. Wt.: 942
Bioactivity: P388: ED_{50} 10^{-7}–10^{-9} μg/ml
Melting Point: >350°C
$[\alpha]_D$: +99 Solvent: Me
Spectral Data: UV, IR, CMR, PMR, Mass Spec.
Organism: *Cephalodiscus gilchristi* (Chordata/Hemichordata)
Location: Indian Ocean
Reference: 884

Cartilage inducing factor A (CIF A)

Mol. Wt.: 24,000
Bioactivity: CCl 64: 50% inhibition at 0.5 ng/ml
A549: 55% inhibition at 10 ng/ml
2981: 52% inhibition at 10 ng/ml
A375: 45% inhibition at 10 ng/ml
MCF7: 58% inhibition at 10 ng/ml
A431: 30% inhibition at 10 ng/ml
Stimulation of DNA synthesis in normal cells
Inhibition of growth of A549 tumor colonies
Organism: *Bos* sp. (Chordata/Vertebrata)
Reference: 913

Cartilage inducing factor B (CIF B)

Mol. Wt.: 24,000
Bioactivity: CCl 64: 50% inhibition at 0.5 ng/ml
A549: 48% inhibition at 10 ng/ml
2981: 46% inhibition at 10 ng/ml
A375: 52% inhibition at 10 ng/ml
A431: 23% inhibition at 10 ng/ml
MCF7: 60% inhibition at 10 ng/ml
Stimulation of DNA synthesis in normal cells
Inhibition of growth of A549 tumor colonies
Organism: *Bos* sp. (Chordata/Vertebrata)
Reference: 913

Sarcophaga lectin

Mol. Wt.:	~94,000
Bioactivity:	Antitumor activity against both ascitic and solid Sarcoma 180 tumors
Organism:	*Sarcophaga peregrina* (Arthropoda)
Reference:	479

Section B

MARINE ANIMAL BIOSYNTHETIC PRODUCTS

Chapter 13 HYDROCARBONS, ALCOHOLS, AND ESTERS

$C_9H_{14}Br_2O_2$ **9,9-Dibromonon-8-enoic acid**

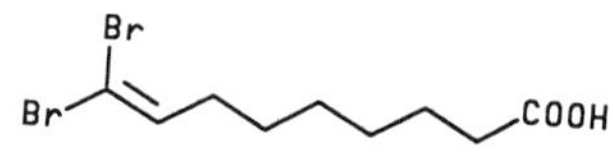

Mol. Wt.: 314
Bioactivity: Antibacterial activity against *Bacillus subtilis*
Spectral Data: UV, IR, CMR, PMR, Mass Spec. (of methyl ester)
Organism: *Xestospongia* sp. (Porifera)
Location: Gulf of Eilat, Red Sea
Reference: 427

$C_{15}H_{19}BrO$ **Cupalaurenol**

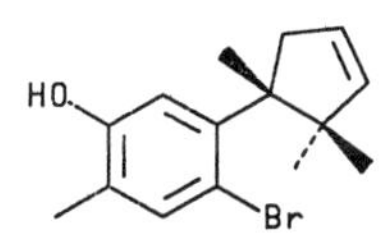

Mol. Wt.: 295
Bioactivity: Antibacterial activity against *Bacillus subtilis*
Antifungal activity against *Aspergillus* sp. and *Trichoderma* sp.
Ichthyotoxicity against guppies at 5–10 ppm
Melting Point: Oil
$[\alpha]_D^{19}$: +87.9 Solvent: Chf
Spectral Data: UV, IR, PMR, Mass Spec.
Organism: *Aplysia dactylomela* (Mollusca)
Laurencia pinnata Yamada (Rhodophyta)
Location: Okinawa and Nagasaki, Japan
Reference: 324, 325, 448

$C_{15}H_{19}BrO$ **Cyclolaurenol**

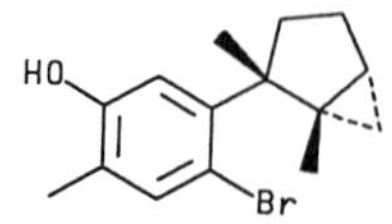

Mol. Wt.: 295
Bioactivity: Antibacterial activity against *Bacillus subtilis*
Antifungal activity against *Aspergillus* sp.
Ichthyotoxicity against guppies at 5–10 ppm
Melting Point: 109–109.5°C
$[\alpha]_D^{21}$: -9.3 Solvent: Chf
Spectral Data: UV, IR, PMR, Mass Spec.
Organism: *Aplysia dactylomela* (Mollusca)
Location: Okinawa, Japan
Reference: 448

$C_{15}H_{20}$ **Cyclolaurene**

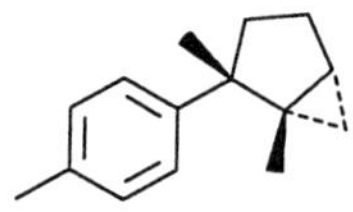

Mol. Wt.: 200
Melting Point: Oil
$[\alpha]_D$: -9.0 Solvent: Chf
Spectral Data: IR, PMR, Mass Spec.
Organism: *Aplysia dactylomela* (Mollusca)
Location: Okinawa, Japan
Reference: 448

$C_{16}H_{17}BrO_2$ **16-Bromohexadeca-7(E),11(E), 15(E)-trien-5,13-diynoic acid**

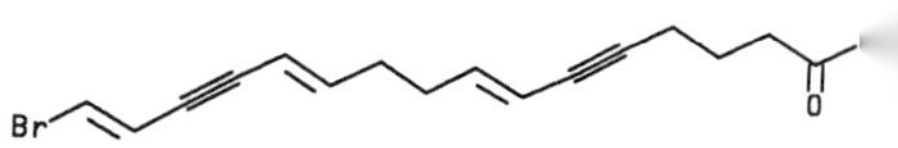

Mol. Wt.: 321
Bioactivity: Antibacterial activity against *Bacillus subtilis*
Spectral Data: IR, CMR, PMR, UV and Mass Spec. of methyl ester
Organism: *Xestospongia* sp. (Porifera)
Location: Gulf of Eilat, Red Sea
Reference: 427

$C_{16}H_{17}BrO_2$ **16-Bromohexadeca-7(E),11(E),15(Z)-trien-5,13-diynoic acid**

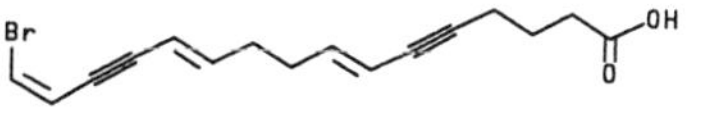

Mol. Wt.: 321
Bioactivity: Antibacterial activity against *Bacillus subtilis*
Spectral Data: UV, IR, CMR, PMR, Mass Spec. (of methyl ester)
Organism: *Xestospongia* sp. (Porifera)
Location: Gulf of Eilat, Red Sea
Reference: 427

$C_{16}H_{19}BrO_2$ **16-Bromohexadeca-7(E),15(E)-dien-5,13-diynoic acid**

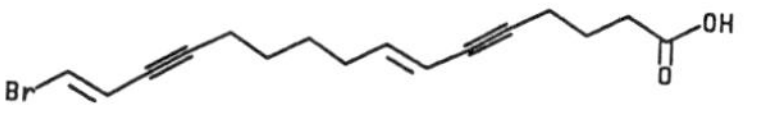

Mol. Wt.: 323
Bioactivity: Antibacterial activity against *Bacillus subtilis*
Spectral Data: UV, IR, CMR, PMR (of methyl ester)
Organism: *Xestospongia* sp. (Porifera)
Location: Gulf of Eilat, Red Sea
Reference: 427

$C_{16}H_{26}O_3$ **Raspailyne B2**

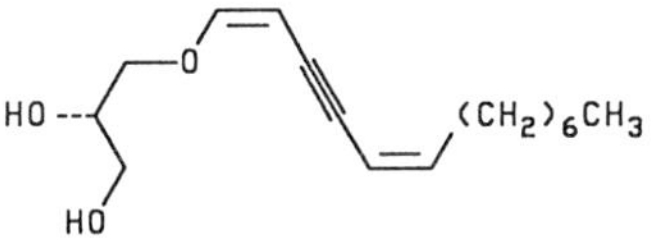

Mol. Wt.: 266
Melting Point: Oil
$[\alpha]_D^{22}$: -10.8 Solvent: Chf
Spectral Data: UV, IR, CMR, PMR, Mass Spec.
Organism: *Raspailia pumila* Bowerbank
R. ramosa Bowerbank
(Porifera)
Location: Brittany, France
Reference: 370

$C_{17}H_{21}BrO_2$ **Cupalaurenol acetate**

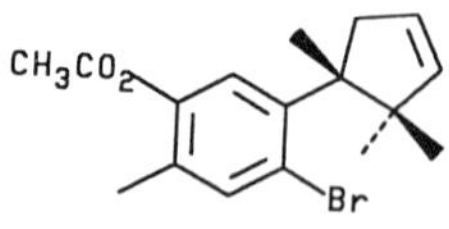

Mol. Wt.: 337
Bioactivity: Antibacterial activity against *Bacillus subtilis*
Antifungal activity against *Aspergillus* sp.
Ichthyotoxicity against guppies at 5–10 ppm
$[\alpha]_D^{19}$: +65.1 Solvent: Chf
Spectral Data: UV, IR, PMR, Mass Spec.
Organism: *Aplysia dactylomela* (Mollusca)
Location: Okinawa, Japan
Reference: 448

$C_{17}H_{21}BrO_2$ **Cyclolaurenol acetate**

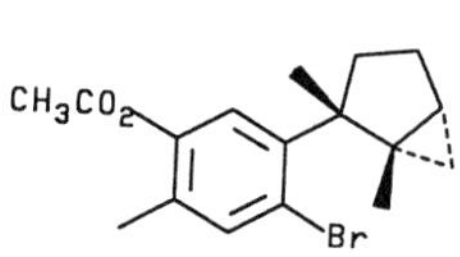

Mol. Wt: 337
Bioactivity: Antibacterial activity against *Bacillus subtilis*
Ichthyotoxicity against guppies at 5–10 ppm
$[\alpha]_D^{19}$: −9.2 Solvent: Chf
Spectral Data: UV, IR, PMR, Mass Spec.
Organism: *Aplysia dactylomela* (Mollusca)
Location: Okinawa, Japan
Reference: 448

$C_{17}H_{24}O_2$ **Tochuinyl acetate**

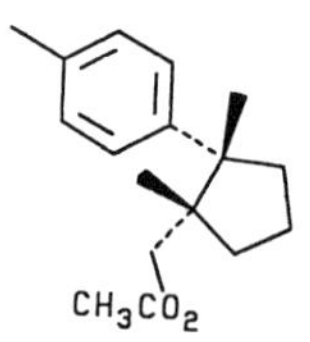

Mol. Wt.: 260
Melting Point: Oil
$[\alpha]_D^{25}$: −42.5 Solvent: Dcm
Spectral Data: IR, CMR, PMR, Mass Spec.
Organism: *Tochuina tetraquetra* (Mollusca)
Gersemia rubiformis (Coelenterata)
Location: British Columbia
Reference: 1179

$C_{17}H_{26}O_2$ **Dihydrotochuinyl acetate**

Mol. Wt.: 262
Melting Point: Oil
$[\alpha]_D^{25}$: −29.3 Solvent: Dcm
Spectral Data: IR, CMR, PMR, Mass Spec.
Organism: *Tochuina tetraquetra* (Mollusca)
Gersemia rubiformis (Coelenterata)
Location: British Columbia
Reference: 1179

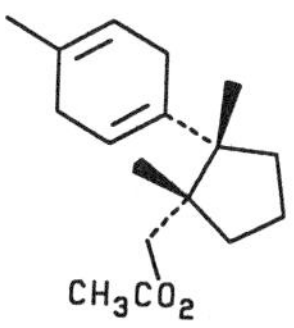

$C_{17}H_{28}O_3$ **Isoraspailyne B1**

Mol. Wt.: 280
Melting Point: Oil
Spectral Data: UV, IR, CMR, PMR, Mass Spec.
Organism: *Raspailia pumila* Bowerbank
R. ramosa Bowerbank
(Porifera)
Location: Brittany, France
Reference: 370

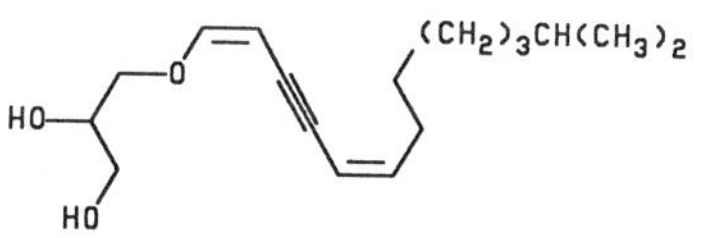

$C_{17}H_{28}O_3$ **Isoraspailyne B1a**

Mol. Wt.: 280
Melting Point: Oil
Spectral Data: UV, IR, CMR, PMR, Mass Spec.
Organism: *Raspailia pumila* Bowerbank
R. ramosa Bowerbank
(Porifera)
Location: Brittany, France
Reference: 370

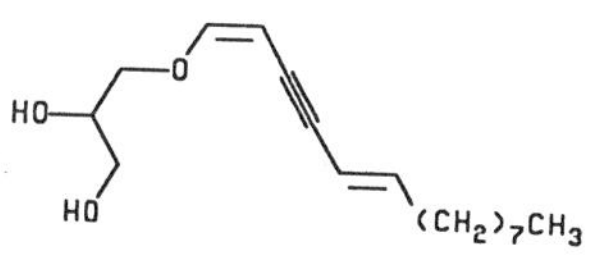

$C_{17}H_{28}O_3$ **Isoraspailyne B1b**

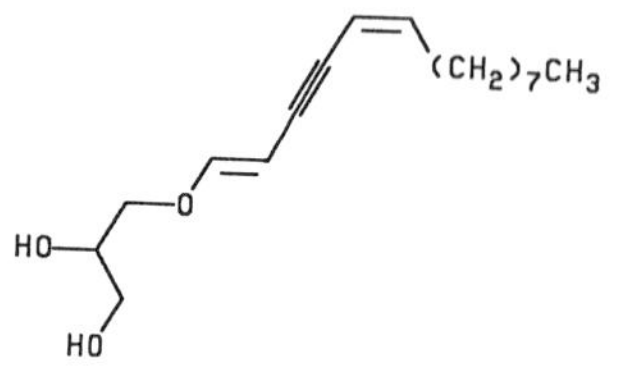

Mol. Wt.: 280
Melting Point: Oil
Spectral Data: UV, IR, PMR, Mass Spec.
Organism: *Raspailia pumila* Bowerbank
R. ramosa Bowerbank
(Porifera)
Location: Brittany, France
Reference: 370

$C_{17}H_{28}O_3$ **Raspailyne B1**

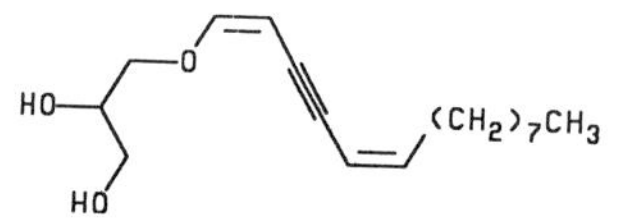

Mol. Wt.: 280
Melting Point: Oil
$[\alpha]_D^{22}$: −4.9 Solvent: Chf
Spectral Data: UV, IR, CMR, PMR, Mass Spec.
Organism: *Raspailia pumila* Bowerbank
R. ramosa Bowerbank
(Porifera)
Location: Brittany, France
Reference: 370, 371

$C_{18}H_{22}Br_2O_2$ **18,18-Dibromooctadeca-9(E), 17(E)-dien-5,7-diynoic acid**

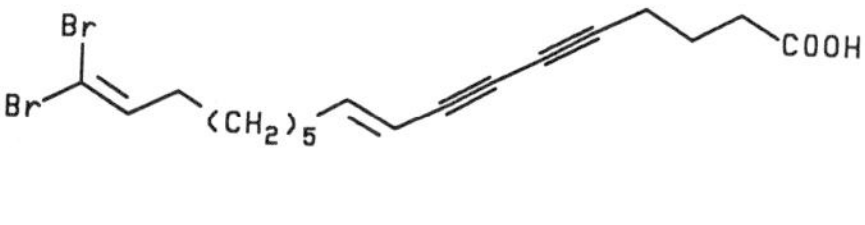

Mol. Wt.: 430
Bioactivity: Antibacterial activity against *Bacillus subtilis*
Spectral Data: UV, IR, CMR, PMR, Mass Spec. (of methyl ester)
Organism: *Xestospongia* sp.
(Porifera)
Location: Gulf of Eilat, Red Sea
Reference: 427

$C_{18}H_{30}O_3$ **Isoraspailyne B**

Mol. Wt.: 294
Melting Point: Oil
Spectral Data: UV, IR, CMR, PMR, Mass Spec.
Organism: *Raspailia pumila* Bowerbank
R. ramosa Bowerbank
(Porifera)
Location: Brittany, France
Reference: 370

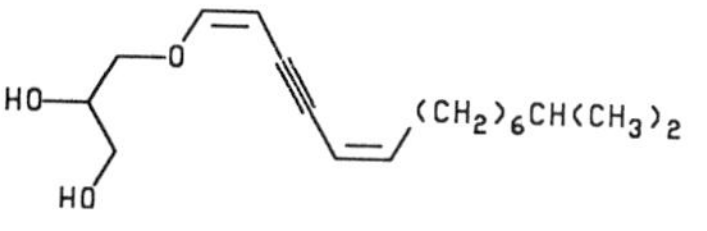

$C_{18}H_{30}O_3$ **Isoraspailyne Ba**

Mol. Wt.: 294
Melting Point: Oil
Spectral Data: UV, IR, CMR, PMR, Mass Spec.
Organism: *Raspailia pumila* Bowerbank
R. ramosa Bowerbank
(Porifera)
Location: Brittany, France
Reference: 370

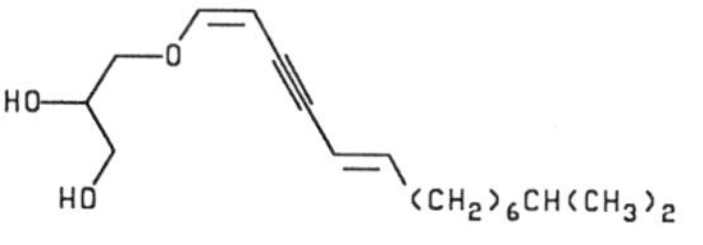

$C_{18}H_{30}O_3$ **Raspailyne B**

Mol. Wt.: 294
Melting Point: Oil
Spectral Data: UV, IR, CMR, PMR, Mass Spec.
Organism: *Raspailia pumila* Bowerbank
R. ramosa Bowerbank
(Porifera)
Location: Brittany, France
Reference: 370

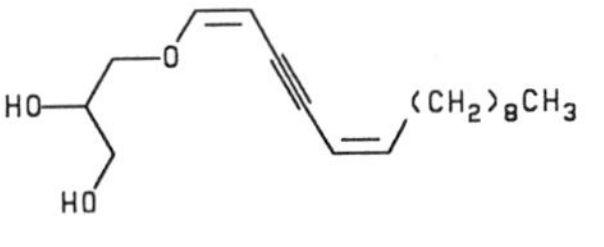

$C_{19}H_{32}O_4$ **Raspailyne A1**

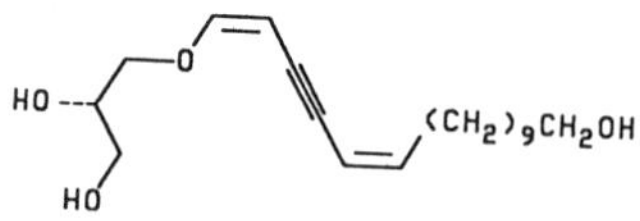

Mol. Wt.: 324
Melting Point: Oil
$[\alpha]_D^{22}$: +1.0 Solvent: Chf
Spectral Data: UV, IR, CMR, PMR, Mass Spec.
Organism: *Raspailia pumila* Bowerbank
R. ramosa Bowerbank
(Porifera)
Location: Brittany, France
Reference: 370

$C_{20}H_{30}O_3$ **8-(R)-Hydroxy-5Z,9E,11Z,14Z,17Z-eicosapentaenoic acid**

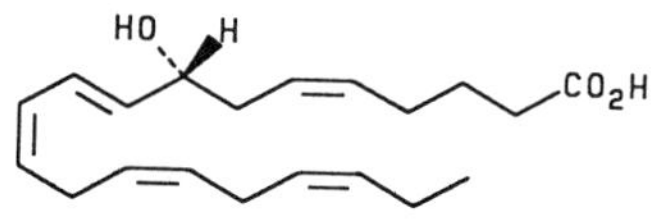

Mol. Wt.: 318
Spectral Data: UV, CD, PMR, Mass Spec.
Organism: *Patiria miniata*
(Echinodermata)
Location: Gulf of California
Reference: 220

$C_{20}H_{30}O_5S$ **Umbraculumin-C**

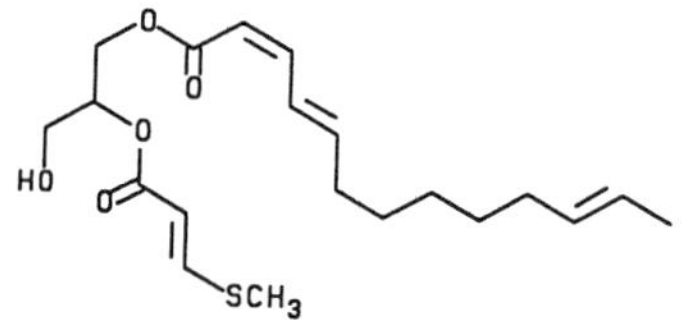

Mol. Wt.: 382
Bioactivity: Ichthyotoxic to *Gambusia affinis* at 0.1 μg/ml
$[\alpha]_D$: +7.0 Solvent: Chf
Spectral Data: UV, CMR, PMR, Mass Spec.
Organism: *Umbraculum mediterraneum* Lamarck
(Mollusca)
Location: Mediterranean
Reference: 182

$C_{20}H_{32}O_3$ **8-(R)-Hydroxy-5Z,9E,11Z,14Z-eicosatetraenoic acid [8-(R)-HETE]**

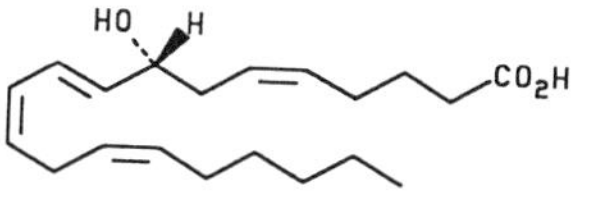

Mol. Wt.: 320
Bioactivity: Triggers oocyte maturation in starfish
Spectral Data: UV, CD, PMR, Mass Spec.
Organism: *Patiria miniata* (Echinodermata)
Location: Gulf of California
Reference: 65, 727

$C_{21}H_{32}O_5$ **Umbraculumin-A**

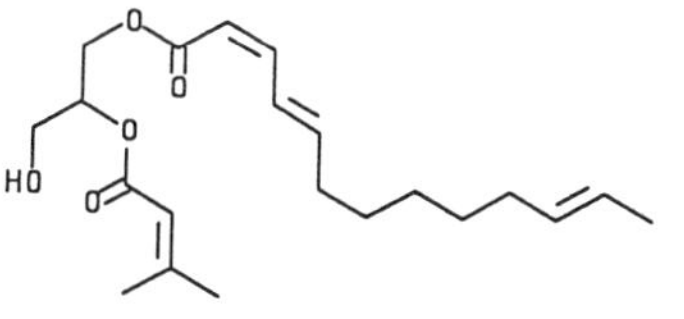

Mol. Wt.: 364
Bioactivity: Ichthyotoxic to *Gambusia affinis* at 10 μg/ml
$[\alpha]_D$: -24.3 Solvent: Chf
Spectral Data: UV, IR, CMR, PMR, Mass Spec.
Organism: *Umbraculum mediterraneum* Lamarck (Mollusca)
Location: Mediterranean
Reference: 182

$C_{21}H_{36}O_4$ **Isoraspailyne A**

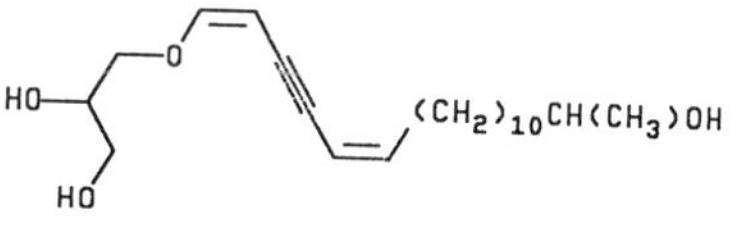

Mol. Wt.: 352
Melting Point: Oil
$[\alpha]_D^{22}$: +2.1 Solvent: Chf
Spectral Data: UV, IR, CMR, PMR, Mass Spec.
Organism: *Raspailia pumila* Bowerbank *R. ramosa* Bowerbank (Porifera)
Location: Brittany, France
Reference: 370

$C_{21}H_{36}O_4$ **(+)-Raspailyne-A**

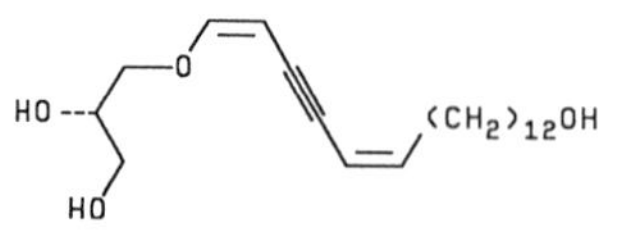

Mol. Wt.: 352
Melting Point: 54–55°C
$[\alpha]_D^{25}$: +5.6 Solvent: Me
Spectral Data: UV, IR, CMR, PMR, Mass Spec.
Organism: *Raspailia pumila* Bowerbank
R. ramosa Bowerbank
(Porifera)
Location: Brittany, France
Reference: 368, 370

$C_{23}H_{24}O_2$ **Siphonodiol**
(previously known)

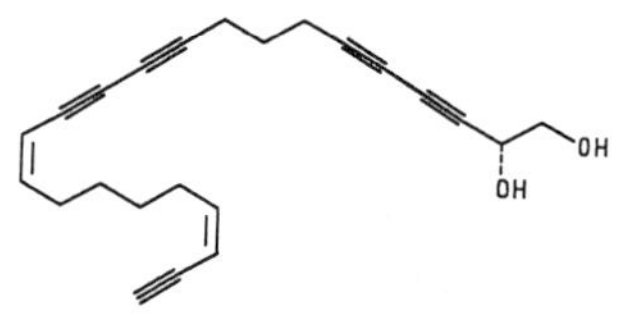

Mol. Wt.: 332
Bioactivity: Antimicrobial activity
H,K–ATPase inhibitor
Melting Point: 31–32°C
$[\alpha]_D$: –6.7 Solvent: Me
Spectral Data: UV, CD, IR, CMR, PMR, Mass Spec.
Organism: *Siphonochalina truncata*
(Porifera)
Location: Gulf of Suruga, Japan
Reference: 335, 1069

$C_{23}H_{26}O_2$ **Dihydrosiphonodiol**

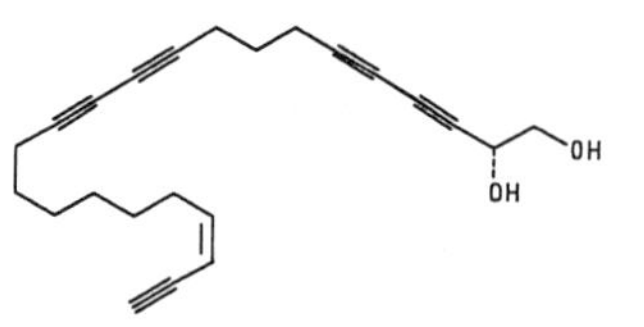

Mol. Wt.: 334
Bioactivity: H,K–ATPase inhibitor
Spectral Data: UV, CD, CMR, PMR, Mass Spec.
Organism: *Siphonochalina truncata*
(Porifera)
Location: Gulf of Suruga, Japan
Reference: 335

$C_{23}H_{28}O_2$ **Tetrahydrosiphonodiol**

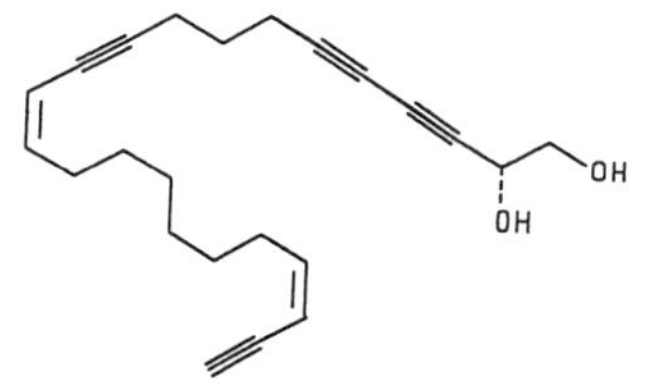

Mol. Wt.: 336
Bioactivity: H,K-ATPase inhibitor
Spectral Data: UV, CD, CMR, PMR, Mass Spec.
Organism: *Siphonochalina truncata* (Porifera)
Location: Gulf of Suruga, Japan
Reference: 335

$C_{24}H_{38}O_4$ **Trunculin A**

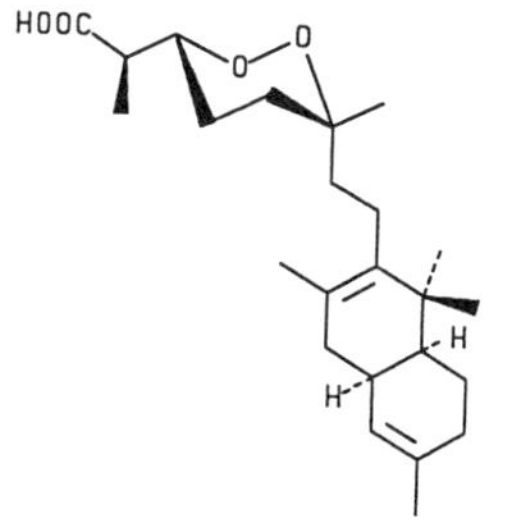

Mol. Wt.: 390
Bioactivity: Antimicrobial activity
Melting Point: 157–158°C
Spectral Data: Characterized as the methyl ester (see p. 225)
Organism: *Latrunculia brevis* (Porifera)
Location: New South Wales, Australia
Reference: 146

$C_{24}H_{38}O_5$ **Trunculin B**

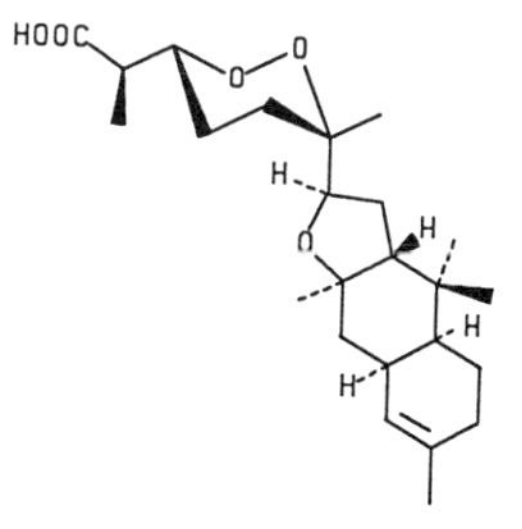

Mol. Wt.: 406
Bioactivity: Antimicrobial activity
Melting Point: 96–98°C
Spectral Data: Characterized as the methyl ester (see below)
Organism: *Latrunculia brevis* (Porifera)
Location: New South Wales, Australia
Reference: 146

$C_{25}H_{40}O_4$ **Trunculin A, methyl ester**

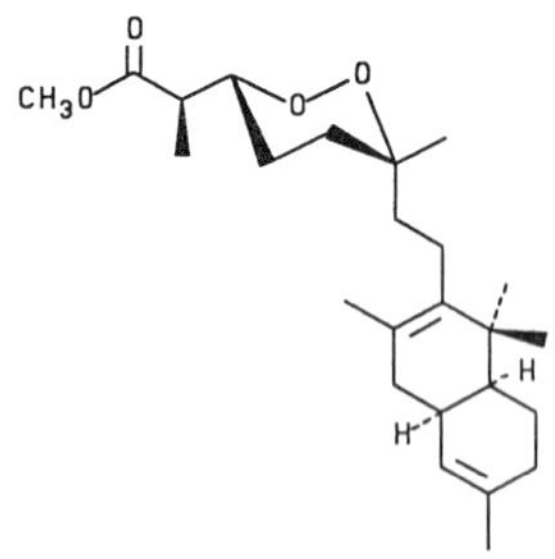

Mol. Wt.: 404
Melting Point: 66.5–67.5°C
$[\alpha]_D$: +158.3 Solvent: Chf
Spectral Data: CMR, PMR, Mass Spec., x-ray c.s.
Organism: *Latrunculia brevis* (Porifera)
Location: New South Wales, Australia
Reference: 146

$C_{25}H_{40}O_5$ **Trunculin B, methyl ester**

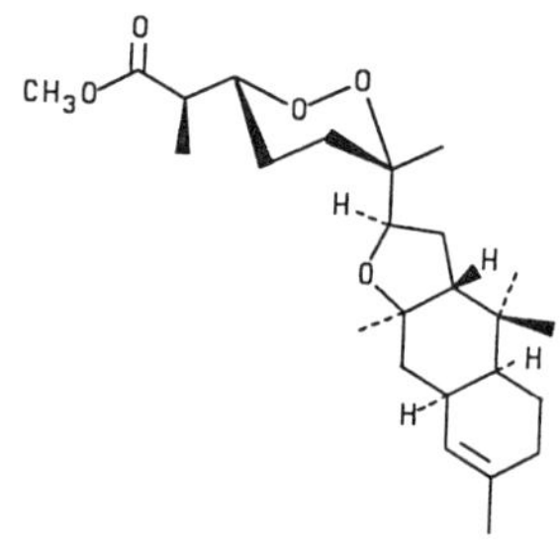

Mol. Wt.: 420
Melting Point: 91–93°C
$[\alpha]_D$: +13.1 Solvent: Chf
Spectral Data: CMR, PMR, Mass Spec., x-ray c.s.
Organism: *Latrunculia brevis* (Porifera)
Location: New South Wales, Australia
Reference: 146

$C_{30}H_{32}O_4$ **Petrosynone**

Mol. Wt.: 456
Bioactivity: Antibacterial activity against *Bacillus subtilis*
Melting Point: Oil
Spectral Data: UV, IR, CMR, PMR, Mass Spec.
Organism: *Petrosia* sp. (Porifera)
Location: Izu Archipelago, Japan
Reference: 333

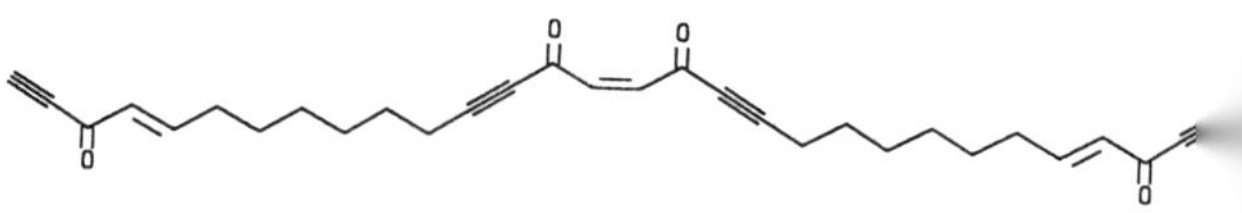

$C_{30}H_{40}O_4$ **Petrosynol**
(previously known)

Mol. Wt.: 464
Bioactivity: Fertilized starfish egg assay: IC_{99} 1 μg/ml
Antifungal activity against *Mortierella ramannianus*
Melting Point: Oil
$[\alpha]_D^{23}$: +107 Solvent: Chf
Spectral Data: UV, CD, IR, PMR, Mass Spec. (of 3-benzoate and 14-benzoate derivatives)
Organism: *Petrosia* sp. (Porifera)
Location: Izu Archipelago, Japan
Reference: 332, 333

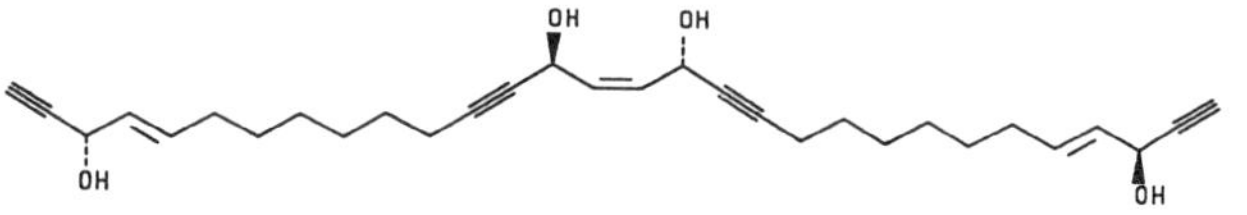

$C_{32}H_{50}O_3$ **Melyne B**

Mol. Wt.: 482
$[\alpha]_D$: -7.2 Solvent: Chf
Spectral Data: UV, IR, CMR, PMR, Mass Spec.
Organism: *Xestospongia* sp. (Porifera)
Location: Vanuatu
Reference: 908

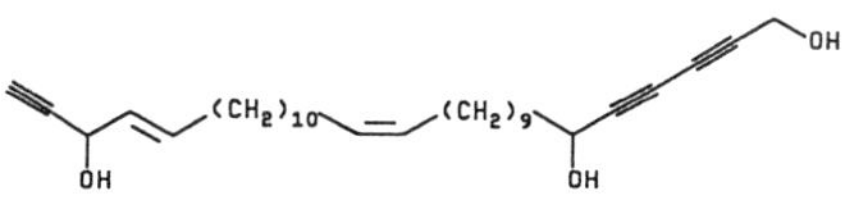

$C_{33}H_{52}O_3$ **Melyne A**

Mol. Wt.: 496
Bioactivity: Activity against *Giardia* (intestinal protozoan)
$[\alpha]_D$: -8.0 Solvent: Chf
Spectral Data: UV, IR, CMR, PMR, Mass Spec.
Organism: *Xestospongia* sp. (Porifera)
Location: Vanuatu
Reference: 908

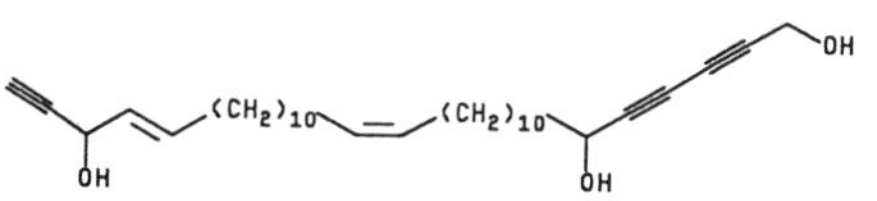

$C_{34}H_{50}O_3$ **Melyne C**

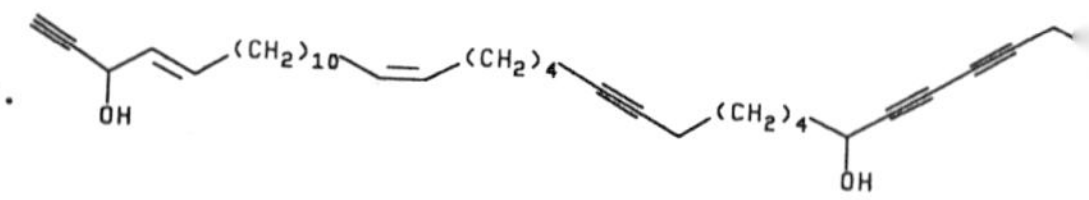

Mol. Wt.: 506
$[\alpha]_D$: −6.0 Solvent: Chf
Spectral Data: UV, IR, CMR, PMR, Mass Spec.
Organism: *Xestospongia* sp. (Porifera)
Location: Vanuatu
Reference: 908

$C_{63}H_{104}O_6$ **Glyceryl trieicosa-8,11,14-trienoate**

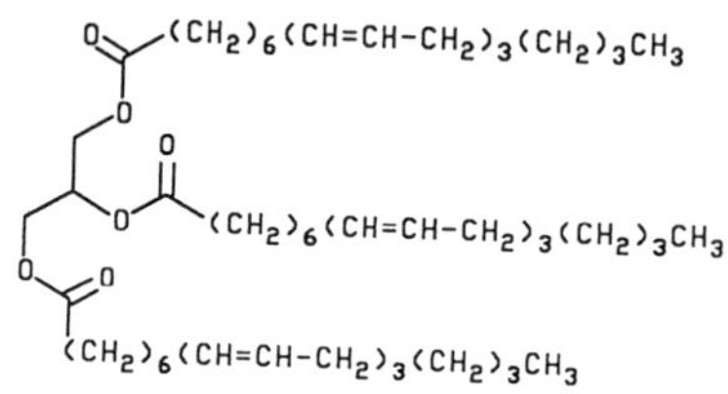

Mol. Wt.: 958
Bioactivity: Inhibition of platelet aggregation
Spectral Data: IR, CMR, PMR,
Organism: *Strongylocentrotus droebachiensis* (Echinodermata)
Location: Maine
Reference: 791

Chapter 14 TERPENOIDS

$C_{10}H_{12}O_3$ **Adriadysiolide**

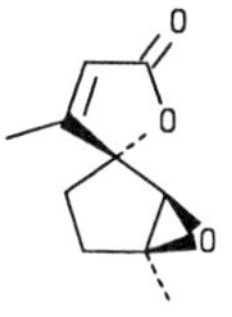

Mol. Wt.:	180
Melting Point:	76-77°C
$[\alpha]_D^{20}$:	0
$[\alpha]_{435}^{20}$:	+2.1 Solvent: Me
Spectral Data:	UV, IR, CMR, PMR, Mass Spec.
Organism:	*Dysidea* sp. (Porifera)
Location:	Venice
Reference:	695

$C_{15}H_{20}O_3$ **Subergoric acid**
(previously known)

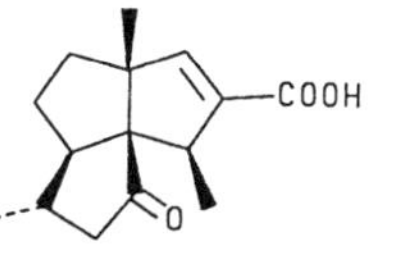

Mol. Wt.:	248
Bioactivity:	Cardiotoxic activity
Melting Point:	179-180°C
$[\alpha]_D$:	-23 Solvent: Chf
Spectral Data:	UV, IR, CMR, PMR, Mass Spec., x-ray c.s.
Organism:	*Subergorgia suberosa* (Coelenterata)
Location:	Guam
Reference:	365, 1194

$C_{15}H_{24}$ **Guaia-1(5),6-diene**

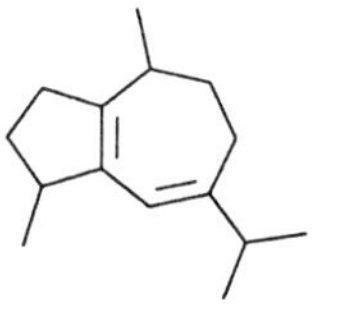

Mol. Wt.:	204
Bioactivity:	Antibacterial activity: growth inhibition of *Staphylococcus aureus* at 25 μg/ml and *Bacillus subtilis* at 100 μg/ml
Melting Point:	Oil
$[\alpha]_D^{20}$:	-30.2 Solvent: Chf
Spectral Data:	UV, IR, CMR, PMR, Mass Spec.
Organism:	*Halichondria* sp. (Porifera)
Location:	Ponape, Marshall Islands
Reference:	1045

$C_{15}H_{24}$ **Nephthene**

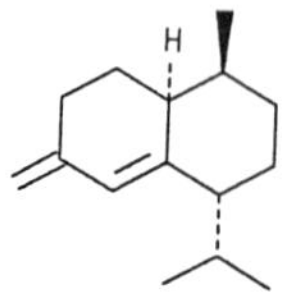

Mol. Wt.: 204
Melting Point: Oil
$[\alpha]_D^{20}$: -9.0 Solvent: Chf
Spectral Data: UV, CD, IR, CMR, PMR, Mass Spec.
Organsism: *Nephthea* sp. (Coelenterata)
Location: Okinawa, Japan
Reference: 563

$C_{15}H_{24}O$ **Coralloidin E**

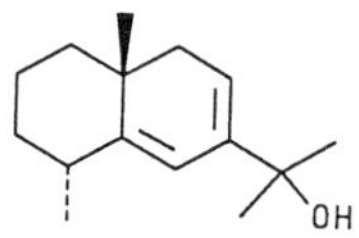

Mol. Wt.: 220
Melting Point: 55°C
$[\alpha]_D^{20}$: +305 Solvent: Alc
Spectral Data: UV, CMR, PMR, Mass Spec.
Organism: *Alcyonium coralloides* (Coelenterata)
Location: Mediterranean Sea
Reference: 214

$C_{15}H_{24}O$ **1,2-Epoxy-4-isopropyl-1,6-dimethyl-1,2,3,4,4a,7,8,8a-octahydronaphthalene**

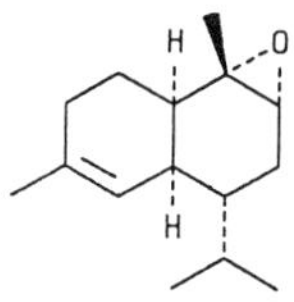

Mol. Wt.: 220
Melting Point: 47-50°C
$[\alpha]_D$: +146 Solvent: Chf
Spectral Data: IR, CMR, PMR, Mass Spec.
Organism: *Xenia crassa* (Coelenterata)
Location: Great Barrier Reef, Australia
Reference: 105

$C_{15}H_{24}O$ **12-Hydroxyzonarene**

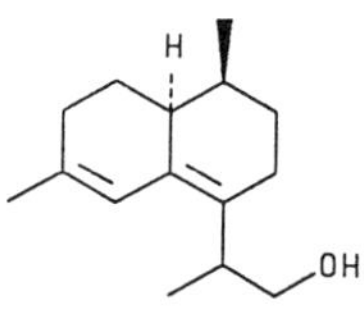

Mol. Wt.: 220
Melting Point: Oil
$[\alpha]_D$: +227.6 Solvent: Chf
Spectral Data: UV, IR, PMR, Mass Spec.
Organism: *Lemnalia cervicornis* (Coelenterata)
Location: Great Barrier Reef, Australia
Reference: 99

$C_{15}H_{24}O$ **4-Isopropyl-6-methyl-3,4,4a,7,8,8a-hexahydro-naphthalene-1-methanol**

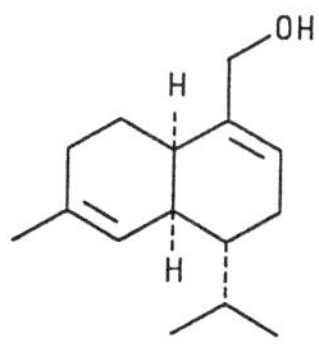

Mol. Wt.: 220
Melting Point: Oil
$[\alpha]_D$: +67 Solvent: Chf
Spectral Data: IR, CMR, PMR, Mass Spec.
Organism: *Xenia mayi* (Coelenterata)
Location: Townsville, Australia
Reference: 105

$C_{15}H_{24}O$ **3,3,7,11-Tetramethyltricyclo [6.3.0.0^{2,4}]un-dec-1(8)-en-4-ol**

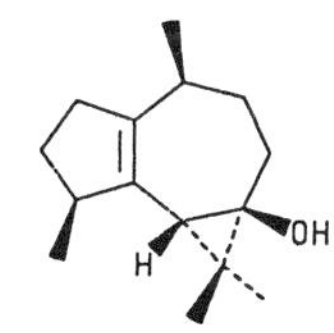

Mol. Wt.: 220
Melting Point: 121-124°C
$[\alpha]_D$: +66
Spectral Data: IR, CMR, PMR, Mass Spec., x-ray c.s.
Organism: *Xenia novae-britanniae* (Coelenterata)
Location: Great Barrier Reef, Australia
Reference: 97

$C_{15}H_{25}BrO$ **Lankalapuol A**

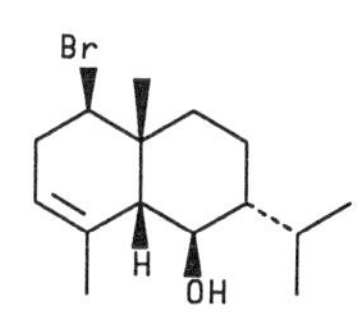

Mol. Wt.: 301
Melting Point: 83.5-84°C (acetate)
$[\alpha]_D$: +96 Solvent: Me (acetate)
Spectral Data: IR, CMR, PMR, Mass Spec., x-ray c.s. (acetate)
Organism: *Aplysia dactylomela* (Mollusca)
Location: Sri Lanka
Reference: 46

$C_{15}H_{25}BrO$ **Lankalapuol B**

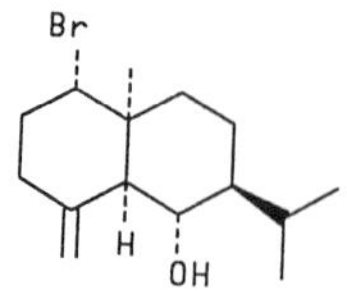

Mol. Wt.: 301
Melting Point: 93.5-94°C (acetate)
$[\alpha]_D$: -93 Solvent: Me (acetate)
Spectral Data: IR, CMR, PMR, Mass Spec. (acetate)
Organism: *Aplysia dactylomela* (Mollusca)
Location: Sri Lanka
Reference: 46

$C_{15}H_{26}O$ **Nephthenol**

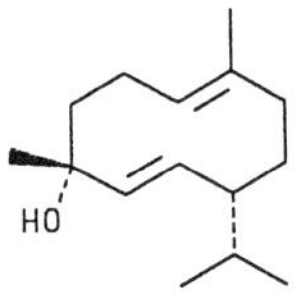

Mol. Wt.: 222
Melting Point: Oil
$[\alpha]_D^{20}$: +184 Solvent: Chf
Spectral Data: CD, IR, CMR, PMR, Mass Spec.
Organism: *Nephthea* sp. (Coelenterata)
Location: Okinawa, Japan
Reference: 563

$C_{15}H_{26}O_2$ **Nephthediol**

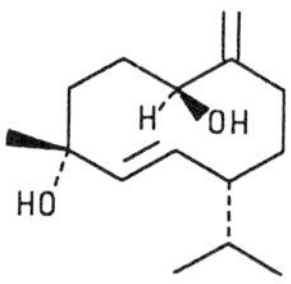

Mol. Wt.: 238
$[\alpha]_D^{21}$: +82 Solvent: Chf
Spectral Data: CD, IR, CMR, PMR, Mass Spec.
Organism: *Nephthea* sp. (Coelenterata)
Location: Okinawa, Japan
Reference: 563

$C_{15}H_{26}O_2$ **ent-Oplopanone**

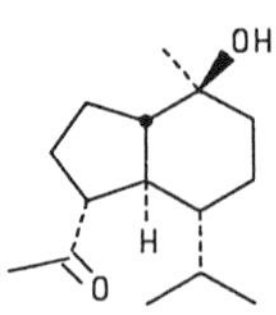

Mol. Wt.: 238
Melting Point: 83-84°C
$[\alpha]_D^{22}$: +19 Solvent: Di
Spectral Data: CD, IR, CMR, PMR, Mass Spec.
Organism: *Nephthea* sp. (Coelenterata)
Location: Okinawa, Japan
Reference: 563

$C_{17}H_{26}O_2$ **12-Acetoxyzonarene**

Mol. Wt.: 262
Melting Point: Oil
$[\alpha]_D$: +241.8
Spectral Data: UV, IR, CMR, PMR, Mass Spec.
Organism: *Lemnalia cervicornis* (Coelenterata)
Location: Great Barrier Reef, Australia
Reference: 99

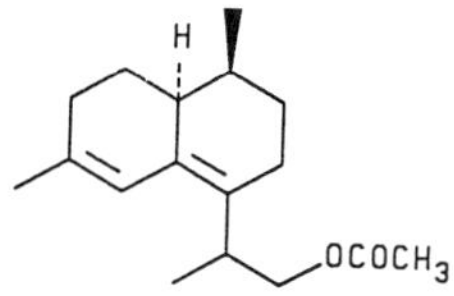

$C_{17}H_{26}O_2$ **Coralloidin A**

Mol. Wt.: 262
Melting Point: Oil
$[\alpha]_D^{20}$: +225 Solvent: Cy
Spectral Data: UV, IR, CMR, PMR, Mass Spec.
Organism: *Alcyonium (=Parerythropodium) coralloides* (Coelenterata)
Location: Mediterranean Sea
Reference: 375

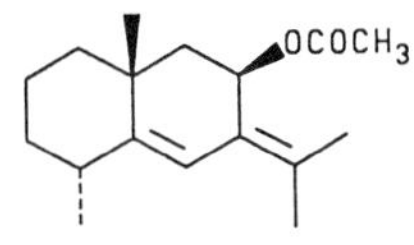

$C_{17}H_{26}O_2$ **Coralloidin B**

Mol. Wt.: 262
Melting Point: Oil
$[\alpha]_D^{20}$: -33.2 Solvent: Cy
Spectral Data: UV, IR, CMR, PMR, Mass Spec.
Organism: *Alcyonium (=Parerythropodium) coralloides* (Coelenterata)
Location: Mediterranean Sea
Reference: 375

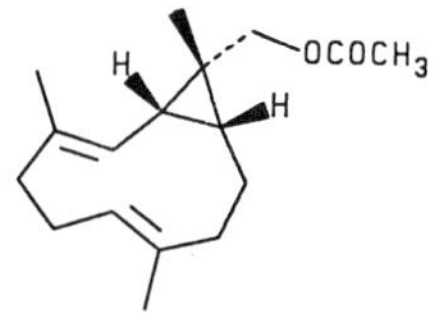

$C_{17}H_{26}O_2$ **Coralloidin C**

Mol. Wt.: 262
Melting Point: Oil
$[\alpha]_D^{20}$: -168.7 Solvent: Chf
Spectral Data: UV, CMR, PMR, Mass Spec.
Organism: *Alcyonium coralloides* (Coelenterata)
Location: Mediterranean Sea, France
Reference: 214

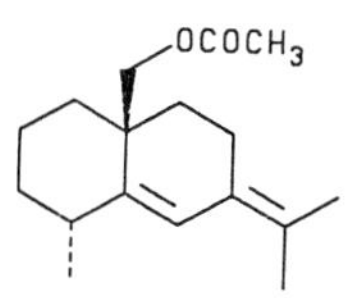

$C_{17}H_{26}O_3$ **5,6-Epoxy-4-isopropyl-6-methyl-3,4,4a,5,6,7,8,8a-octahydro-naphthalene-1-methanol acetate**

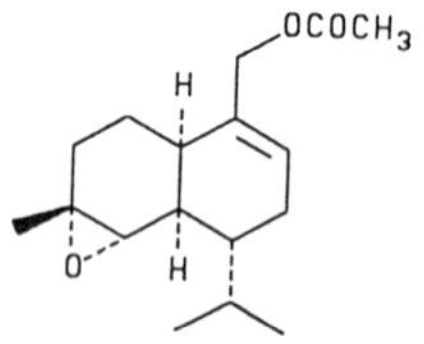

Mol. Wt.: 278
Melting Point: Oil
$[\alpha]_D$: -19 Solvent: Chf
Spectral Data: CMR, PMR, Mass Spec.
Organism: *Xenia mayi* (Coelenterata)
Location: Townsville, Australia
Reference: 105

$C_{18}H_{28}O_4$ **Xestodiol**

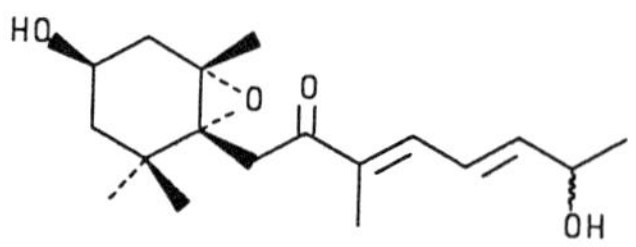

Mol. Wt.: 308
Melting Point: Oil
$[\alpha]_D$: -27 Solvent: Me
Spectral Data: UV, IR, CMR, PMR, Mass Spec.
Organism: *Xestospongia vanilla* (Porifera)
Location: British Columbia, Canada
Reference: 829

$C_{19}H_{26}O_2$ **Acalycixeniolide B**

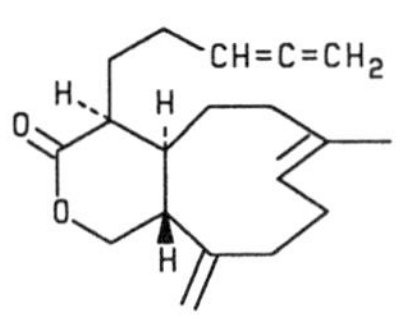

Mol. Wt.: 286
Bioactivity: Inhibition of fertilized starfish egg cell division: ED_{50} 5 μg/ml
Spectral Data: IR, CMR, PMR, Mass Spec.
Organism: *Acalycigorgia inermis* (Hedlund) (Coelenterata)
Location: Gulf of Suruga, Japan
Reference: 330

$C_{19}H_{28}O_2$ **Acalycixeniolide A**

Mol. Wt.: 288
Bioactivity: Inhibition of fertilized starfish egg cell division: ED_{50} 20 μg/ml
$[\alpha]_D^{23}$: +143 Solvent: Dcm
Spectral Data: IR, CMR, PMR, Mass Spec.
Organism: *Acalycigorgia inermis* (Hedlund) (Coelenterata)
Location: Gulf of Suruga, Japan
Reference: 330

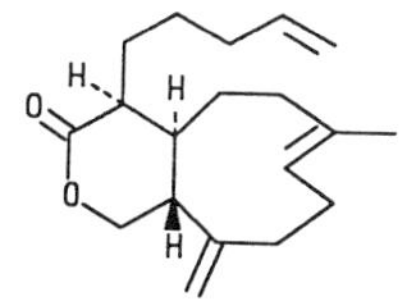

$C_{19}H_{28}O_2$ **Xestenone**

Mol. Wt.: 288
Melting Point: Oil
$[\alpha]_D$: 0 Solvent: Me
Spectral Data: UV, CD, IR, CMR, PMR, Mass Spec.
Organism: *Xestospongia vanilla* (Porifera)
Location: British Columbia, Canada
Reference: 830

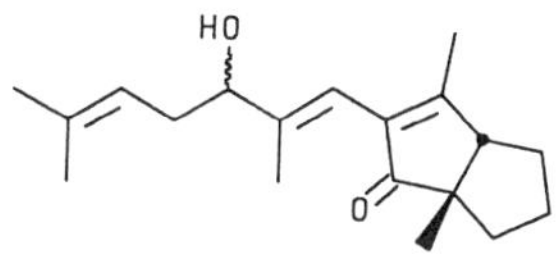

$C_{19}H_{28}O_4$ **Coralloidin D**

Mol. Wt.: 320
Melting Point: Oil
$[\alpha]_D^{20}$: -14.1 Solvent: Alc
Spectral Data: UV, CMR, PMR, Mass Spec.
Organism: *Alcyonium coralloides* (Coelenterata)
Location: Mediterranean Sea
Reference: 214

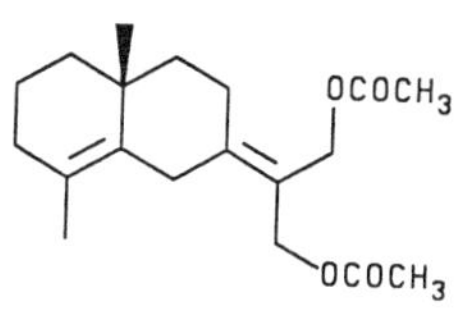

$C_{20}H_{24}O_4$ **Epilophodione**

Mol. Wt.: 328
Melting Point: 153-155°C
$[\alpha]_D^{25}$: +136.2 Solvent: Dcm
Spectral Data: UV, IR, CMR, PMR, Mass Spec.
Organism: *Gersemia rubiformis* (Coelenterata)
Location: British Columbia, Canada
Reference: 1181

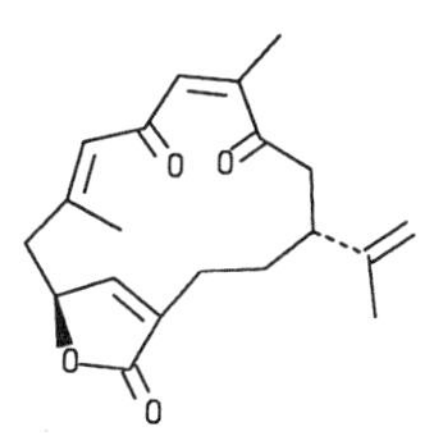

$C_{20}H_{24}O_4$ **Gersemolide**

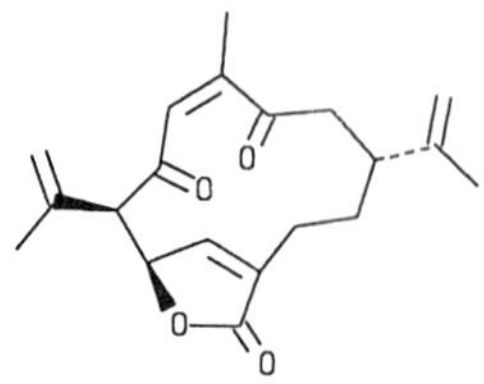

Mol. Wt.: 328
Spectral Data: CMR, PMR, Mass Spec., x-ray c.s.
Organism: *Gersemia rubiformis* (Coelenterata)
Location: British Columbia, Canada
Reference: 1181

$C_{20}H_{24}O_4$ **Gersolide**

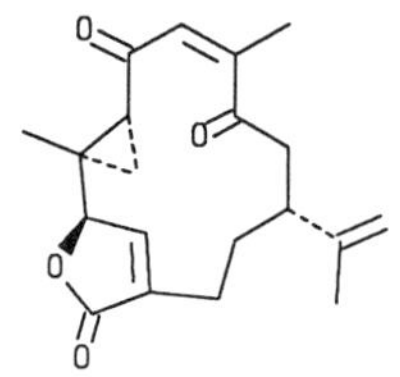

Mol. Wt.: 328
Melting Point: 176-178°C
$[\alpha]_D$: -51.9 Solvent: Dcm
Spectral Data: PMR, Mass Spec., x-ray c.s.
Organism: *Gersemia rubiformis* (Coelenterata)
Location: British Columbia, Canada
Reference: 1180

$C_{20}H_{26}O_3$ (previously known)

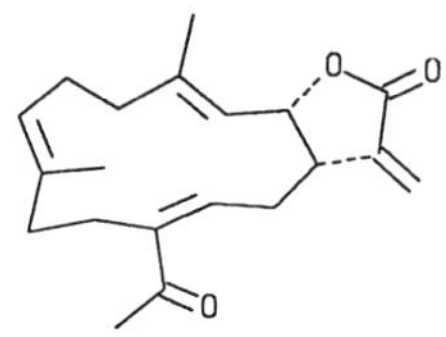

Mol. Wt.: 314
Melting Point: Oil
$[\alpha]_D$: +28 Solvent: Chf
Spectral Data: UV, IR, PMR, Mass Spec.
Organism: *Sinularia mayi* (Coelenterata)
Location: Okinawa, Japan
Reference: 102, 589

$C_{20}H_{26}O_5$ **Mayolide D**

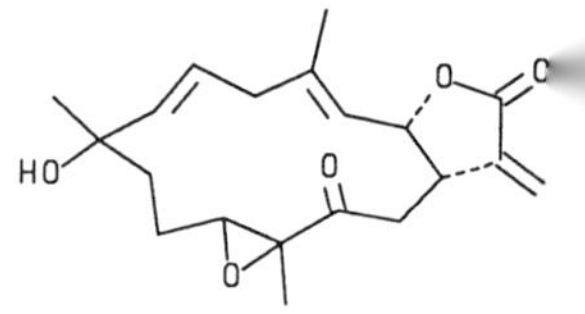

Mol. Wt.: 346
Melting Point: Oil
$[\alpha]_D$: +33 Solvent: Chf
Spectral Data: UV, IR, CMR, PMR, Mass Spec.
Organism: *Sinularia mayi* (Coelenterata)
Location: Okinawa, Japan
Reference: 588

$C_{20}H_{28}O_3$ | **(2R,7R,8R)-7,8-Epoxycembra-3,11,15-trien-16,2-olide**

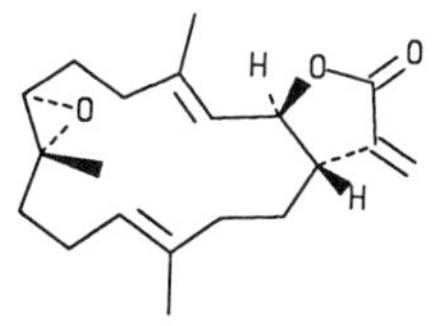

Mol. Wt.: 316
[α]D: +48.1 Solvent: Chf
Spectral Data: UV, IR, CMR, PMR, Mass Spec.
Organism: *Efflatounaria variabilis* (Coelenterata)
Location: Townsville, Australia
Reference: 98

$C_{20}H_{28}O_3$ | **(2S,7S,8S)-7,8-Epoxycembra-3,11,15-trien-16,2-olide**

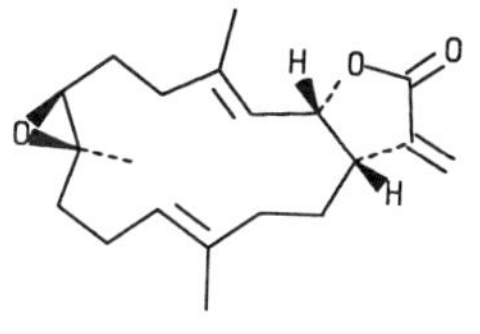

Mol. Wt.: 316
Melting Point: 171-172°C
[α]D: +3.0 Solvent: Chf
Spectral Data: UV, IR, CMR, PMR, Mass Spec., x-ray c.s.
Organism: *Efflatounaria* sp. (Coelenterata)
Location: Townsville, Australia
Reference: 98

$C_{20}H_{28}O_4$ | **Mayolide B**

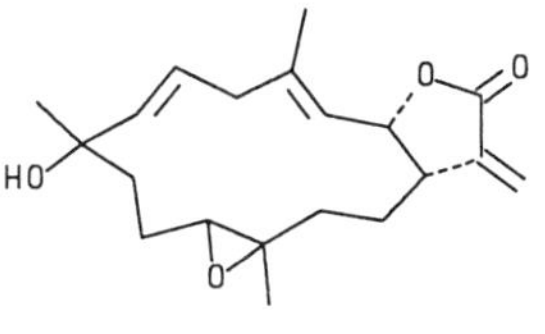

Mol. Wt.: 332
Melting Point: Oil
[α]D: +35 Solvent: Chf
Spectral Data: UV, IR, CMR, PMR, Mass Spec.
Organism: *Sinularia mayi* (Coelenterata)
Location: Okinawa, Japan
Reference: 588

$C_{20}H_{30}O_2$

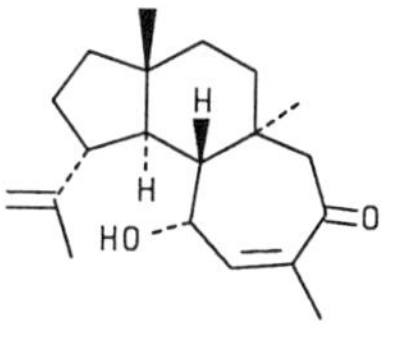

Mol. Wt.: 302
Melting Point: Oil
[α]D: +35 Solvent: Chf
Spectral Data: UV, IR, CMR, PMR, Mass Spec.
Organism: *Higginsia* sp. (unidentified) (Porifera)
Location: Lancelin, Western Australia
Reference: 157

$C_{20}H_{30}O_2$ **(2<u>R</u>,11<u>R</u>,12<u>R</u>)-Isosarcophytoxide**
(previously known)

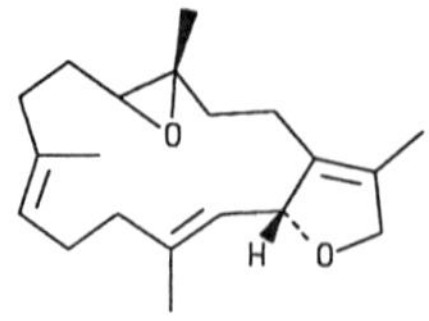

Mol. Wt.: 302
$[\alpha]_D$: -161±5 Solvent: Chf
Spectral Data: CMR, PMR
Organism: *Sarcophyton* cf. *birklandi* Veseveldt
Sarcophyton glaucum Quoy and Gaimard
(Coelenterata)
Location: Australia; Guam
Reference: 101, 103

$C_{20}H_{30}O_2$ **(2<u>S</u>,11<u>R</u>,12<u>R</u>)-Isosarcophytoxide**

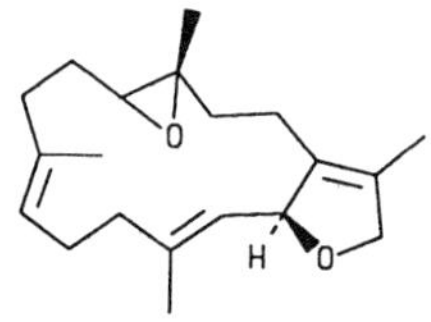

Mol. Wt.: 302
Melting Point: 70-71°C
$[\alpha]_D$: +203±7 Solvent: Chf
Spectral Data: IR, CMR, PMR, Mass Spec., x-ray c.s.
Organism: *Sarcophyton* cf. *birklandi* Veseveldt
Sarcophyton glaucum Quoy and Gaimard
(Coelenterata)
Location: Australia; Guam
Reference: 101

$C_{20}H_{30}O_2$ **Reiswigin B**

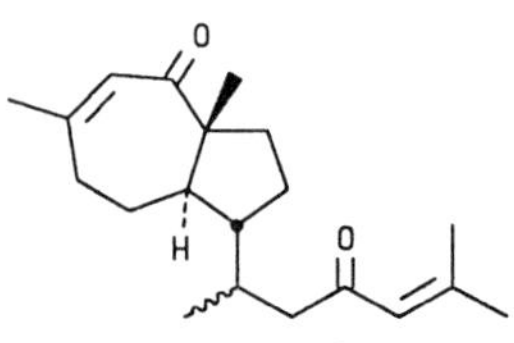

Mol. Wt.: 302
Bioactivity: Inhibition of HSV-1 at 2 μg
Partial inhibition of A59 at 20 μg
$[\alpha]_D^{20}$: -20 Solvent: Chf
Spectral Data: UV, IR, CMR, PMR, Mass Spec.
Organism: *Eipolasis reiswigi*
(Porifera)
Location: Venezuela
Reference: 521

$C_{20}H_{30}O_2$ **(2<u>R</u>,7<u>S</u>,8<u>S</u>)-Sarcophytoxide**

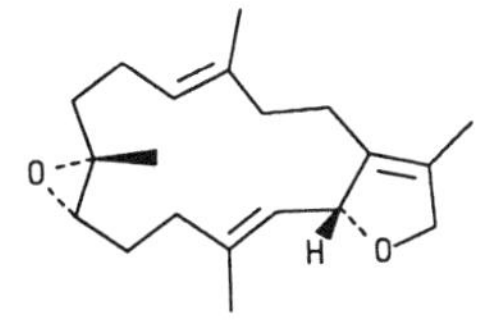

Mol. Wt.: 302
Melting Point: 52-56°C
[α]$_D$: -64 Solvent: Chf
Spectral Data: IR, CMR, PMR, Mass Spec.
Organism: *Lobophytum pauciflorum* Ehrenberg (Coelenterata)
Location: North Queensland, Australia
Reference: 101

$C_{20}H_{30}O_3$

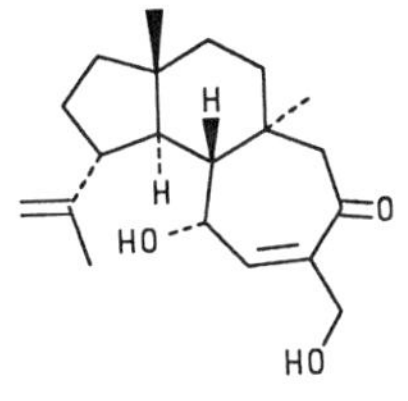

Mol. Wt.: 318
Melting Point: 104-105°C
[α]$_D$: +58.8 Solvent: Chf
Spectral Data: UV, IR, CMR, PMR, Mass Spec., x-ray c.s.
Organism: *Higginsia* sp. (unclassified) (Porifera)
Location: Lancelin, Western Australia
Reference: 157

$C_{20}H_{30}O_3$ **4,5-Deoxyneodolabelline**

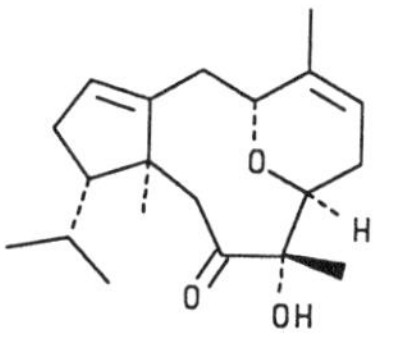

Mol. Wt.: 318
Melting Point: 116.5-117.5°C
[α]$_D$: +29 Solvent: Chf
Spectral Data: IR, CMR, PMR, Mass Spec.
Organism: *Cespitularia* sp. (Coelenterata)
Location: North Queensland, Australia
Reference: 100

$C_{20}H_{30}O_3$ **Spongian-17-al-16-one**

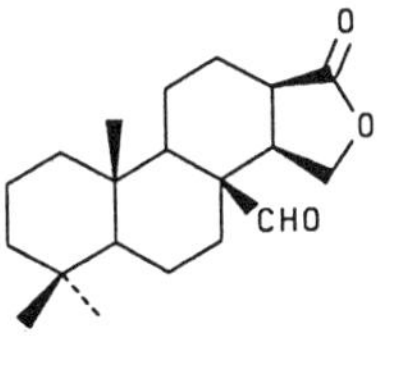

Mol. Wt.: 318
Melting Point: Oil
Spectral Data: IR, CMR, PMR, Mass Spec.
Organism: *Chromodoris epicuria* (Mollusca)
Location: South Australia
Reference: 615, 616

$C_{20}H_{30}O_4$

Dendrillol-1
(17β-Hydroxy-15,17-oxido-spongian-16-one)

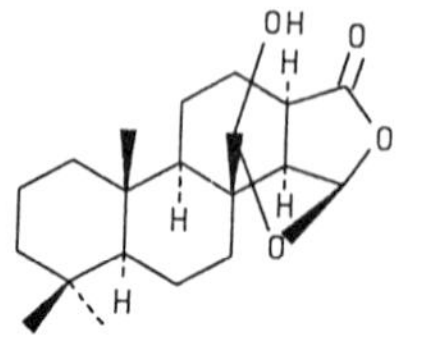

Mol. Wt.: 334
Melting Point: 229-231°C
$[\alpha]_D^{20}$: -31.8 Solvent: Chf
Spectral Data: IR, CMR, PMR, Mass Spec., x-ray c.s.
Organism: *Dendrilla rosea* (Porifera)
Chromodoris epicuria (Mollusca)
Location: Leigh, New Zealand; South Australia
Reference: 513, 615, 616

$C_{20}H_{30}O_4$

Mayolide A

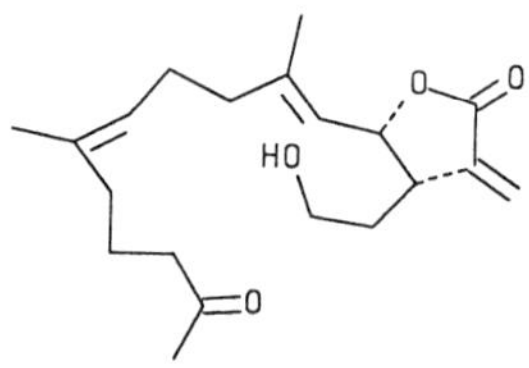

Mol. Wt.: 334
Melting Point: Oil
$[\alpha]_D$: -52 Solvent: Chf
Spectral Data: UV, IR, CMR, PMR, Mass Spec.
Organism: *Sinularia mayi* (Coelenterata)
Location: Okinawa, Japan
Reference: 588

$C_{20}H_{32}O$

Germacrexeniolone

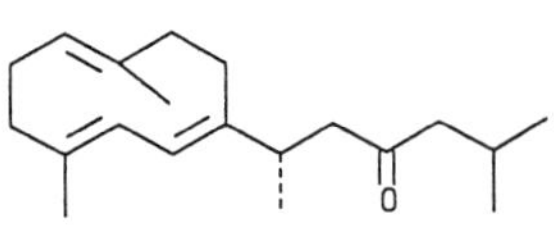

Mol. Wt.: 288
Melting Point: Oil
$[\alpha]_D^{20}$: +33 Solvent: Chf
Spectral Data: UV, IR, CMR, PMR, Mass Spec.
Organism: *Xenia* sp. (Coelenterata)
Location: Okinawa, Japan
Reference: 562

$C_{20}H_{32}O$ **(14<u>S</u>)-Hydroxycembra-1,3,7,11-tetraene**

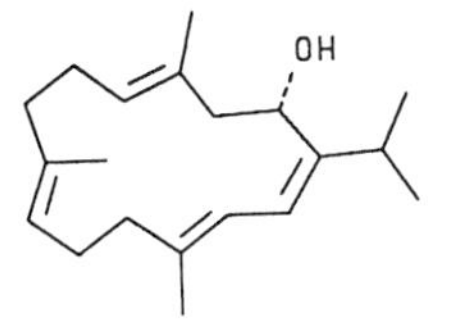

Mol. Wt.: 288
Melting Point: Oil
$[\alpha]_D$: +115 Solvent: Chf
Spectral Data: UV, IR, CMR, PMR, Mass Spec.
Organism: *Lobophytum pauciflorum* Ehrenberg
Sarcophyton sp.
(Coelenterata)
Location: North Queensland, Australia
Reference: 71, 101

$C_{20}H_{32}O$ **15-Hydroxycembra-1,3,7,11-tetraene**

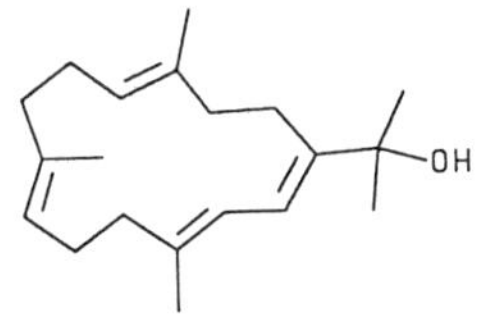

Mol. Wt.: 288
Melting Point: 81-83°C
Spectral Data: UV, IR, CMR, PMR, Mass Spec.
Organism: *Lobophytum pauciflorum* Ehrenberg
(Coelenterata)
Location: North Queensland, Australia
Reference: 101

$C_{20}H_{32}O$ **(4<u>E</u>,7<u>E</u>,11<u>E</u>)-11-Isopropyl-1,4,8-trimethyl-1,2,3,3a,6,9,10,12a-octahydrocyclopentacycloundecen-1-ol**

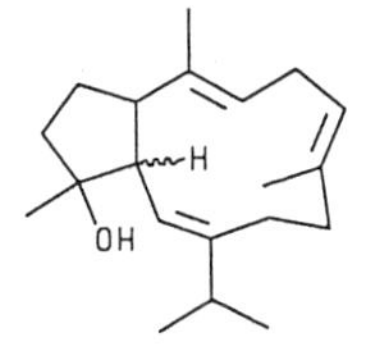

Mol. Wt.: 288
Melting Point: Oil
Spectral Data: IR, CMR, PMR, Mass Spec.
Organism: *Cespitularia* sp.
(Coelenterata)
Location: North Queensland, Australia
Reference: 100

$C_{20}H_{32}O_2$ **Reiswigin A**

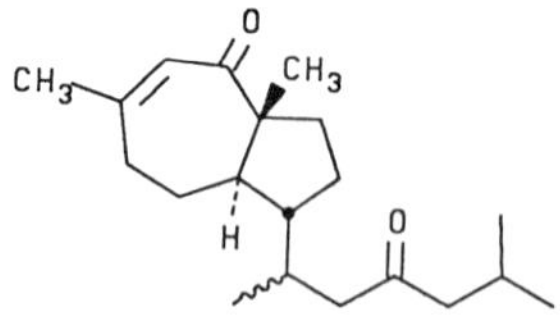

Mol. Wt.: 304
Bioactivity: Antiviral activity: inhibition of HSV-1 and VSV at 2 μg
Partial inhibition of A59 at 20 μg
$[\alpha]_D^{20}$: -10 Solvent: Chf
Spectral Data: UV, IR, CMR, PMR, Mass Spec.
Organism: *Epipolasis reiswigi* (Porifera)
Location: Venezuela
Reference; 521

$C_{20}H_{32}O_2$ **Sinulariol A**
(previously known)

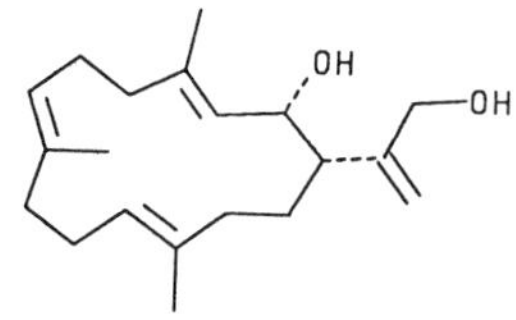

Mol. Wt.: 304
Melting Point: 116-117.5°C
$[\alpha]_D$: +101 Solvent: Chf
Spectral Data: IR, PMR, Mass Spec.
Organism: *Sinularia mayi* (Coelenterata)
Location: Okinawa, Japan
Reference: 589, 1119

$C_{20}H_{32}O_3$ **Aplykurodin B**

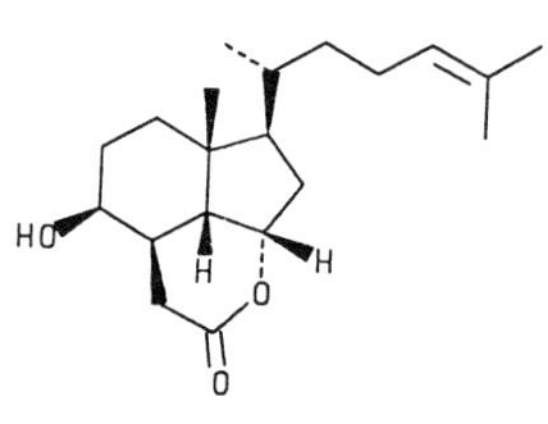

Mol. Wt.: 320
Melting Point: 130-131°C
$[\alpha]_D$: -36 Solvent: Chf
Spectral Data: CMR, PMR, Mass Spec.
Organism: *Aplysia kurodai* (Mollusca)
Reference: 748

$C_{20}H_{32}O_4$ **Shahamin E**

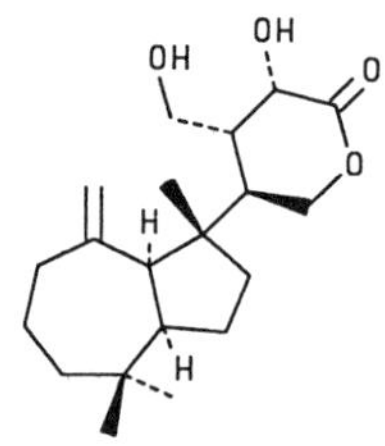

Mol. Wt.: 336
Melting Point: Oil
$[\alpha]_D$: +72 Solvent: Chf
Spectral Data: IR, CMR, PMR, Mass Spec.
Organism: *Dysidea* sp. (Porifera)
Location: Red Sea
Reference: 150

$C_{20}H_{34}O_2$ **11-Isopropyl-1,4,8-trimethyl-1,2,3,3a,4,5,6,9,10,12a-decahydro-cyclopentacycloundecene-1,4-diol**

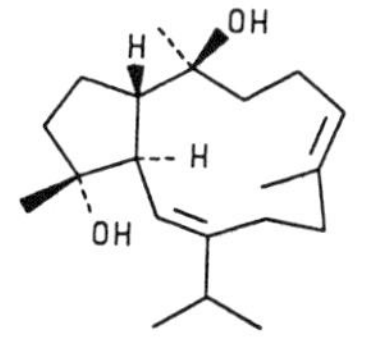

Mol. Wt.: 306
Melting Point: 109-110°C
[α]D: +93 Solvent: Chf
Spectral Data: IR, CMR, PMR, Mass Spec,. x-ray c.s.
Organism: *Cespitularia* sp. (Coelenterata)
Location: North Queensland, Australia
Reference: 100

$C_{20}H_{34}O_2$ **Sinulariol B**

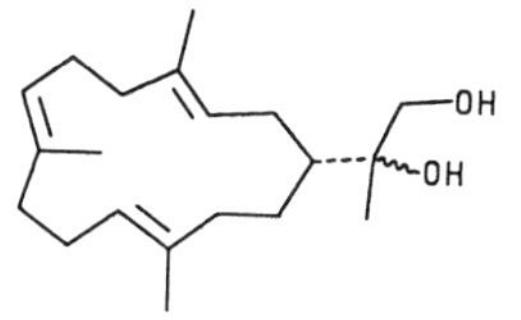

Mol. Wt.: 306
Melting Point: 61-63°C
[α]D: -52 Solvent: Chf
Spectral Data: IR, PMR, Mass Spec.
Organism: *Sinularia mayi* (Coelenterata)
Location: Okinawa, Japan
Reference: 589

$C_{20}H_{34}O_3$ **Aplykurodin A**

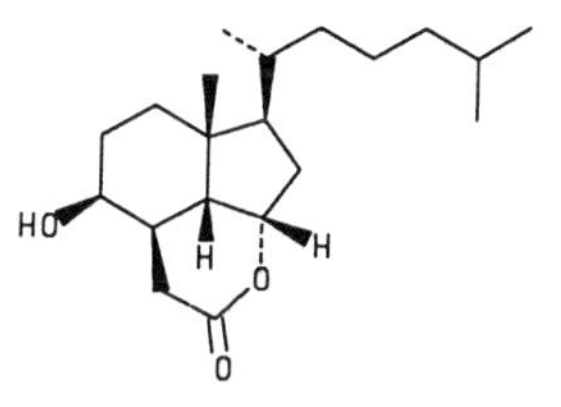

Mol. Wt.: 322
Melting Point: 138°C
[α]D: -44 Solvent: Chf
Spectral Data: IR, CMR, PMR, Mass Spec., x-ray c.s.
Organism: *Aplysia kurodai* (Mollusca)
Reference: 748

$C_{20}H_{34}O_3$ **Hydratoisoxeniolone**

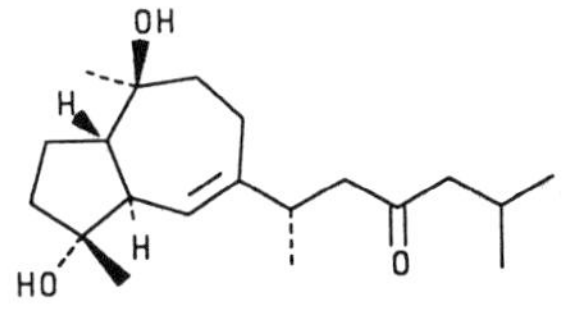

Mol. Wt.: 322
Melting Point: Oil
$[\alpha]_D^{22}$: -4.7 Solvent: Chf
Spectral Data: IR, CMR, PMR, Mass Spec.
Organism: *Xenia* sp. (Coelenterata)
Location: Okinawa, Japan
Reference: 562

$C_{20}H_{34}O_3$ **Hydratoxeniolone**

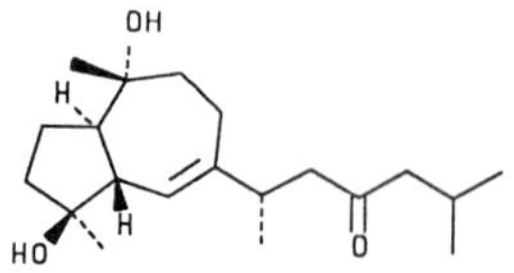

Mol. Wt.: 322
Melting Point: Oil
$[\alpha]_D^{22}$: +8.0 Solvent: Chf
Spectral Data: IR, CMR, PMR, Mass Spec.
Organism: *Xenia* sp.
(Coelenterata)
Location: Okinawa, Japan
Reference: 562

$C_{20}H_{34}O_4$

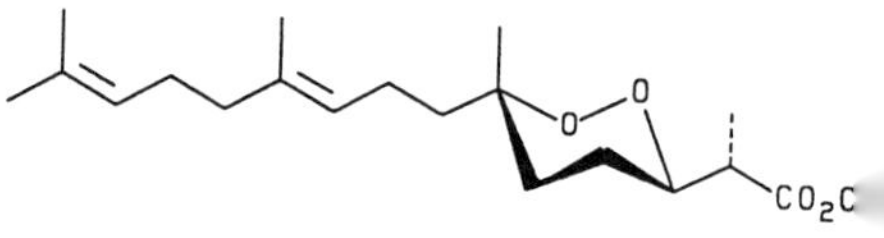

Mol. Wt.: 338
Melting Point: Oil
$[\alpha]_D^{25}$: +52.2 Solvent: Chf
Spectral Data: CMR, PMR, Mass Spec.
Organism: *Latrunculia* sp.
(Porifera)
Location: New South Wales, Australia
Reference: 141

$C_{21}H_{28}O_4$ **Membranolide**

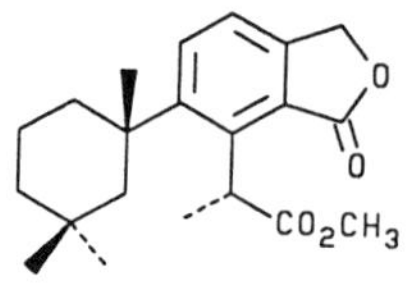

Mol. Wt.: 344
Bioactivity: *Bacillus subtilis*: growth inhibition at 100 μg/disk
Staphylococcus aureus: mildly active
$[\alpha]_D$: -28.8 Solvent: Chf
Spectral Data: UV, IR, CMR, PMR, Mass Spec.
Organism: *Dendrilla membranosa*
(Porifera)
Location: McMurdo, Antarctica
Reference: 755

$C_{21}H_{32}O_4$ **Dendrillol-3**

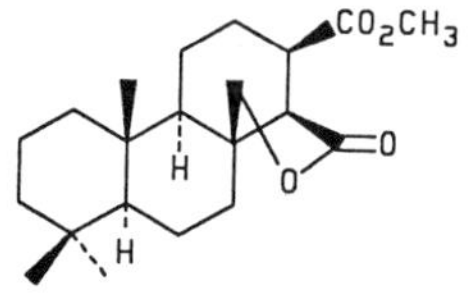

Mol. Wt.: 348
Melting Point: 162-164°C
Spectral Data: IR, CMR, PMR, Mass Spec.
Organism: *Dendrilla rosea* (Porifera)
Location: Leigh, New Zealand
Reference: 513

$C_{21}H_{32}O_6$ **Dendrillol-4**

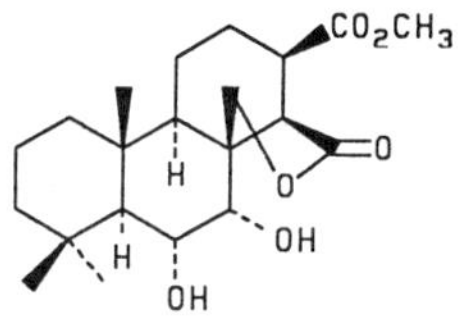

Mol. Wt.: 380
Melting Point: 235-237°C
$[\alpha]_D^{20}$: +40 Solvent: Chf
Spectral Data: UV, IR, CMR, PMR, Mass Spec.
Organism: *Dendrilla rosea* (Porifera)
Location: Leigh, New Zealand
Reference: 513

$C_{21}H_{34}O_5$ **Shahamin B**

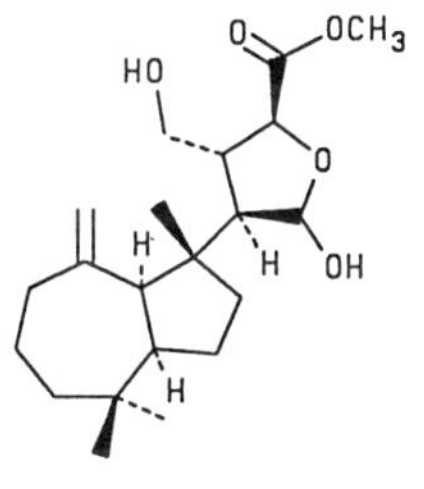

Mol. Wt.: 366
Melting Point: Oil
Spectral Data: IR, PMR, Mass Spec.
Organism: *Dysidea* sp. (Porifera)
Location: Red Sea
Reference: 150

$C_{22}H_{28}O_5$ **Aplysulphurin**
(previously known)

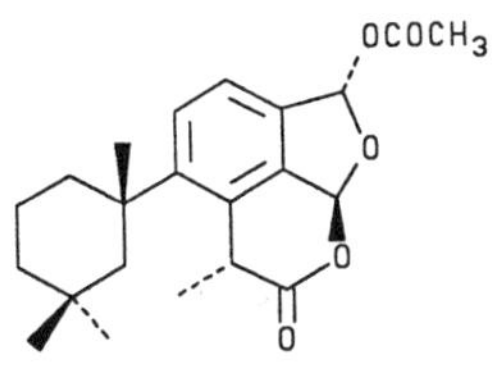

Mol. Wt.: 372
Melting Point: 195°C
Organism: *Darwinella* sp. (formerly *Aplysilla rosea*) *Darwinella oxeata* Bergquist (Porifera)
Location: Leigh, New Zealand
Reference: 513, 515

$C_{22}H_{29}ClO_7$ **Solenolide E**

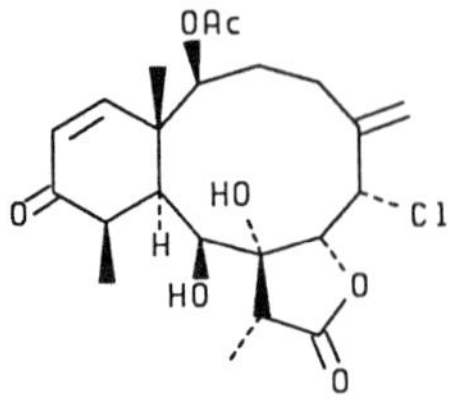

Mol. Wt.: 440
Bioactivity: Antiinflammatory activity:
mouse ear assay: >70% reduction of edema at ~15 μg
Inhibition of cyclooxygenase
Rhinovirus: IC_{50} 12.5 μg/ml
Inhibition of Herpes and Ann Arbor viruses
Larvicidal against Blowfly larvae: ED_{100} 30-35 ppm.
Melting Point: Oil
$[\alpha]_D^{20}$: +11 Solvent: Chf
Spectral Data: UV, IR, CMR, PMR, Mass Spec.
Organism: *Solenopodium* sp. (Coelenterata)
Location: Palau
Reference: 366

$C_{22}H_{30}O_4$ (previously known)

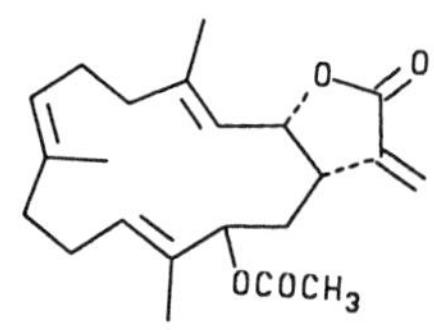

Mol. Wt.: 358
Melting Point: Oil
$[\alpha]_D$: +29 Solvent: Chf
Spectral Data: UV, IR, PMR, Mass Spec.
Organism: *Sinularia mayi* (Coelenterata)
Location: Okinawa, Japan
Reference: 589, 1120

$C_{22}H_{30}O_6$ **Mayolide C**

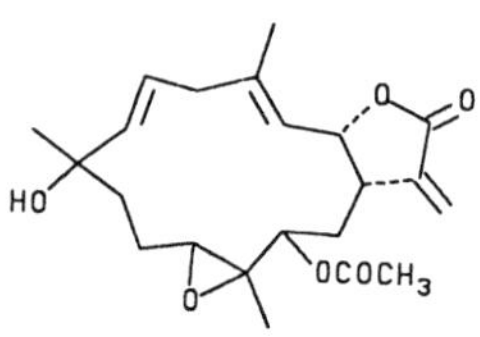

Mol. Wt.: 390
Melting Point: Oil
$[\alpha]_D$: +19 Solvent: Chf
Spectral Data: UV, IR, CMR, PMR, Mass Spec.
Organism: *Sinularia mayi* (Coelenterata)
Location: Okinawa, Japan
Reference: 588

$C_{22}H_{32}O_4$

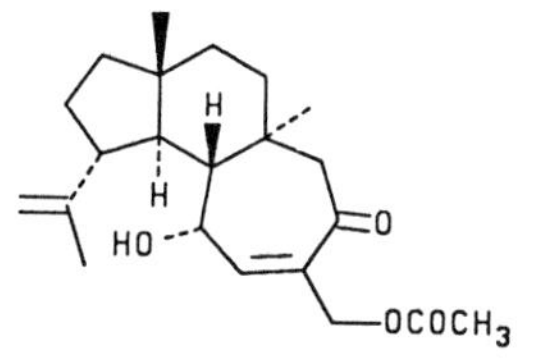

Mol. Wt.: 360
Melting Point: Oil
[α]$_D$: +52 Solvent: Chf
Spectral Data: UV, IR, CMR, PMR, Mass Spec.
Organism: *Higginsia* sp. (unidentified) (Porifera)
Location: Lancelin, Western Australia
Reference: 157

$C_{22}H_{32}O_4$ **Dictyodendrillolide**

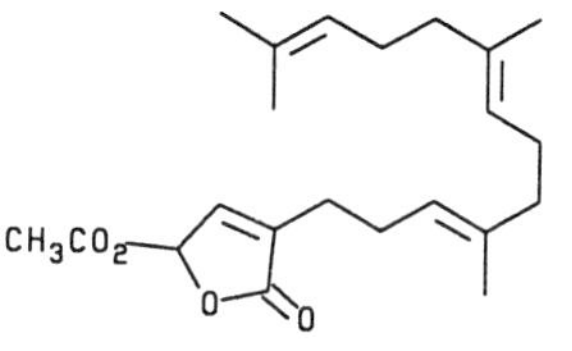

Mol. Wt.: 360
Melting Point: Oil
[α]$_D^{23}$: +21.9 Solvent: Chf
Spectral Data: UV, IR, CMR, PMR, Mass Spec.
Organism: *Dictyodendrilla nov.* sp. (Porifera)
Location: Great Barrier Reef, Australia
Reference: 132

$C_{22}H_{32}O_5$ **Shahamin F**

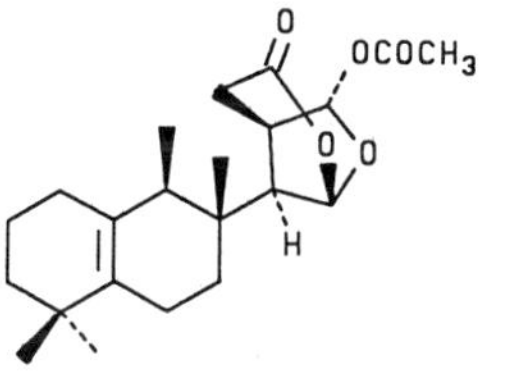

Mol. Wt.: 376
Melting Point: Oil
[α]$_D$: -49.6 Solvent: Chf
Spectral Data: IR, CMR, PMR, Mass Spec.
Organism: *Dysidea* spp. (Porifera)
Location: Red Sea
Reference: 150

$C_{22}H_{32}O_5$ **Styelolide**

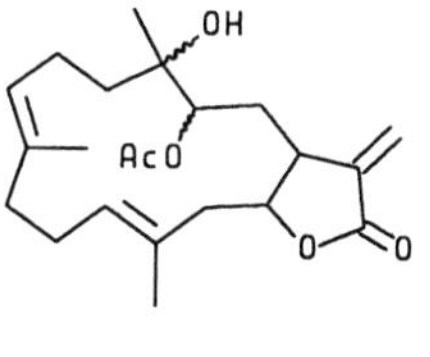

Mol. Wt.: 376
Spectral Data: CMR, PMR
Organism: *Styela plicata* (Chordata/Tunicata)
Reference: 1163

$C_{22}H_{32}O_5$ **Tetrahydroaplysulphurin-1**

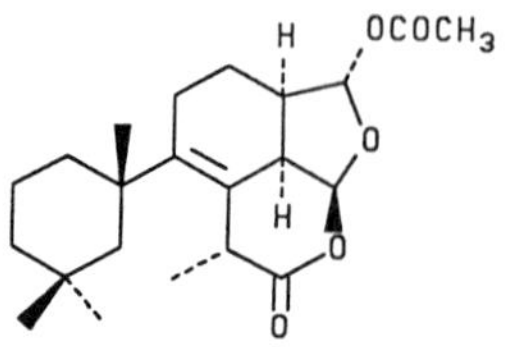

Mol. Wt.: 376
Melting Point: 109°C
$[\alpha]_D^{21}$: +169 Solvent: Chf
Spectral Data: UV, IR, CMR, PMR, Mass Spec.
Organism: *Darwinella* sp. (formerly *Aplysilla rosea*)
Darwinella oxeata Bergquist (Porifera)
Location: Leigh, New Zealand
Reference: 513

$C_{22}H_{32}O_5$ **Tetrahydroaplysulphurin-2**

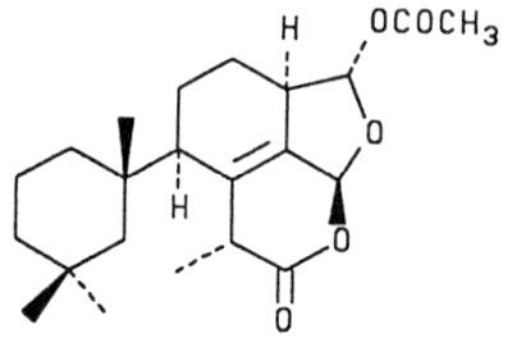

Mol. Wt.: 376
Melting Point: 181-183°C
Spectral Data: UV, IR, PMR, Mass Spec.
Organism: *Darwinella oxeata* Bergquist (Porifera)
Location: Leigh, New Zealand
Reference: 513

$C_{22}H_{32}O_5$ **Tetrahydroaplysulphurin-3**
(tentative structure)

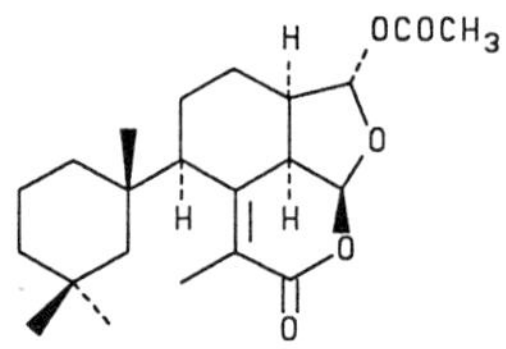

Mol. Wt.: 376
Melting Point: Oil
$[\alpha]_D^{20}$: +11.6 Solvent: Chf
Spectral Data: UV, IR, PMR, Mass Spec.
Organism: *Darwinella oxeata* Bergquist (Porifera)
Location: Leigh, New Zealand
Reference: 513

$C_{22}H_{32}O_6$ **6α,17β-Dihydroxy-15,17-oxidospongian-16-one 6-acetate**

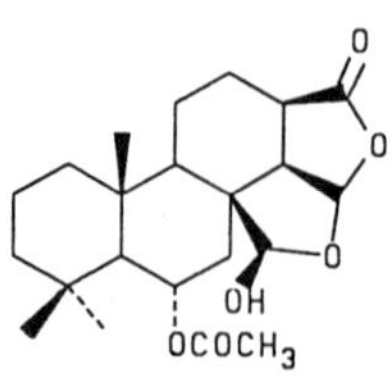

Mol. Wt.: 392
Melting Point: Oil
Spectral Data: IR, CMR, PMR, Mass Spec.
Organism: *Chromodoris epicuria* (Mollusca)
Location: South Australia
Reference: 615, 616

$C_{22}H_{32}O_6$ **Shahamin G**

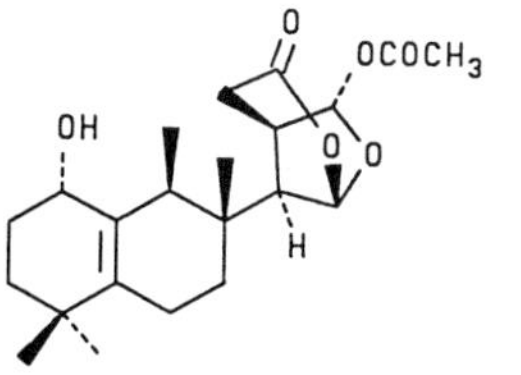

Mol. Wt.: 392
Melting Point: Oil
Spectral Data: IR, PMR, Mass Spec.
Organism: *Dysidea* sp. (Porifera)
Location: Red Sea
Reference: 150

$C_{22}H_{32}O_6$ **Shahamin H**

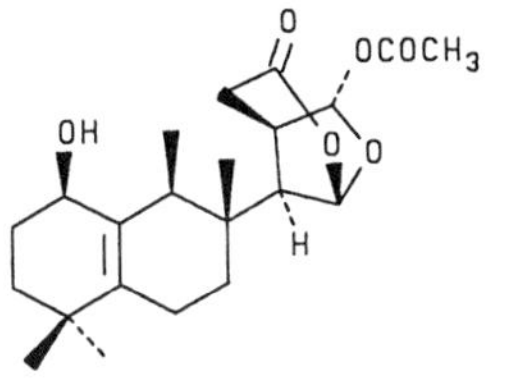

Mol. Wt.: 392
Melting Point: Oil
Spectral Data: IR, PMR, Mass Spec.
Organism: *Dysidea* sp. (Porifera)
Location: Red Sea
Reference: 150

$C_{22}H_{34}O_4$ **16-Oxospongian-7-yl acetate**

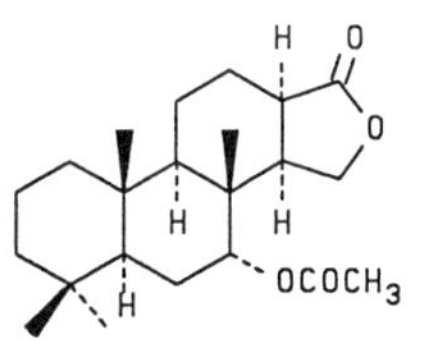

Mol. Wt.: 362
Melting Point: Oil
Spectral Data: UV, PMR, Mass Spec.
Organism: *Aplysilla rosea* Barrois (Porifera)
Location: Sydney, Australia
Reference: 516

$C_{22}H_{34}O_4$ **Sclerophytin B**

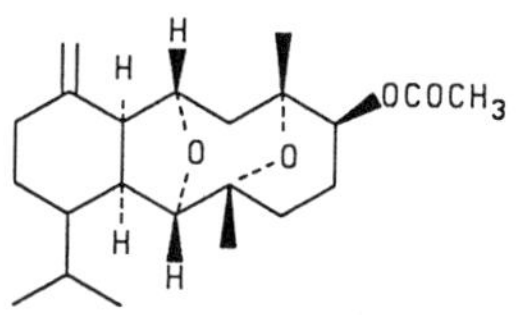

Mol. Wt.: 362
Melting Point: 191°C
Spectral Data: IR, CMR, PMR, Mass Spec.
Organism: *Sclerophytum capitalis* (Coelenterata)
Location: Enewetak, Micronesia
Reference: 998

$C_{22}H_{34}O_5$ **Shahamin D**

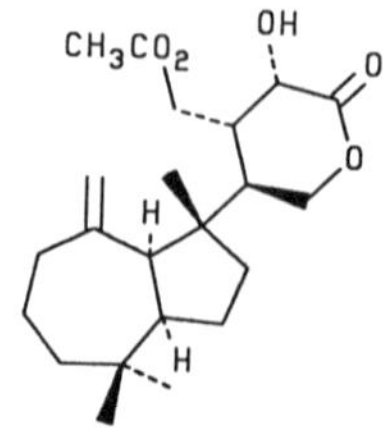

Mol. Wt.: 378
Melting Point: Oil
Spectral Data: IR, PMR, Mass Spec.
Organism: *Dysidea* sp.
(Porifera)
Location: Red Sea
Reference: 150

$C_{23}H_{34}O_5$ **Shahamin A**

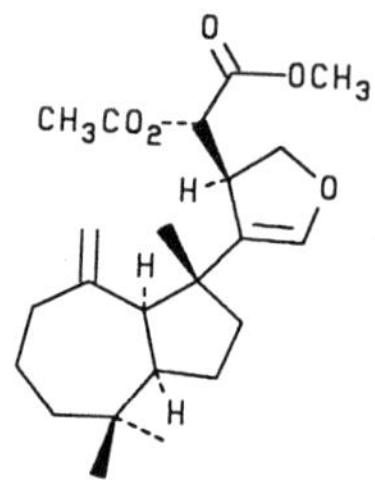

Mol. Wt.: 390
Melting Point: Oil
$[\alpha]_D$: +25 Solvent: Chf
Spectral Data: IR, CMR, PMR, Mass Spec.
Organism: *Dysidea* sp.
(Porifera)
Location: Red Sea
Reference: 150

$C_{24}H_{29}ClO_8$ **Ptilosarcenone**
(previously known)

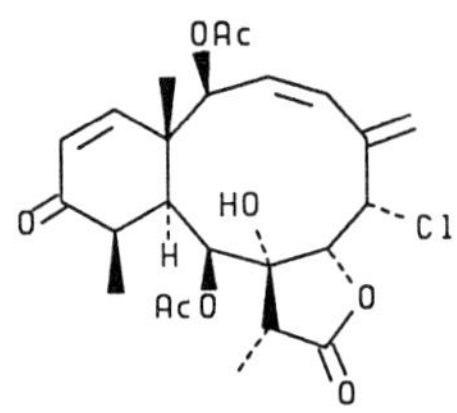

Mol. Wt.: 480
Bioactivity: Toxic to tobacco hornworm larvae at 250 ppm
Melting Point: 153-155°C
$[\alpha]_D^{26}$: -72.4 Solvent: DCM
Spectral Data: IR, CMR, Mass Spec.
Organism: *Tochuina tetraquetra*
(Mollusca)
Ptilosarcus gurneyi
(Coelenterata)
Location: British Columbia, Canada
Reference: 411, 1179

$C_{24}H_{29}ClO_9$ **11-Hydroxyptilosarcenone**

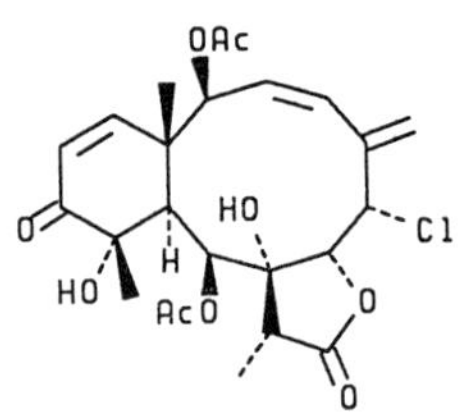

Mol. Wt.: 496
$[\alpha]_D^{26}$: -62.5 Solvent: Dcm
Spectral Data: UV, IR, CMR, PMR, Mass Spec.
Organism: *Ptilosarcus gurneyi*
(Coelenterata)
Location: British Columbia, Canada
Reference: 411

$C_{24}H_{29}ClO_9$ **Minabein-1**

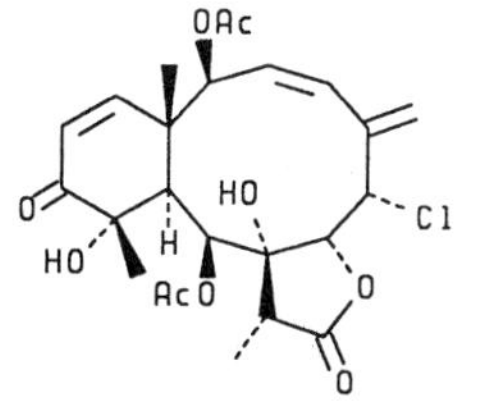

Mol. Wt.: 496
Melting Point: 190-192°C
$[\alpha]_D$: -48 Solvent: Chf
Spectral Data: UV, IR, CMR, PMR, Mass Spec.
Organism: *Minabea* sp. (Coelenterata)
Location: Truk
Reference: 614

$C_{24}H_{31}ClO_8$ **Ptilosarcen-12-ol**

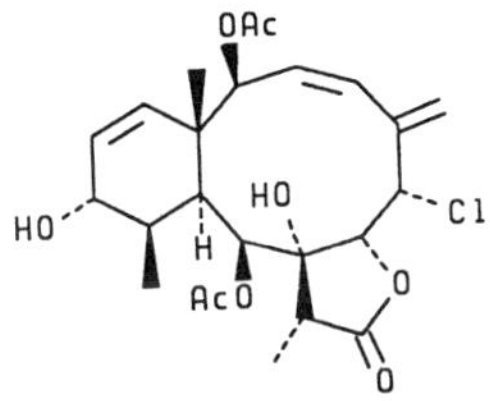

Mol. Wt.: 482
$[\alpha]_D^{26}$: -62.9 Solvent: Dcm
Spectral Data: UV, IR, PMR, Mass Spec.
Organism: *Ptilosarcus gurneyi* (Coelenterata)
Location: Seattle, Washington
Reference: 411

$C_{24}H_{31}ClO_9$ **Brianthein X**

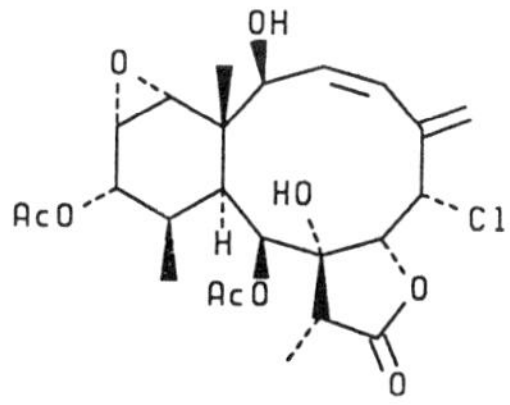

Mol. Wt.: 498
Melting Point: 230-232°C (dec.)
Spectral Data: UV, IR, CMR, PMR, Mass Spec.
Organism: *Briareum polyanthes* (Coelenterata)
Location: Bermuda
Reference: 364

$C_{24}H_{31}ClO_9$ **Minabein-2**

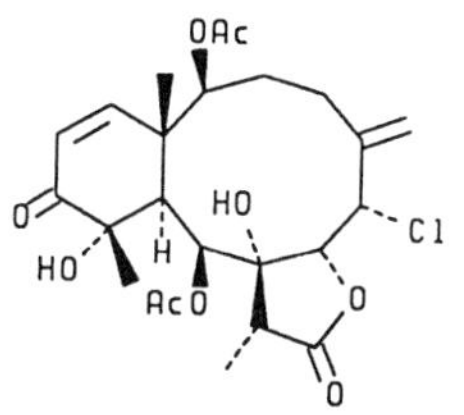

Mol. Wt.: 498
Melting Point: Oil
Spectral Data: UV, IR, CMR, PMR, Mass Spec.
Organism: *Minabea* sp. (Coelenterata)
Location: Truk
Reference: 614

$C_{24}H_{31}ClO_9$ **Minabein-5**

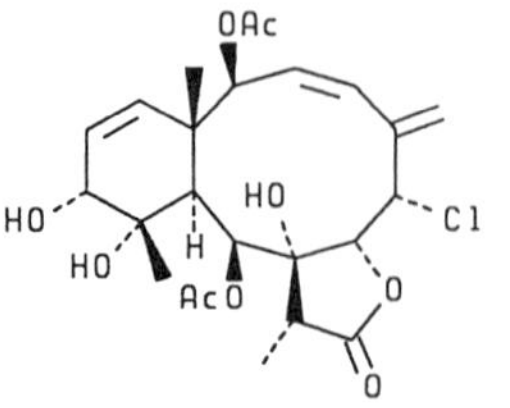

Mol. Wt.: 498
Melting Point: 155-158°C
Spectral Data: UV, IR, CMR, PMR, Mass Spec.
Organism: *Minabea* sp.
(Coelenterata)
Location: Truk
Reference: 614

$C_{24}H_{31}ClO_{10}$ **Solenolide C**

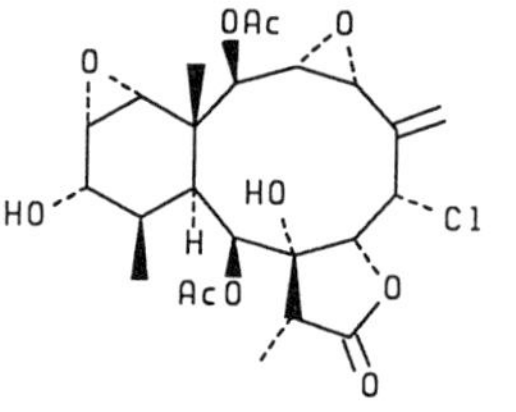

Mol. Wt.: 514
Bioactivity: Larvicidal towards Blowfly larvae: ED_{100} 30-35 ppm
Melting Point: 196-198°C (dec.)
$[\alpha]_D^{20}$: -25 Solvent: Me
Spectral Data: IR, CMR, PMR, Mass Spec.
Organism: *Solenopodium* sp.
(Coelenterata)
Location: Palau
Reference: 366

$C_{24}H_{32}O_9$ **Renillafoulin A**
(Minabein-8)

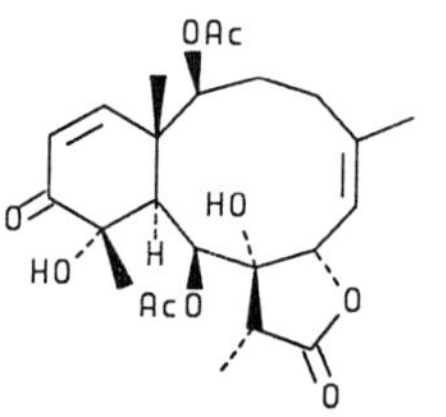

Mol. Wt.: 464
Bioactivity: Inhibition of barnacle larval settlement
Melting Point: 241-245°C
$[\alpha]_D$: -63 Solvent: Chf
Spectral Data: UV, IR, CMR, PMR, Mass Spec.
Organism: *Renilla reniformis*
Minabea sp.
(Coelenterata)
Location: North Carolina, Truk
Reference: 538, 614

$C_{24}H_{33}ClO_9$ **13-Desacetyl-11(19)-havannachlorhydrin**

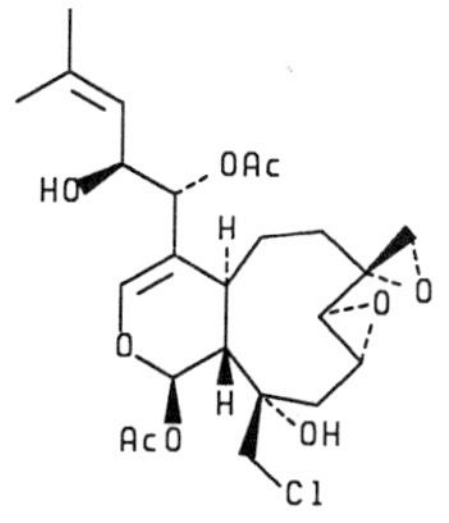

Mol. Wt.: 500
Spectral Data: IR, CMR, PMR, Mass Spec.
Organism: *Xenia membranacea* Schenk (Coelenterata)
Location: New Caledonia
Reference: 14

$C_{24}H_{33}ClO_9$ **Solenolide B**

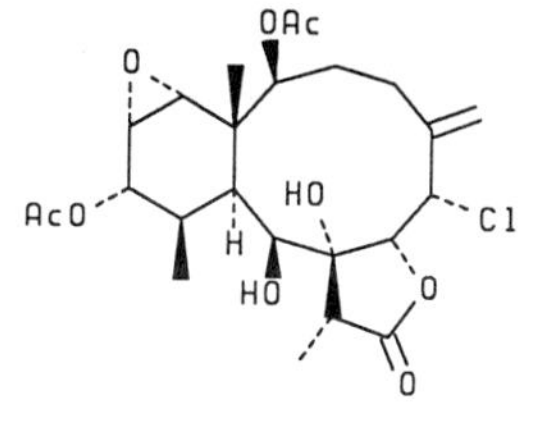

Mol. Wt.: 500
Bioactivity: Larvicidal towards Blowfly larvae: ED_{100} 30-35 ppm
Melting Point: Oil
$[\alpha]_D^{20}$: -5.0 Solvent: Chf
Spectral Data: IR, CMR, PMR, Mass Spec.
Organism: *Solenopodium* sp. (Coelenterata)
Location: Palau
Reference: 366

$C_{24}H_{34}O_7$ **6α,17α-Dihydroxy-15,17-oxidospongian-16-one 6,17-diacetate**

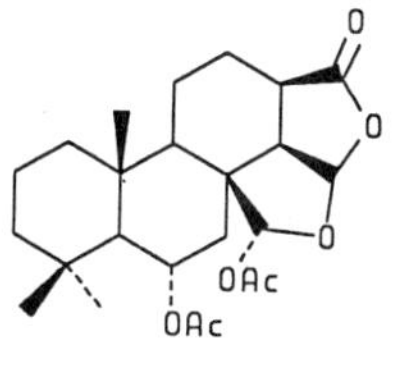

Mol. Wt.: 434
Melting Point: Oil
Spectral Data: IR, CMR, PMR, Mass Spec.
Organism: *Chromodoris epicuria* (Mollusca)
Location: South Australia
Reference: 615, 616

$C_{24}H_{34}O_7$ **Shahamin I**

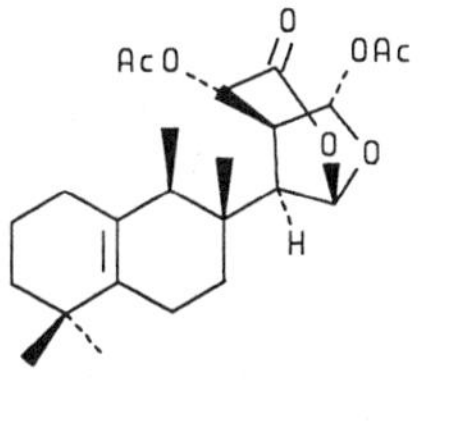

Mol. Wt.: 434
Melting Point: Oil
$[\alpha]_D$: -48.3 Solvent: Chf
Spectral Data: IR, CMR, PMR, Mass Spec.
Organism: *Dysidea* sp. (Porifera)
Location: Red Sea
Reference: 150

$C_{24}H_{34}O_8$ **Dendrillol-2**

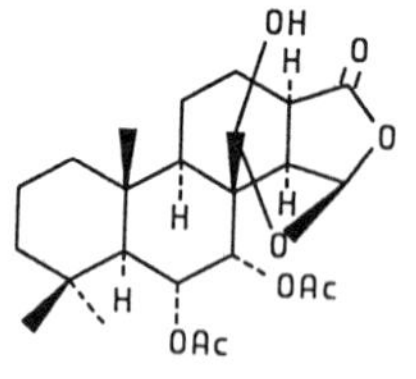

Mol. Wt.: 450
Spectral Data: UV, IR, CMR, PMR, Mass Spec.
Organism: *Dendrilla rosea* (Porifera)
Location: Leigh, New Zealand
Reference: 513

$C_{24}H_{34}O_8$ **Shahamin J**

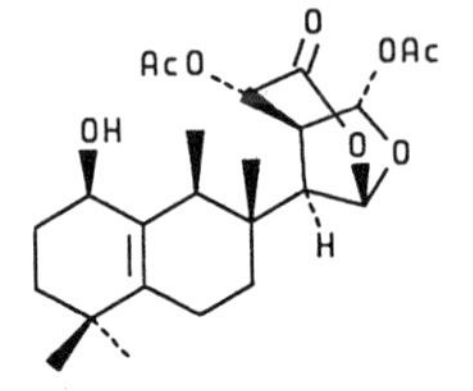

Mol. Wt.: 450
Melting Point: Oil
Spectral Data: IR, PMR, Mass Spec.
Organism: *Dysidea* sp. (Porifera)
Location: Red Sea
Reference: 150

$C_{24}H_{34}O_8$ **Solenolide F**

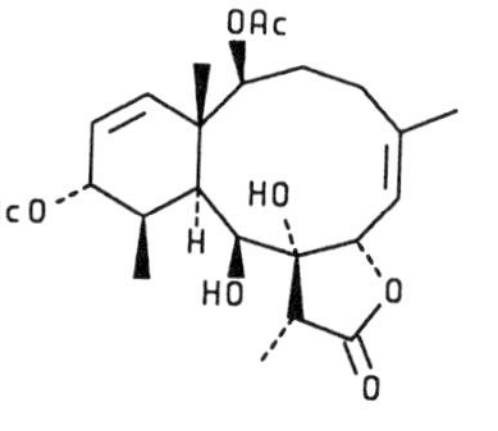

Mol. Wt.: 450
Bioactivity: Antiinflammatory activity: mouse ear assay: >70% reduction of edema at ~15 μg; Larvicidal activity against Blowfly larvae: ED_{100} 30-35 ppm
Melting Point: Oil
$[\alpha]_D^{20}$: -45 Solvent: Chf
Spectral Data: IR, CMR, PMR, Mass Spec.
Organism: *Solenopodium* sp. (Coelenterata)
Location: Palau
Reference: 366

$C_{24}H_{34}O_9$ **Minabein-7**

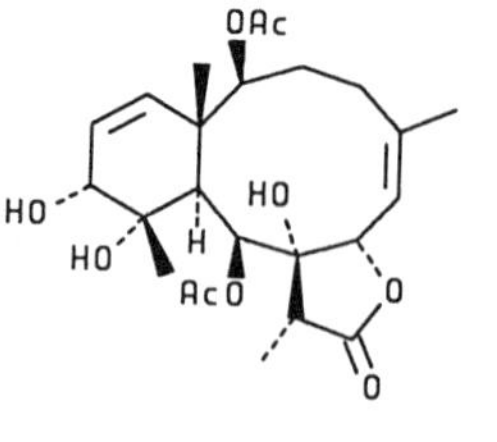

Mol. Wt.: 466
Melting Point: 278-280°C
Spectral Data: IR, CMR, PMR, Mass Spec.
Organism: *Minabea* sp. (Coelenterata)
Location: Truk
Reference: 614

$C_{24}H_{36}O_6$ **6α,17β-Dihydroxy-15,17-oxidospongian-16-one 6-butyrate**

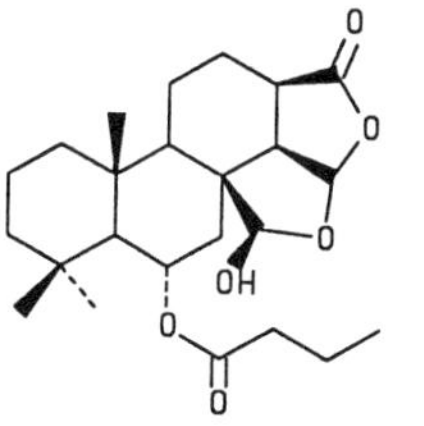

Mol. Wt.: 420
Melting Point: Oil
Spectral Data: IR, CMR, PMR, Mass Spec.
Organism: *Chromodoris epicuria* (Mollusca)
Location: South Australia
Reference: 615, 616

$C_{24}H_{36}O_6$ **16-Oxospongian-7,17-diyl diacetate**

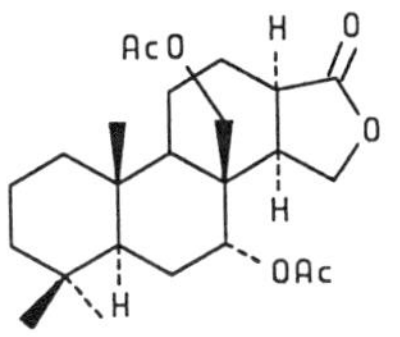

Mol. Wt.: 420
Spectral Data: UV, IR, CMR, PMR, Mass Spec.
Organism: *Aplysilla rosea* Barrois (Porifera)
Location: Sydney, Australia
Reference: 516

$C_{24}H_{36}O_6$ **Shahamin C**

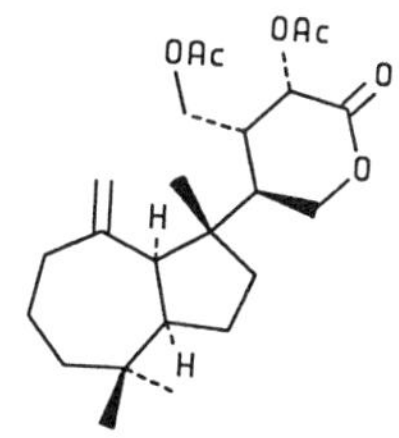

Mol. Wt.: 420
Melting Point: Oil
$[\alpha]_D$: +81 Solvent: Chf
Spectral Data: IR, CMR, PMR, Mass Spec.
Organism: *Dysidea* sp. (Porifera)
Location: Red Sea
Reference: 150

$C_{24}H_{36}O_7$ **Aplyroseol-3**

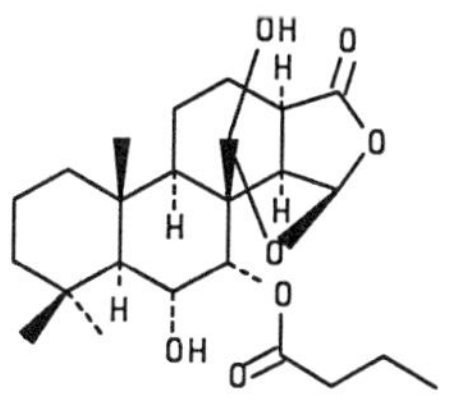

Mol. Wt.: 436
Melting Point: 214-215°C
$[\alpha]_D^{25}$: -0.6 Solvent: Chf
Spectral Data: UV, IR, CMR, PMR, Mass Spec.
Organism: *Dendrilla rosea*
Aplysilla rosea Barrois (Porifera)
Location: Leigh, New Zealand; Sydney, Australia
Reference: 513, 516

$C_{24}H_{36}O_7$ **Aplyroseol-5**

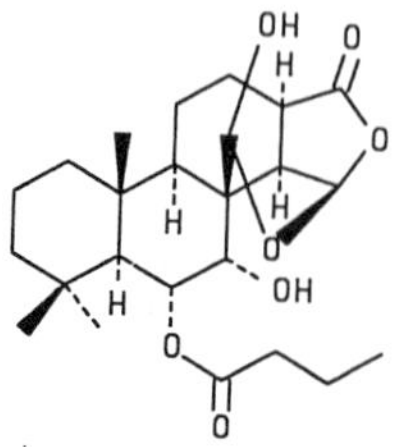

Mol. Wt.: 436
Melting Point: 214-217°C
$[\alpha]_D^{25}$: -3.4 Solvent: Chf
Spectral Data: UV, IR, CMR, PMR, Mass Spec.
Organism: *Aplysilla rosea* Barrois
Dendrilla rosea
(Porifera)
Location: Sydney, Australia; Leigh, New Zealand
Reference: 513, 516

$C_{24}H_{36}O_7$ **6α,7α,17β-Trihydroxy-15β,17-oxidospongian-16-one 7-butyrate**

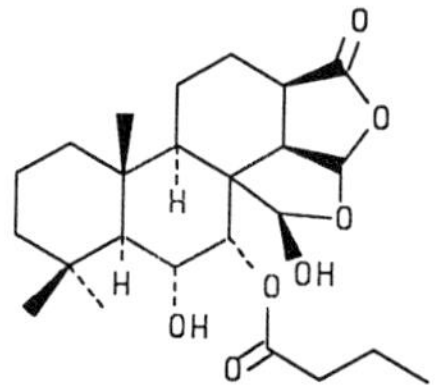

Mol. Wt.: 436
Melting Point: 212-213°C
Spectral Data: CD, IR, CMR, PMR, Mass Spec.
Organism: *Aplysilla* sp.
(Porifera)
Location: Australia
Reference: 753

$C_{24}H_{40}O_4$

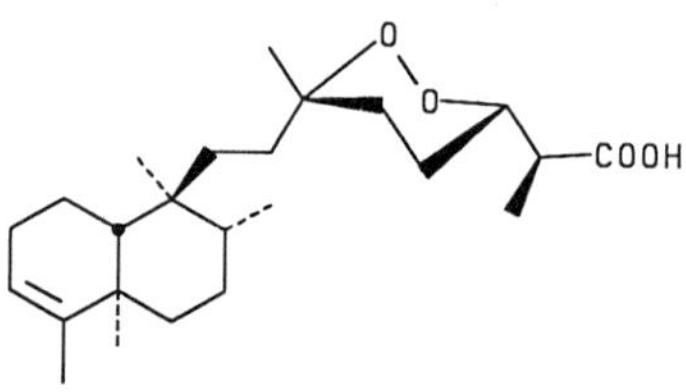

Mol. Wt.: 392
$[\alpha]_D$: -106.7 Solvent: Chf (methyl ester)
Spectral Data: CMR, PMR, Mass Spec. (methyl ester)
Organism: *Mycale ancorina* Whitelegge
(Porifera)
Location: Australia
Reference: 142

$C_{24}H_{40}O_4$

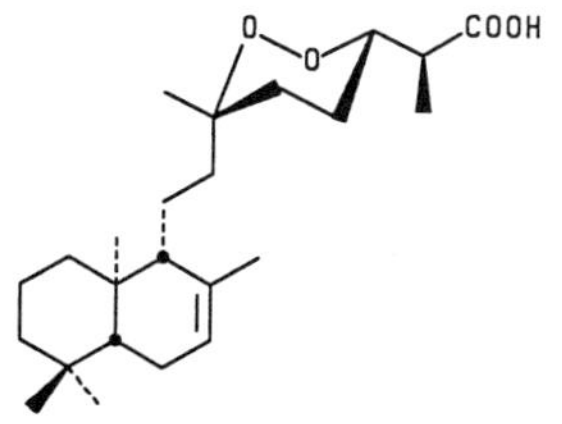

Mol. Wt.: 392
$[\alpha]_D$: -91 Solvent: Chf (methyl ester)
Spectral Data: CMR, PMR, Mass Spec. (methyl ester)
Organism: *Mycale ancorina* Whitelegge (Porifera)
Location: Australia
Reference: 142

$C_{24}H_{40}O_4$

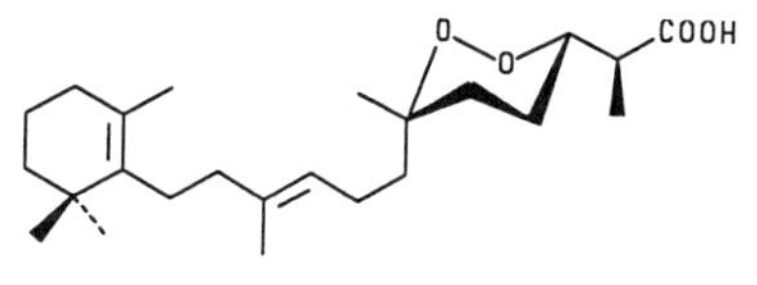

Mol. Wt.: 392
Bioactivity: Antimicrobial activity
Melting Point: Oil
$[\alpha]_D^{25}$: -59.2 Solvent: Chf (methyl ester)
Spectral Data: CMR, PMR, Mass Spec. (methyl ester)
Organism: *Latrunculia* sp. (Porifera)
Location: New South Wales, Australia
Reference: 141

$C_{24}H_{40}O_4$

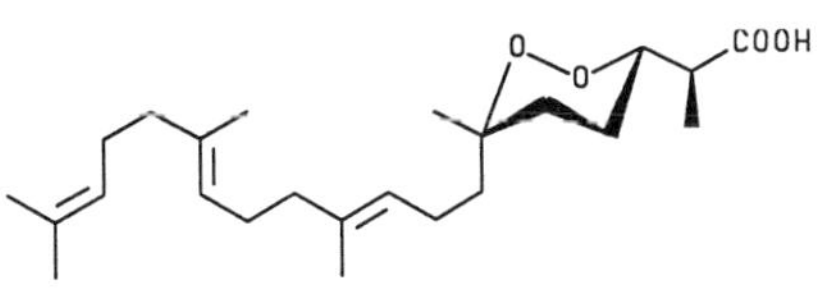

Mol. Wt.: 392
Bioactivity: Antimicrobial activity
Melting Point: Oil
$[\alpha]_D^{25}$: -60.0 Solvent: Chf (methyl ester)
Spectral Data: CMR, PMR, Mass Spec. (methyl ester)
Organism: *Latrunculia* sp. (Porifera)
Location: New South Wales, Australia
Reference: 141

$C_{24}H_{40}O_5$ **3,11-Diacetoxy-15,16-dehydrocembran-6-one**

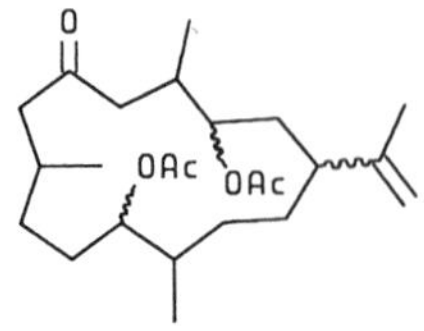

Mol. Wt.: 408
Melting Point: 145°C
$[\alpha]_D^{22}$: -4.0
Spectral Data: CMR, PMR
Organism: *Planaxis sulcatus* (Mollusca)
Location: Australia
Reference: 663

$C_{25}H_{34}O_9$ **Renillafoulin B**

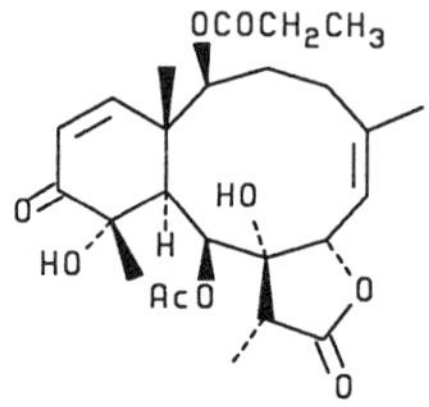

Mol. Wt.: 478
Bioactivity: Inhibition of barnacle larval settlement
Melting Point: Oil
Spectral Data: UV, IR, CMR, PMR, Mass Spec.
Organism: *Renilla reniformis* (Coelenterata)
Location: North Carolina
Reference: 538

$C_{25}H_{36}O_4$ **25-Nor-24-methyl-12,24-dioxoscalar-16-en-22-oic acid**

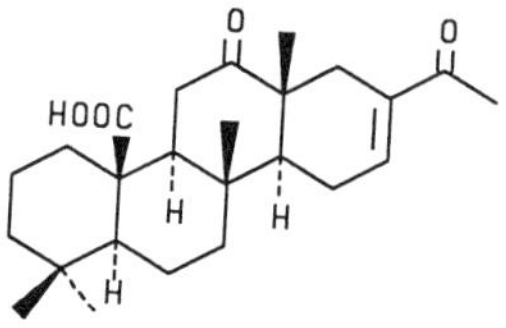

Mol. Wt.: 400
Spectral Data: IR, CMR, PMR, Mass Spec.
Organism: *Dictyoceratida* sp.
Halichondria sp.
(Porifera)
Location: Palau
Reference: 794

$C_{25}H_{38}O_3$ **12-Desacetyl-12-epi-scalaradial**

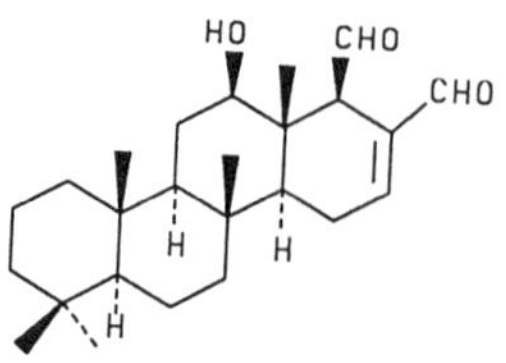

Mol. Wt.: 386
Melting Point: 165-167°C
$[\alpha]_D$: +9.2 Solvent: Chf
Spectral Data: CMR, PMR, Mass Spec.
Orgnism: *Hyrtios erecta* Keller (Porifera)
Location: Tonga
Reference: 209

$C_{25}H_{38}O_7$

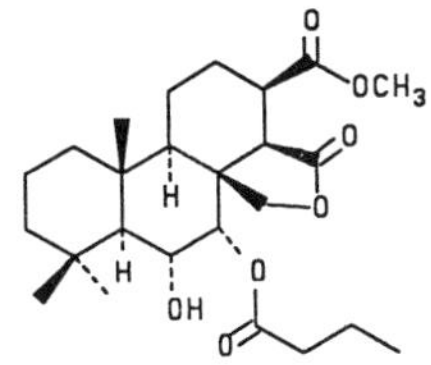

Mol. Wt.:	450
Melting Point:	Oil
Spectral Data:	IR, CMR, PMR, Mass Spec.
Organism:	*Aplysilla* sp. (Porifera)
Location:	Australia
Reference:	753

$C_{25}H_{38}O_7$ **Methyl 15,16-dideoxy-15α,17β-dihydroxy-15,17-oxidospongian-16-carboxylate 15,17-diacetate**

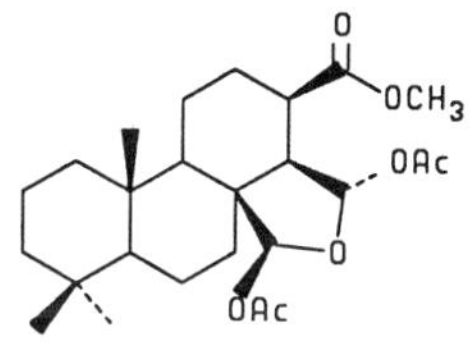

Mol. Wt.:	450
Melting Point:	Oil
Spectral Data:	IR, CMR, PMR, Mass Spec.
Organism:	*Chromodoris epicuria* (Mollusca)
Location:	South Australia
Reference:	615, 616

$C_{25}H_{40}O_2$

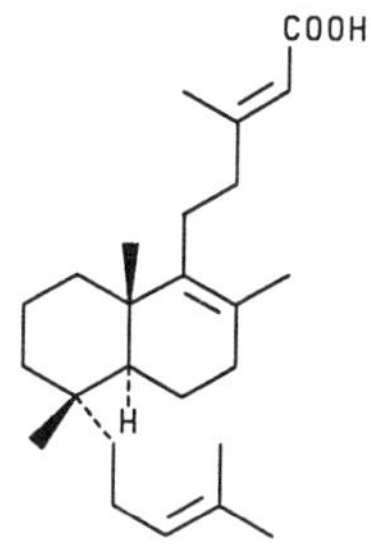

Mol. Wt.:	372
Bioactivity:	Aldose reductase inhibitory activity
Melting Point:	Oil
Spectral Data:	IR, CMR, PMR, Mass Spec.
Organism:	*Dysidea* sp. (Porifera)
Location:	Palau
Reference:	795

$C_{25}H_{40}O_5$ **Verrucosin-A**

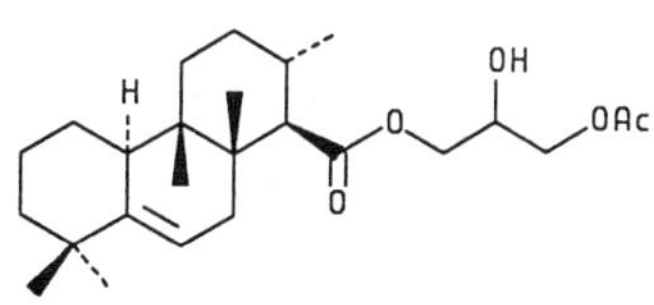

Mol. Wt.:	420
Bioactivity:	Toxic to *Gambusia affinis* at 1.0 μg/ml
$[\alpha]_D$:	+37.3 Solvent: Chf
Spectral Data:	IR, CMR, PMR, Mass Spec.
Organism:	*Doris verrucosa* Cuvier (Mollusca)
Location:	Naples
Reference:	187

$C_{25}H_{40}O_5$ **Verrucosin-B**

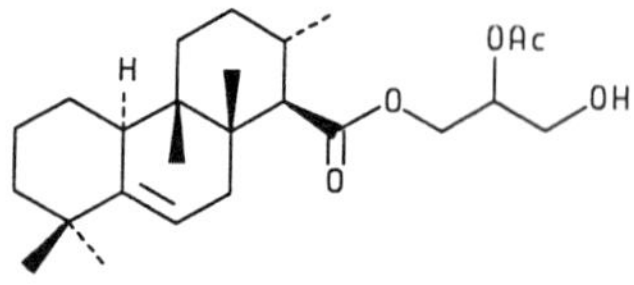

Mol. Wt.:	420
Bioactivity:	Toxic to *Gambusia affinis* at 0.1 μg/ml
Melting Point:	118-120°C
[α]$_D$:	+19.2 Solvent: Chf
Spectral Data:	IR, CMR, PMR, Mass Spec., x-ray c.s.
Organism:	*Doris verrucosa* Cuvier (Mollusca)
Location:	Naples
Reference:	187

$C_{25}H_{42}O_4$ **6β-Isovaleroxylabda-8,13-dien-7α,15-diol**

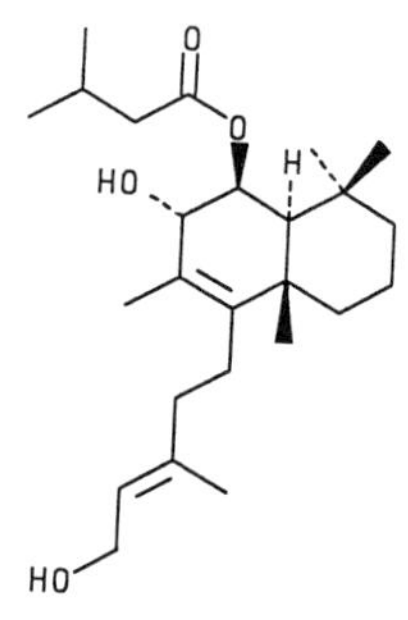

Mol. Wt.:	406
Melting Point:	Oil
[α]$_D$:	+38.7
Spectral Data:	IR, CMR, PMR, Mass Spec.
Organism:	*Trimusculus reticulatus* (Mollusca)
Location:	California
Reference:	696

$C_{26}H_{33}ClO_8$ **Ptilosarcenone butanoate**

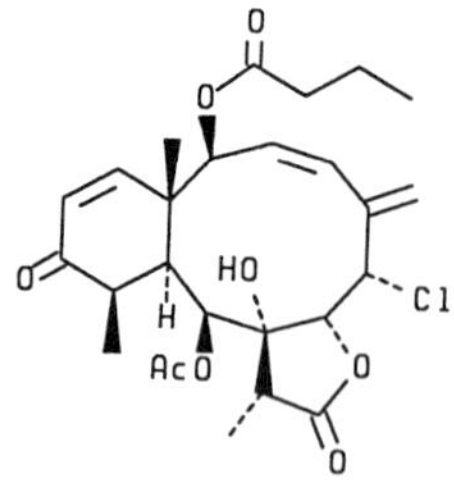

Mol. Wt.:	508
Melting Point:	Oil
[α]$_D^{25}$:	-49.2 Solvent: Dcm
Spectral Data:	UV, IR, PMR, Mass Spec.
Organism:	*Tochuina tetraquetra* (Mollusca)
Location:	British Columbia, Canada
Reference:	1179

$C_{26}H_{33}ClO_9$ **Ptilosarcen-12-acetate**

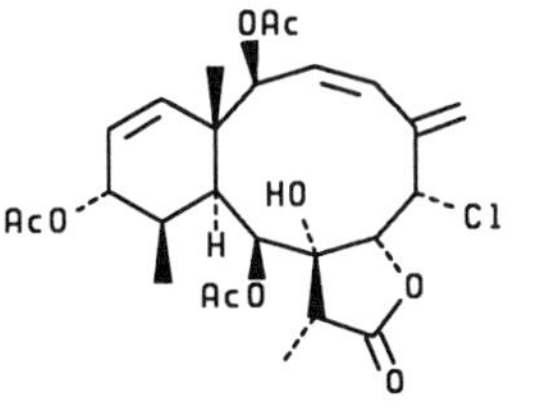

Mol. Wt.: 524
$[\alpha]_D^{26}$: -82.4 Solvent: Dcm
Spectral Data: UV, IR, PMR, Mass Spec.
Organism: *Ptilosarcus gurneyi* (Coelenterata)
Location: Seattle, Washington
Reference: 411

$C_{26}H_{33}ClO_{10}$ **Minabein-4**

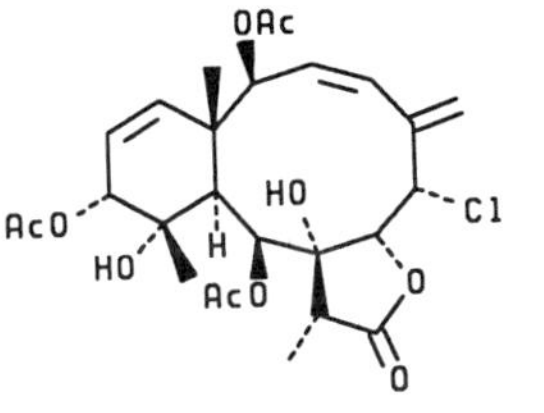

Mol. Wt.: 540
Melting Point: 227-230°C
$[\alpha]_D$: -299 Solvent: Chf
Spectral Data: UV, IR, CMR, PMR, Mass Spec.
Organism: *Minabea* sp. (Coelenterata)
Location: Truk
Reference: 614

$C_{26}H_{33}ClO_{11}$ **Solenolide D**

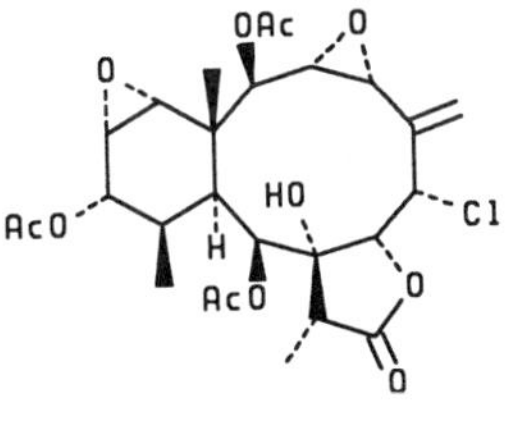

Mol. Wt.: 556
Bioactivity: Antiinflammatory activity: mouse ear assay: >70% reduction of edema at ~15 μg
Antiviral activity: inhibition of Semiliki Forest and Ann Arbor viruses
Larvicidal activity toward Blowfly larvae: ED_{100} 30-35 ppm
Melting Point: 183-185°C
$[\alpha]_D$: -16 Solvent: Chf
Spectral Data: IR, CMR, PMR, Mass Spec.
Organism: *Solenopodium* sp. (Coelenterata)
Location: Palau
Reference: 366

$C_{26}H_{34}O_9$ **Desoxyhavannahine**

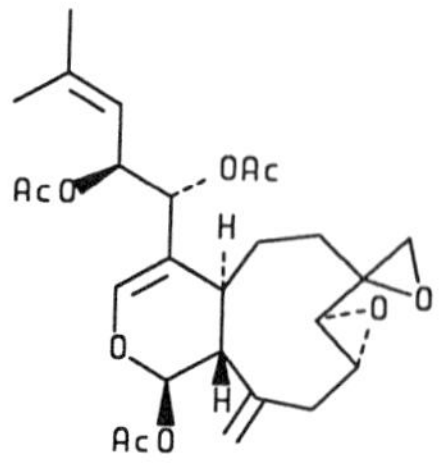

Mol. Wt.: 490
$[\alpha]_D$: +37 Solvent: Chf
Spectral Data: IR, CMR, PMR, Mass Spec.
Organism: *Xenia membranacea* Schenk (Coelenterata)
Location: New Caledonia
Reference: 14, 650

$C_{26}H_{34}O_{10}$ **Havannahine**

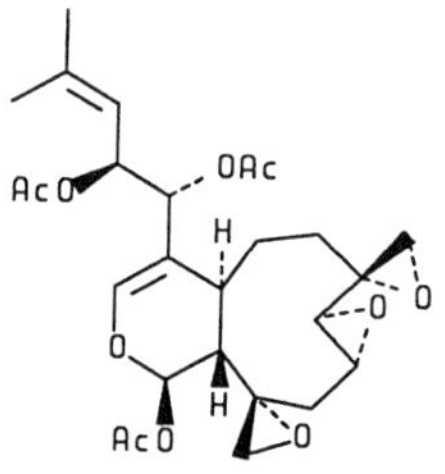

Mol. Wt.: 506
Melting Point: 181°C
$[\alpha]_D$: +33 Solvent: Chf
Spectral Data: IR, CMR, PMR, Mass Spec., x-ray c.s.
Organism: *Xenia membranacea* Schenk (Coelenterata)
Location: New Caledonia
Reference: 14, 650

$C_{26}H_{34}O_{11}$ **Minabein-10**

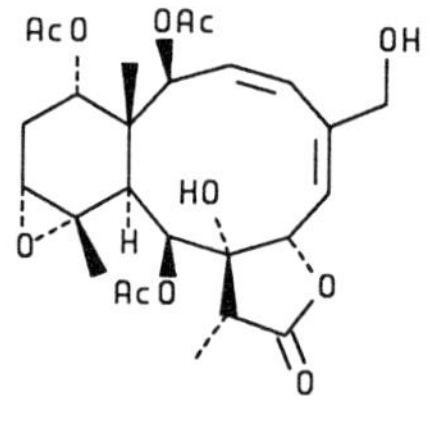

Mol. Wt.: 522
Melting Point: 135-138°C
Spectral Data: IR, CMR, PMR, Mass Spec.
Organism: *Minabea* sp. (Coelenterata)
Location: Truk
Reference: 614

$C_{26}H_{35}ClO_{10}$ **7(18)-Havannachlorhydrin**

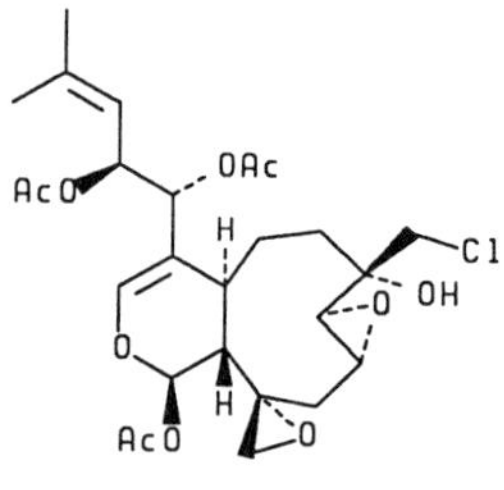

Mol. Wt.: 542
$[\alpha]_D$: +22 Solvent: Chf
Spectral Data: IR, CMR, PMR, Mass Spec.
Organism: *Xenia membranacea* Schenk (Coelenterata)
Location: New Caledonia
Reference: 14

$C_{26}H_{35}ClO_{10}$ **11(19)-Havannachlorhydrin**

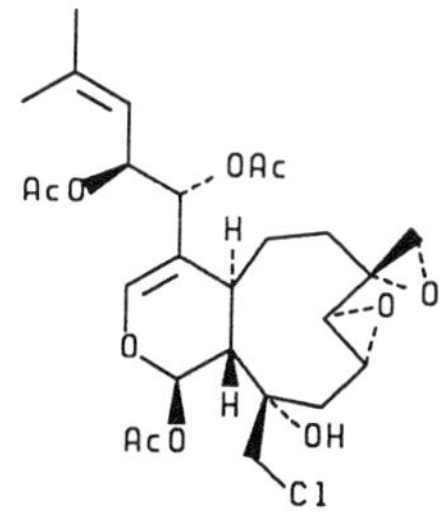

Mol. Wt.:	542
Melting Point:	145°C
$[\alpha]_D$:	-1.0 Solvent: Chf
Spectral Data:	IR, CMR, PMR, Mass Spec.
Organism:	*Xenia membranacea* Schenk (Coelenterata)
Location:	New Caledonia
Reference:	14

$C_{26}H_{35}ClO_{10}$ **Minabein-3**

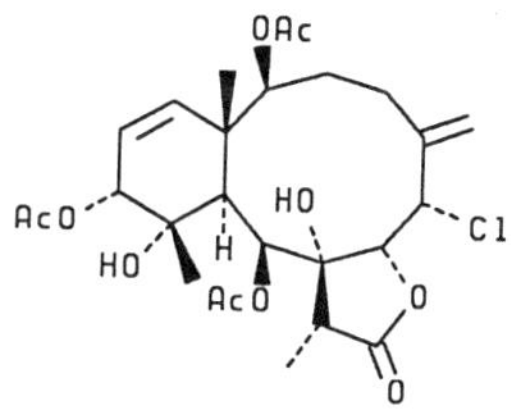

Mol. Wt.:	542
Melting Point:	241-243°C
Spectral Data:	IR, CMR, PMR, Mass Spec.
Organism:	*Minabea* sp. (Coelenterata)
Location:	Truk
Reference:	614

$C_{26}H_{36}O_7$ **14-Acetoxy-11,12-epoxy-18-oxobriara-5,8(17)-dien-2-yl butanoate**

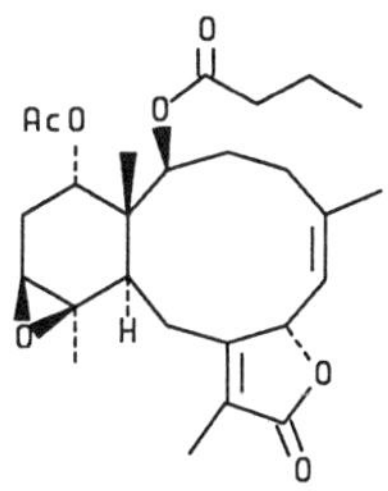

Mol. Wt.:	460
Melting Point:	158-160°C
$[\alpha]_D$:	+55.2 Solvent: Chf
Spectral Data:	IR, CMR, PMR, Mass Spec.
Organism:	*Briareum steckei* (Coelenterata)
Location:	Great Barrier Reef, Australia
Reference:	104

$C_{26}H_{36}O_7$ **Waixenicin-A**

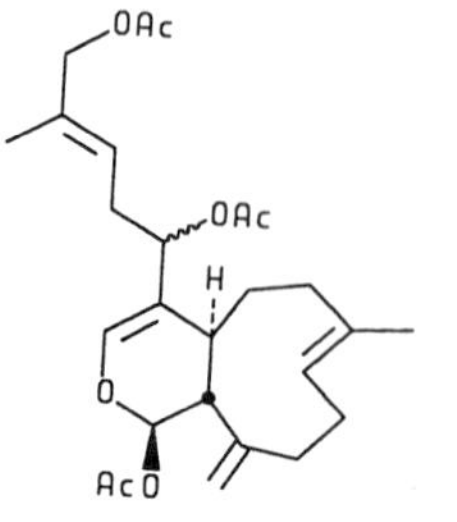

Mol. Wt.:	460
Melting Point:	Oil
$[\alpha]_D$:	+62.7 Solvent: Me
Spectral Data:	UV, IR, CMR, PMR, Mass Spec.
Organism:	*Anthelia edmondsoni* *Xenia* sp. (Coelenterata)
Location:	Hawaii; Great Barrier Reef, Australia
Reference:	97, 205

$C_{26}H_{36}O_8$ **Waixenicin-B**

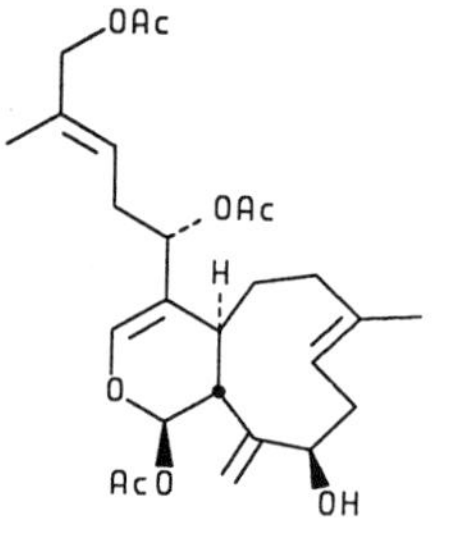

Mol. Wt.:	476
Melting Point:	124-125°C
$[\alpha]_D$:	+17.5 Solvent: Me
Spectral Data:	UV, IR, CMR, PMR, Mass Spec., x-ray c.s.
Organism:	*Anthelia edmondsoni* (Coelenterata)
Location:	Hawaii
Reference:	205

$C_{26}H_{36}O_9$ **Renillafoulin C**

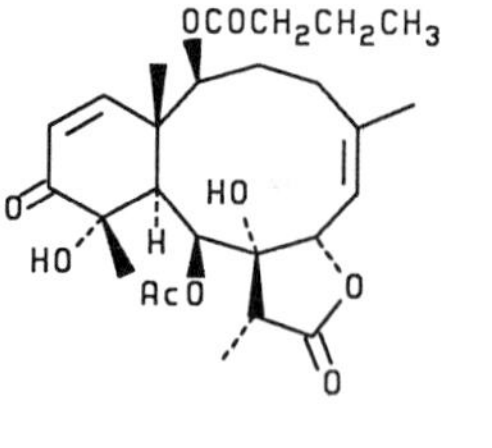

Mol. Wt.:	492
Bioactivity:	Inhibition of barnacle larval settlement
Spectral Data:	UV, IR, CMR, PMR, Mass Spec., x-ray c.s.
Organism:	*Renilla reniformis* (Coelenterata)
Location:	North Carolina
Reference:	538

$C_{26}H_{36}Cl_2O_{10}$ **7(18),11(19)-Havanna-dichlorhydrin**

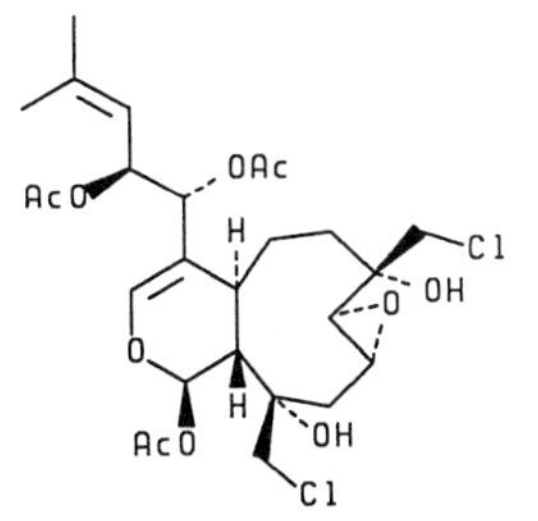

Mol. Wt.: 579
$[\alpha]_D$: -5.0 Solvent: Chf
Spectral Data: IR, CMR, PMR, Mass Spec., x-ray c.s. of bromohydrin derivative
Organism: *Xenia membranacea* (Coelenterata)
Location: New Caledonia
Reference: 14

$C_{26}H_{36}O_{10}$ **Minabein-6**

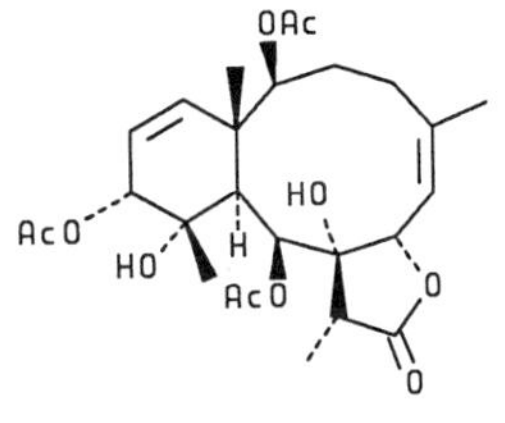

Mol. Wt.: 508
Melting Point: 259-262°C
$[\alpha]_D$: -204 Solvent: Chf
Spectral Data: IR, CMR, PMR, Mass Spec.
Organism: *Minabea* sp. (Coelenterata)
Location: Truk
Reference: 614

$C_{26}H_{36}O_{11}$ **Minabein-9**

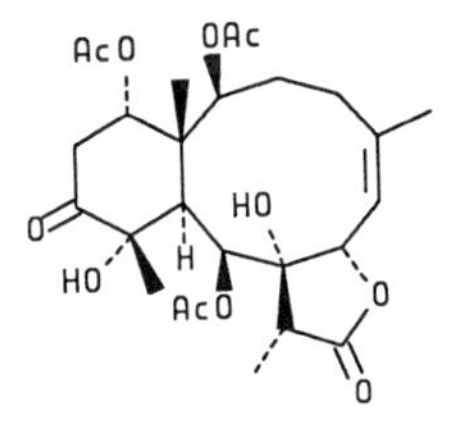

Mol. Wt.: 524
Melting Point: 190-193°C
Spectral Data: IR, CMR, PMR, Mass Spec.
Organism: *Minabea* sp. (Coelenterata)
Location: Truk
Reference: 614

$C_{26}H_{38}O_5$ **12α-Hydroxy-24-methyl-24,25-dioxoscalar-16-en-22-oic acid**

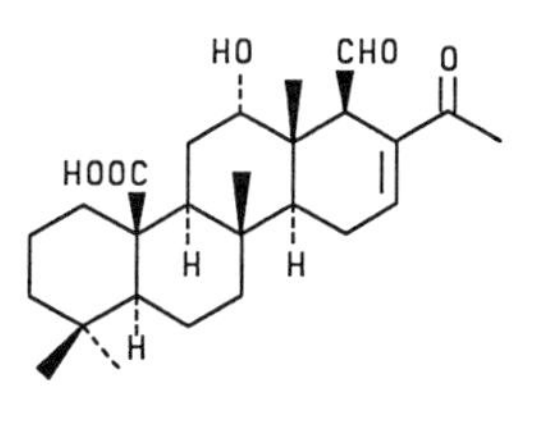

Mol. Wt.: 430
Spectral Data: IR, CMR, PMR, Mass Spec.
Organism: *Dictyoceratida* sp. *Halichondria* sp. (Porifera)
Location: Palau
Reference: 794

$C_{26}H_{38}O_7$ **6α,17α-Dihydroxy-15,17-oxidospongian-16-one 6-butyrate 17-acetate**

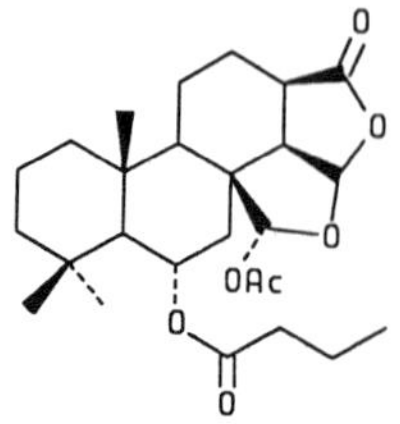

Mol. Wt.: 462
Melting Point: Oil
Spectral Data: IR, CMR, PMR, Mass Spec.
Organism: *Chromodoris epicuria* (Mollusca)
Location: South Australia
Reference: 615, 616

$C_{26}H_{38}O_8$ **Aplyroseol-4**

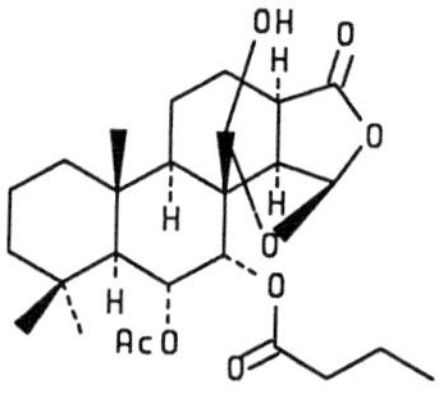

Mol. Wt.: 478
Melting Point: 125-127°C
Spectral Data: UV, IR, CMR, PMR, Mass Spec.
Organism: *Aplysilla rosea* Barrois (Porifera)
Location: Sydney, Australia
Reference: 516

$C_{26}H_{38}O_8$ **Aplyroseol-6**

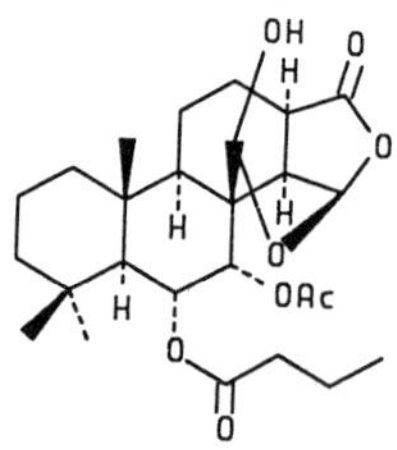

Mol. Wt.: 478
Melting Point: 133-135°C
$[\alpha]_D^{25}$: -10.9 Solvent: Chf
Spectral Data: UV, IR, CMR, PMR, Mass Spec.
Organism: *Dendrilla rosea*
Aplysilla rosea Barrois (Porifera)
Location: Leigh, New Zealand; Sydney, Australia
Reference: 513, 516

$C_{27}H_{35}ClO_9$ **Ptilosarcen-12-propionate**

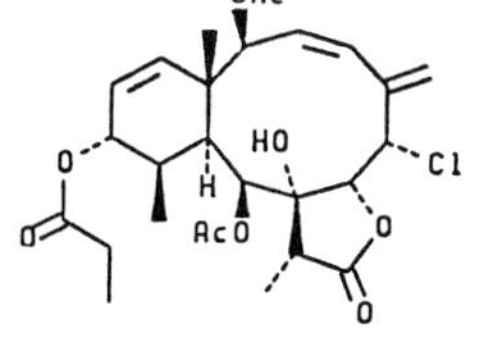

Mol. Wt.: 538
Bioactivity: Larvae of *Manduca sexta* (tobacco hornworm): reduction of weight gain
$[\alpha]_D^{26}$: -117 Solvent: Dcm
Spectral Data: UV, IR, CMR, PMR, Mass Spec.
Organism: *Ptilosarcus gurneyi* (Coelenterata)
Location: British Columbia, Canada; Seattle, Washington
Reference: 411

$C_{27}H_{36}O_9$ **4,14-Diacetoxy-11,12-epoxy-18-oxobriara-5,8(17)-dien-2-yl propanoate**

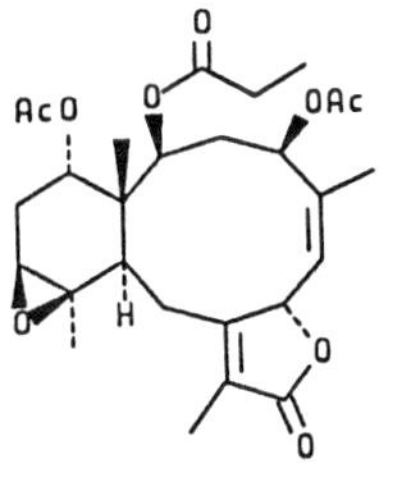

Mol. Wt.: 504
Spectral Data: PMR, CMR, x-ray c.s.
Organism: *Briareum steckei* (Coelenterata)
Location: Great Barrier Reef, Australia
Reference: 104

$C_{27}H_{38}O_6$ **Manoalide 25-monoacetate**

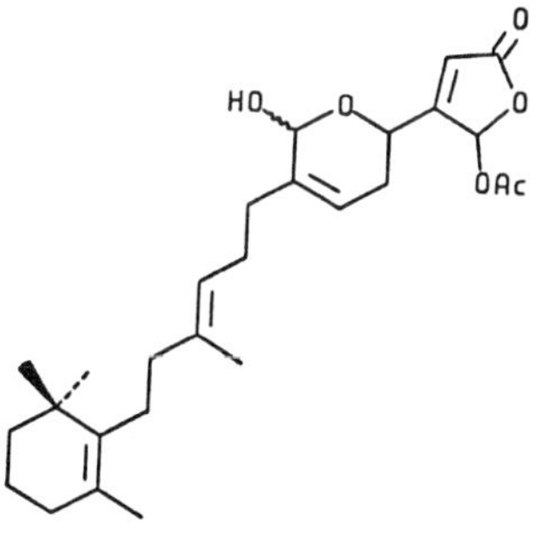

Mol. Wt.: 458
Melting Point: 117-119°C
$[\alpha]_D^{17}$: +34 Solvent: Chf
Spectral Data: UV, IR, CMR, PMR, Mass Spec.
Organism: *Thorectandra excavatus* (Ridley) *Stelospongus excavatus* (Porifera)
Location: Darwin, Australia
Reference: 134

$C_{27}H_{38}O_6$ **Thorectolide 25-monoacetate**

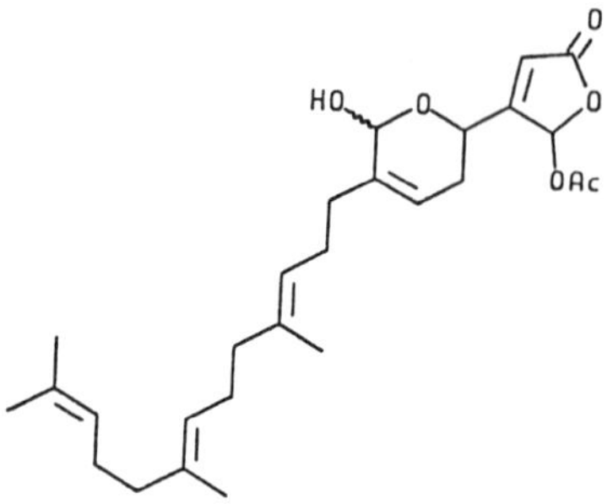

Mol. Wt.: 458
$[\alpha]_D^{23}$: +33 Solvent: Chf
Spectral Data: UV, IR, CMR, PMR, Mass Spec.
Organism: *Thorectandra excavatus* (Ridley)
Stelospongus excavatus
(Porifera)
Location: Darwin, Australia
Reference: 134

$C_{27}H_{40}O_4$ **12-epi-Scalaradial**
(previously known)

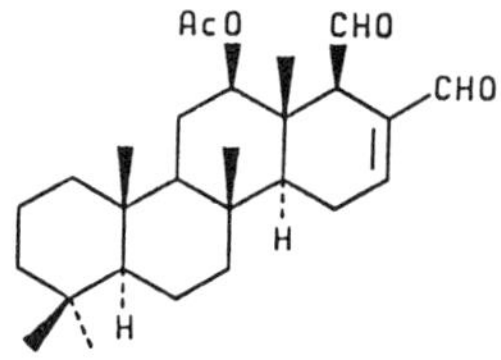

Mol. Wt.: 428
Bioactivity: Hypotensive effect
Organism: *Hyrtios erecta*
(Porifera)
Location: Palau
Reference: 185, 270

$C_{27}H_{40}O_9$ **Methyl 15,16-dideoxy-6α,15α,-17β-trihydroxy-15,17-oxidospongian-16-carboxylate 6,15,17-triacetate**

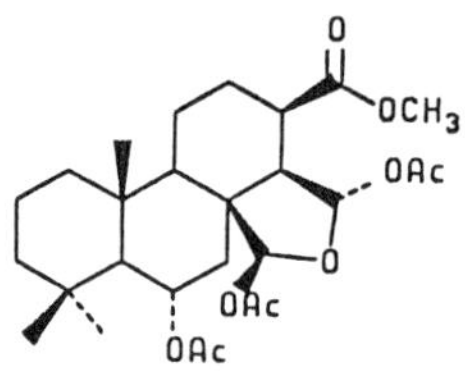

Mol. Wt.: 508
Melting Point: Oil
Spectral Data: IR, CMR, PMR, Mass Spec.
Organsism: *Chromodoris epicuria*
(Mollusca)
Location: South Australia
Reference: 615, 616

$C_{27}H_{44}O_4$ **12-Desacetyl-trans-24,25-dimethyoxyscalaran**

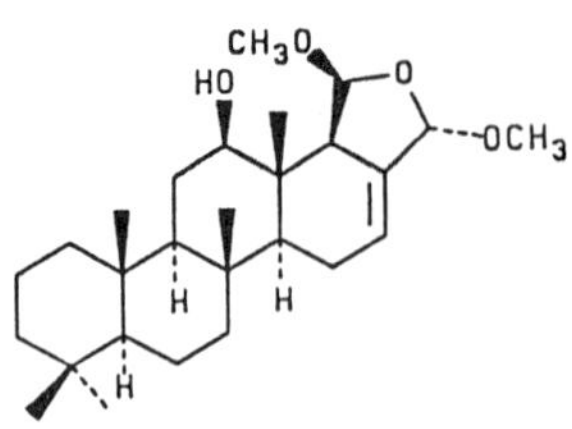

Mol. Wt.: 432
Spectral Data: CMR, PMR, Mass Spec.
Organism; *Hyrtios erecta* Keller
(Porifera)
Location: Tonga
Reference: 209

$C_{28}H_{37}ClO_{10}$	**Brianthein Y**	
Mol. Wt.:	568	
Bioactivity:	Antiviral to mouse corona virus at 400 μg/ml	
Melting Point:	233-235°C	
Spectral Data:	UV, IR, CMR, PMR, Mass Spec., x-ray c.s.	
Organism:	*Briareum polyanthes* *B. asbestinum* (Coelenterata)	
Location:	Bermuda, Bahamas	
Reference:	204, 364	

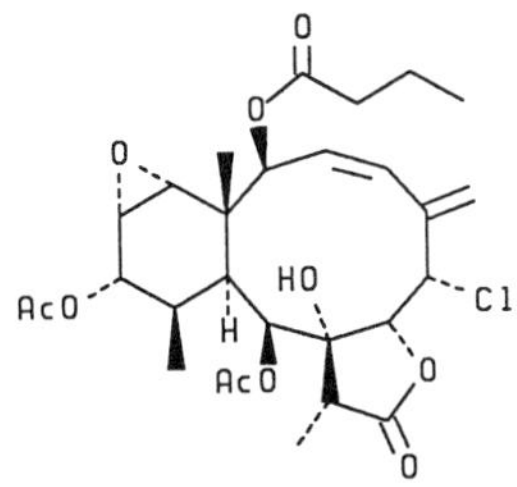

$C_{28}H_{38}O_9$	**3,14-Diacetoxy-11,12-epoxy-18-oxobriara-5,8(17)-dien-2-yl butanoate**	
Mol. Wt.:	518	
Melting Point:	Glass	
$[\alpha]_D$:	+155	Solvent: Chf
Spectral Data:	IR, CMR, PMR, Mass Spec.	
Organism:	*Briareum steckei* (Coelenterata)	
Location:	Great Barrier Reef, Australia	
Reference:	104	

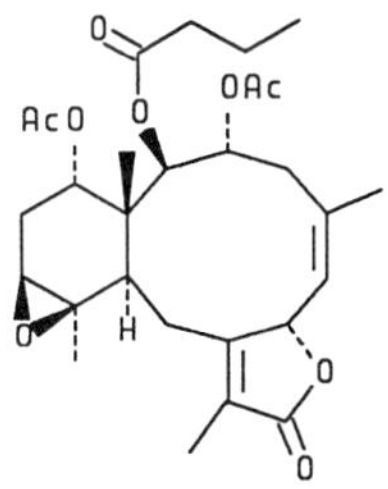

$C_{28}H_{38}O_9$	**4,14-Diacetoxy-11,12-epoxy-18-oxobriara-5,8(17)-dien-2-yl butanoate**	
Mol. Wt.:	518	
Melting Point:	183-186°C	
$[\alpha]_D$:	+101	Solvent: Chf
Spectal Data:	IR, CMR, PMR, Mass Spec., x-ray c.s.	
Organism:	*Briareum steckei* (Coelenterata)	
Location:	Great Barrier Reef, Australia	
Reference:	104	

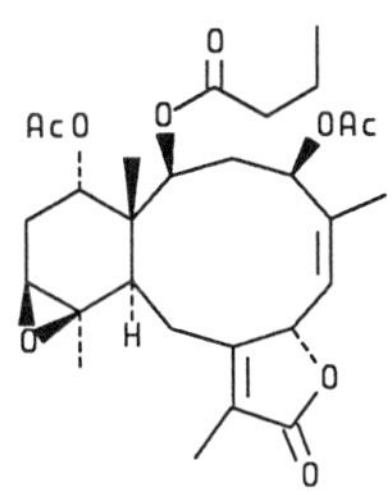

$C_{28}H_{39}ClO_{10}$ **Ptilosarcol**

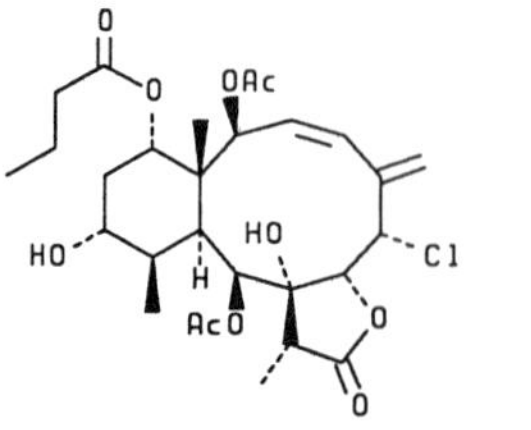

Mol. Wt.: 570
$[\alpha]_D^{26}$: -55.8 Solvent: Dcm
Spectral Data: UV, IR, PMR, Mass Spec.
Organism: *Ptilosarcus gurneyi* (Coelenterata)
Location: British Columbia, Canada
Reference: 411

$C_{28}H_{40}O_5$ **12α-Acetoxy-24-methyl-24-oxoscalar-16-en-22,25-dial**

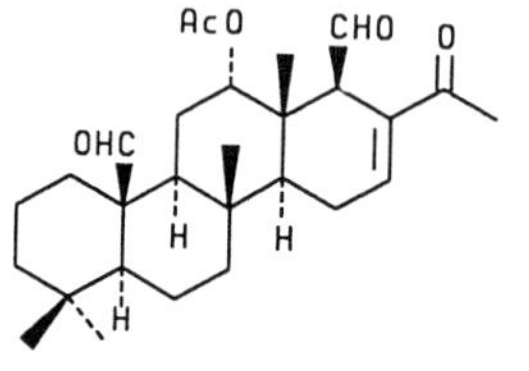

Mol. Wt.: 456
Bioactivity: Inhibition of platelet aggregation
Spectral Data: IR, CMR, PMR, Mass Spec.
Organism: *Dictyoceratida* sp.
Halichondria sp.
(Porifera)
Location: Palau
Reference: 794

$C_{28}H_{41}ClO_9$ **Solenolide A**

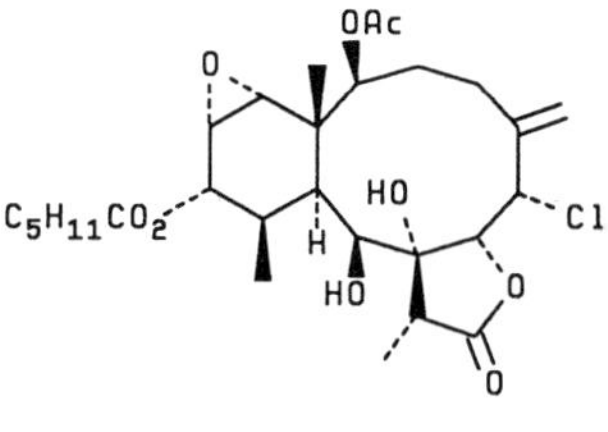

Mol. Wt.: 556
Bioactivity: Antiinflammatory activity:
mouse ear assay: >70% reduction of edema at ~15 μg
Inhibition of 5-lipoxygenase
Antiviral activity: Rhinovirus: IC_{50} 0.39 μg/ml
Inhibition of Polio III, Herpes, Ann Arbor and Maryland viruses
Larvicidal against Blowfly larvae: ED_{100} 30-35 ppm
Melting Point: 132-133°C
$[\alpha]_D^{20}$: -56 Solvent: Chf
Spectral Data: IR, CMR, PMR, Mass Spec.
Organism: *Solenopodium* sp. (Coelenterata)
Location: Palau
Reference: 366

$C_{28}H_{42}O_5$ **16β-Acetoxy-24-methyl-12,24-dioxoscalaran-25-al**

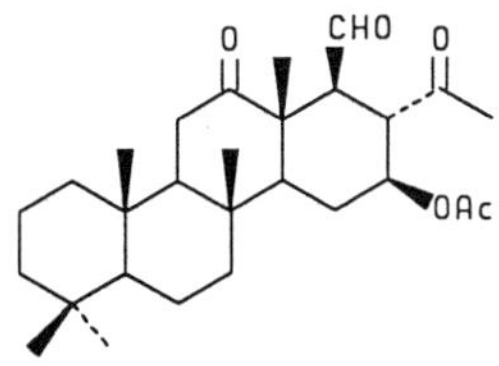

Mol. Wt.: 458
Melting Point: 227-229°C
[α]$_D$: +135 Solvent: Chf
Spectral Data: IR, CMR, PMR, Mass Spec.
Organism: *Carteriospongia flabellifera* (syn. *Phyllospongia flabellifera*) (Porifera)
Location: Great Barrier Reef, Australia
Reference: 983

$C_{29}H_{44}O_9$ **Methyl 15,16-dideoxy-6α,15α,17β-trihydroxy-15,17-oxidospongian-16-carboxylate 6-butyrate 15,17-diacetate**

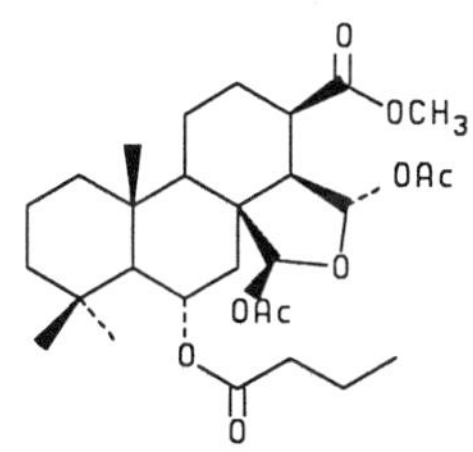

Mol. Wt.: 536
Melting Point: Oil
Spectral Data: IR, CMR, PMR, Mass Spec.
Organism: *Chromodoris epicuria* (Mollusca)
Location: South Australia
Reference: 615, 616

$C_{29}H_{46}O_5$ **12-<u>epi</u>-<u>cis</u>-24,25-Dimethoxyscalaran**

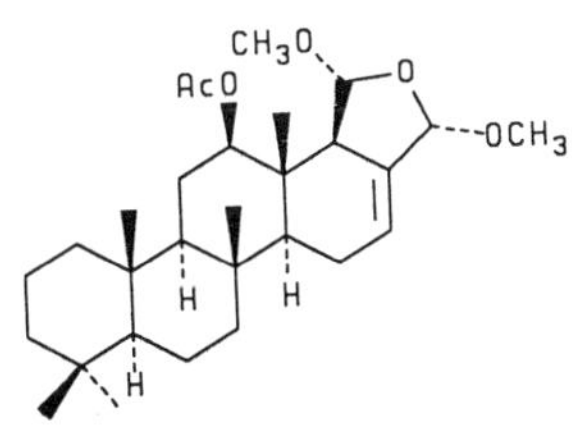

Mol. Wt.: 474
Melting Point: 196-198.5°C
[α]$_D$: -72 Solvent: Chf
Spectral Data: CMR, PMR, Mass Spec.
Organism: *Hyrtios erecta* Keller (Porifera)
Location: Tonga
Reference: 209

$C_{29}H_{46}O_7$ **2α,7α-Diacetoxy-6β-isovaleroxy-labda-8,13-dien-15-ol**

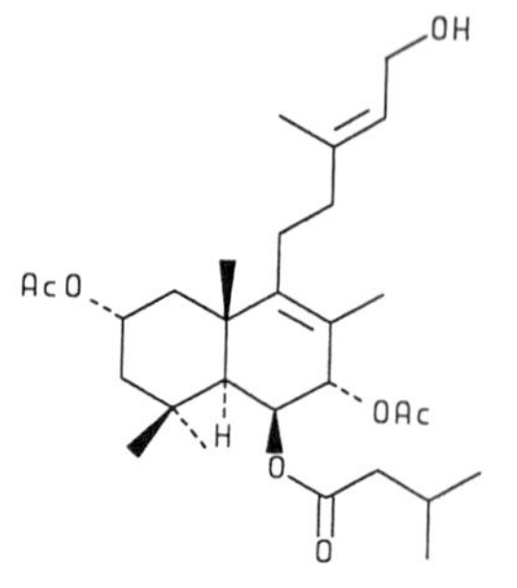

Mol. Wt.: 506
$[\alpha]_D$: +41.2 Solvent: Chf
Spectral Data: IR, CMR, PMR, Mass Spec.
Organism: *Trimusculus reticulatus* (Mollusca)
Location: California
Reference: 696

$C_{30}H_{46}O_4$ **Limatulone**

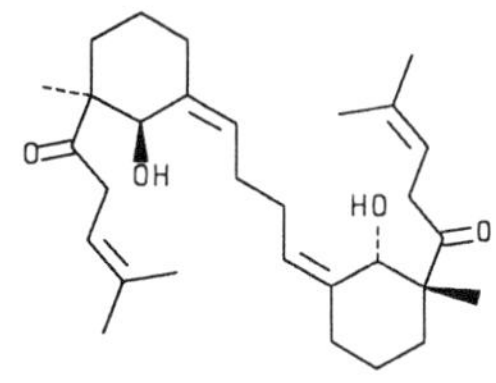

Mol. Wt.: 470
Bioactivity: Potent inhibitor of fish feeding
Spectral Data: IR, CMR, PMR, Mass Spec.
Organism: *Collisella limatula* (Mollusca)
Location: Southern California
Reference: 11

$C_{30}H_{50}O_6$ **Neviotine-A**

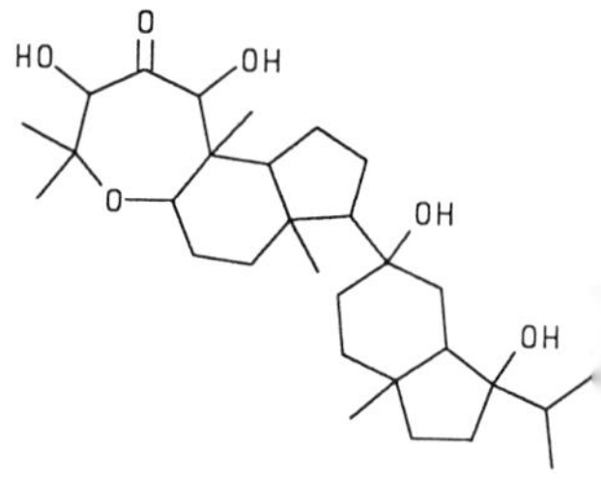

Mol. Wt.: 506
Melting Point: 231-233°C
$[\alpha]_D^{24}$: -50 Solvent: Chf
Spectral Data: IR, CMR, PMR, Mass Spec.
Organism: *Siphonochalina siphonella* (Porifera)
Location: Red Sea
Reference: 151

$C_{31}H_{46}O_7$ **12-<u>epi</u>-Heteronemin acetate**

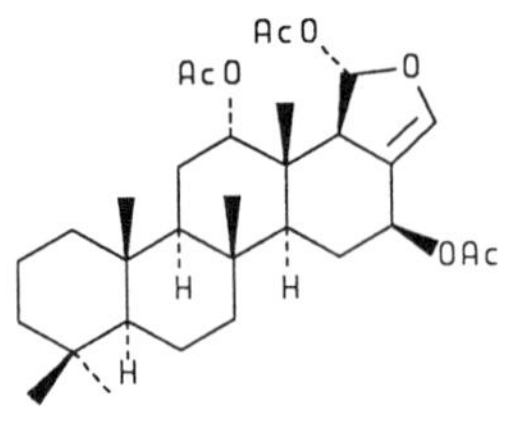

Mol. Wt.: 530
Spectral Data: CMR, PMR, Mass Spec.
Organism: *Hyrtios erecta* Keller (Porifera)
Location: Tonga
Reference: 209

$C_{31}H_{46}O_7$ **Heteronemin acetate**

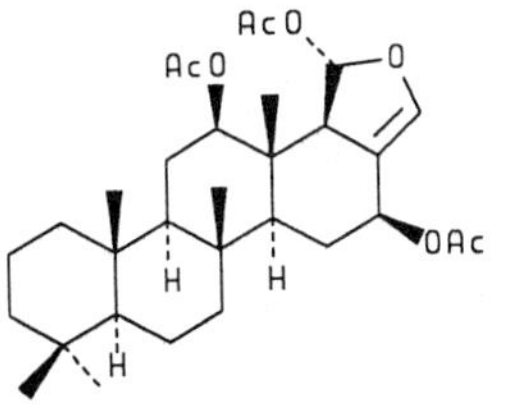

Mol. Wt.: 530
Melting Point: 211-212°C
$[\alpha]_D$: -30 Solvent: Chf
Spectral Data: CMR, PMR, Mass Spec.
Organism: *Hyrtios erecta* Keller (Porifera)
Location: Tonga
Reference: 209

$C_{40}H_{50}$ **3,4-Didehydro-γ,χ-carotene**

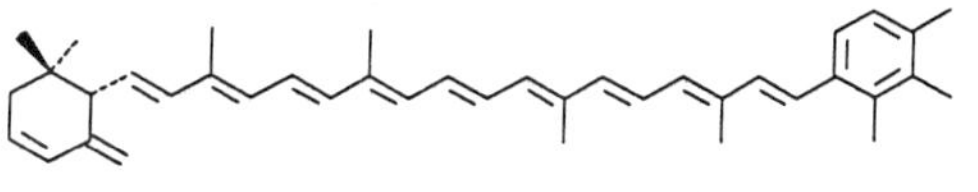

Mol. Wt.: 530
Spectral Data: UV, CD, IR, PMR, Mass Spec.
Organism: *Microciona prolifera* (Porifera)
Location: Massachusetts
Reference: 667, 1022

$C_{40}H_{50}O$ **Allopurpurin (Tedaniaxanthin)** (previously known)

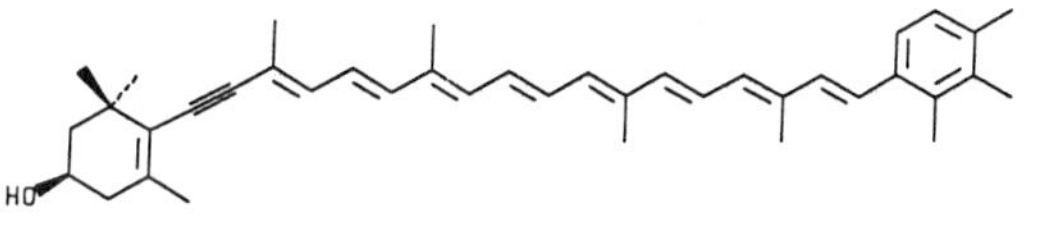

Mol. Wt.: 546
Spectral Data: UV, IR, PMR, Mass Spec.
Organism: *Microciona prolifera* (Porifera)
Location: Massachusetts
Reference: 667, 1080

$C_{40}H_{52}O_2$ **Alloxanthin** (previously known)

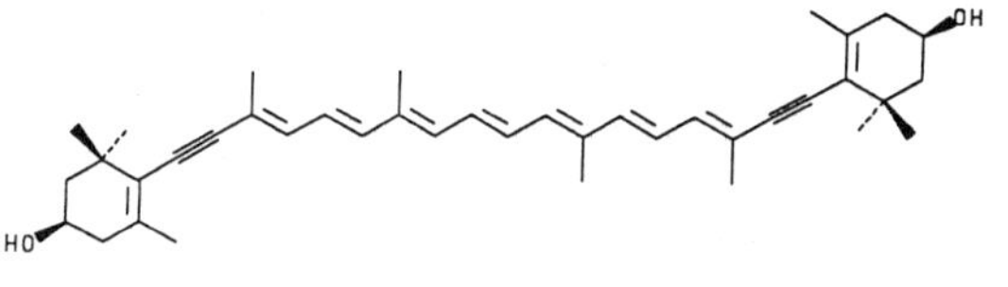

Mol. Wt.: 564
Melting Point: 186-188°C
Spectral Data: UV, CD, IR, PMR, Mass Spec.
Organism: *Microciona prolifera* (Porifera)
Location: Massachusetts.
Reference: 165, 262, 667, 693

$C_{40}H_{52}O_3$ **Trikentriophidin**

Mol. Wt.: 580
Spectral Data: UV, CD, PMR, Mass Spec.
Organism: *Microciona prolifera* (Porifera)
Location: Massachusetts
Reference: 667

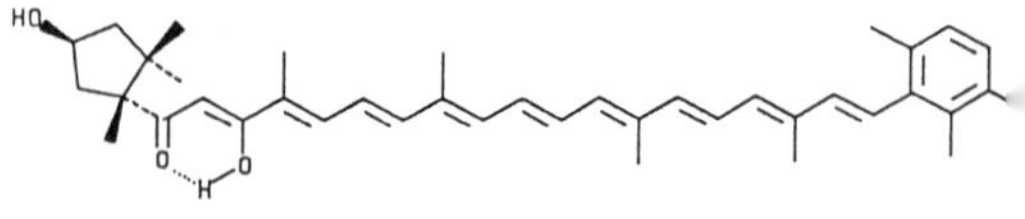

$C_{40}H_{64}O_{11}$ **Pouoside C**

Mol. Wt.: 721
Melting Point: Oil
Spectral Data: IR, CMR, PMR, Mass Spec.
Organism: *Asteropus* sp. (Porifera)
Location: Truk
Reference: 618

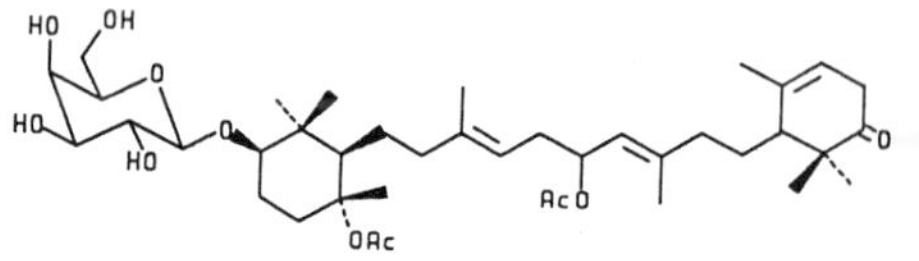

$C_{40}H_{64}O_{12}$ **Pouoside B**

Mol. Wt.: 737
Melting Point: Oil
Spectral Data: IR, CMR, PMR, Mass Spec.
Organism: *Asteropus* sp. (Porifera)
Location: Truk
Reference: 618

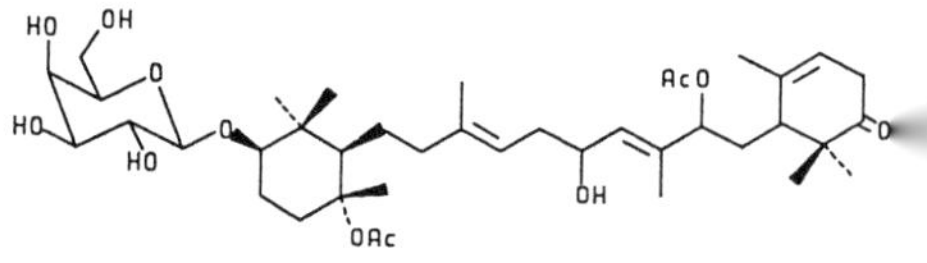

$C_{41}H_{62}O_9$ **Methyl isosartortuoate**

Mol. Wt.: 698
Melting Point: 194-195°C
Spectral Data: IR, CMR, PMR, Mass Spec., x-ray c.s.
Organism: *Sarcophyton tortuosum* Tixier-Durivault (Coelenterata)
Location: South China Sea
Reference: 1038

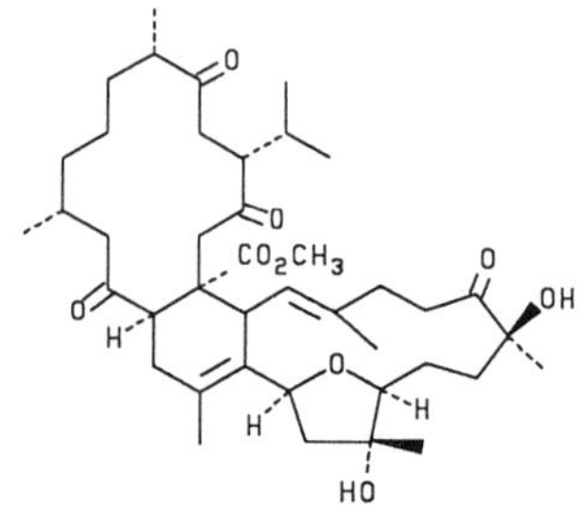

$C_{44}H_{68}O_{14}$ **Pouoside D**

Mol. Wt.: 821
Melting Point: Oil
Spectral Data: IR, PMR, Mass Spec.
Organism: *Asteropus* sp. (Porifera)
Location: Truk
Reference: 618

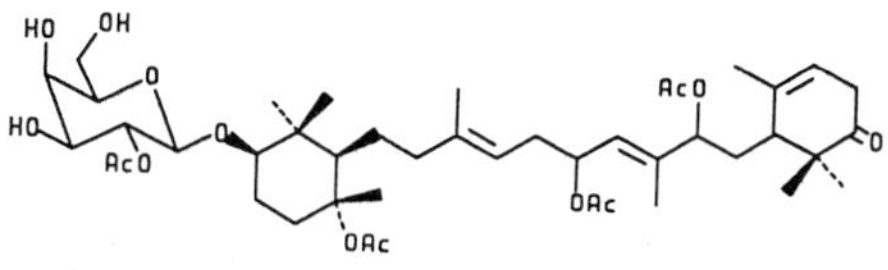

$C_{44}H_{68}O_{14}$ **Pouoside E**

Mol. Wt.: 821
Melting Point: Oil
Spectral Data: IR, PMR, Mass Spec.
Organism: *Asteropus* sp. (Porifera)
Location: Truk
Reference: 618

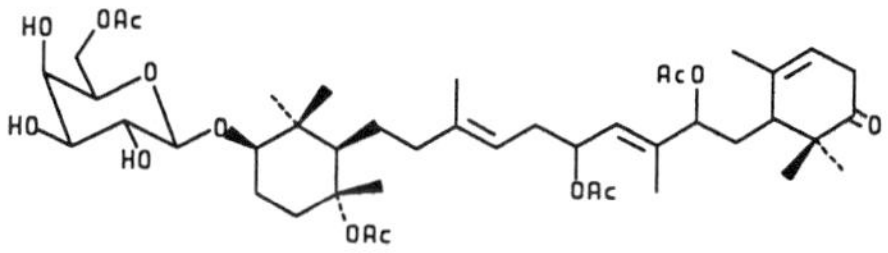

Chapter 15 STEROLS AND STEROIDS

$C_{21}H_{28}O_2$

Agnatasterone A

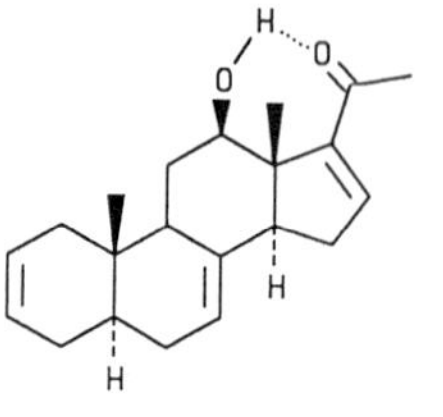

Mol. Wt.: 312
Melting Point: 123–124°C
$[\alpha]_D^{20}$: +63.5 Solvent: Chf
Spectral Data: UV, IR, CMR, PMR, Mass Spec.
Organism: *Axinella agnata* (Porifera)
Location: Brittany
Reference: 372

$C_{21}H_{28}O_2$

Agnatasterone B

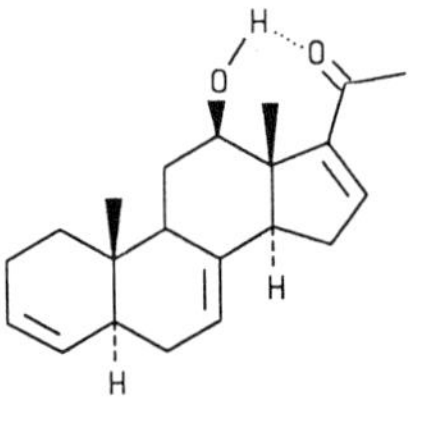

Mol. Wt.: 312
Melting Point: 104–105°C
$[\alpha]_D^{20}$: +17.6 Solvent: Chf
Spectral Data: UV, IR, CMR, PMR, Mass Spec.
Organism: *Axinella agnata* (Porifera)
Location: Brittany
Reference: 372

$C_{26}H_{42}O_3$

(22E)-24-Nor-5α-cholesta-7,22-diene-3β,5,6β-triol

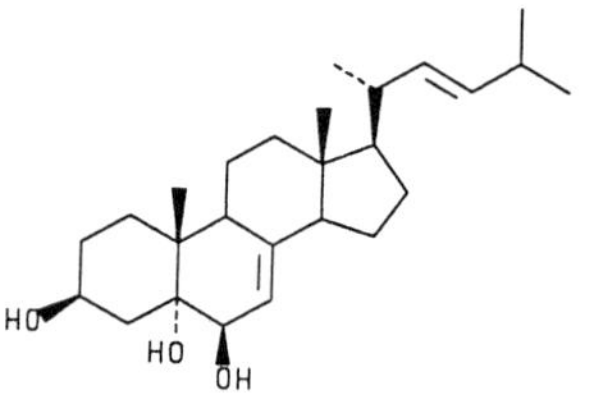

Mol. Wt.: 402
Melting Point: 215–217°C
Spectral Data: IR, PMR, Mass Spec.
Organism: *Spongionella gracilis* Vosmaer (Porifera)
Location: Naples, Italy
Reference: 895

$C_{26}H_{44}O$

(E)-24-Norcholest-22-en-3α-ol

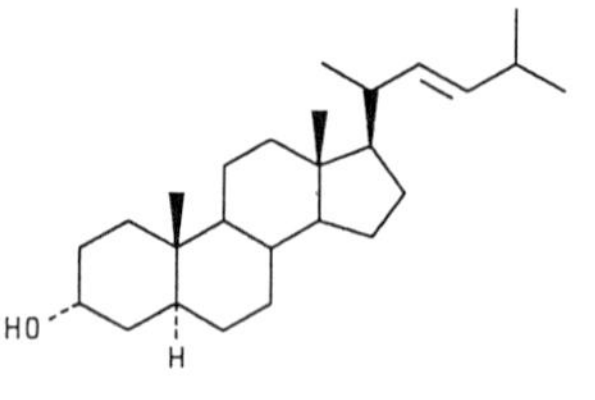

Mol. Wt.: 372
Spectral Data: PMR, Mass Spec.
Organism: *Esperiopsis edwardii* (Porifera)
Location: Chile
Reference: 994

$C_{26}H_{44}O_8$

3β,4β,5,6α,8,14,15α-Heptahydroxy-27-nor-5α-cholestan-24-one

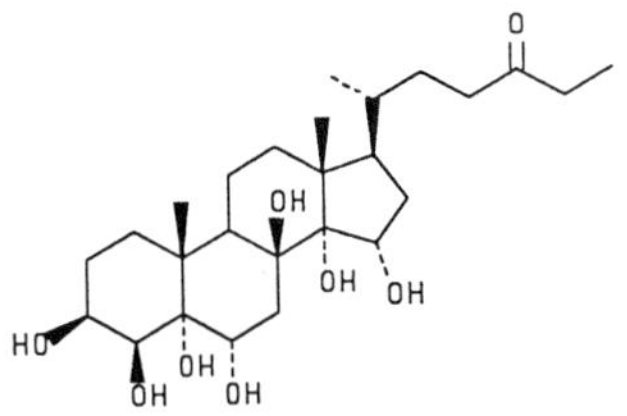

Mol. Wt.: 484
[α]$_D$: +40 Solvent: Me
Spectral Data: IR, CMR, PMR, Mass Spec.
Organism: *Archaster typicus* (Echinodermata)
Location: New Caledonia
Reference: 933

$C_{26}H_{45}NaO_{12}S$

(24R)-27-Nor-5α-cholestane-3β,4β,-5,6α,7β,8,14,15α,24-nonaol 6-sulfate

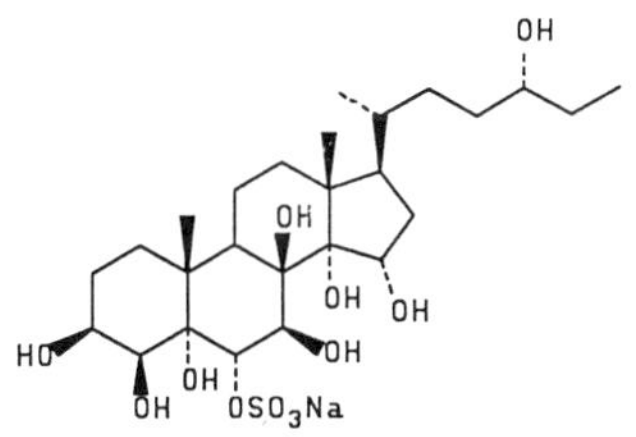

Mol. Wt.: 604
[α]$_D$: +56.2 Solvent: Me
Spectral Data: CMR, PMR, Mass Spec.
Organism: *Archaster typicus* (Echinodermata)
Location: Sweden
Reference: 933

$C_{26}H_{46}O_8$

(24R)-27-Nor-5α-cholestane-3β,4β,5,6α,8,14,15α,24-octaol

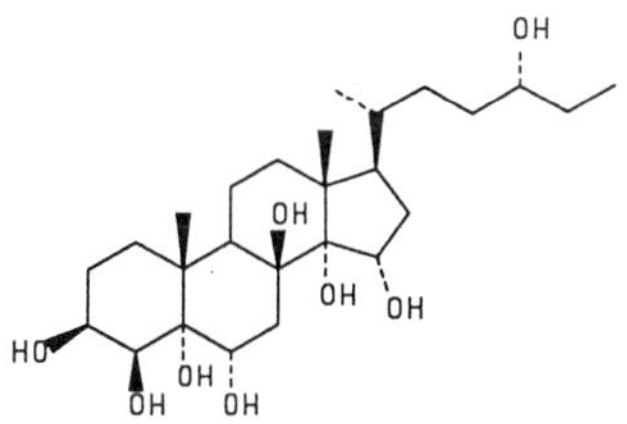

Mol. Wt.: 486
Melting Point: 294°C
[α]$_D$: +43.4 Solvent: Me
Spectral Data: CMR, PMR, Mass Spec.
Organism: *Archaster typicus* (Echinodermata)
Location: New Caledonia
Reference: 933

$C_{26}H_{46}O_9$ **(24R)-27-Nor-5α-cholestane-3β,4β,5,6α,7β,8,14,15α,24-nonaol**

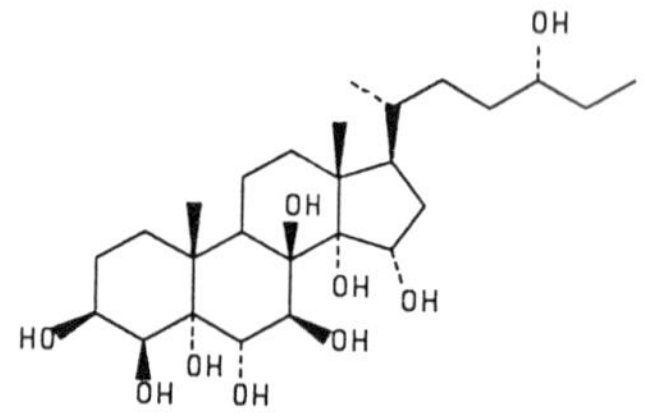

Mol. Wt.: 502
Melting Point: 288–290°C
$[\alpha]_D$: +37.6 Solvent: Me
Spectral Data: CMR, PMR, Mass Spec.
Organism: *Archaster typicus* (Echinodermata)
Location: New Caledonia
Reference: 933

$C_{27}H_{38}O_3$ **Minabeolide-4**

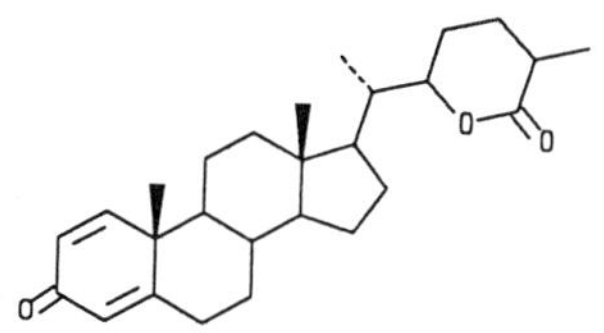

Mol. Wt.: 410
Melting Point: Oil
Spectral Data: UV, IR, CMR, PMR, Mass Spec.
Organism: *Minabea* sp. (Porifera)
Location: Truk
Reference: 617

$C_{27}H_{40}O_3$ **Minabeolide-6**

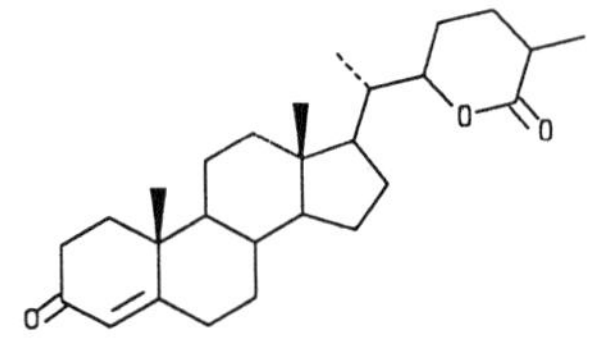

Mol. Wt.: 412
Melting Point: Oil
Spectral Data: UV, IR, CMR, PMR, Mass Spec.
Organism: *Minabea* sp. (Porifera)
Location: Truk
Reference: 617

$C_{27}H_{42}O_3$ **5α,8α-Epidioxycholesta-6,24-dien-3β-ol**

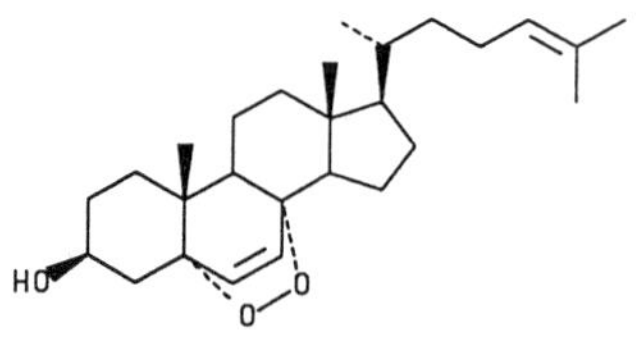

Mol. Wt.: 414
Spectral Data: CMR, PMR, Mass Spec.
Organism: *Dendrodoa grossularia* Von Beneden (Chordata/Tunicata)
Aplysia punctata Cuvier (Mollusca)
Location: Spain
Reference: 497

$C_{27}H_{42}O_4$ **Diaulusterol B**

Mol. Wt.: 430
Melting Point: Oil
Spectral Data: PMR, Mass Spec.
Organism: *Diaulula sandiegensis* (Mollusca)
Location: British Columbia, Canada
Reference: 1182

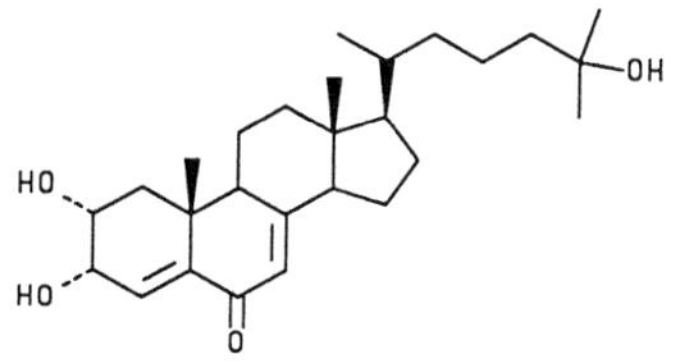

$C_{27}H_{42}Na_2O_8S_2$ **(20R,22E)-Cholesta-5,22-diene-3α,21-diyl sodium sulfate**

Mol. Wt.: 604
Spectral Data: PMR
Organism: *Ophioderma longicaudum* (Echinodermata)
Location: Naples, Italy
Reference: 924

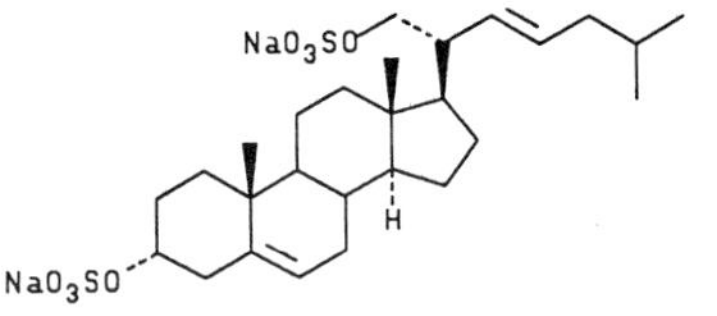

$C_{27}H_{43}Na_3O_{12}S_3$ **Cholest-5-ene-2β,3α,26-triyl sulfate**

Mol. Wt.: 724
Spectral Data: IR, CMR, PMR, Mass Spec.
Organism: *Ophiarachna incrassata* (Echinodermata)
Location: New Caledonia
Reference: 221

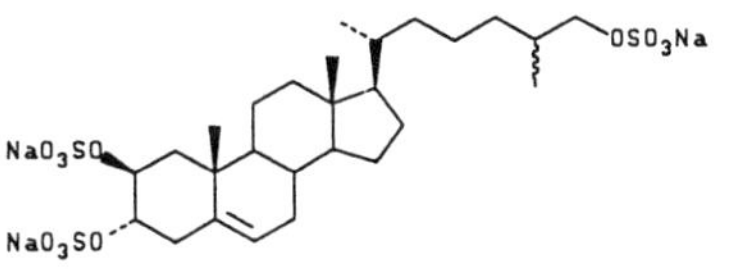

$C_{27}H_{43}O_7S$ **Thornasterol A sulfate**

Mol. Wt.: 511
Spectral Data: PMR, Mass Spec., CMR of the free sterol
Organism: *Asterias rubens* (Echinodermata)
Location: Scotland
Reference: 1141

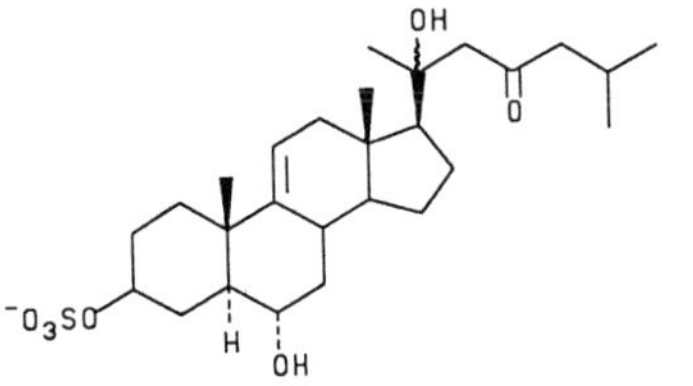

$C_{27}H_{44}O_2$

5α-Cholest-7,24-diene-3β,6α-diol

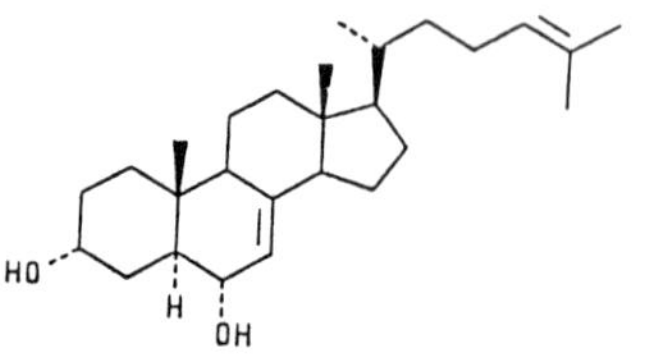

Mol. Wt.: 400
Spectral Data: IR, CMR, PMR, Mass Spec.
Organism: *Spongionella gracilis* Vosmaer (Porifera)
Location: Naples, Italy
Reference: 894

$C_{27}H_{44}O_3$

(22E)-5α-Cholesta-7,22-diene-3β,-5,6β-triol

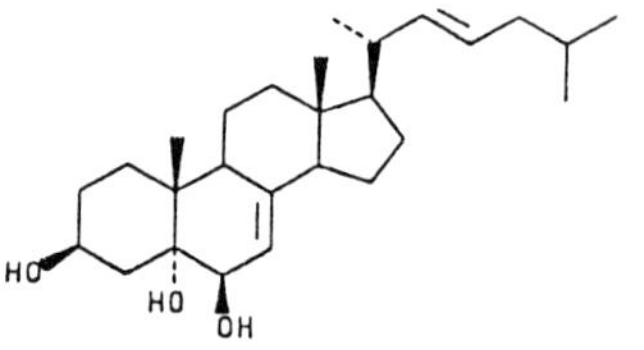

Mol. Wt.: 416
$[\alpha]_D$: −25 Solvent: Me
Melting Point: 234–236°C
Spectral Data: IR, PMR, Mass Spec.
Organism: *Patinopecten yessoensis* Jay (Mollusca)
Myriapora truncata Pallas (Bryozoa)
Spongionella gracilis Vosmaer (Porifera)
Location: Japan; Naples, Italy
Reference: 128, 460, 895

$C_{27}H_{44}O_3$

(22E)-27-Nor-24-methyl-5α-cholesta-7,22-diene-3β,5,6β-triol

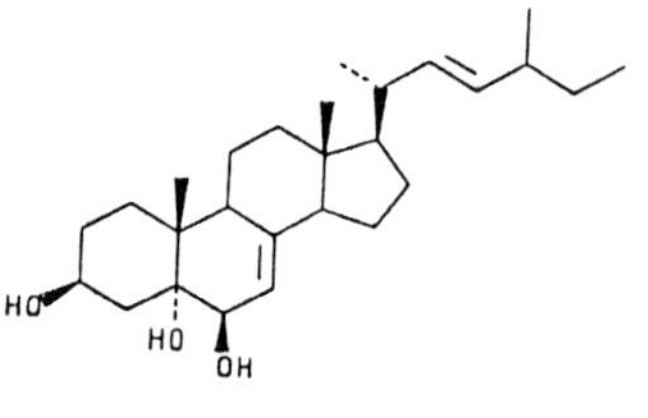

Mol. Wt.: 416
Melting Point: 235–237°C
Spectral Data: IR, PMR, Mass Spec.
Organism: *Spongionella gracilis* Vosmaer (Porifera)
Location: Naples, Italy
Reference: 895

$C_{27}H_{44}O_7$ **5α-Cholesta-7,22-diene-2α,3β,5α,-6β,9α,11α,19-heptol**

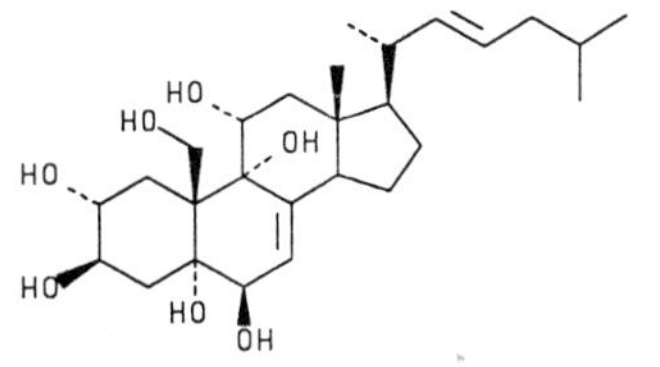

Mol. Wt.: 480
Melting Point: 260°C (dec.)
$[\alpha]_D^{25}$: -28.6 Solvent: Alc
Spectral Data: CMR, PMR, Mass Spec.
Organism: *Dysidea etheria* (Porifera)
Location: Bermuda
Reference: 1173

$C_{27}H_{44}Na_2O_8S_2$ **(20R)-Cholest-5-en-3α,21-diyl sodium sulfate**

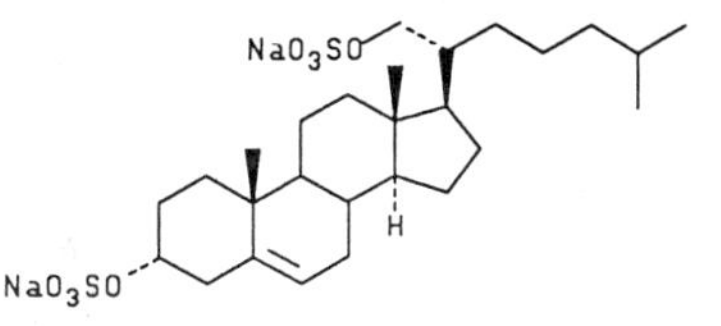

Mol. Wt.: 606
Spectral Data: PMR
Organism: *Ophioderma longicaudum* (Echinodermata)
Location: Naples, Italy
Reference: 924

$C_{27}H_{44}O_8$ **Gerardiasterone**

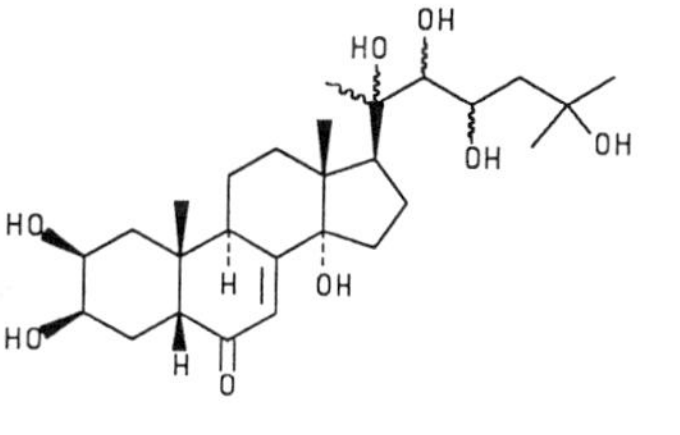

Mol. Wt.: 496
Melting Point: 143–146°C
$[\alpha]_D^{22}$: +52.3 Solvent: Me
Spectral Data: UV, CMR, PMR, Mass Spec.
Organism: *Gerardia savaglia* (Coelenterata)
Location: Mediterranean
Reference: 376

$C_{27}H_{44}Na_2O_{10}S_2$ **5β-Cholest-22-ene-3α,4α,11β,21-tetrol 3,21-disulfate**

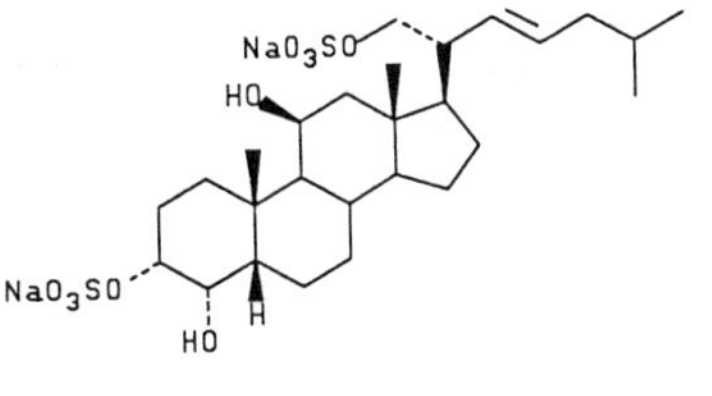

Mol. Wt.: 638
$[\alpha]_D$: -24.5 Solvent: Me
Spectral Data: CMR, PMR, Mass Spec.
Organism: *Ophiocoma dentata* *Ophiarthrum elegans* (Echinodermata)
Location: New Caledonia
Reference: 221

$C_{27}H_{44}Na_2O_{10}S_2$ **11-Keto-5β-cholestane-3α,4α,21-triol 3,21-disulfate**

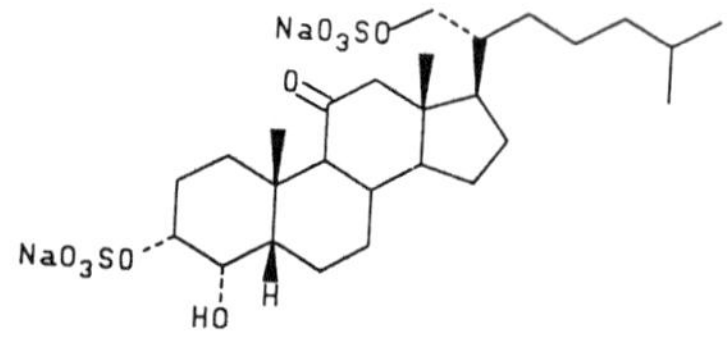

Mol. Wt.: 638
[α]D: +25 Solvent: Me
Spectral Data: CD, CMR, PMR, Mass Spec.
Organism: *Ophiarthrum elegans* (Echinodermata)
Location: New Caledonia
Reference: 221

$C_{27}H_{45}NaO_9S$ **(24E)-5α-Cholest-24-ene-3β,6α,8,14,15α,26-hexaol 15-sulfate**

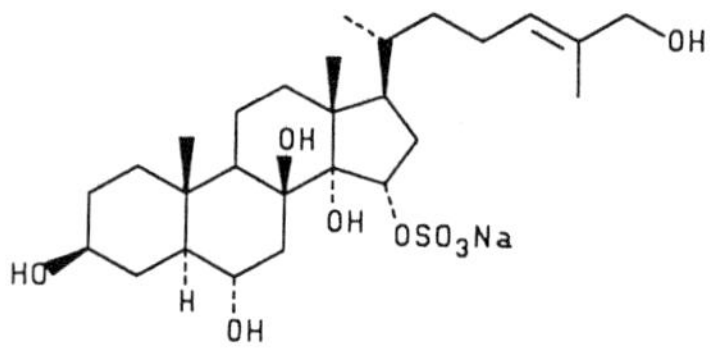

Mol. Wt.: 568
[α]D: +54.5 Solvent: Me
Spectral Data: CMR, PMR, Mass Spec.
Organism: *Archaster typicus* (Echinodermata)
Location: New Caledonia
Reference: 933

$C_{27}H_{45}NaO_{10}S$ **(24E)-5α-Cholest-24-ene-3β,4β,6α,8,14,15α,26-heptaol 15-sulfate**

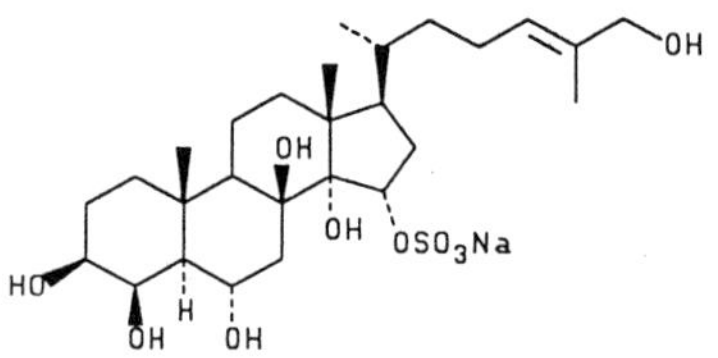

Mol. Wt.: 584
[α]D: +43.6 Solvent: Me
Spectral Data: CMR, PMR, Mass Spec.
Organism: *Archaster typicus* (Echinodermata)
Location: New Caledonia
Reference: 933

$C_{27}H_{45}NaO_{12}S$

(24E)-5α-Cholest-24-ene-3β,-4β,5,6α,7β,8,14,15α,26-nonaol 6-sulfate

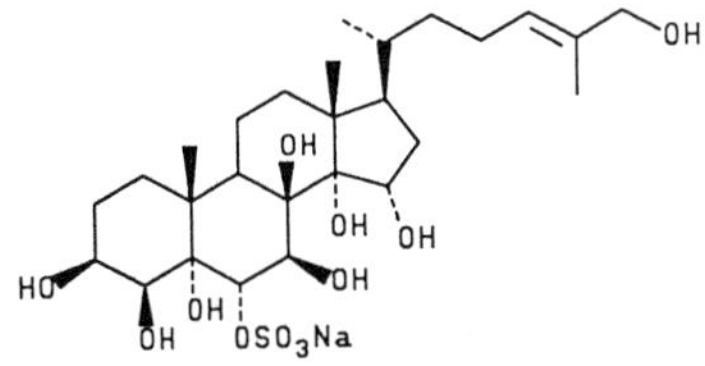

Mol. Wt.: 616
[α]$_D$: +47.4 Solvent: Me
Spectral Data: CMR, PMR, Mass Spec.
Organism: *Archaster typicus* (Echinodermata)
Location: New Caledonia
Reference: 933

$C_{27}H_{45}Na_3O_{12}S_3$

5α-Cholestane-2β,3α,26-triyl sulfate

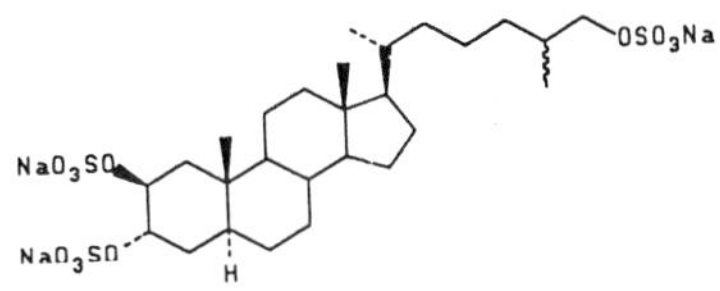

Mol. Wt.: 726
Spectral Data: IR, CMR, PMR, Mass Spec.
Organism: *Ophiarachna incrassata* (Echinodermata)
Location: New Caledonia
Reference: 221

$C_{27}H_{46}O$

(E)-Cholest-22-en-3α-ol

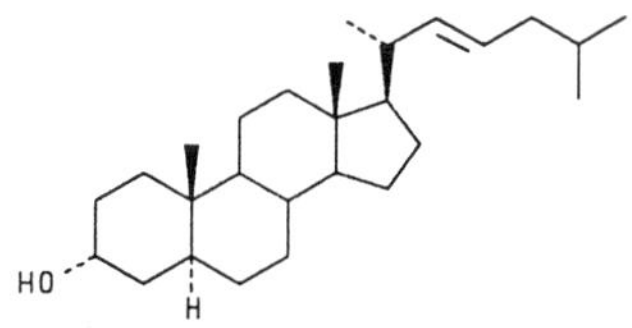

Mol. Wt.: 386
Spectral Data: PMR, Mass Spec.
Organism: *Esperiopsis edwardii* (Porifera)
Location: Chile
Reference: 994

$C_{27}H_{46}O$

(E)-27-Nor-24(S)-methylcholest-22-en-3α-ol

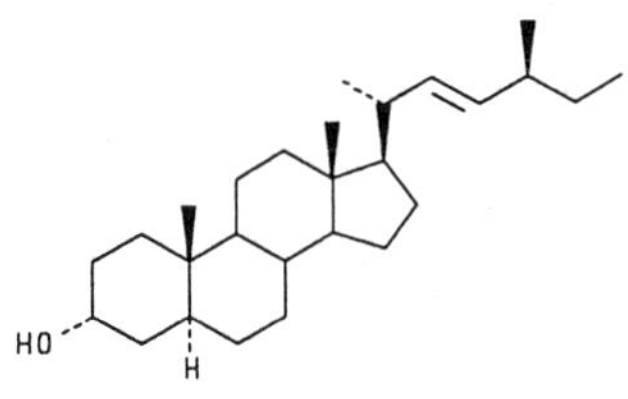

Mol. Wt.: 386
Spectral Data: PMR, Mass Spec.
Organism: *Esperiopsis edwardii* (Porifera)
Location: Chile
Reference: 994

$C_{27}H_{46}O_2$

5α-Cholest-7-ene-3β,6α-diol
(previously known)

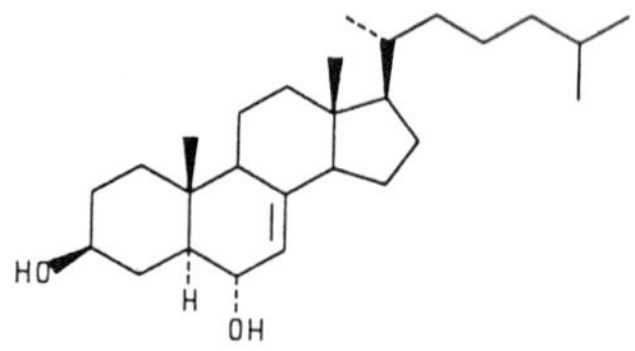

Mol. Wt.: 402
Spectral Data: IR, PMR, Mass Spec.
Organism: *Spongionella gracilis* Vosmaer (Porifera)
Location: Naples, Italy
Reference: 130, 237, 894

$C_{27}H_{46}O_3$

5α-Cholest-7-ene-3β,5,6β-triol
(previously known)

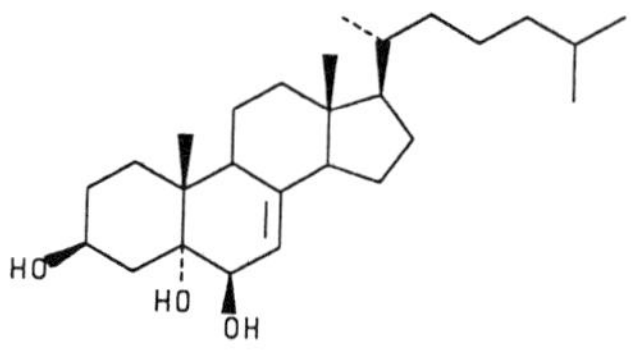

Mol. Wt.: 418
[α]$_D$: −20.8 Solvent: Me
Melting Point: 227–229°C
Spectral Data: IR, PMR, Mass Spec.
Organism: *Patinopecten yessoensis* Jay (Mollusca)
Myriapora truncata Pallas (Bryozoa)
Spongionella gracilis Vosmaer (Porifera)
Location: Japan; Naples, Italy
Reference: 128, 460, 895, 955

$C_{27}H_{46}O_7$

5α-Cholest-7-ene-2α,3β,5α,6β,9α,11α,-19-heptol

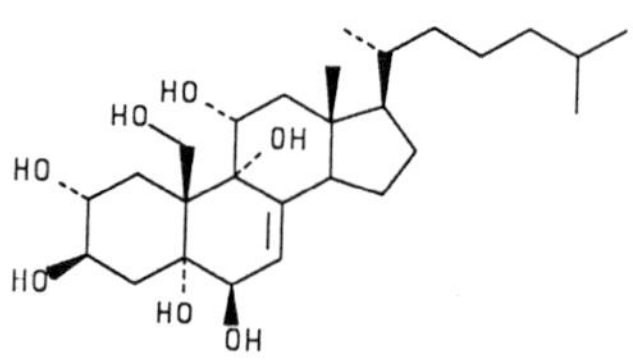

Mol. Wt.: 482
Melting Point: 250°C dec.
[α]$_D^{25}$: −24.2 Solvent: Alc
Spectral Data: CMR, PMR, Mass Spec.
Organism: *Dysidea etheria* (Porifera)
Location: Bermuda
Reference: 1173

$C_{27}H_{46}Na_2O_8S_2$

(20R)-5α-Cholestane-3α,21-diyl sodium sulfate

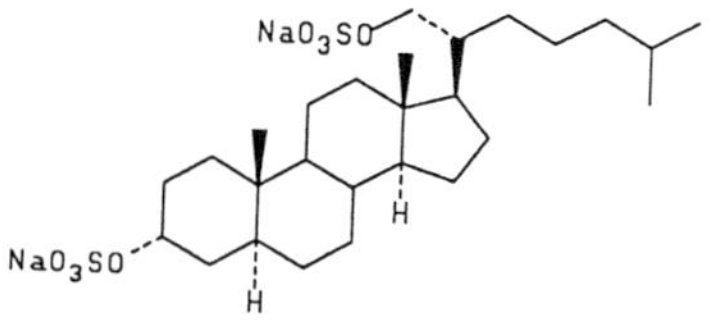

Mol. Wt.: 608
Spectral Data: CMR, PMR
Organism: *Ophioderma longicaudum* (Echinodermata)
Location: Naples, Italy
Reference: 924

$C_{27}H_{46}Na_2O_{11}S_2$

5β-Cholestane-3α,4α,11β,-12β,21-pentol 3,21-disulfate

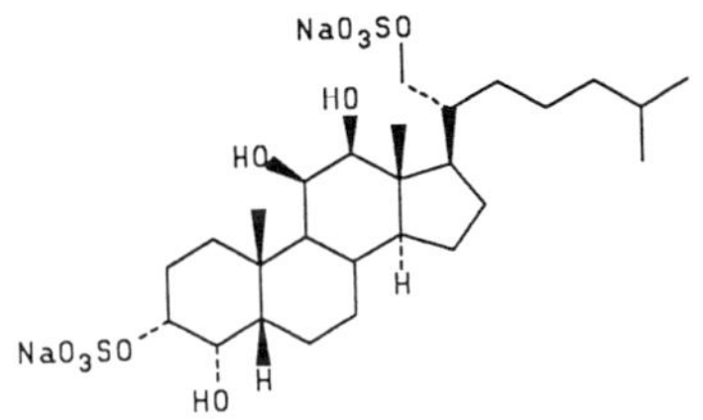

Mol. Wt.: 656
Melting Point: 192–195°C
[α]D: +10.8 Solvent: Me
Spectral Data: CMR, PMR, Mass Spec.
Organism: *Ophioderma longicaudum* (Echinodermata)
Location: Naples, Italy
Reference: 924

$C_{27}H_{48}O$

Cholestan-3α-ol

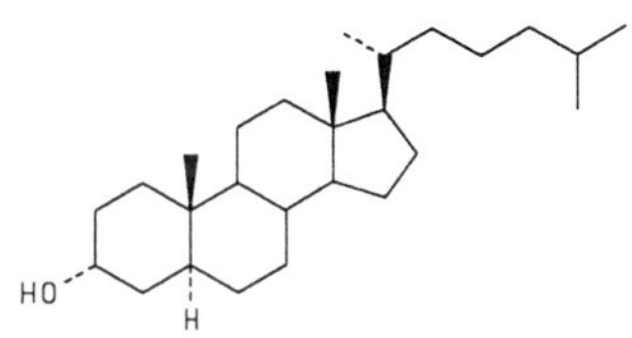

Mol. Wt.: 388
Spectral Data: PMR, Mass Spec.
Organism: *Esperiopsis edwardii* (Porifera)
Location: Chile
Reference: 994

$C_{27}H_{48}O_5$

(24S)-5α-Cholestane-3β,6α,8,15β,24-pentol

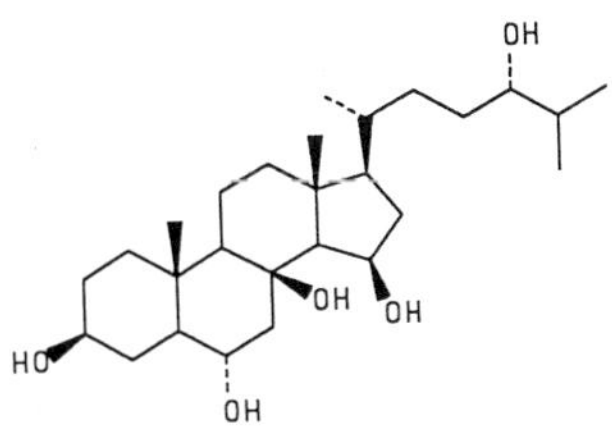

Mol. Wt.: 452
[α]D: +12 Solvent: Me
Spectral Data: CMR, PMR, Mass Spec.
Organism: *Nardoa gomophia* Gray *Gomophia watsoni* (Echinodermata)
Location: New Caledonia
Reference: 923, 931

$C_{27}H_{48}O_6$ **(24S)-5α-Cholestane-3β,4β,6α,8,15β,-24-hexol**

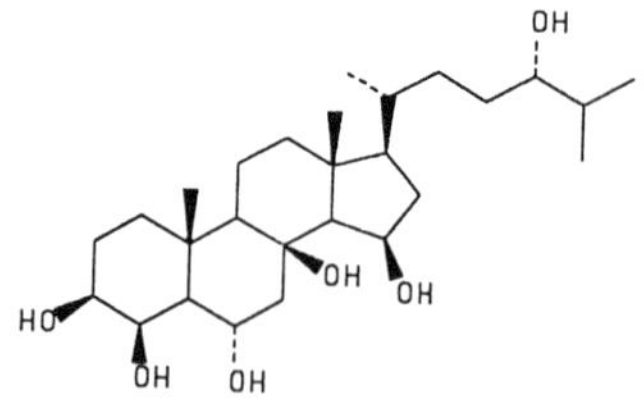

Mol. Wt.: 468
$[\alpha]_D$: +7.2 Solvent: Me
Spectral Data: CMR, PMR, Mass Spec.
Organism: *Gomophia watsoni* (Echinodermata)
Location: New Caledonia
Reference: 923

$C_{27}H_{48}O_6$ **(25S)-5α-Cholestane-3β,6α,8,15α,-16β,26-hexol** (previously known)

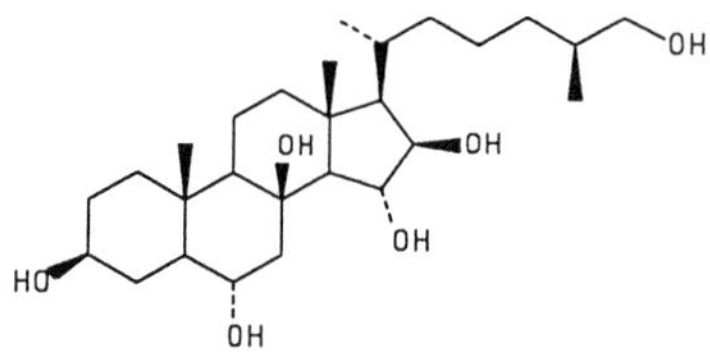

Mol. Wt.: 468
Melting Point: 285–287°C
$[\alpha]_D$: +14 Solvent: Me
Spectral Data: CMR, PMR
Organism: *Poraster superbus* *Protoreaster nodosus* (Echinodermata)
Location: New Caledonia
Reference: 219, 926, 929

$C_{27}H_{48}O_6$ **(25S)-5α-Cholestane-3β,6α,8,15β,-16β,26-hexol**

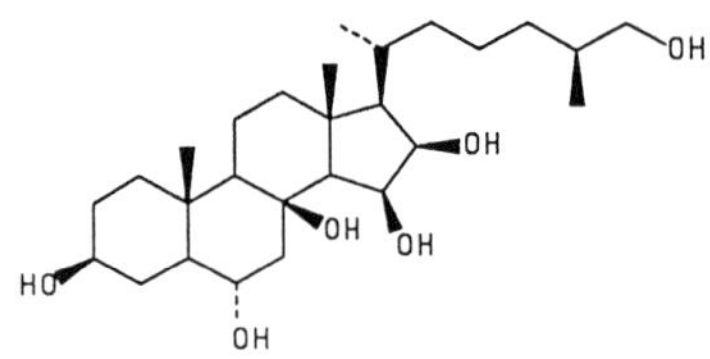

Mol. Wt.: 468
$[\alpha]_D$: –0 Solvent: Me
Spectral Data: PMR, Mass Spec.
Organism: *Halityle regularis* Fisher *Nardoa gomophia* Gray (Echinodermata)
Location: New Caledonia
Reference: 459, 931

$C_{27}H_{48}O_6$ **(25S)-5α-Cholestane-3β,6β,8,15α,-16β,26-hexol**

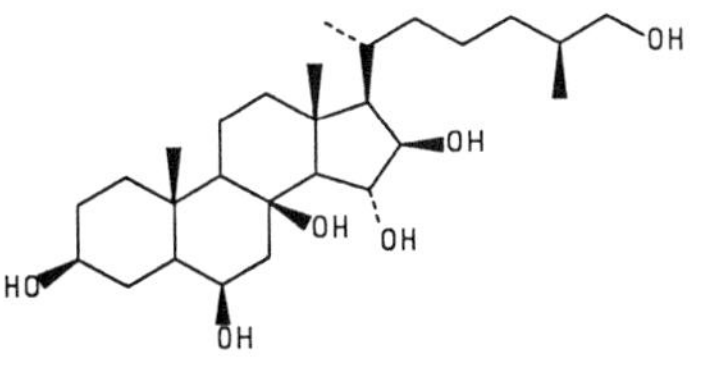

Mol. Wt.: 468
Spectral Data: PMR, Mass Spec.
Organism: *Sphaerodiscus placenta* Muller–Troshel (Echinodermata)
Location: Palinuro, Italy
Reference: 1225

$C_{27}H_{48}O_7$ **(25S)-5α-Cholestane-3β,4β,6α,-8,15β,16β,26-heptol**

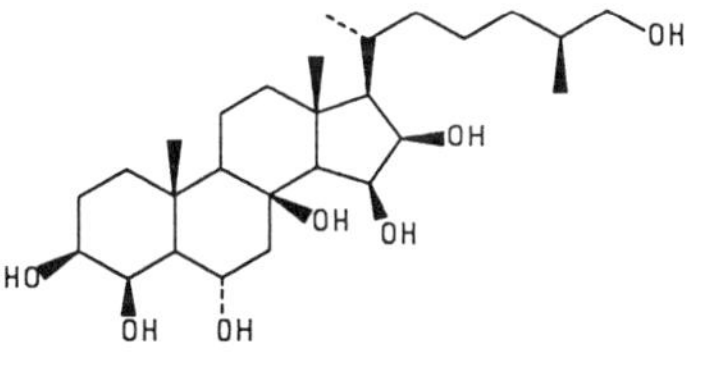

Mol. Wt.: 484
[α]$_D$: +6.3 Solvent: Me
Spectral Data: CMR, PMR, Mass Spec.
Organism: *Halityle regularis* Fisher (Echinodermata)
Location: New Caledonia
Reference: 459

$C_{27}H_{48}O_7$ **(25S)-5α-Cholestane-3β,6α,7α,8,-15α,16β,26-heptol**
(previously known)

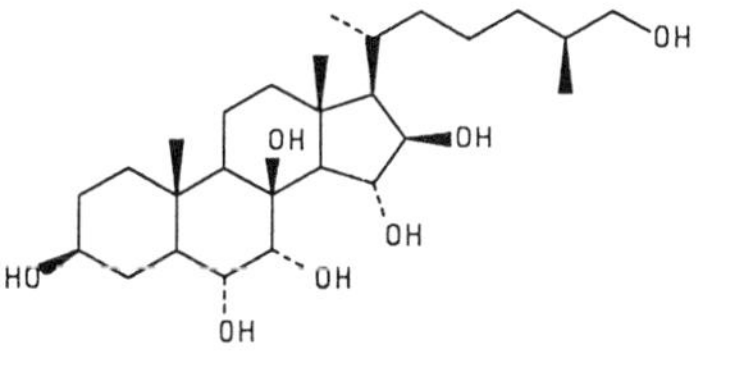

Mol. Wt.: 484
Melting point: 255–258°C
[α]$_D$: +32 Solvent: Me
Spectral Data: CMR, PMR
Organism: *Poraster superbus* *Protoreaster nodosus* (Echinodermata)
Location: New Caledonia
Reference: 926, 929

$C_{28}H_{38}O_3$ **Minabeolide-1**

Mol. Wt.: 422
Melting Point: Oil
Spectral Data: UV, IR, CMR, PMR, Mass Spec.
Organism: *Minabea* sp.
(Porifera)
Location: Truk
Reference: 617

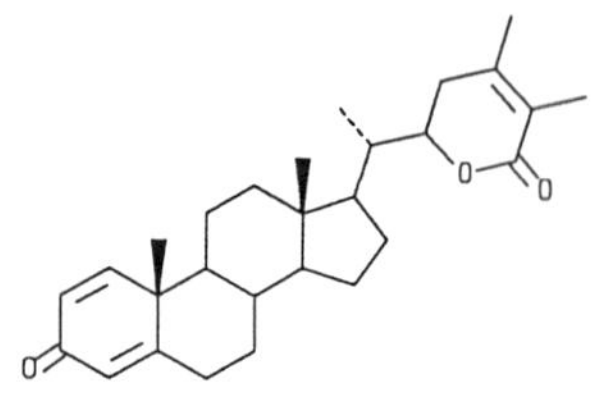

$C_{28}H_{40}O_3$ **Minabeolide-3**

Mol. Wt.: 424
Melting Point: Oil
Spectral Data: IR, CMR, PMR, Mass Spec.
Organism: *Minabea* sp.
(Porifera)
Location: Truk
Reference: 617

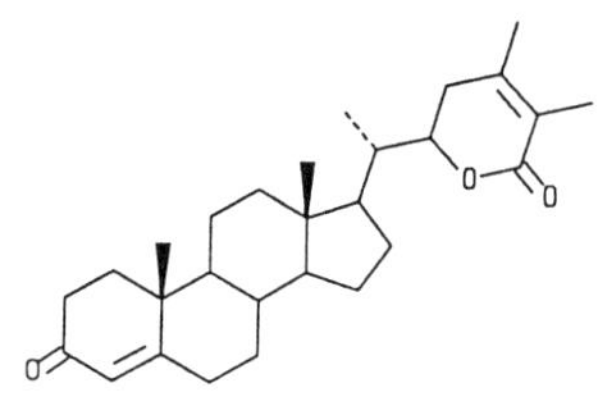

$C_{28}H_{44}O$

Mol. Wt.: 396
Spectral Data: Mass Spec.
Organism: *Actinia equina*
Edwarsia sp
(Coelenterata)
Location: Black Sea
Reference: 732

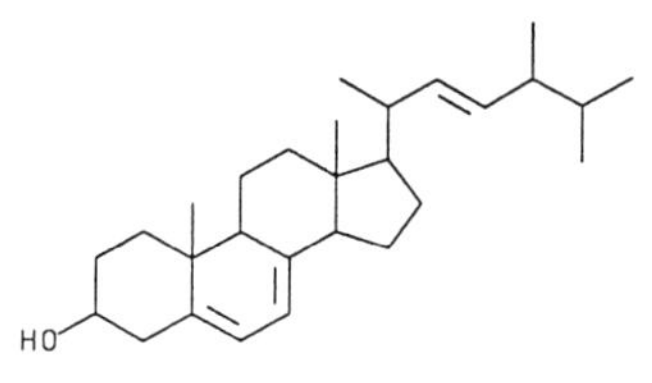

$C_{28}H_{44}Na_2O_8S_2$ **(20R)-24-Methylcholesta-5,24(28)-diene-3α,21-diyl sodium sulfate**

Mol. Wt.: 618
Spectral Data: PMR
Organism: *Ophioderma longicaudum*
(Echinodermata)
Location: Naples, Italy
Reference: 924

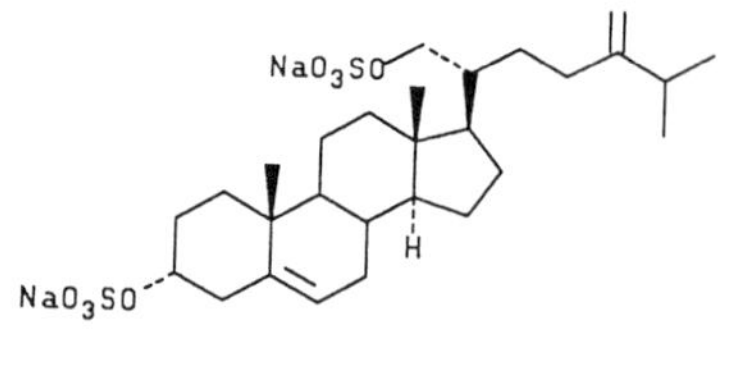

$C_{28}H_{46}O_2$

24-Methylene-5α-cholest-7-ene-3β,6α-diol

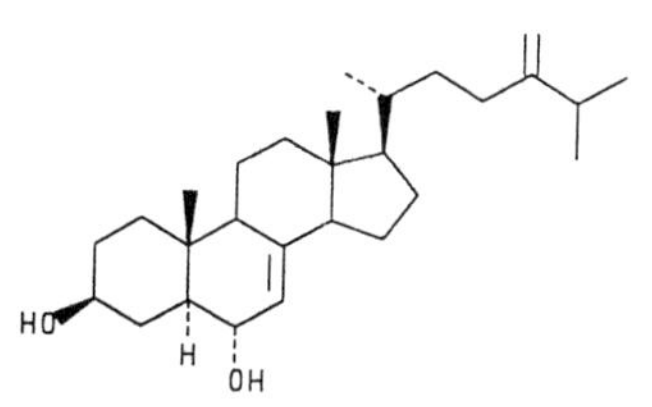

Mol. Wt.: 414
Spectral Data: IR, CMR, PMR, Mass Spec.
Organism: *Spongionella gracilis* Vosmaer (Porifera)
Location: Naples, Italy
Reference: 894

$C_{28}H_{46}O_3$

(22E)-3β,5α-Dihydroxy-6β-methoxycholesta-7,22-diene

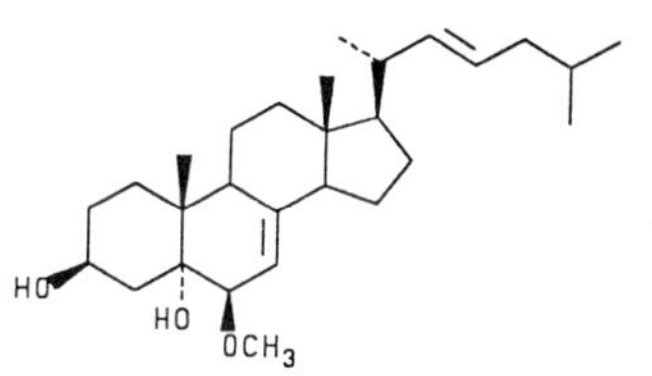

Mol. Wt.: 430
$[\alpha]_D$: −159 Solvent: Chf
Spectral Data: PMR, Mass Spec.
Organism: *Spongia agaricina* Pallas (Porifera)
Location: Naples, Italy
Reference: 7

$C_{28}H_{46}O_3$

(22E,24R)-24-Methyl-5α-cholesta-7,22-diene-3β,5,6β-triol (Cerevisterol)
(previously known)

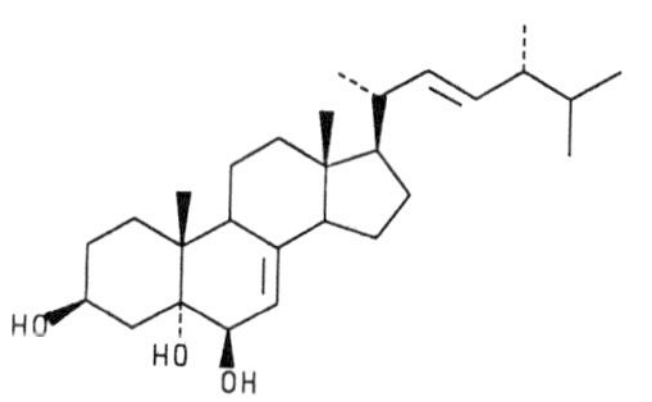

Mol. Wt.: 430
Melting Point: 253–255°C (synthetic sample)
$[\alpha]_D$: −16.5 Solvent: Me
$[\alpha]_D^{25}$: −75 Solvent: Py
Spectral Data: IR, CMR, PMR, Mass Spec.
Organism: *Patinopecten yessoensis* Jay (Mollusca)
Spongionella gracilis Vosmaer (Porifera)
Myriapora truncata Pallas (Bryozoa)
Location: Japan; Naples, Italy
Reference: 128, 460, 895

$C_{28}H_{46}O_3$

(22E,24S)-24-Methyl-5α-cholesta-7,22-diene-3β,5,6β-triol
(previously known)

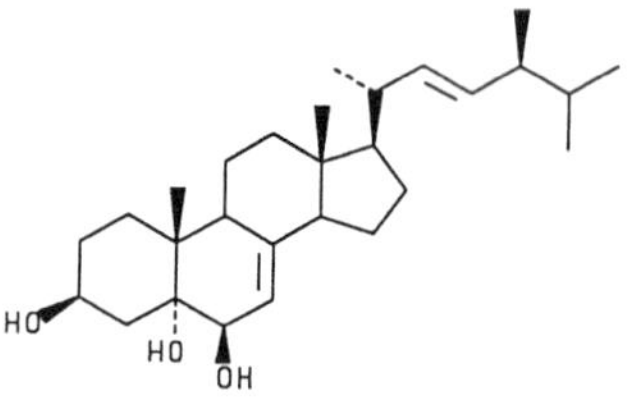

Mol. Wt.: 430
Melting Point: 245–247°C
Spectral Data: IR, PMR, Mass Spec.
Organism: *Spongionella gracilis* Vosmaer (Porifera)
Myriapora truncata (Bryozoa)
Location: Naples, Italy
Reference: 128, 895

$C_{28}H_{46}O_3$

24-Methylene-5α-cholest-7-ene-3β,5,6β-triol

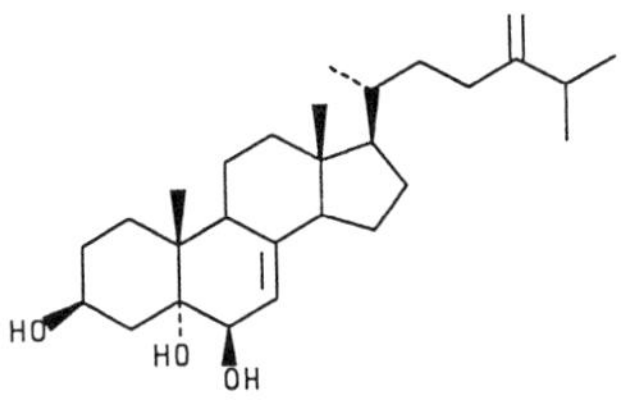

Mol. Wt.: 430
Melting Point: 244–246°C
$[\alpha]_D$: −26 Solvent: Me
Spectral Data: IR, CMR, PMR, Mass Spec.
Organism: *Spongionella gracilis* Vosmaer (Porifera)
Patinopecten yessoensis Jay (Mollusca)
Location: Naples, Italy; Japan
Reference: 460, 895

$C_{28}H_{46}O_6$

2-Desacetyl-22-epi-hippurin-1

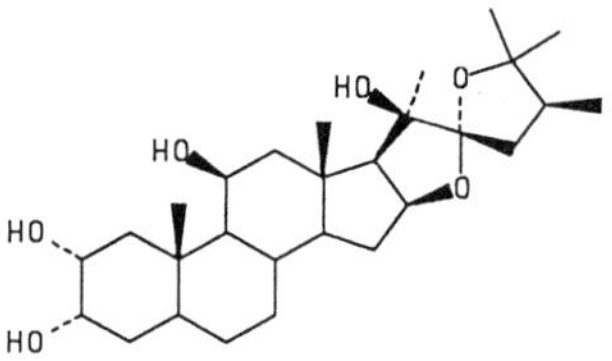

Mol. Wt.: 478
Melting Point: 260–261°C
Spectral Data: IR, CMR, PMR, Mass Spec.
Organism: *Isis hippuris* (Coelenterata)
Location: Bay of Bengal
Reference: 916

$C_{28}H_{46}O_7$ **24-Methyl-5α-cholesta-7,22-diene-2α,3β,5α,6β,9α,11α,19-heptol**

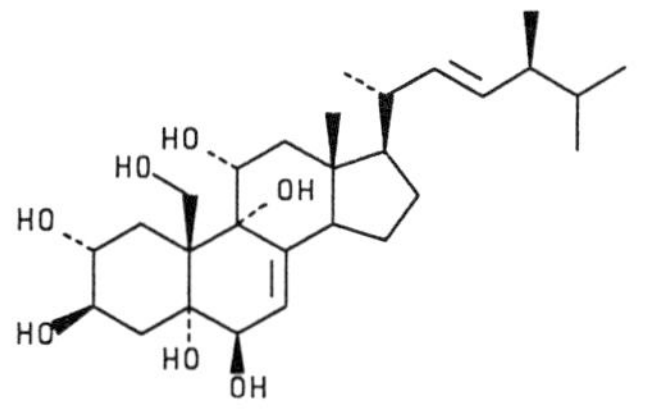

Mol. Wt.: 494
Melting Point: 260–270°C (dec.)
$[\alpha]_D^{25}$: −24.4 Solvent: Alc
Spectral Data: CMR, PMR, Mass Spec.
Organism: *Dysidea etheria* (Porifera)
Location: Bermuda
Reference: 1173

$C_{28}H_{46}Na_2O_{10}S_2$ **24-Methylene-5β-cholestane-3α,4α,-11β,21-tetrol 3,21-disulfate**

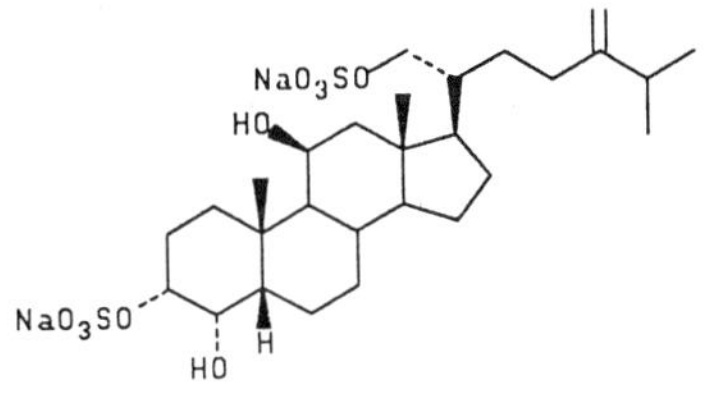

Mol. Wt.: 652
$[\alpha]_D$: +15.8 Solvent: Me
Spectral Data: CMR, PMR, Mass Spec.
Organism: *Ophiocoma dentata* (Echinodermata)
Location: New Caledonia
Reference: 221

$C_{28}H_{48}O$ **24-Methylcholest-24(28)-en-3α-ol**

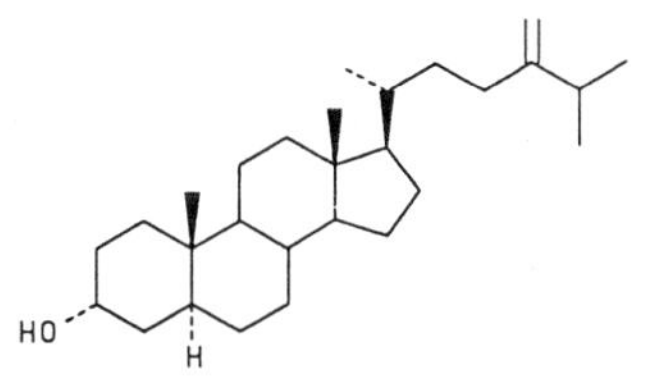

Mol. Wt.: 400
Spectral Data: PMR, Mass Spec.
Organism: *Esperiopsis edwardii* (Porifera)
Location: Chile
Reference: 994

$C_{28}H_{48}O$ **(E)-24-Methylcholest-22-en-3α-ol**

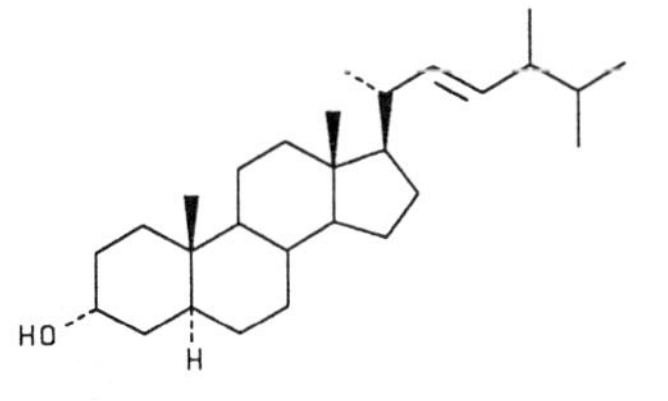

Mol. Wt.: 400
Spectral Data: PMR, Mass spec.
Organism: *Esperiopsis edwardii* (Porifera)
Location: Chile
Reference: 994

$C_{28}H_{48}O_3$ **3β,5α-Dihydroxy-6β-methoxycholest-7-ene**

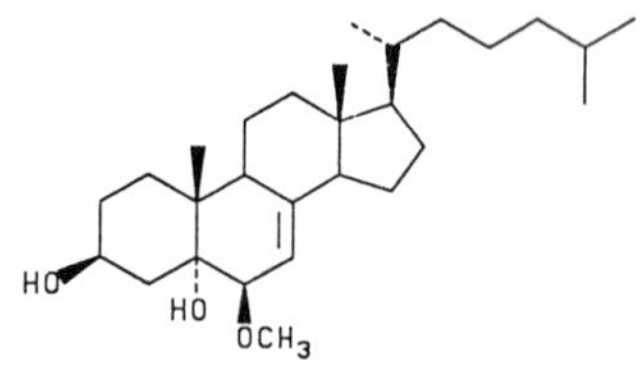

Mol. Wt.: 432
[α]D: −83 Solvent: Chf
Spectral Data: CMR, PMR, Mass Spec.
Organism: *Spongia agaricina* Pallas (Porifera)
Location: Naples, Italy
Reference: 7

$C_{28}H_{48}O_3$ **(24S)-24-Methylcholest-7-ene-3β,5α,6β-triol**

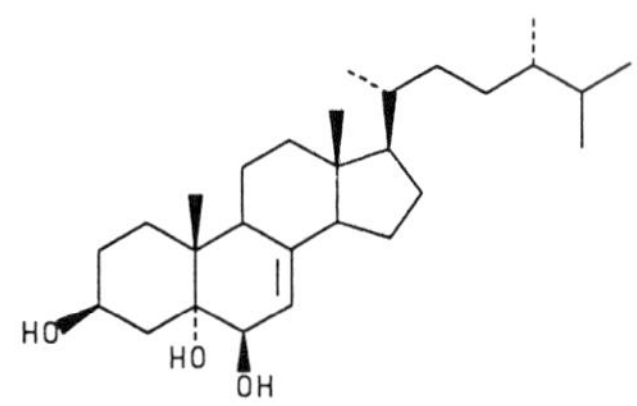

Mol. Wt.: 432
[α]D: −10 Solvent: Me
Spectral Data: PMR, Mass Spec.
Organism: *Patinopecten yessoensis* Jay (Mollusca)
Location: Japan
Reference: 460

$C_{28}H_{48}O_5$ **(25R)-24-Methyl-5α-cholest-24(28)-en-3β,6β,15α,16β,26-pentol**

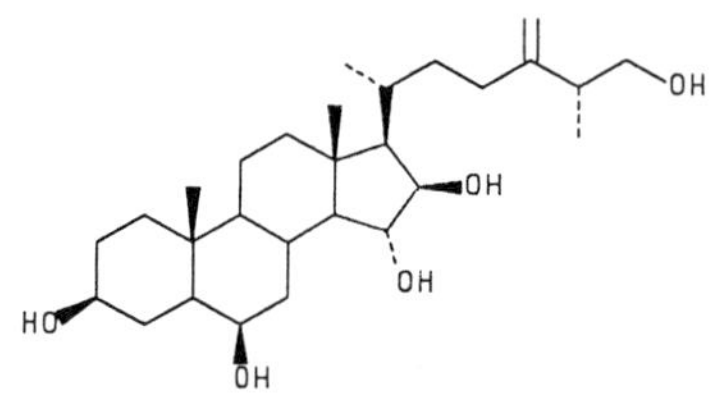

Mol. Wt.: 464
[α]D: +28.1 Solvent: Me
Spectral Data: CMR, PMR, Mass Spec.
Organism: *Sphaerodiscus placenta* Muller–Troshel (Echinodermata)
Location: Palinuro, Italy
Reference: 1225

$C_{28}H_{48}O_6$ **(25R)-24-Methyl-5α-cholest-24(28)-en-3β,6β,8,15α,16β,26-hexol**

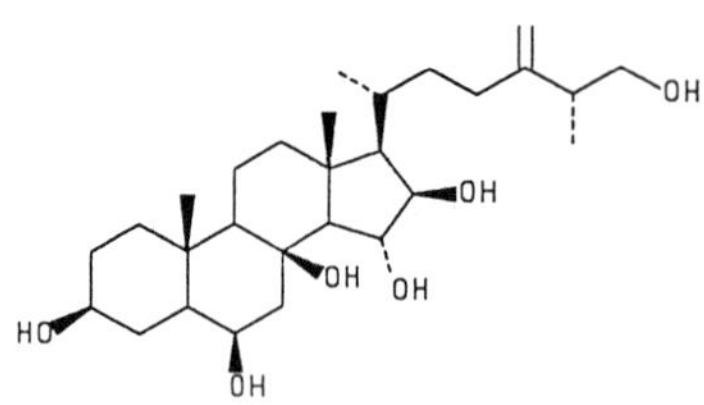

Mol. Wt.: 480
[α]D: +11.7 Solvent: Me
Spectral Data: CMR, PMR, Mass Spec.
Organism: *Sphaerodiscus placenta* Muller–Troshel (Echinodermata)
Location: Palinuro, Italy
Reference: 1225

$C_{28}H_{50}O$ **24ξ-Methylcholestan-3α-ol**

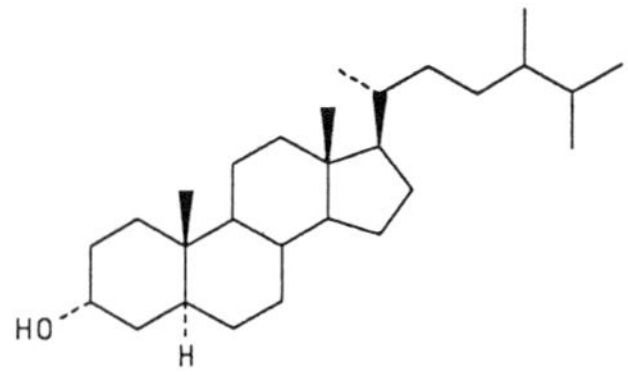

Mol. Wt.: 402
Spectral Data: PMR, Mass Spec.
Organism: *Esperiopsis edwardii* (Porifera)
Location: Chile
Reference: 994

$C_{29}H_{40}O_5$ **Minabeolide-5**

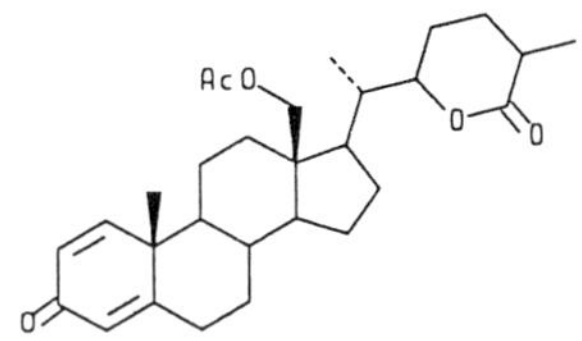

Mol. Wt.: 468
Melting Point: Oil
Spectral Data: UV, IR, CMR, PMR, Mass Spec.
Organism: *Minabea* sp. (Porifera)
Location: Truk
Reference: 617

$C_{29}H_{42}O_5$ **Minabeolide-7**

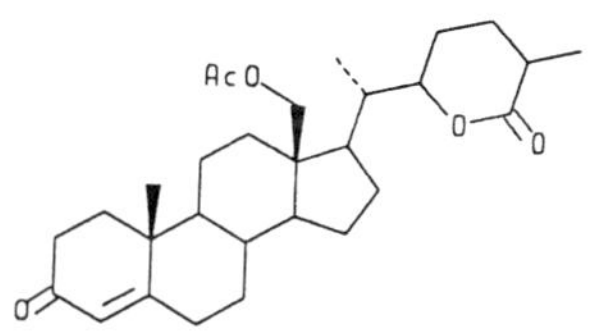

Mol. Wt.: 470
Melting Point: Oil
Spectral Data: IR, CMR, PMR, Mass Spec.
Organism: *Minabea* sp. (Porifera)
Location: Truk
Reference: 617

$C_{29}H_{42}O_5$ **Minabeolide-8**

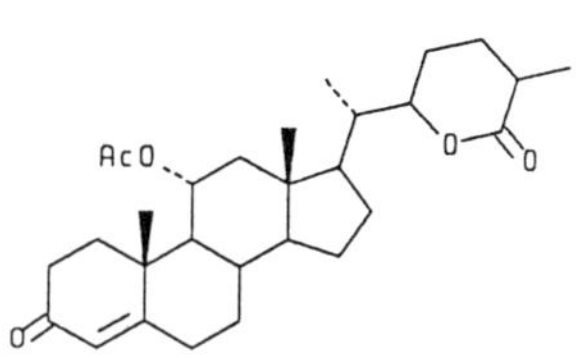

Mol. Wt.: 470
Melting Point: Oil
Spectral Data: UV, IR, CMR, PMR, Mass Spec.
Organism: *Minabea* sp. (Porifera)
Location: Truk
Reference: 617

$C_{29}H_{44}O$

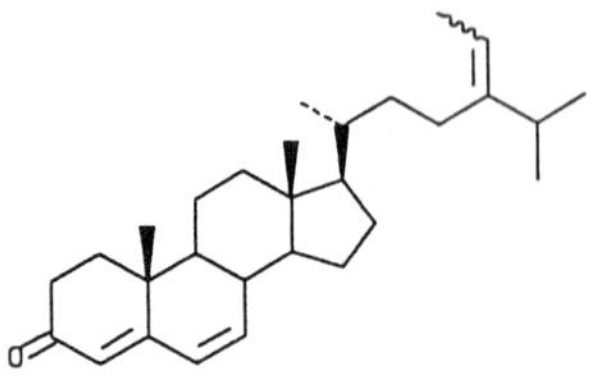

Mol. Wt.: 408
Spectral Data: PMR, Mass Spec.
Organism: *Esperiopsis edwardii* (Porifera)
Location: Chile
Reference: 994

$C_{29}H_{46}O$ **(23<u>S</u>)-23<u>H</u>-Isocalysterol**

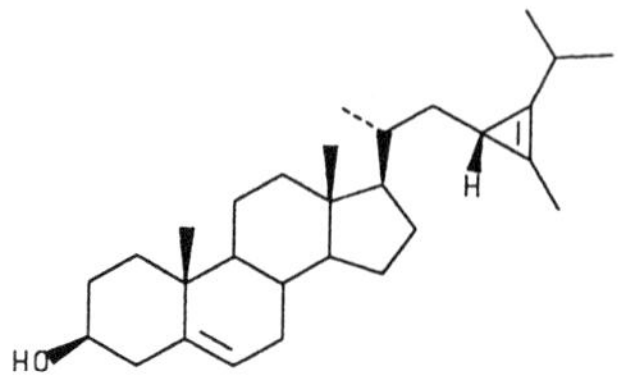

Mol. Wt.: 410
Melting Point: 112–113°C
Spectral Data: CMR, PMR, Mass Spec.
Organism: *Calyx podatypa* (Porifera)
Location: Bahamas
Reference: 245

$C_{29}H_{48}O$ **5α-Calystanol**

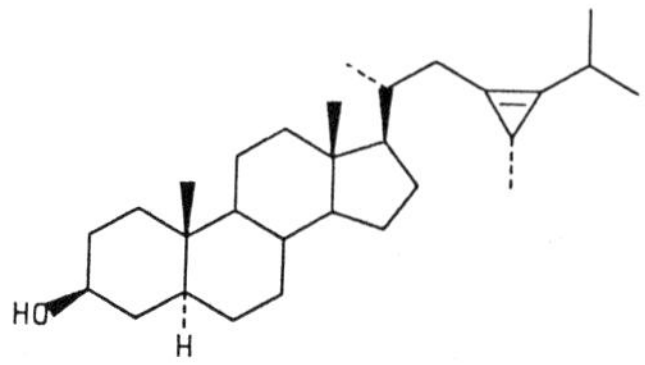

Mol. Wt.: 412
Spectral Data: PMR, Mass Spec.
Organism: *Calyx podatypa* (Porifera)
Location: Bahamas
Reference: 245

$C_{29}H_{48}O$ **Hebesterol**

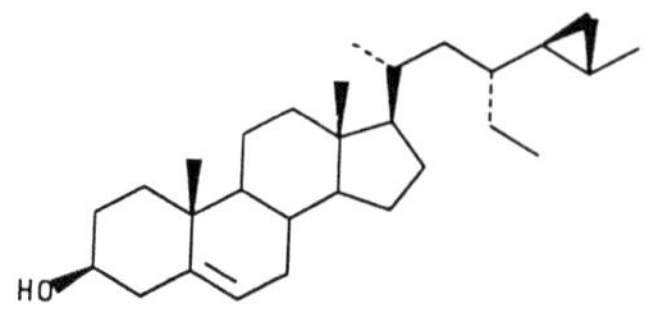

Mol. Wt.: 412
Melting Point: 133–134°C (synthetic sterol)
$[\alpha]_D^{20}$: −2.1 Solvent: Chf (synthetic sterol)
Spectral Data: PMR, Mass Spec.
Organism: *Petrosia hebes* (Porifera)
Location: New Zealand
Reference: 173

$C_{29}H_{48}O$ **(23S)-23H-5α-Isocalystanol**

Mol. Wt.: 412
Spectral Data: PMR, Mass Spec.
Organism: *Calyx podatypa* (Porifera)
Location: Bahamas
Reference: 245

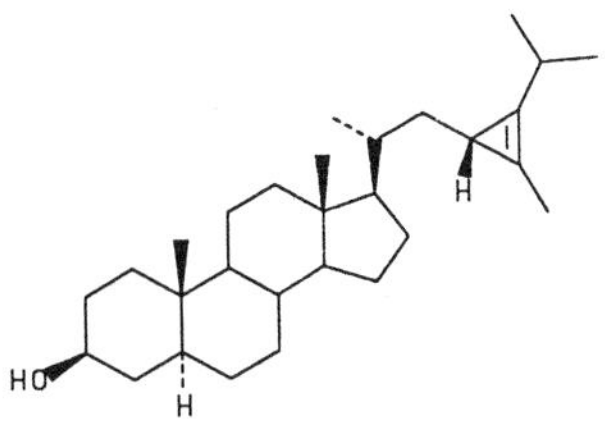

$C_{29}H_{48}O$ **(24S)-24H-5α-Isocalystanol**

Mol. Wt.: 412
Spectral Data: PMR, Mass Spec.
Organism: *Calyx podatypa* (Porifera)
Location: Bahamas
Reference: 245

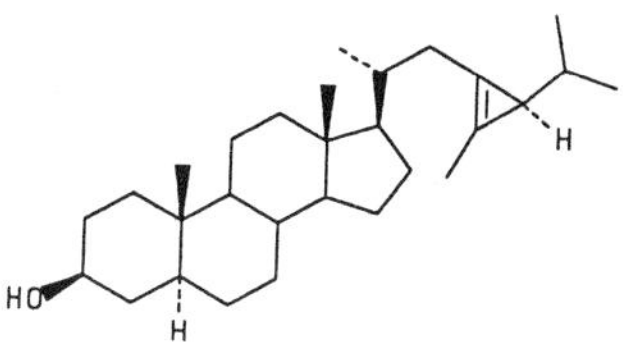

$C_{29}H_{48}O$ **Isojaspisterol**

Mol. Wt.: 412
Melting Point: 130–131°C (synthetic sterol)
$[\alpha]_D^{20}$: −52.8 Solvent: Chf (synthetic sterol)
Spectral Data: CMR, PMR, Mass Spec. (synthetic sterol)
Organism: *Jaspis stellifera* (Porifera)
Location: Australia
Reference: 174

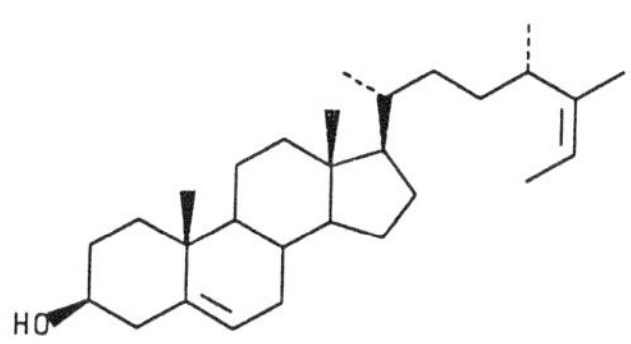

$C_{29}H_{48}O$ **Jaspisterol**

Mol. Wt.: 412
Melting Point: 113–114°C (synthetic sterol)
$[\alpha]_D^{20}$: −44.1 Solvent: Chf (synthetic sterol)
Spectral Data: CMR, PMR, Mass Spec. (synthetic sterol)
Organism: *Jaspis stellifera* (Porifera)
Location: Australia
Reference: 174

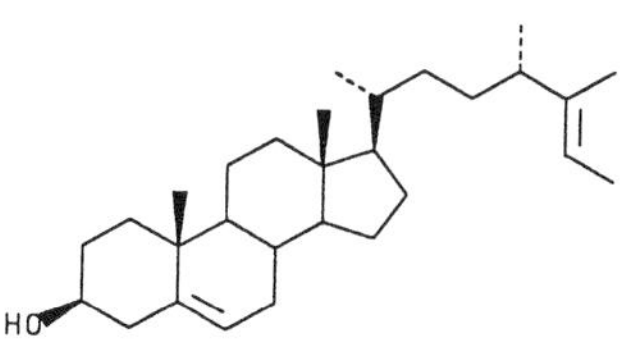

$C_{29}H_{48}O_3$

(22E,24ξ)-3β,5α-Dihydroxy-6β-methoxy-24-methylcholesta-7,22-diene

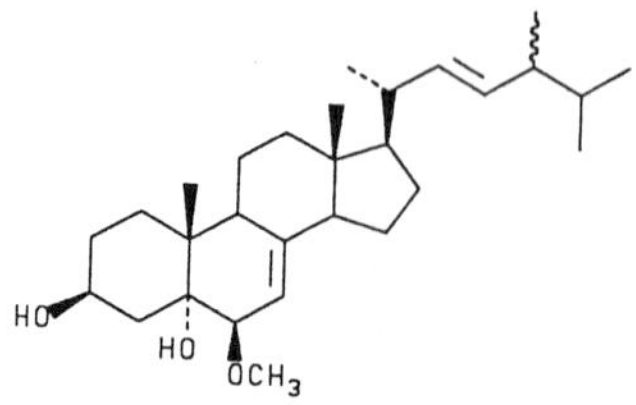

Mol. Wt.: 444
[α]D: -160 Solvent: Chf
Spectral Data: PMR, Mass Spec.
Organism: *Spongia agaricina* Pallas (Porifera)
Location: Naples, Italy
Reference 7

$C_{29}H_{48}O_3$

(22E,24ξ)-24-Ethylcholesta-7,22-diene-3β,5α,6β-triol

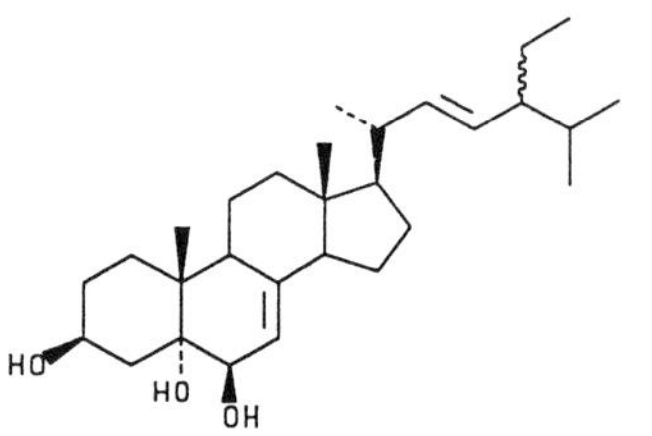

Mol. Wt.: 444
[α]D: -4.6 Solvent: Me
Spectral Data: PMR, Mass Spec.
Organism: *Patinopecten yessoensis* Jay (Mollusca)
Myriapora truncata Pallas (Bryozoa)
Location: Japan; Naples, Italy
Reference: 128, 460

$C_{29}H_{48}O_4$

(22E,24ξ)-24-Ethylcholesta-7,22-diene-3β,5α,6β,9α-tetraol

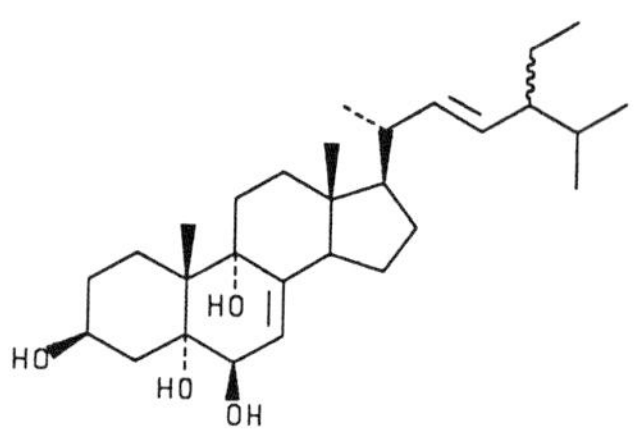

Mol. Wt.: 460
[α]D: -66.5 Solvent: Me
Spectral Data: PMR, Mass Spec.
Organism: *Patinopecten yessoensis* Jay (Mollusca)
Location: Japan
Reference: 460

$C_{29}H_{48}O_8$

5α-Cholest-7-ene-2α,3β,5α,6β,9α,11α,-19-heptol 11-acetate

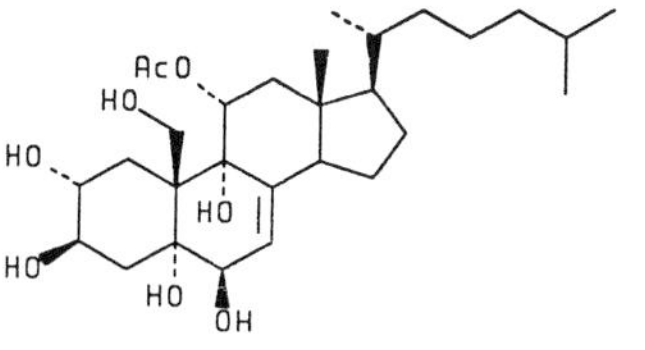

Mol. Wt.: 524
Melting Point: 211–220°C
$[\alpha]_D^{25}$: −40.9 Solvent: Alc
Spectral Data: CMR, PMR, Mass Spec.
Organism: *Dysidea etheria* (Porifera)
Location: Bermuda
Reference: 1173

$C_{29}H_{50}O$

(23S,24S,28R)-5α-Dihydrocalystanol

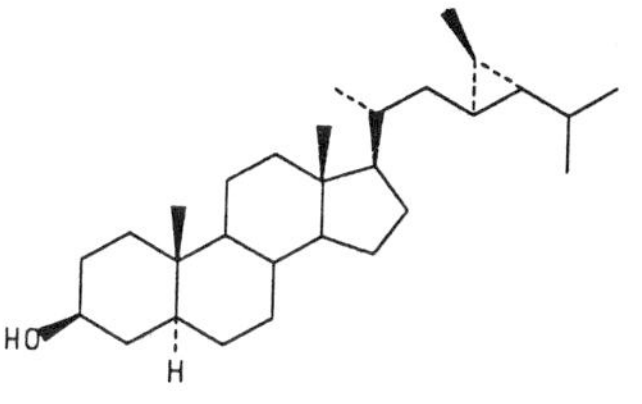

Mol. Wt.: 414
Melting Point: 119–120°C (synthetic sterol)
Spectral Data: PMR, Mass Spec.
Organism: *Petrosia hebes* (Porifera)
Location: New Zealand
Reference: 173

$C_{29}H_{50}O$

(23S,24R)-23,24-Dimethylcholest-5-en-3β-ol

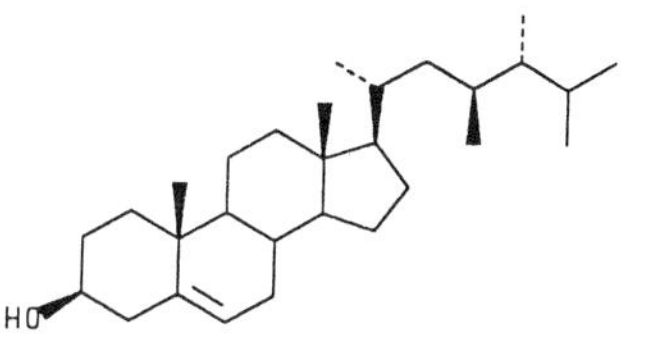

Mol. Wt.: 414
Spectral Data: PMR
Organism: *Stelleta conulosa* (Porifera)
Location: New Zealand
Reference: 1223

$C_{29}H_{50}O$

(22E,24ξ)-24-Ethylcholest-22-en-3α-ol

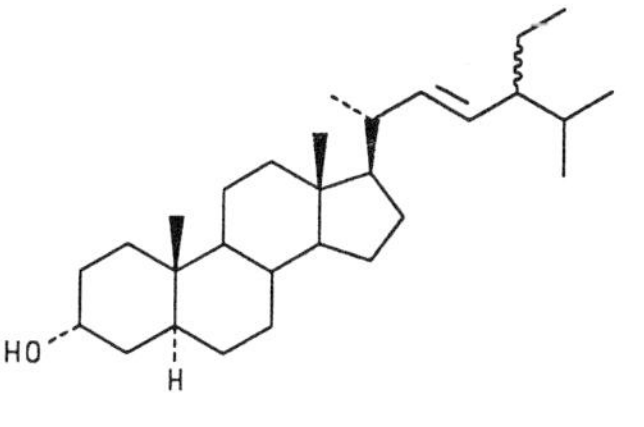

Mol. Wt.: 414
Spectral Data: PMR, Mass Spec.
Organism: *Esperiopsis edwardii* (Porifera)
Location: Chile
Reference: 994

$C_{29}H_{50}O$ **24-Ethylcholest-24(28)-en-3α-ol**

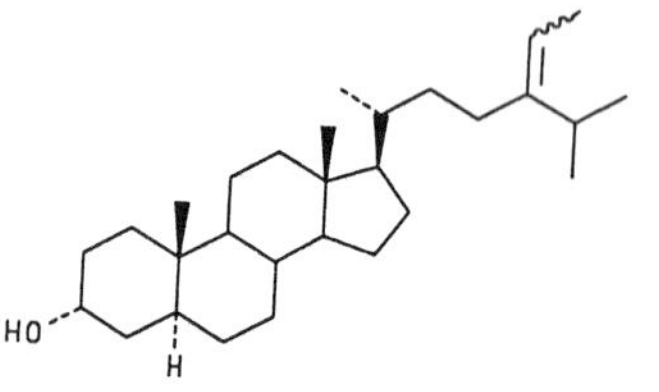

Mol. Wt.: 414
Spectral Data: PMR, Mass Spec.
Organism: *Esperiopsis edwardii* (Porifera)
Location: Chile
Reference: 994

$C_{29}H_{50}O$ **5α-Petrostanol**

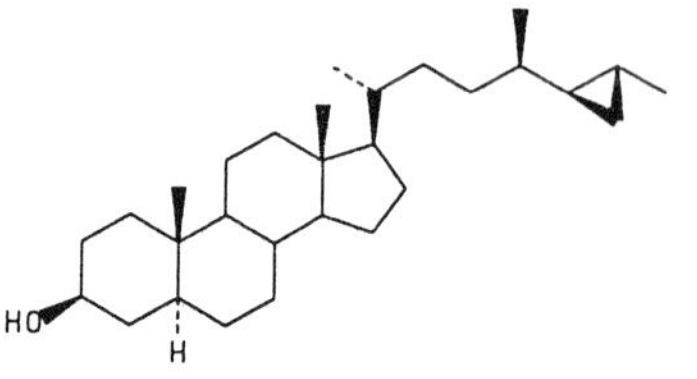

Mol. Wt.: 414
Melting Point: 122–123°C (synthetic sterol)
Spectral Data: PMR, Mass Spec.
Organism: *Petrosia hebes* (Porifera)
Location: New Zealand
Reference: 173

$C_{29}H_{50}O_3$ **(24R)-24-Ethyl-5α-cholest-7-ene-3β,5,6β-triol**

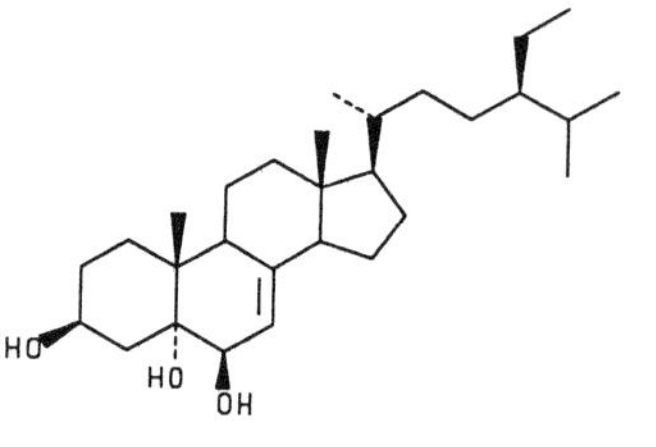

Mol. Wt.: 446
Melting Point: 254–256°C
Spectral Data: IR, PMR, Mass Spec.
Organism: *Spongionella gracilis* Vosmaer (Porifera)
Location: Naples, Italy
Reference: 895

$C_{29}H_{50}O_3$ **(24ξ)-24-Ethyl-5α-cholest-7-ene-3β,5,6β-triol**

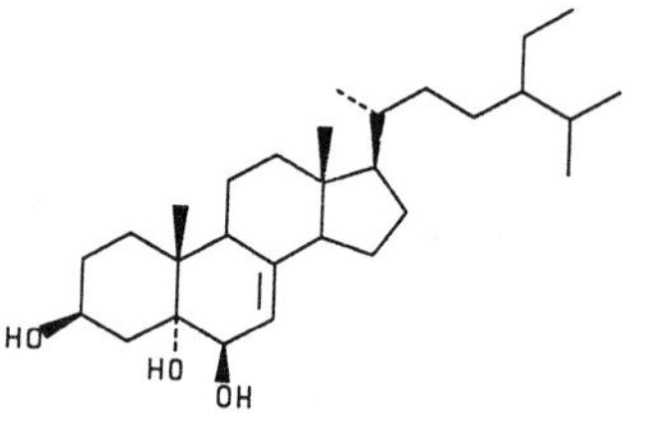

Mol. Wt.: 446
$[\alpha]_D$: −12.7 Solvent: Me
Spectral Data: PMR, Mass Spec.
Organism: *Patinopecten yessoensis* Jay (Mollusca)
Location: Japan
Reference: 460

$C_{29}H_{51}NaO_9S$ **(24R)-24-Ethyl-5α-cholestane-3β,6α,8,15α,16β,29-hexol 29-sulfate**

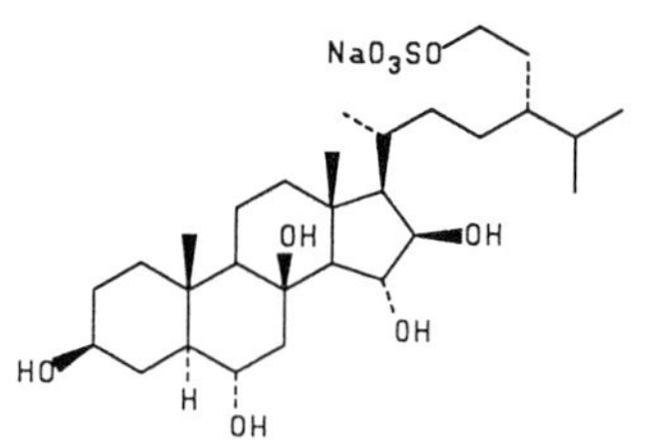

Mol. Wt.: 598
[α]D: +4.9 Solvent: Me
Spectral Data: CMR, PMR, Mass Spec.
Organism: *Poraster superbus* (Echinodomata)
Location: New Caledonia
Reference: 926

$C_{29}H_{52}O$ **(23S,24R)-23,24-Dimethyl-5α-cholestan-3β-ol** (previously known)

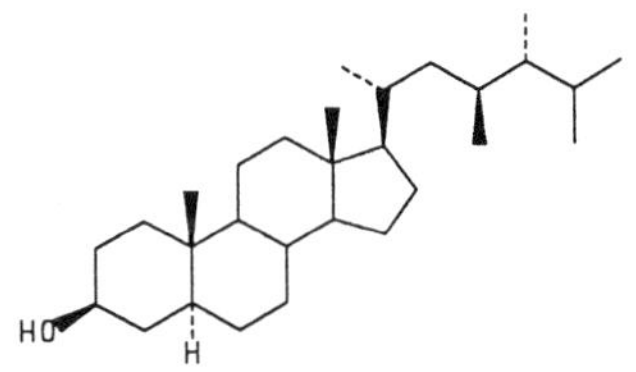

Mol. Wt.: 416
Spectral Data: PMR, Mass Spec.
Organism: *Bugula neritina* (Bryozoa)
Location: Gulf of Mexico
Reference: 344, 1223

$C_{29}H_{52}O$ **24ξ-Ethylcholestan-3α-ol**

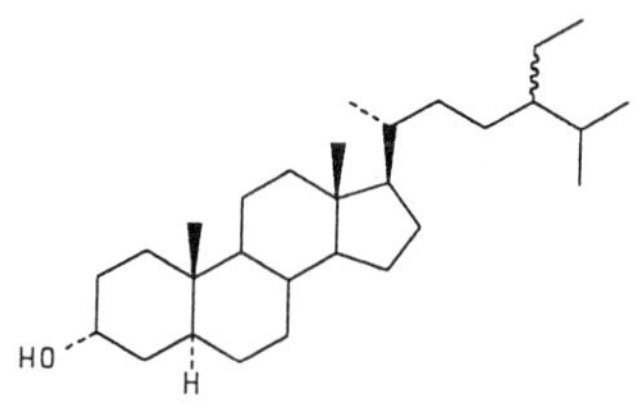

Mol. Wt.: 416
Spectral Data: PMR, Mass Spec.
Organism: *Esperiopsis edwardii* (Porifera)
Location: Chile
Reference: 994

$C_{30}H_{40}O_5$ **Minabeolide-2**

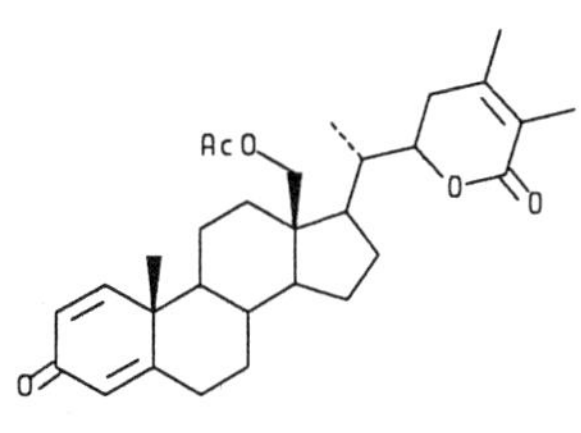

Mol. Wt.: 480
Melting Point: Oil
Spectral Data: UV, IR, CMR, PMR, Mass Spec.
Organism: *Minabea* sp. (Porifera)
Location: Truk
Reference: 617

$C_{30}H_{48}O$	**24-Ethyl-25-methylcholesta-5,22,-24(28)-trien-3β-ol**	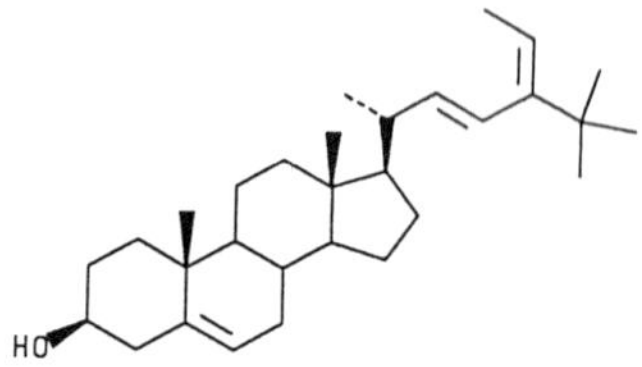
Mol. Wt.:	424	
Spectral Data:	PMR, Mass Spec.	
Organism:	*Pseudaxinyssa* sp. (Porifera)	
Location:	Great Barrier Reef, Australia	
Reference:	383	

$C_{30}H_{48}O$	**24(R)-Isopropylcholesta-5,22,25-trien-3β-ol**	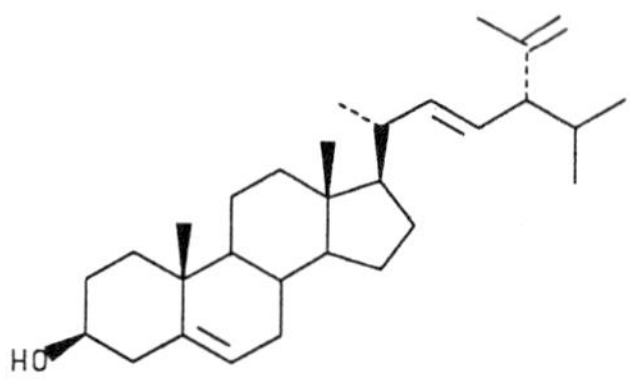
Mol. Wt.:	424	
Spectral Data:	PMR, Mass Spec.	
Organism:	*Pseudaxinyssa* sp. (Porifera)	
Location:	Great Barrier Reef, Australia	
Reference:	383	

$C_{30}H_{48}O$	**24(S)-Isopropylcholesta-5,22,25-trien-3β-ol**	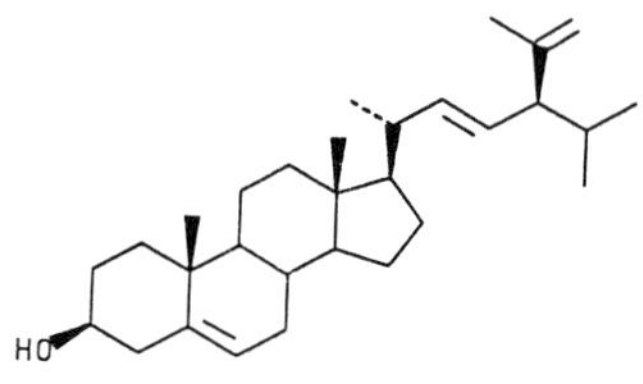
Mol. Wt.:	424	
Spectral Data:	PMR, Mass Spec.	
Organism:	*Pseudaxinyssa* sp. (Porifera)	
Location:	Great Barrier Reef, Australia	
Reference:	383	

$C_{30}H_{48}O$	**24(S)-24-Methyl-24-ethylcholesta-5,22,25-trien-3β-ol**	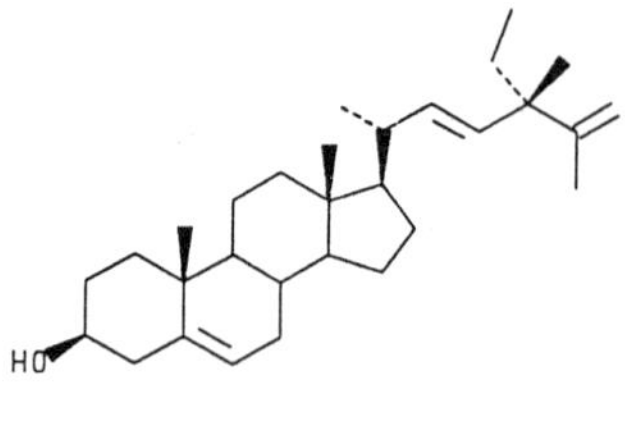
Mol. Wt.:	424	
Spectral Data:	PMR, Mass Spec.	
Organism:	*Pseudaxinyssa* sp. (Porifera)	
Location:	Great Barrier Reef, Australia	
Reference:	383	

$C_{30}H_{48}O_7$

3-Acetyl-2-desacetyl-22-epi-hippurin-1

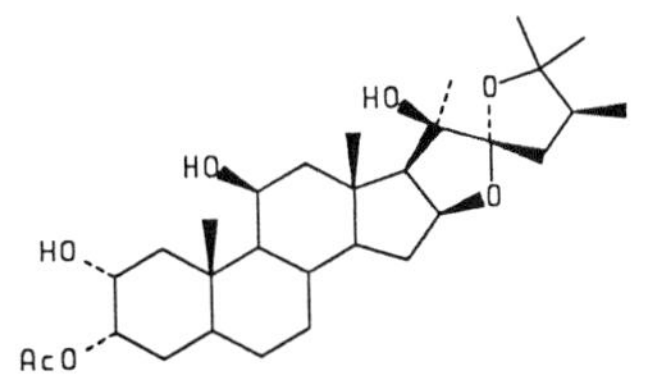

Mol. Wt.: 520
Melting Point: 248–250°C
Spectral Data: IR, CMR, PMR, Mass Spec.
Organism: *Isis hippuris* (Coelenterata)
Location: Bay of Bengal
Reference: 916

$C_{30}H_{48}O_8$

24-Methyl-5α-cholesta-7,22-diene-2α,3β,5α,6β,9α,11α,19-heptol 11-acetate

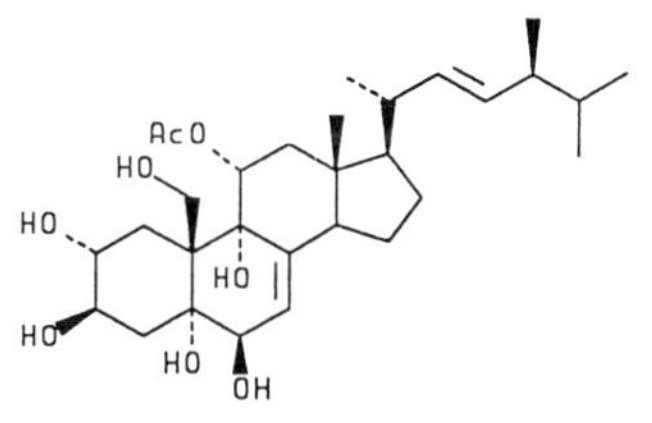

Mol. Wt.: 536
Melting Point: 213°C
$[\alpha]_D^{25}$: −32.2 Solvent: Alc
Spectral Data: CMR, PMR, Mass Spec.
Organism: *Dysidea etheria* (Porifera)
Location: Bermuda
Reference: 1173

$C_{30}H_{50}O$

24(R)-24-Methyl-24-ethylcholesta-5,22-dien-3β-ol

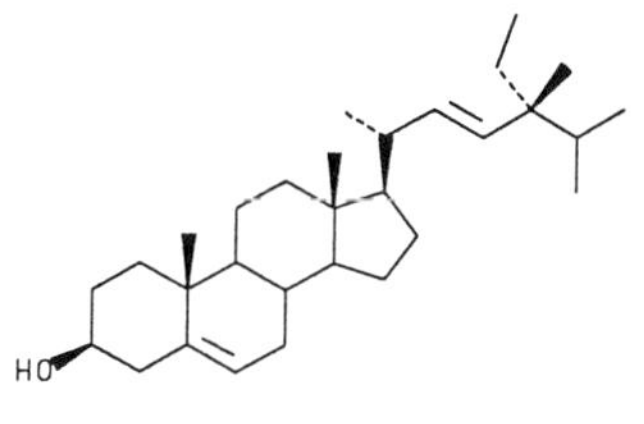

Mol. Wt.: 426
Spectral Data: PMR, Mass Spec.
Organism: *Pseudaxinyssa* sp. (Porifera)
Location: Great Barrier Reef, Australia
Reference: 383

$C_{30}H_{50}O$ **Strongylosterol**
[(24R)-24-Ethyl-27-methyl-cholesta-5,25-dien-3β-ol]

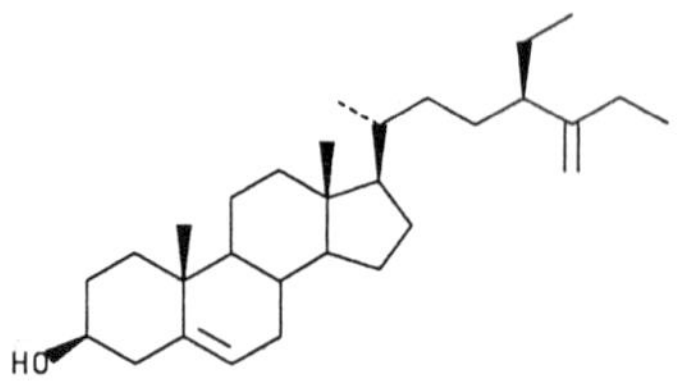

Mol. Wt.: 426
Melting Point: 112–112.5°C
$[\alpha]_D$: −43 Solvent: Dcm
Spectral Data: IR, CMR, PMR, Mass Spec.
Organism: *Strongylophora durissima* (Porifera)
Location: Papua, New Guinea
Reference: 92, 1035

$C_{30}H_{50}O_5$ **Xeniasterol-a**

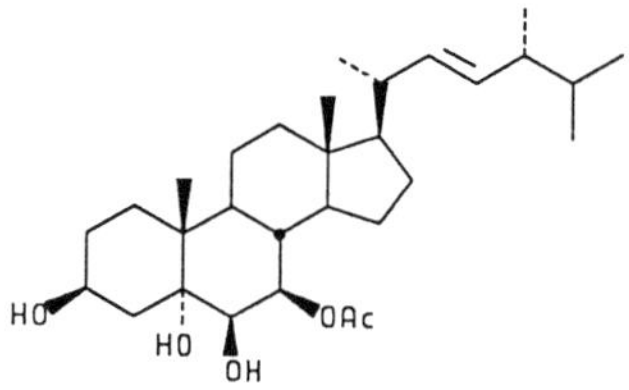

Mol. Wt.: 490
Melting Point: 208–209°C
$[\alpha]_D^{20}$: +12 Solvent: Py
Spectral Data: IR, CMR, PMR, Mass Spec.
Organism: *Xenia* sp. (Coelenterata)
Location: Okinawa, Japan
Reference: 564

$C_{30}H_{52}O$ **24(R)-24-Methyl-24-ethyl-5α-cholest-22-en-3β-ol**

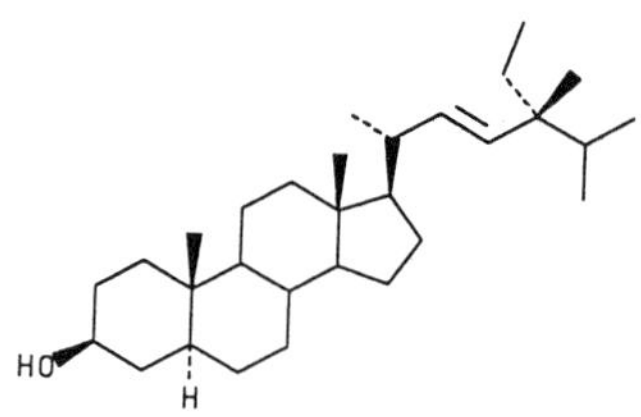

Mol. Wt.: 428
Spectral Data: PMR, Mass Spec.
Organism: *Pseudaxinyssa* sp. (Porifera)
Location: Great Barrier Reef, Australia
Reference: 383

$C_{30}H_{52}O_3$ **Xeniasterol-c**

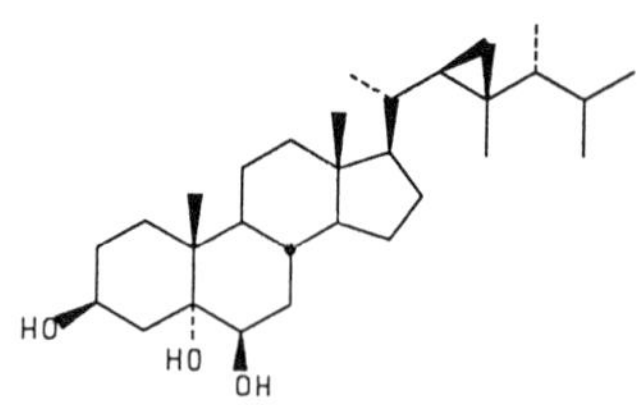

Mol. Wt.: 460
Melting Point: 255–256°C
$[\alpha]_D^{22}$: −3.0 Solvent: Chf-Me 1:1
Spectral Data: IR, CMR, PMR, Mass Spec.
Organism: *Xenia* sp. (Coelenterata)
Location: Okinawa, Japan
Reference: 564

$C_{30}H_{52}O_5$

Gorgostane-1α,3β,5α,6β,11α-pentaol

Mol. Wt.: 492
Melting Point: 295–297°C
Spectral Data: IR, CMR, PMR, Mass Spec.
Organism: *Isis hippuris* (Coelenterata)
Location: Bay of Bengal
Reference: 916

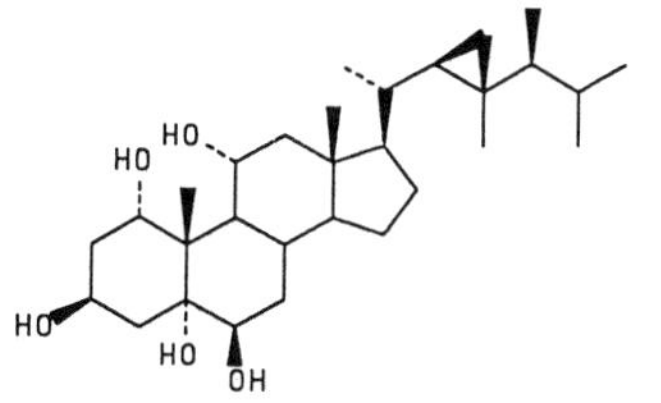

$C_{30}H_{52}O_5$

Xeniasterol-b

Mol. Wt.: 492
Melting Point: 218–220°C
$[\alpha]_D^{22}$: +50 Solvent: Py
Spectral Data: IR, CMR, PMR, Mass Spec.
Organism: *Xenia* sp. (Coelenterata)
Location: Okinawa, Japan
Reference: 564

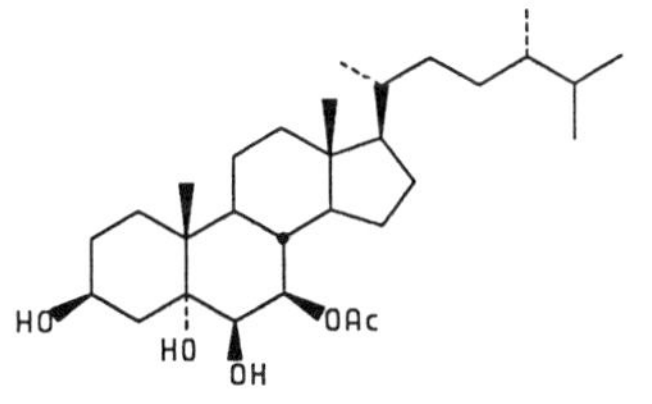

$C_{30}H_{54}O$

24-Isopropyl-5α-cholestan-3β-ol

Mol. Wt.: 430
Spectral Data: PMR, Mass Spec.
Organism: *Pseudaxinyssa* sp. (Porifera)
Location: Great Barrier Reef, Australia
Reference: 383

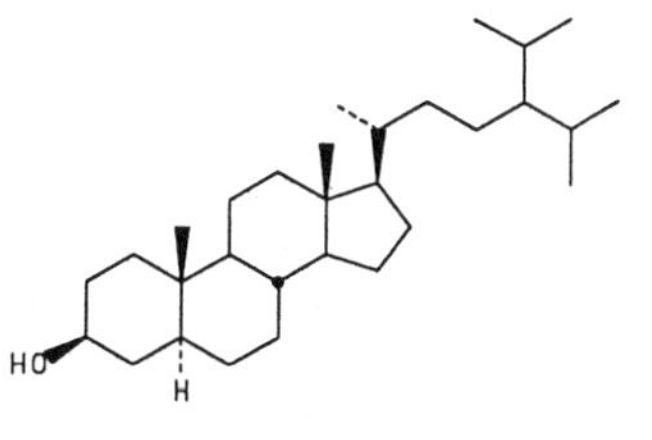

$C_{30}H_{54}O$

(23R,24R)-4α,23,24-Trimethyl-5α-cholestan-3β-ol

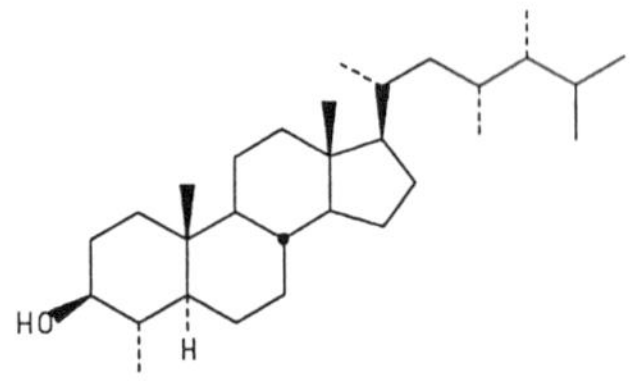

Mol. Wt.: 430
Spectral Data: PMR, Mass Spec.
Organism: *Protoceratium reticulatum* (Pyrrophyta, cultured)
Orbulina universa (Pyrrophyta, cultured)
Ascidia nigra (Chordata/Tunicata)
Location: Florida
Reference: 1223

$C_{30}H_{54}O$

(23S,24R)-4α,23,24-Trimethyl-5α-cholestan-3β-ol

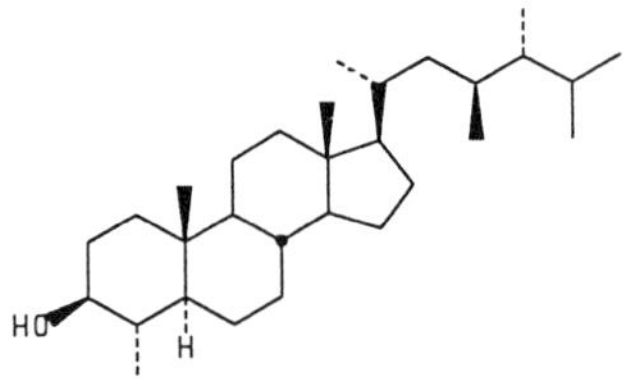

Mol. Wt.: 430
Spectral Data: PMR
Organism: *Siphonogorgia* sp. (Coelenterata)
Location: Papua, New Guinea
Reference: 1223

$C_{31}H_{48}O_6$

Diaulusterol A

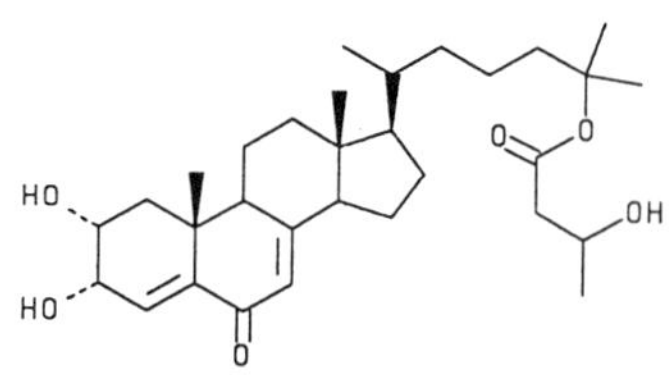

Mol. Wt.: 516
Melting Point: Oil
Spectral Data: IR, CMR, PMR; UV, Mass Spec. of the triacetate
Organism: *Diaulula sandiegensis* (Mollusca)
Location: British Columbia, Canada
Reference: 1182

$C_{31}H_{48}O_9$

5α-Cholesta-7,22-diene-2α,3β,5α,-6β,9α,11α,19-heptol 11,19-diacetate

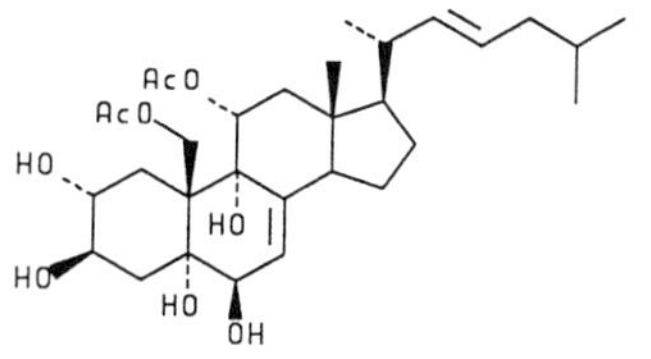

Mol. Wt.: 564
Melting Point: 150°C
$[\alpha]_D^{25}$: −53.3 Solvent: Alc
Spectral Data: CMR, PMR, Mass Spec.
Organism: *Dysidea etheria* (Porifera)
Location: Bermuda
Reference: 1173

$C_{31}H_{50}O$

24-Methyl-24-isopropylcholesta-5,22,25-trien-3β-ol

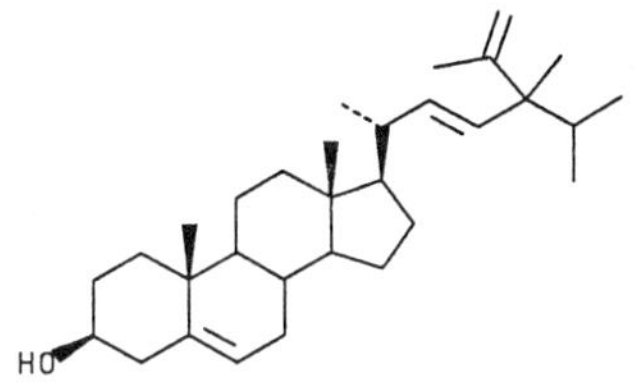

Mol. Wt.: 438
Spectral Data: PMR, Mass Spec.
Organism: *Pseudaxinyssa* sp. (Porifera)
Location: Great Barrier Reef, Australia
Reference: 383

$C_{31}H_{52}O$

24-Methyl-24-isopropylcholesta-5,25-dien-3β-ol

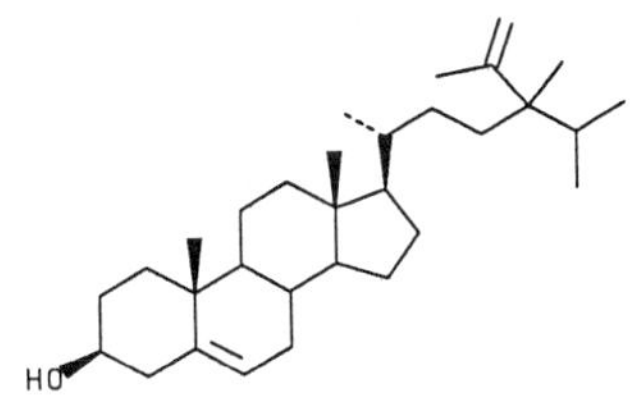

Mol. Wt.: 440
Spectral Data: PMR, Mass Spec.
Organism: *Pseudaxinyssa* sp. (Porifera)
Location: Great Barrier Reef, Australia
Reference: 383

$C_{31}H_{54}O$

24-Methyl-24-isopropylcholest-5-en-3β-ol

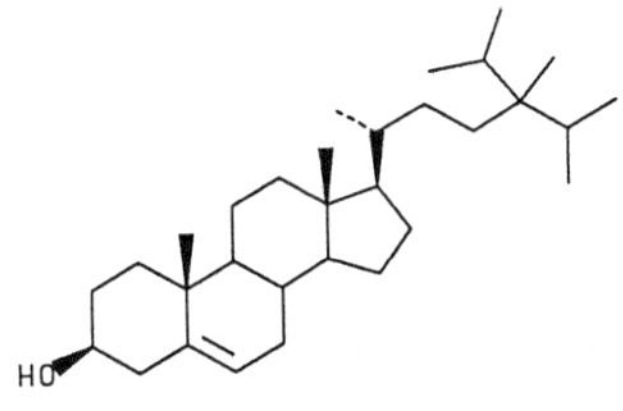

Mol. Wt.: 442
Spectral Data: PMR, Mass Spec.
Organism: *Pseudaxinyssa* sp. (Porifera)
Location: Great Barrier Reef, Australia
Reference: 383

$C_{32}H_{50}O_8$ **3-Acetyl-22-epi-hippurin-1**

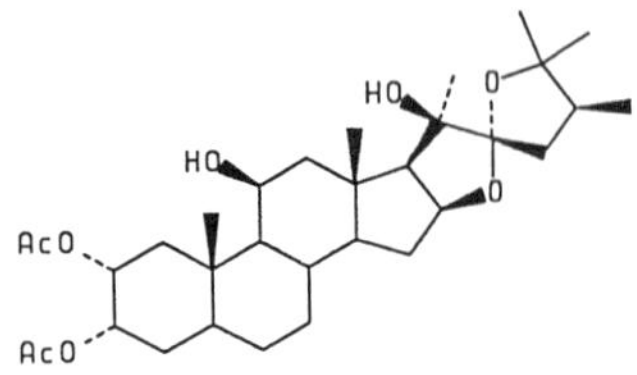

Mol. Wt.: 562
Melting Point: 240–243°C
Spectral Data: IR, CMR, PMR, Mass Spec.
Organism: *Isis hippuris* (Coelenterata)
Location: Bay of Bengal
Reference: 916

$C_{32}H_{54}O_5$ **Xeniasterol-d**

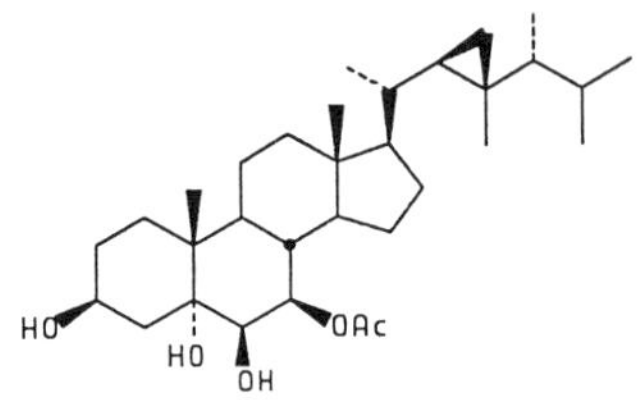

Mol. Wt.: 518
Melting Point: 285–286°C
$[\alpha]_D^{22}$: +32 Solvent: Py
Spectral Data: IR, CMR, PMR, Mass Spec.
Organism: *Xenia* sp. (Coelenterata)
Location: Okinawa, Japan
Reference: 564

$C_{32}H_{55}NaO_{11}S$ **Longicaudoside-A**

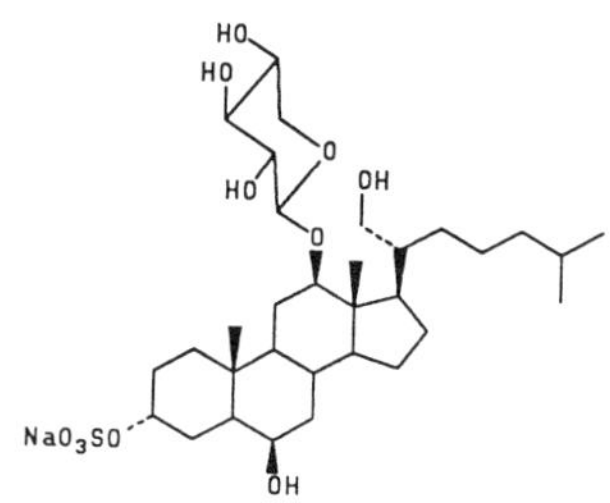

Mol. Wt.: 670
$[\alpha]_D$: ±0 Solvent: Me
Spectral Data: CMR, PMR, Mass Spec.
Organism: *Ophioderma longicaudum* (Echinodermata)
Location: Naples, Italy
Reference: 925

$C_{32}H_{55}NaO_{12}S$ **Glacialoside A**

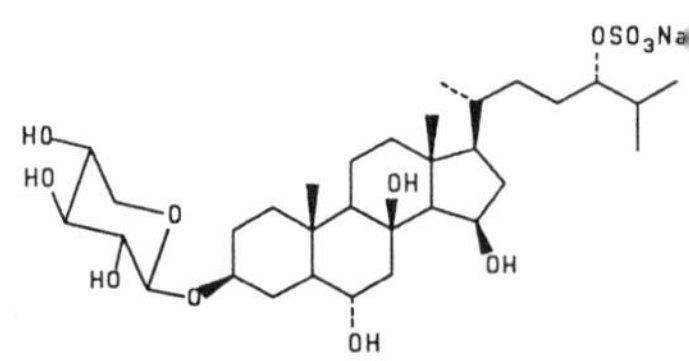

Mol. Wt.: 686
$[\alpha]_D$: +3.0 Solvent: Me
Spectral Data: CMR, PMR, Mass Spec.
Organism: *Marthasterias glacialis* (Echinodermata)
Location: Naples, Italy
Reference: 930

$C_{32}H_{55}NaO_{13}S$ **Glacialoside B**

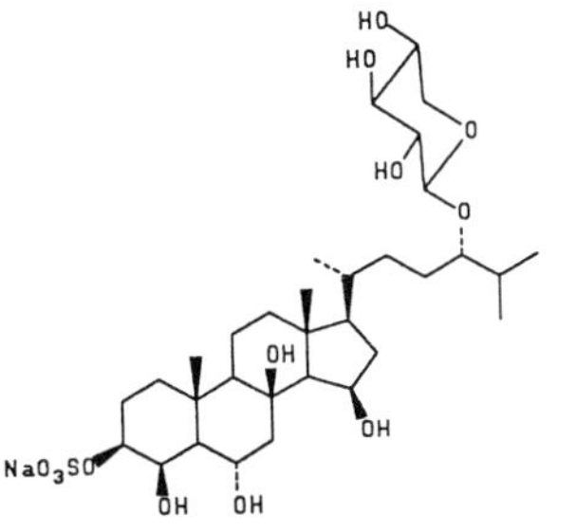

Mol. Wt.: 702
$[\alpha]_D$: +2.0 Solvent: Me
Spectral Data: CMR, PMR, Mass Spec.
Organism: *Marthasterias glacialis* (Echinodermata)
Location: Naples, Italy
Reference: 930

$C_{33}H_{52}O_7$ **Cholest-5-ene-2α,3α,16β,18-tetrol 2,16,18-triacetate**

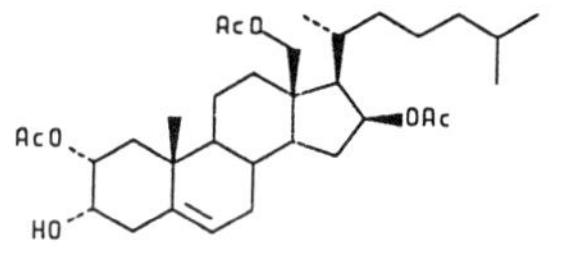

Mol. Wt.: 560
$[\alpha]_D^{26}$: +17.2 Solvent: Chf
Spectral Data: IR, PMR, Mass Spec.
Organism: *Eudendrium glomeratum* Picard (Coelenterata)
Location: Naples, Italy
Reference: 8

$C_{33}H_{52}O_7$ **Cholest-5-ene-3α,7β,15β,18-tetrol 7,15,18-triacetate**

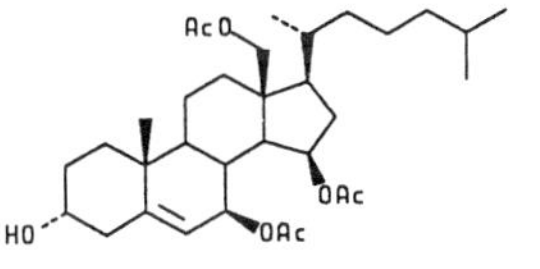

Mol. Wt.: 560
$[\alpha]_D^{26}$: +23 Solvent: Chf
Spectral Data: IR, PMR, Mass Spec.
Organism: *Eudendrium glomeratum* Picard (Coelenterata)
Location: Naples, Italy
Reference: 8

$C_{33}H_{52}O_9$ **(24S)-24-Ethyl-5α-cholesta-7,22-diene-2α,3β,5α,-6β,9α,11α,19-heptol 11,19-diacetate**

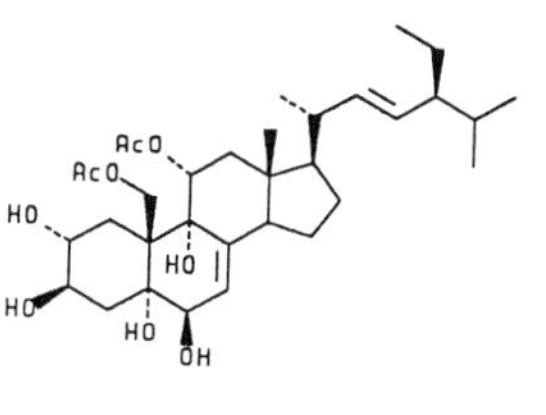

Mol. Wt.: 592
Melting Point: 147°C
$[\alpha]_D^{25}$: −47.5 Solvent: Alc
Spectral Data: CMR, PMR, Mass Spec.
Organism: *Dysidea etheria* (Porifera)
Location: Bermuda
Reference: 1173

$C_{33}H_{57}NaO_{12}S$ **Indicoside B**

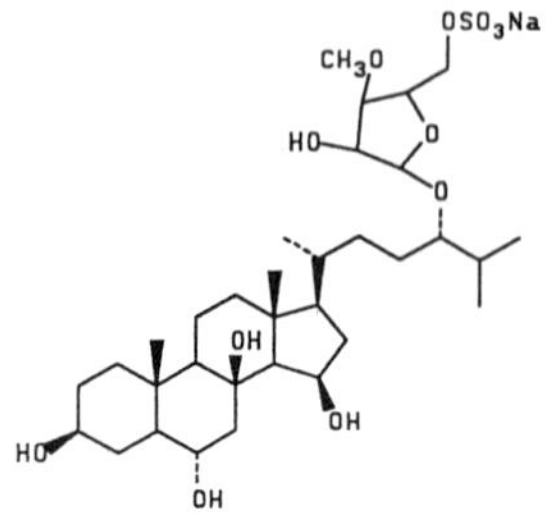

Mol. Wt.: 700
$[\alpha]_D$: −3.0 Solvent: Me
Spectral Data: CMR, PMR, Mass Spec.
Organism: *Astropecten indicus* (Echinodermata)
Location: Karachi
Reference: 928

$C_{33}H_{57}NaO_{12}S$ **Longicaudoside-B**

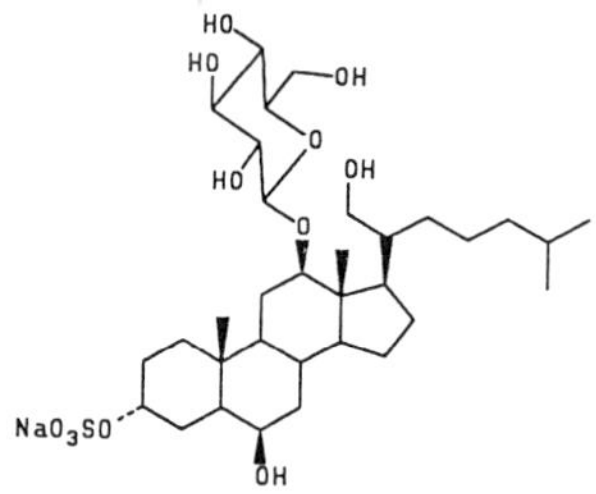

Mol. Wt.: 700
$[\alpha]_D$: +3.8 Solvent: Me
Spectral Data: CMR, PMR, Mass Spec.
Organism: *Ophioderma longicaudum* (Echinodermata)
Location: Naples, Italy
Reference: 925

$C_{33}H_{57}NaO_{13}S$ **Indicoside C**

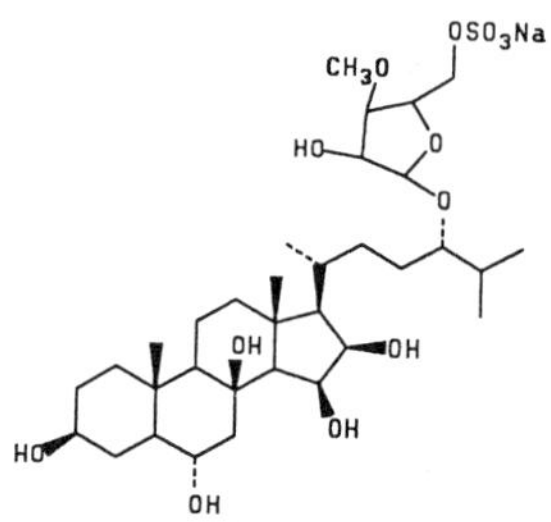

Mol. Wt.: 716
$[\alpha]_D$: −3.8 Solvent: Me
Spectral Data: CMR, PMR, Mass Spec.
Organism: *Astropecten indicus* (Echinodermata)
Location: Karachi
Reference: 928

$C_{33}H_{58}O_{10}$ **(25S)-5α-Cholestane-3β,6α,8,15α,16β,-26-hexol 3-O-2′-O-methyl-β-D-xylopyranoside**

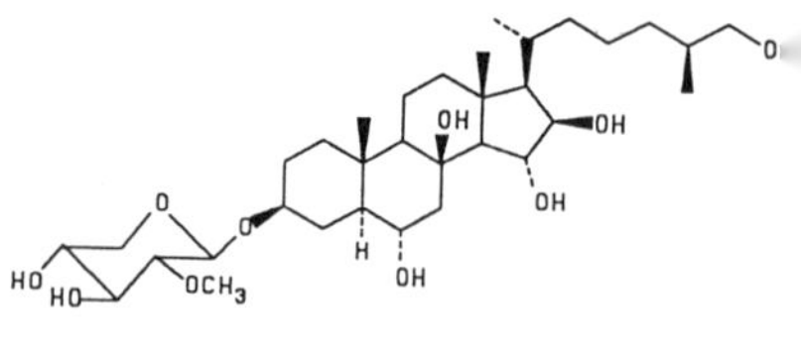

Mol. Wt.: 614
$[\alpha]_D$: +10.4 Solvent: Me
Spectral Data: CMR, PMR, Mass Spec.
Organism: *Poraster superbus* (Echinodermata)
Location: New Caledonia
Reference: 926

$C_{33}H_{58}O_{11}$ **(25S)-5α-Cholestane-3β,6α,7α,8,-15α,16β,26-heptol 3-O-2′-O-methyl-β-D-xylopyranoside**

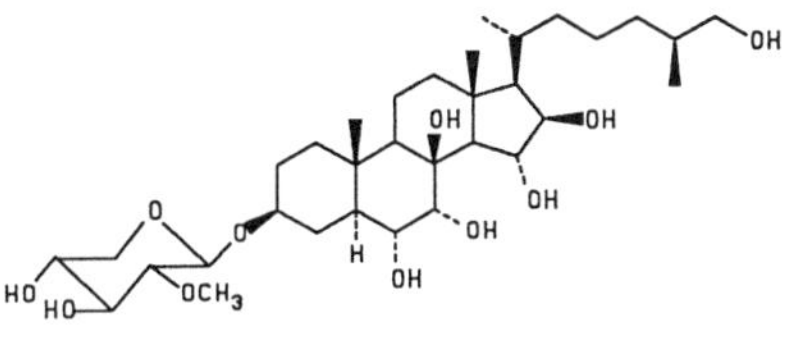

Mol. Wt.: 630
[α]D: +3.4 Solvent: Me
Spectral Data: CMR, PMR, Mass Spec.
Organism: *Poraster superbus* (Echinodermata)
Location: New Caledonia
Reference: 926

$C_{34}H_{52}O_9$ **3,11-Diacetyl-22-epi-hippurin-1**

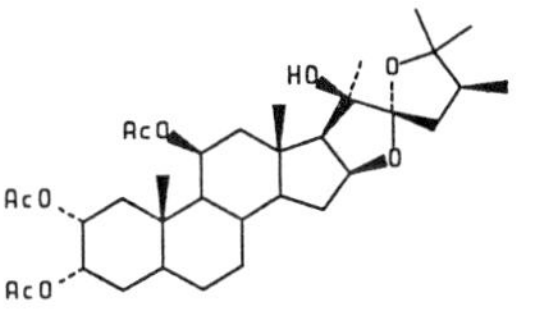

Mol. Wt.: 604
Melting Point: 178–180°C
Spectral Data: IR, CMR, PMR, Mass Spec.
Organism: *Isis hippuris* (Coelenterata)
Location: Bay of Bengal
Reference: 916

$C_{34}H_{52}O_9$ **3,11-Diacetylhippurin-1**

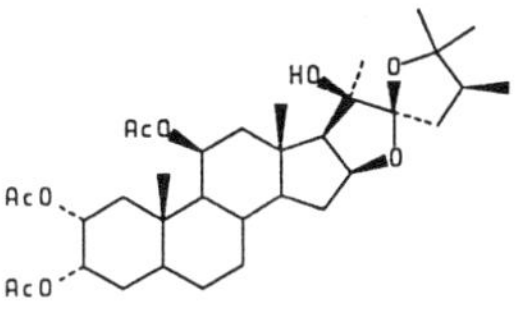

Mol. Wt.: 604
Melting Point: Oil
Spectral Data: IR, CMR, PMR, Mass Spec.
Organism: *Isis hippuris* (Coelenterata)
Location: Bay of Bengal
Reference: 916

$C_{34}H_{55}NaO_{13}S$ **Echinasteroside A**

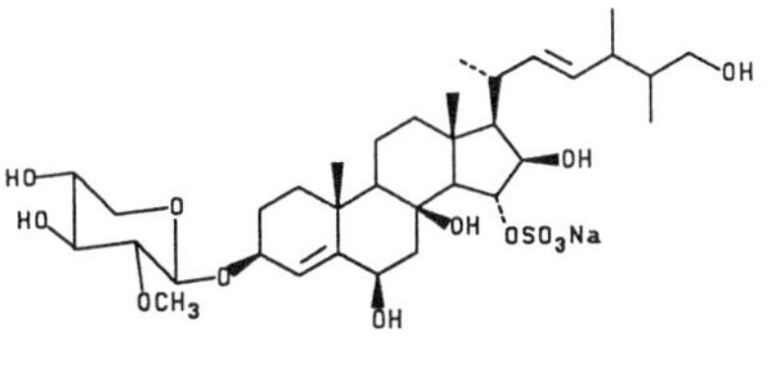

Mol. Wt.: 726
Spectral Data: CMR, PMR, Mass Spec.
Organism: *Echinaster sepositus*
Choriaster granulatus (Echinodermata)
Location: Naples, Italy; New Caledonia
Reference: 897, 1224

$C_{34}H_{56}O_{10}$ **15-Desulfated echinasteroside A**

Mol. Wt.: 624
Spectral Data: PMR
Organism: *Poraster superbus* (Echinodermata)
Location: New Caledonia
Reference: 926, 1224

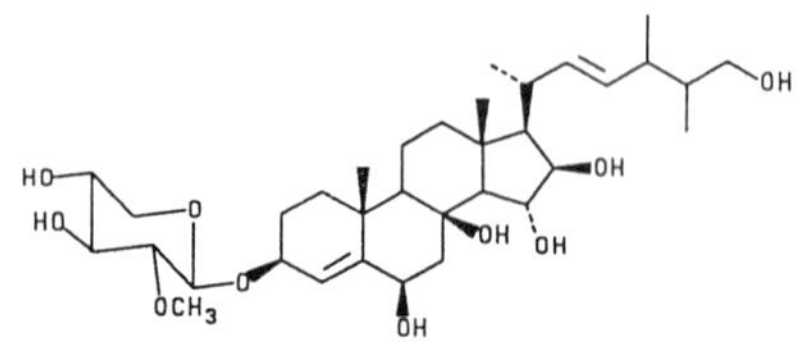

$C_{34}H_{57}NaO_{13}S$ **Attenuatoside S-II**

Mol. Wt.: 728
$[\alpha]_D$: +7.4 Solvent: Me
Spectral Data: PMR, Mass Spec.
Organism: *Hacelia attenuata* (Echinodermata)
Location: Naples, Italy
Reference: 740

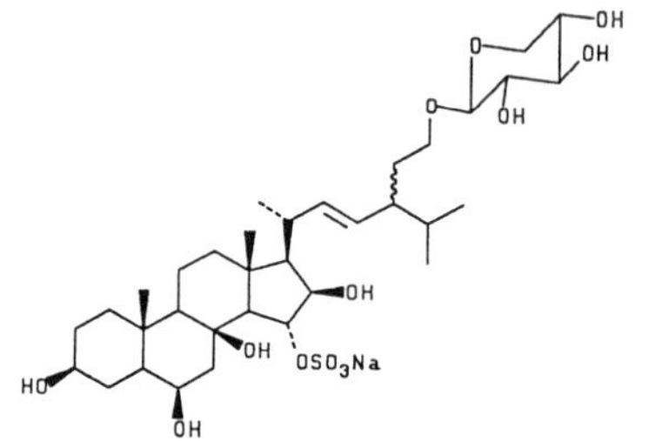

$C_{34}H_{58}O_{10}$ **24-Methyl-5α-cholest-24(28)-en-3β,6β,8,15α,16β,26-hexol 3-O-2'-O-methyl-β-D-xylopyranoside**

Mol. Wt.: 626
$[\alpha]_D$: -67.1 Solvent: Me
Spectral Data: CMR, PMR, Mass Spec.
Organism: *Poraster superbus* (Echinodermata)
Location: New Caledonia
Reference: 926, 932

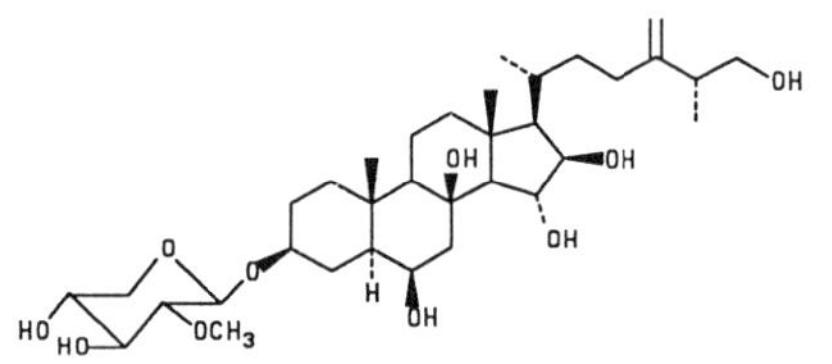

$C_{34}H_{58}O_{11}$ **Thromidioside**

Mol. Wt.: 642
$[\alpha]_D$: +10 Solvent: Me
Spectral Data: CMR, PMR, Mass Spec.
Organism: *Thromidia catalai* (Echinodermata)
Location: New Caledonia
Reference: 932

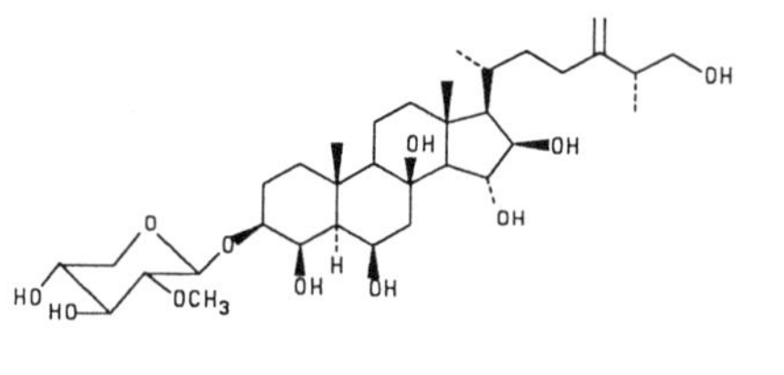

$C_{34}H_{59}NaO_{13}S$ **Attenuatoside S-I**

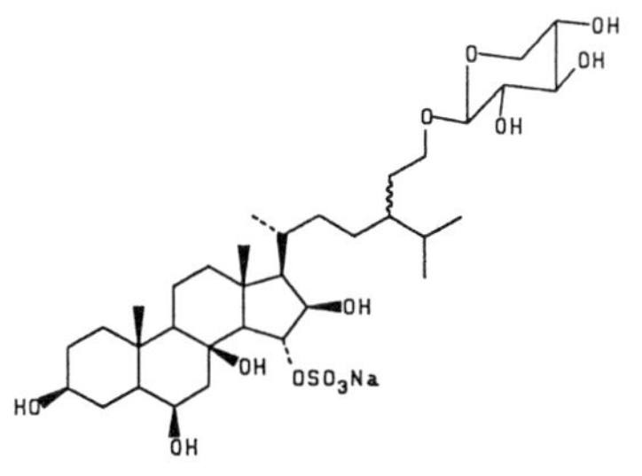

Mol. Wt.: 730
$[\alpha]_D$: +10 Solvent: Me
Spectral Data: CMR, PMR, Mass Spec.
Organism: *Hacelia attenuata* (Echinodermata)
Location: Naples, Italy
Reference: 740

$C_{34}H_{59}NaO_{13}S$ **Attenuatoside S-III**

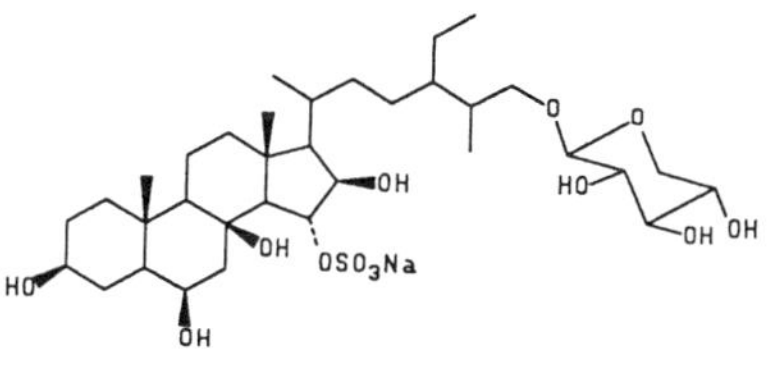

Mol. Wt.: 730
$[\alpha]_D$: +3.0 Solvent: Me
Spectral Data: PMR, Mass Spec.
Organism: *Hacelia attenuata* (Echinodermata)
Location: Naples, Italy
Reference: 740

$C_{34}H_{60}O_{10}$ **29-(α-L-Arabinofuranosyloxy)-5α-stigmastane-3β,6α,8,15α,16β-pentaol**

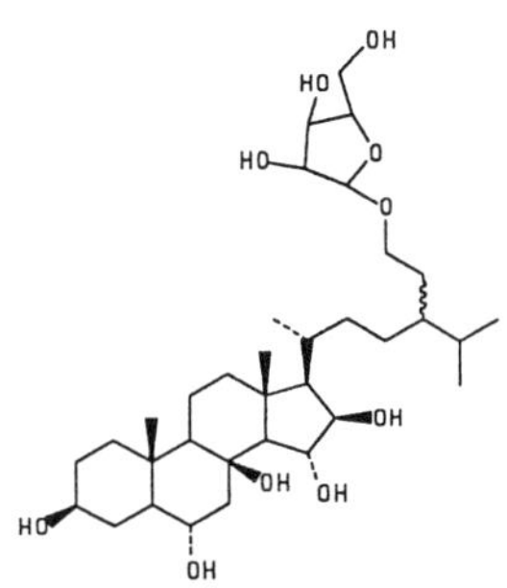

Mol. Wt.: 628
Melting Point: 248–249°C
$[\alpha]_D$: +3.8 Solvent: Me
Spectral Data: CMR, PMR, Mass Spec.
Organism: *Patiria pectinifera* (Echinodermata) (Desulfated extract)
Location: Sea of Japan
Reference: 553

$C_{35}H_{58}O_{10}$ **Mosesin-2**

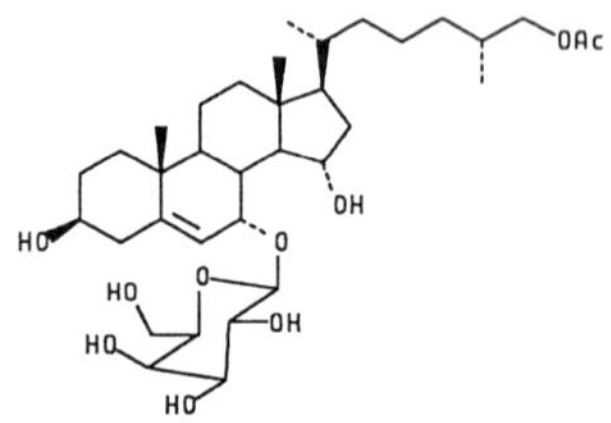

Mol. Wt.: 638
Bioactivity: Shark repellency: LC_{1hr} 14.6–19.6 μg/ml
Melting Point: 202–203°C
$[\alpha]_D^{24}$: −93 Solvent: Alc
Spectral Data: CMR, PMR, Mass Spec.
Organism: *Pardachirus marmoratus* (Chordata/Pisces)
Location: Red Sea
Reference: 1066

$C_{35}H_{58}O_{10}$ **Mosesin-5**

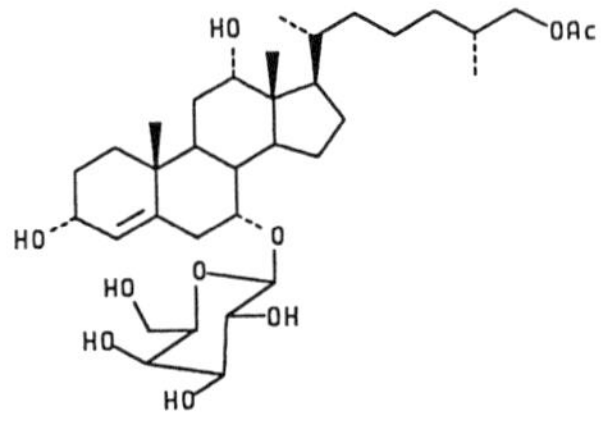

Mol. Wt.: 638
Spectral Data: PMR, Mass Spec.
Organism: *Pardachirus marmoratus* (Chordata/Pisces)
Location: Red Sea
Reference: 1066

$C_{35}H_{59}NaO_{13}S$ **Echinasteroside B**

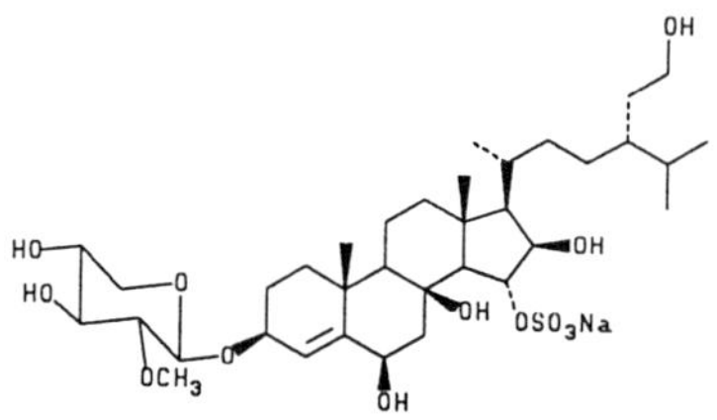

Mol. Wt.: 742
Spectral Data: CMR, PMR, Mass Spec.
Organism: *Echinaster sepositus* *Choriaster granulatus* (Echinodermata)
Location: Naples, Italy; New Caledonia
Reference: 897, 1224

$C_{35}H_{60}O_{10}$ **Mosesin-4**

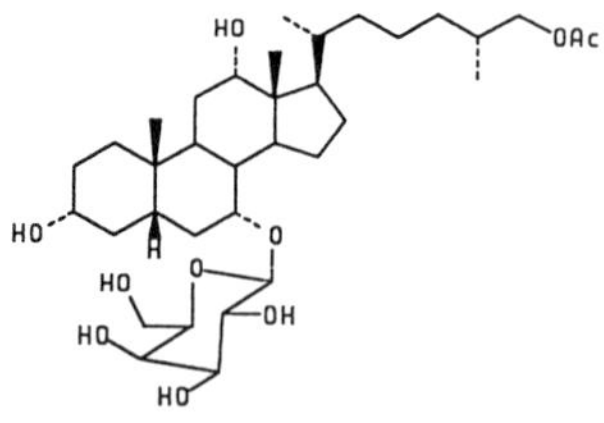

Mol. Wt.: 640
Bioactivity: Shark repellency: LC_{1hr} 11.0–17.4 μg/ml
$[\alpha]_D^{23}$: +3.0 Solvent: Alc
Spectral Data: PMR, Mass Spec.
Organism: *Pardachirus marmoratus* (Chordata/Pisces)
Location: Red Sea
Reference: 1066

$C_{35}H_{62}O_{12}$ **Indicoside A**

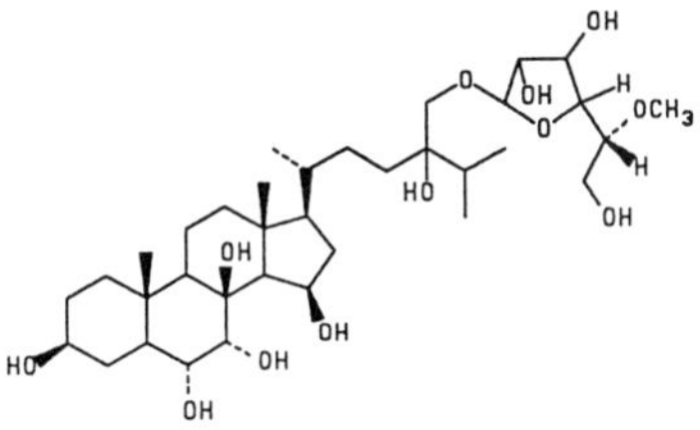

Mol. Wt.: 674
Melting Point: Glass
$[\alpha]_D$: −69.4 Solvent: Me
Spectral Data: CMR, PMR, Mass Spec.
Organism: *Astropecten indicus* (Echinodermata)
Location: Karachi
Reference: 927

$C_{37}H_{60}O_{11}$ **Mosesin-1**

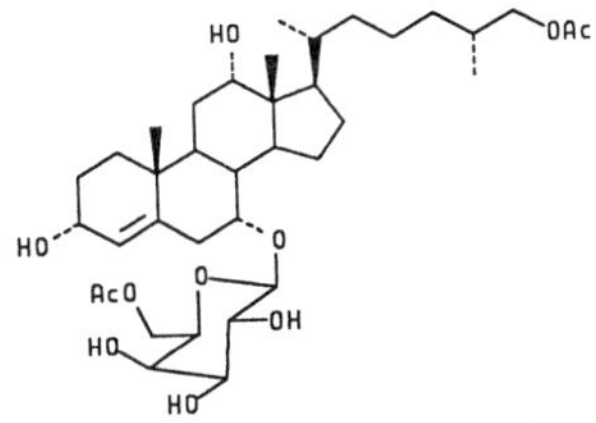

Mol. Wt.: 680
Bioactivity: Shark repellency: LC_{1hr} 6.0–11.7 μg/ml
Melting Point: 101–103°C
$[\alpha]_D^{21}$: +53 Solvent: Alc
Spectral Data: IR, CMR, PMR, Mass Spec.
Organism: *Pardachirus marmoratus* (Chordata/Pisces)
Location: Red Sea
Reference: 1066

$C_{37}H_{62}O_{11}$ **Mosesin-3**

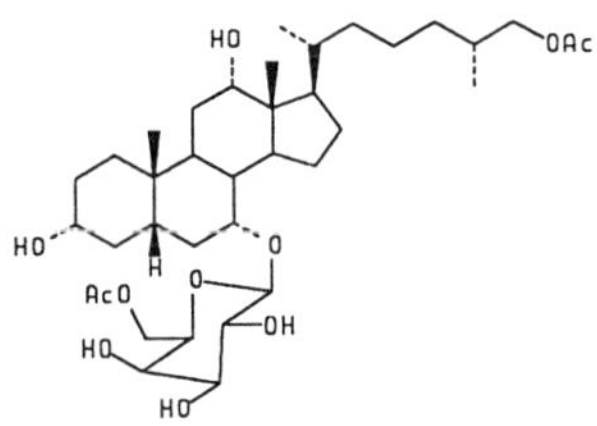

Mol. Wt.: 682
Bioactivity: Shark repellency: LC_{1hr} 8.5–13.0 μg/ml
$[\alpha]_D^{22}$: +15 Solvent: Alc
Spectral Data: CMR, PMR, Mass Spec.
Organism: *Pardachirus marmoratus* (Chordata/Pisces)
Location: Red Sea
Reference: 1066

$C_{38}H_{62}O_{13}$ **Dimorphoside A**

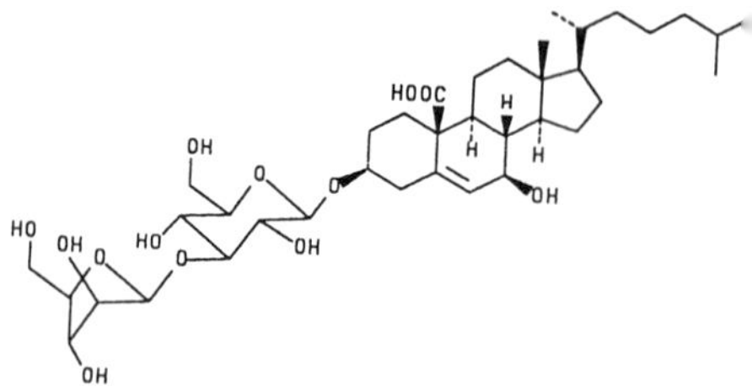

Mol. Wt.: 726
Bioactivity: Fertilized sea urchin egg assay: activity at 6 μg/ml
$[\alpha]_D^{23}$: -59 Solvent: Me
Spectral Data: IR, CMR, PMR, Mass Spec.
Organism: *Anthoplexaura dimorpha* (Coelenterata)
Location: Japan
Reference: 339

$C_{38}H_{64}O_{14}$ **Placentoside A**

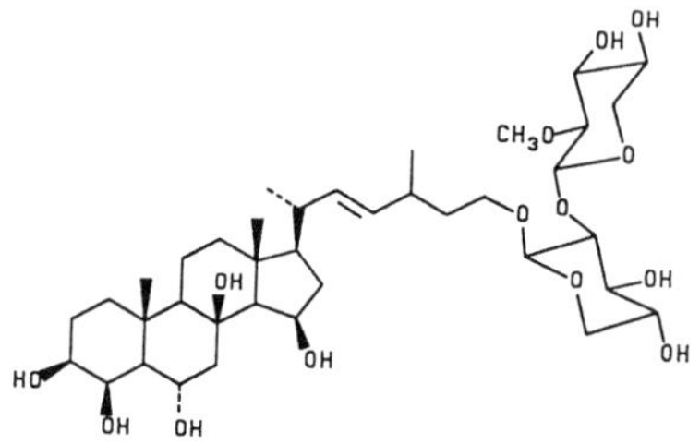

Mol. Wt.: 745
Spectral Data: CMR, PMR, Mass Spec.
Organism: *Sphaerodiscus placenta* Muller-Troshel (Echinodermata)
Location: Palinuro, Italy
Reference: 1225

$C_{38}H_{66}O_{12}$ **Granulatoside B**

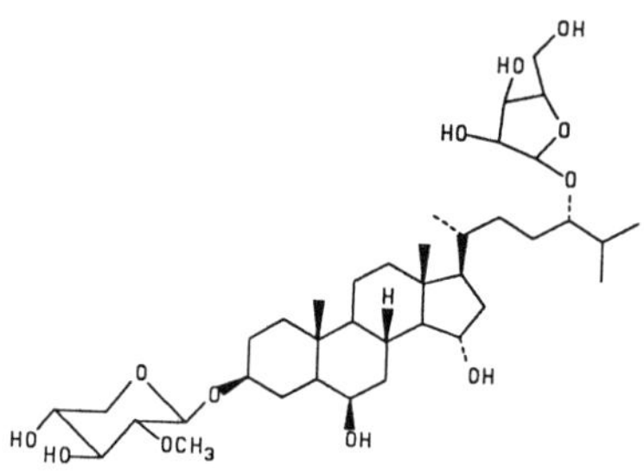

Mol. Wt.: 715
$[\alpha]_D$: -12 Solvent: Me
Spectral Data: CMR, PMR, Mass Spec.
Organism: *Choriaster granulatus* (Echinodermata)
Location: New Caledonia
Reference: 897

$C_{38}H_{66}O_{13}$ **Attenuatoside A-1** (previously known)

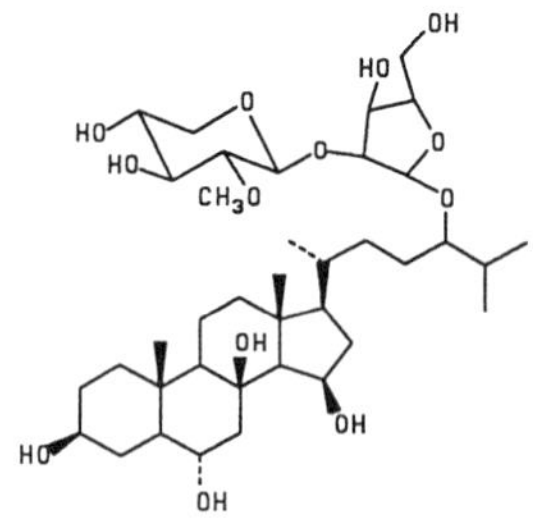

Mol. Wt.: 731
Organism: *Porania pulvillus* O.F. Müller (Echinodermata)
Location: Koster Fjord, Sweden
Reference: 25, 741

$C_{38}H_{66}O_{14}$ **6-*epi*-Nodososide**

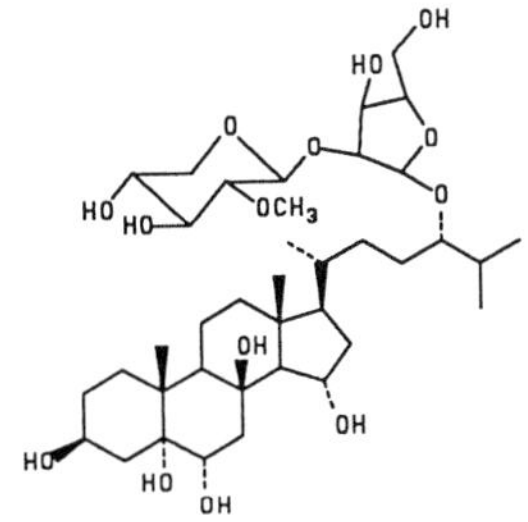

Mol. Wt.: 747
$[\alpha]_D$: ±0
Spectral Data: CMR (aglycone), PMR (aglycone), Mass Spec.
Organism: *Pentaceraster alveolatus* Perrier (Echinodermata)
Location: New Caledonia
Reference: 1226

$C_{38}H_{66}O_{14}$ **Granulatoside A**

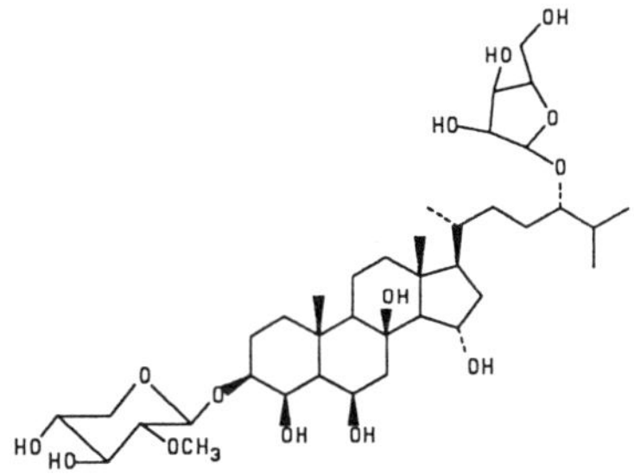

Mol. Wt.: 747
$[\alpha]_D$: −16 Solvent: Me
Spectral Data: CMR, PMR, Mass Spec.
Organism: *Choriaster granulatus* *Thromidia catalai* (Echinodermata)
Location: New Caledonia
Reference: 897, 932

$C_{39}H_{65}NaO_{17}S$ **Halityloside I**

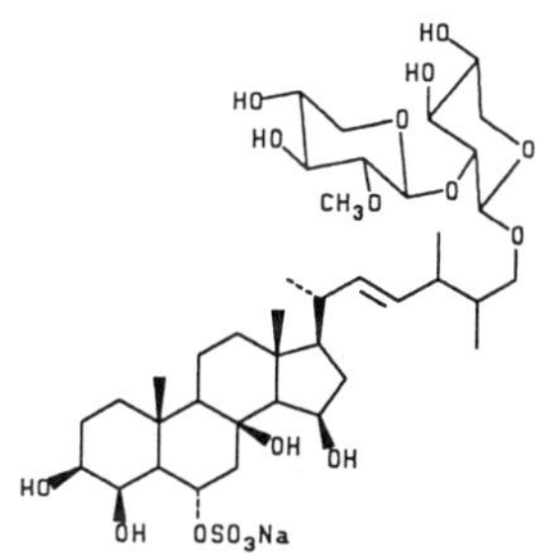

Mol. Wt.: 861
Spectral Data: CMR, PMR, Mass Spec.
Organism: *Halityle regularis* Fisher *Nardoa gomophia* Gray (Echinodermata)
Location: New Caledonia
Reference: 459, 931

$C_{39}H_{66}O_{13}$ **22-Dehydrohalityloside E**

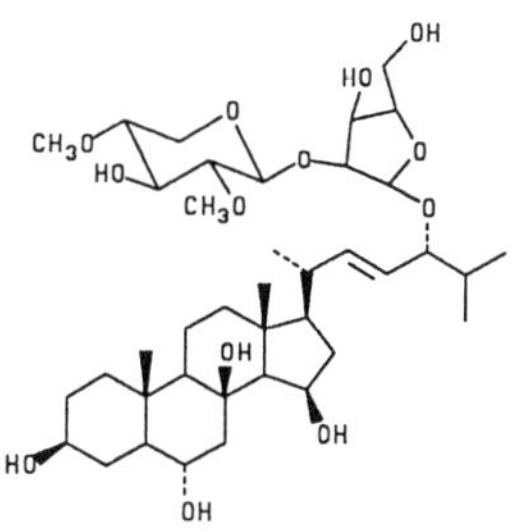

Mol. Wt.: 743
Spectral Data: PMR, Mass Spec.
Organism: *Sphaerodiscus placenta* Muller–Troshel (Echinodermata)
Location: Palinuro, Italy
Reference: 1225

$C_{39}H_{66}O_{13}$ **Poranoside A**

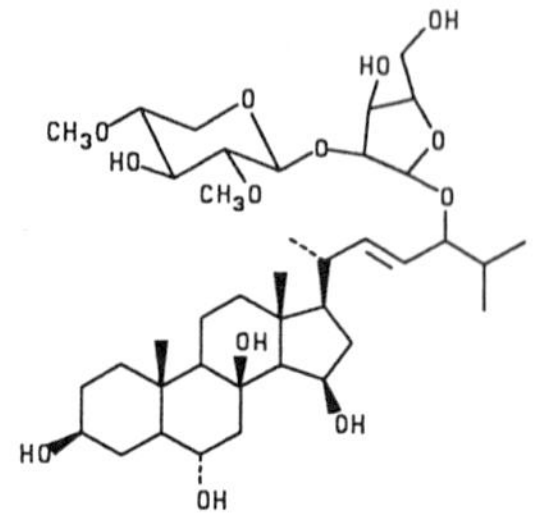

Mol. Wt.: 743
$[\alpha]_D^{22}$: −9.0 Solvent: Me
Spectral Data: PMR, Mass Spec.
Organism: *Porania pulvillus* O. F. Müller (Echinodermata)
Location: Koster Fjord, Sweden
Reference: 25

$C_{39}H_{66}O_{14}$ **22-Dehydrohalityloside D**

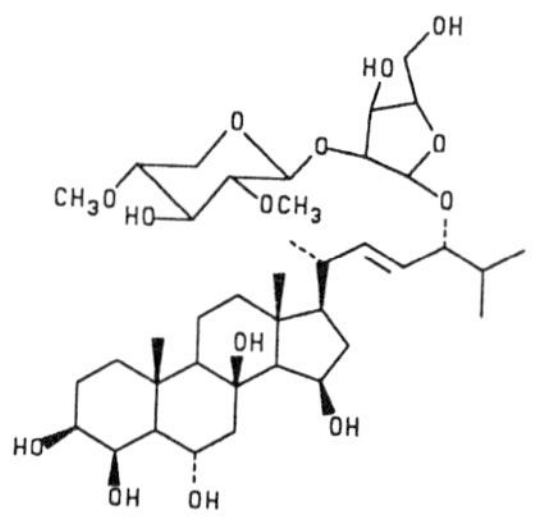

Mol. Wt.: 759
Spectral Data: PMR, Mass Spec.
Organism: *Sphaerodiscus placenta* Muller–Troshel (Echinodermata)
Location: Palinura, Italy
Reference: 1225

$C_{39}H_{68}O_{13}$ **Halityloside E**

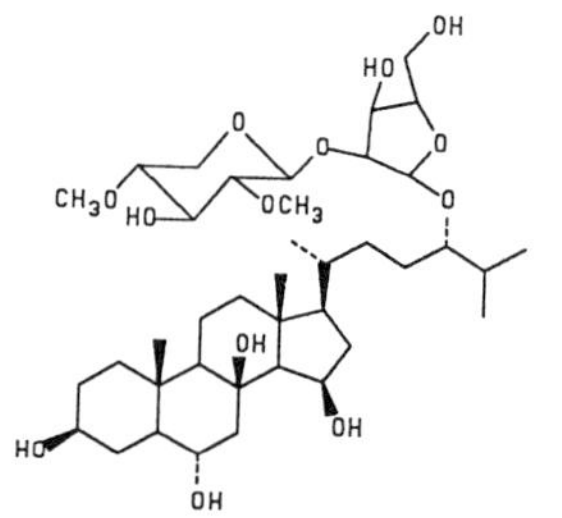

Mol. Wt.: 745
$[\alpha]_D$: −20 Solvent: Me
Spectral Data: CMR, PMR, Mass Spec.
Organism: *Sphaerodiscus placenta* Muller–Troshel
Nardoa gomophia Gray
Porania pulvillus O.F. Müller
Halityle regularis Fisher
(Echinodermata)
Location: Palinuro, Italy; New Caledonia; Koster Fjord, Sweden
Reference: 25, 459, 931, 1225

$C_{39}H_{68}O_{13}$ **Halityloside F**

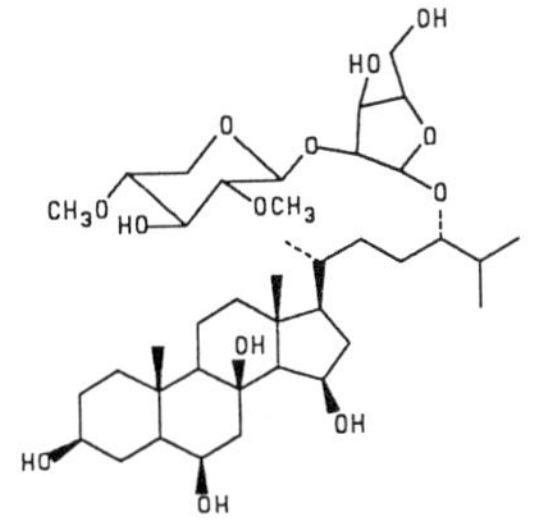

Mol. Wt.: 745
$[\alpha]_D$: -14.1 Solvent: Me
Spectral Data: CMR, PMR, Mass Spec.
Organism: *Halityle regularis* Fisher
Gomophia watsoni
(Echinodermata)
Location: New Caledonia
Reference: 459, 923

$C_{39}H_{68}O_{14}$ **Crossasteroside A**

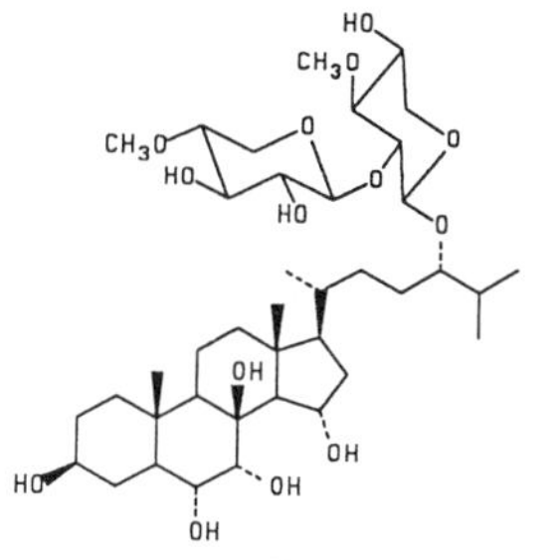

Mol. Wt.: 761
Bioactivity: Guinea pig ileum: 80% inhibition of contractions at 100 μg/ml
$[\alpha]_D$: -19.5 Solvent: Me
Spectral Data: CMR, Mass Spec., PMR of acetate
Organism: *Crossaster papposus*
(Echinodermata)
Location: Sweden
Reference: 24

$C_{39}H_{68}O_{14}$ **Culcitoside C_1**

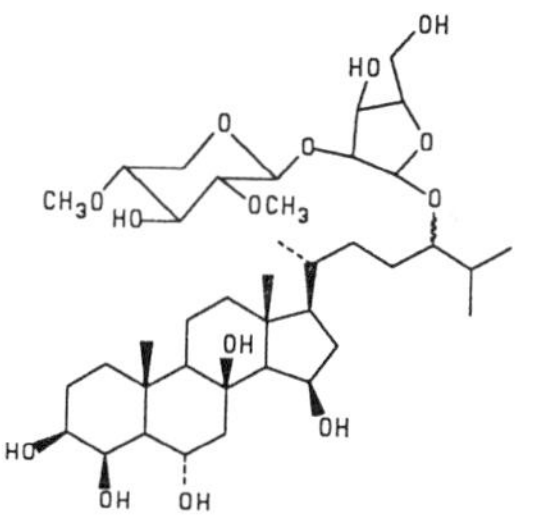

Mol. Wt.: 761
Melting Point: 245-248°C
$[\alpha]_D$: -35.8 Solvent: Me
Spectral Data: CMR, PMR
Organism: *Culcita novaeguineae*
Linckia guildingi
(Echinodermata)
Location: Madagascar
Reference: 552

$C_{39}H_{68}O_{14}$ **Gomophioside A**

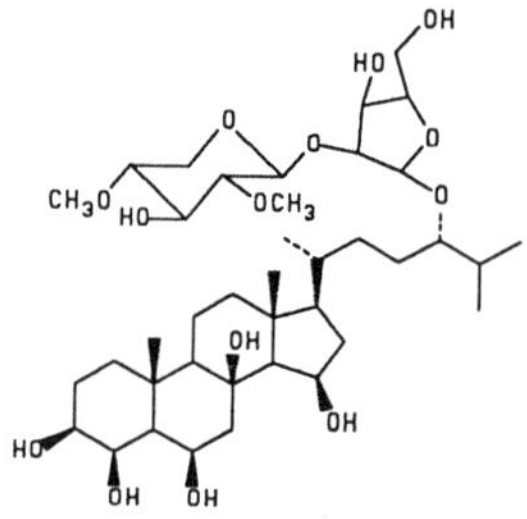

Mol. Wt.: 760
$[\alpha]_D$: -31.3 Solvent: Me
Spectral Data: CMR, PMR, Mass Spec.
Organism: *Gomophia watsoni* (Echinodermata)
Location: New Caledonia
Reference: 923

$C_{39}H_{68}O_{14}$ **Halityloside D**

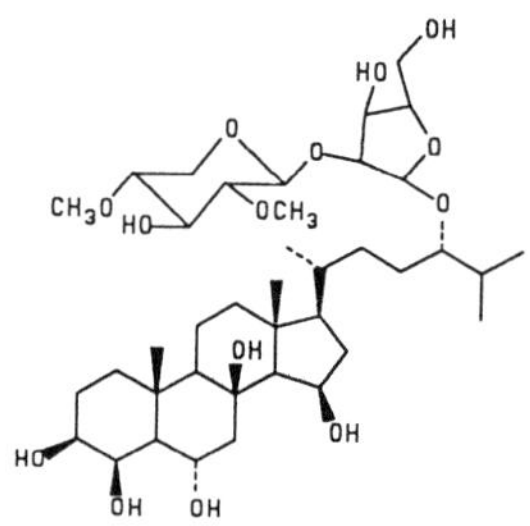

Mol. Wt.: 761
$[\alpha]_D$: -13.7 Solvent: Me
Spectral Data: CD (arabinose), CMR, PMR, Mass Spec.
Organism: *Nardoa novaecaledonia* Perrier
Nardoa gomophia Gray
Halityle regularis Fisher
Porania pulvillus O.F. Müller
(Echinodermata)
Location: New Caledonia;
Koster Fjord, Sweden
Reference: 25, 459, 931

$C_{40}H_{64}O_{13}$ **Dimorphoside B**

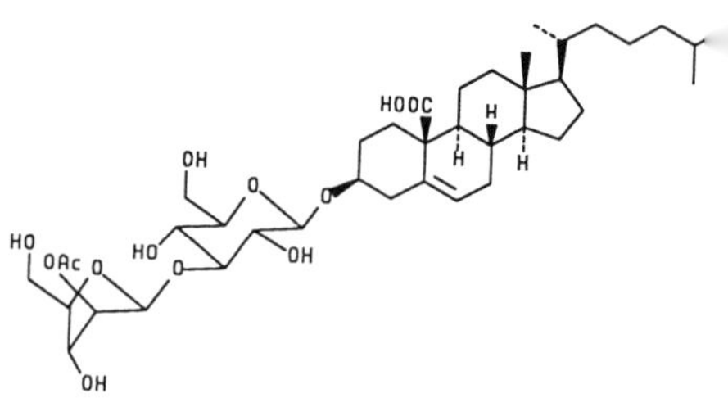

Mol. Wt.: 753
Bioactivity: Fertilized sea urchin egg assay: activity at 6 $\mu g/ml$
$[\alpha]_D^{20}$: -12 Solvent: Me
Spectral Data: CMR, PMR, Mass Spec.
Organism: *Anthoplexaura dimorpha* (Coelenterata)
Location: Japan
Reference: 339

$C_{40}H_{70}O_{14}$ **Culcitoside C_3**

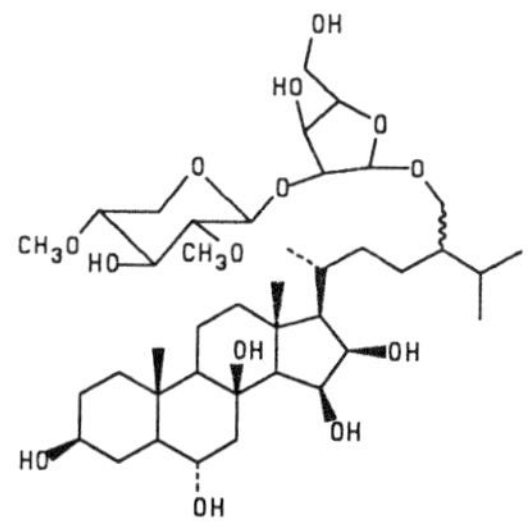

Mol. Wt.: 775
Melting Point: 228–230°C
$[\alpha]_D^{20}$: −19.1 Solvent: Alc
Spectral Data: CMR, PMR
Organism: *Culcita novaeguineae* (Echinodermata)
Location: Madagascar
Reference: 551

$C_{40}H_{70}O_{14}$ **Halityloside B**

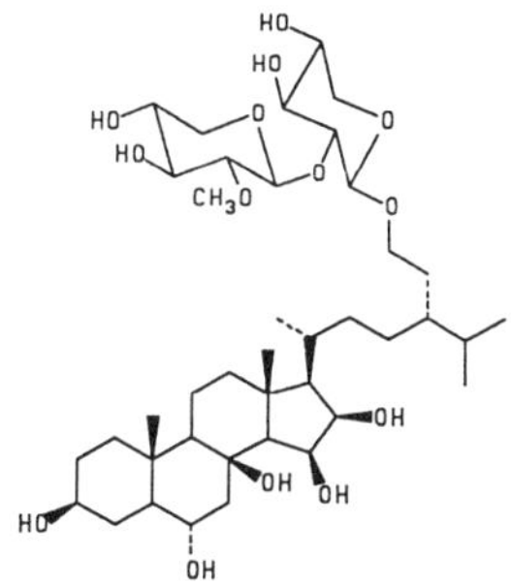

Mol. Wt.: 775
$[\alpha]_D$: −5.0 Solvent: Me
Spectral Data: CMR, PMR, Mass Spec.
Organism: *Sphaerodiscus placenta* Muller-Troshel
Nardoa novaecaledonia Perrier
Nardoa gomophia Gray
Halityle regularis Fisher
(Echinodermata)
Location: Palinuro, Italy; New Caledonia
Reference: 459, 931, 1225

$C_{40}H_{70}O_{15}$ **Culcitoside C_2**

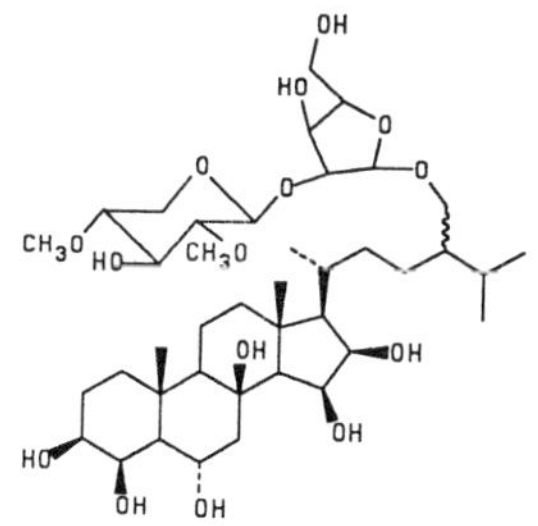

Mol. Wt.: 791
Melting Point: 226–228°C
$[\alpha]_D^{20}$: −18 Solvent: Alc
Spectral Data: CMR, PMR
Organism: *Culcita novaeguiniae* (Echinodermata)
Location: Madagascar
Reference: 551

$C_{40}H_{70}O_{15}$ **Halityloside A**

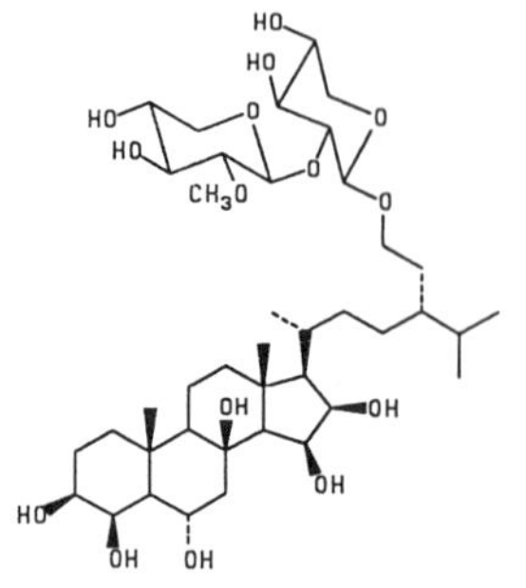

Mol. Wt.: 791
$[\alpha]_D$: -3.1 Solvent: Me
Spectral Data: CD (methylxylose), CMR, PMR, Mass Spec.
Organism: *Nardoa novaecaledonia* Perrier
Nardoa gomophia Gray
Halityle regularis Fisher
Sphaerodiscus placenta Muller-Troshel
(Echinodermata)
Location: New Caledonia;
Palinuro, Italy
Reference: 459, 931, 1225

$C_{41}H_{71}NaO_{18}S$ **Halityloside H, 6-O-sulfate**

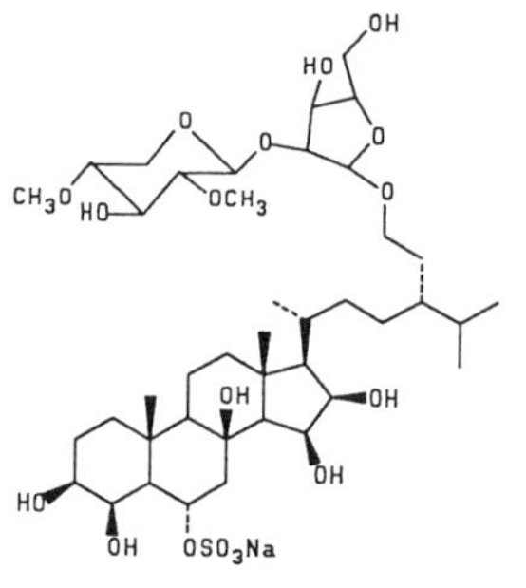

Mol. Wt.: 907
Spectral Data: PMR, Mass Spec.
Organism: *Halityle regularis* Fisher
(Echinodermata)
Location: New Caledonia
Reference: 459

$C_{41}H_{72}O_{14}$ **Gomophioside B**

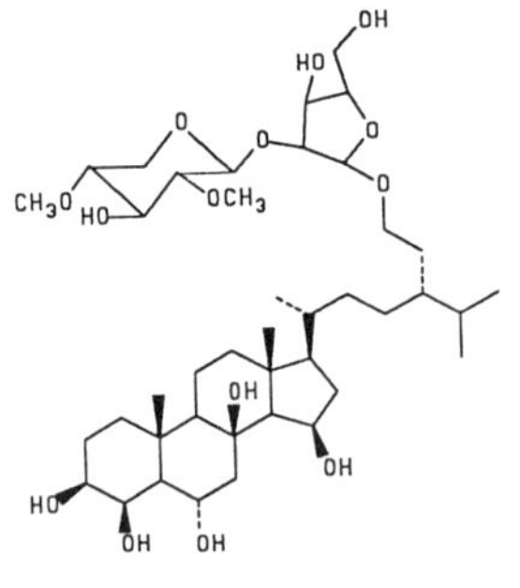

Mol. Wt.: 789
$[\alpha]_D$: -21.5 Solvent: Me
Spectral Data: CMR, PMR, Mass Spec.
Organism: *Gomophia watsoni*
(Echinodermata)
Location: New Caledonia
Reference: 923

$C_{41}H_{72}O_{15}$ **Halityloside H**

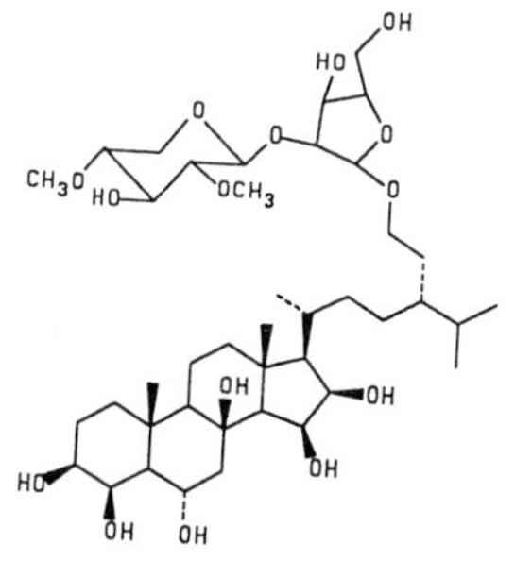

Mol. Wt.:	805
$[\alpha]_D$:	−5.0 Solvent: Me
Spectral Data:	CMR, PMR, Mass Spec.
Organism:	*Halityle regularis* Fisher *Nardoa gomophia* Gray (Echinodermata)
Location:	New Caledonia
Reference:	459, 931

$C_{47}H_{78}O_2$ **Cholesterol 8,11,14-eicosatrienoate**

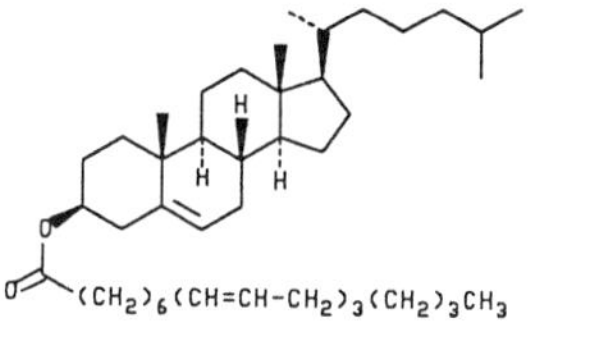

Mol. Wt.:	676
Bioactivity:	Inhibition of platelet aggregation
Spectral Data:	IR, PMR
Organism:	*Strongylocentrotus droebachiensis* (Echinodermata)
Location:	Maine
Reference:	791

$C_{51}H_{81}NaO_{27}S$ **Pectinioside D**

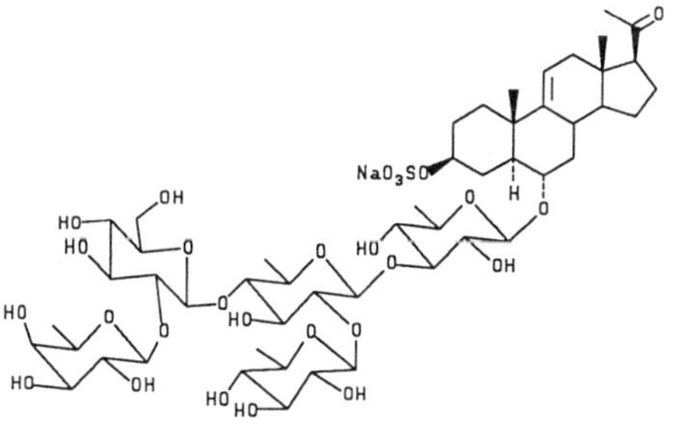

Mol. Wt.:	1182
Melting Point:	230–235°C
$[\alpha]_D$:	+15.6 Solvent: Me
Spectral Data:	IR, CMR, Mass Spec.
Organism:	*Asterina pectinifera* (Echinodermata)
Location:	Fukuoka, Japan
Reference:	248

$C_{53}H_{81}NaO_{24}S$ **Neothyonidioside**

Mol. Wt.: 1158
Melting Point: 241–243°C
$[\alpha]_D$: −73 Solvent: Py
Spectral Data: IR, CMR, PMR, Mass Spec.
Organism: *Neothyonidium magnum* (Echinodermata)
Location: New Caledonia
Reference: 1227

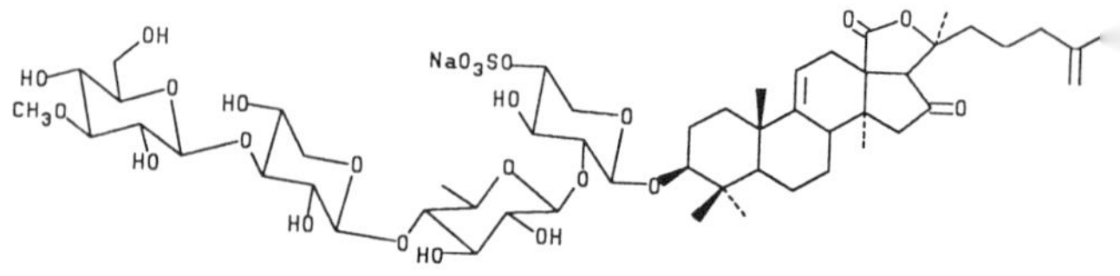

$C_{55}H_{85}NaO_{25}S$ **Cucumarioside G_1**

Mol. Wt.: 1202
Melting Point: 216–218°C
$[\alpha]_D^{20}$: −21.8 Solvent: Me/Aq
Spectral Data: IR, CMR, Mass Spec.
Organism: *Cucumaria fraudatrix* (Echinodermata)
Location: Sea of Japan
Reference: 6

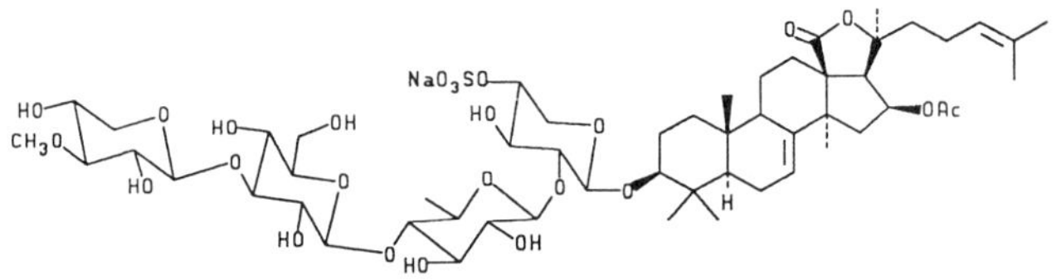

$C_{55}H_{86}N_2O_{20}$ **Sarasinoside C_2**

Mol. Wt.: 1096
Spectral Data: UV, CMR; PMR of the aglycone
Organism: *Asteropus sarasinosum* (Porifera)
Location: Palau
Reference: 567

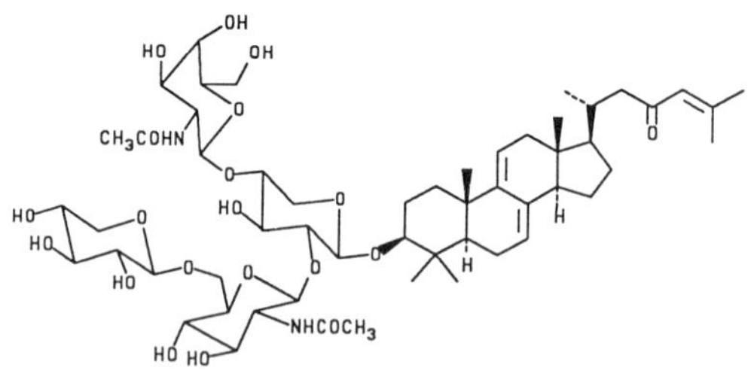

$C_{55}H_{86}N_2O_{20}$ **Sarasinoside C_3**

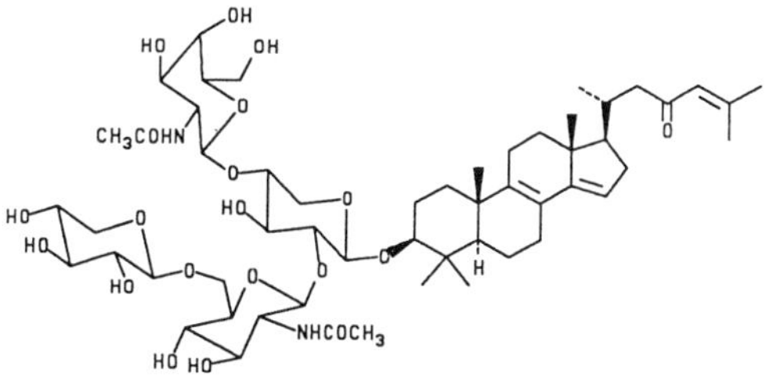

Mol. Wt.: 1096
Spectral Data: UV, CMR; PMR of the aglycone
Organism: *Asteropus sarasinosum* (Porifera)
Location: Palau
Reference: 567

$C_{55}H_{88}N_2O_{20}$ **Sarasinoside C_1**

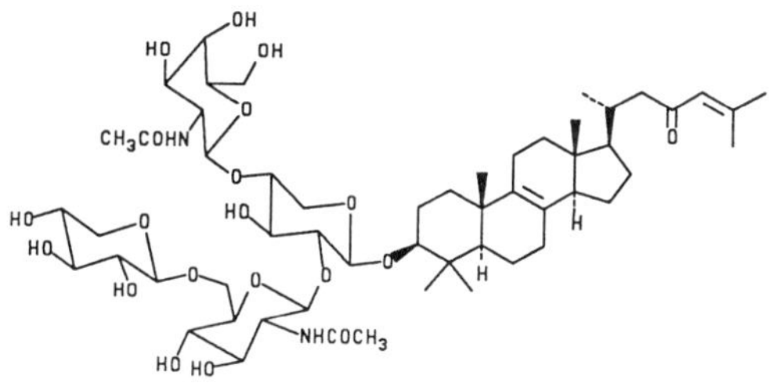

Mol. Wt.: 1098
Spectral Data: UV, CMR, x-ray c.s.; IR, PMR of the aglycone
Organism: *Asteropus sarasinosum* (Porifera)
Location: Palau
Reference: 567, 568

$C_{56}H_{89}NaO_{28}S$ **Acanthaglycoside B**

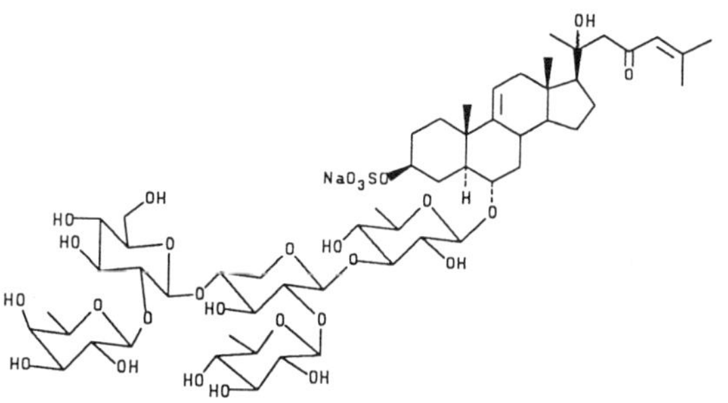

Mol. Wt.: 1266
Melting Point: 230°C (dec.)
$[\alpha]_D$: -7.2 Solvent: Aq
Spectral Data: IR, CMR, Mass Spec.
Organism: *Acanthaster planci* (Echinodermata)
Location: Okinawa, Japan
Reference: 478

$C_{56}H_{89}NaO_{28}S$ **Acanthaglycoside D**

Mol. Wt.: 1266
Bioactivity: Sea urchin assay: ED_{50} 15μg/ml; LD_{99} 5 μg/ml; Starfish assay: ED_{50} 100 μg/ml
Melting Point: 226–227°C (dec.)
$[\alpha]_D$: +1.3 Solvent: Aq
Spectral Data: CD, IR, CMR, Mass Spec.
Organism: *Acanthaster planci* (Echinodermata)
Location: Okinawa, Japan
Reference: 331, 478

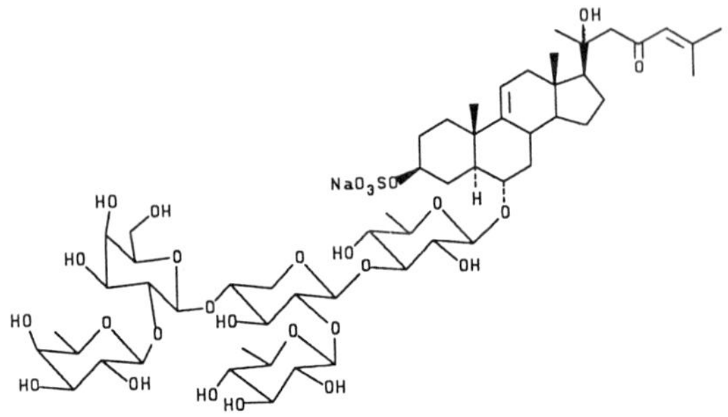

$C_{56}H_{91}NaO_{27}S$ **Asterosaponin-4**

Mol. Wt.: 1252
Bioactivity: Inhibition of spontaneous oocyte maturation (in *A. amurensis*)
Melting Point: 207–209°C
$[\alpha]_D^{27}$: −1.5 Solvent: Aq
Spectral Data: CMR, Mass Spec.; PMR of aglycone
Organism: *Asterias amurensis* (Echinodermata)
Location: Japan
Reference: 848

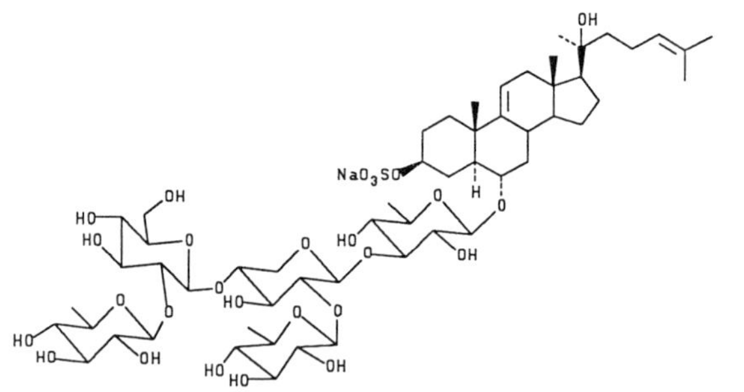

$C_{56}H_{91}NaO_{28}S$ **Acanthaglycoside C**

Mol. Wt.: 1268
Bioactivity: Sea urchin assay: ED_{50} 15 μg/ml; LD_{99}: 2 μg/ml; Starfish assay: ED_{50} 200 μg/ml
Melting Point: 225–230°C (dec.)
$[\alpha]_D$: −6.4; −7.0 Solvent: Aq; Me
Spectral Data: CD, IR, CMR, Mass Spec.
Organism: *Acanthaster planci*
Asterina pectinifera
(Echinodermata)
Location: Fukuoka; Okinawa, Japan
Reference: 248, 331, 478

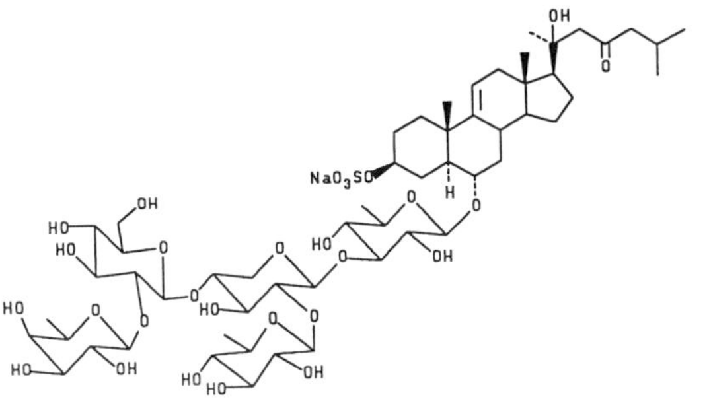

$C_{57}H_{93}NaO_{28}S$ **Versicoside C**

Mol. Wt.: 1282
Bioactivity: Sea urchin assay: ED_{50} 5 μg/ml; LD_{99} 2 μg/ml; Starfish assay: ED_{50} 50 μg/ml
Hemolytic activity
Melting Point: 224.0–226.0°C
$[\alpha]_D$: −9.6 Solvent: Aq
Spectral Data: CD, IR, CMR, Mass Spec.
Organism: *Asterias amurensis* [cf.] *versicolor* Sladen
(Echinodermata)
Location: Nagasaki, Japan
Reference: 331, 434, 477

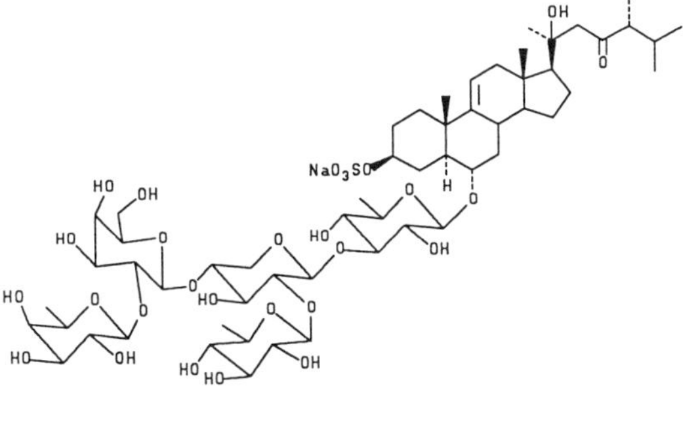

$C_{61}H_{96}N_2O_{25}$ **Sarasinoside B_2**

Mol. Wt.: 1258
Spectral Data: UV, CMR; PMR of the aglycone
Organism: *Asteropus sarasinosum* (Porifera)
Location: Palau
Reference: 567

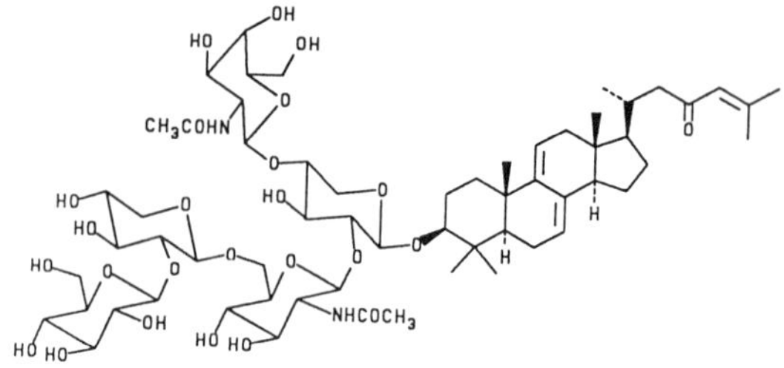

$C_{61}H_{96}N_2O_{25}$ **Sarasinoside B_3**

Mol. Wt.: 1258
Spectral Data: UV, CMR; PMR of the aglycone
Organism: *Asteropus sarasinosum* (Porifera)
Location: Palau
Reference: 567

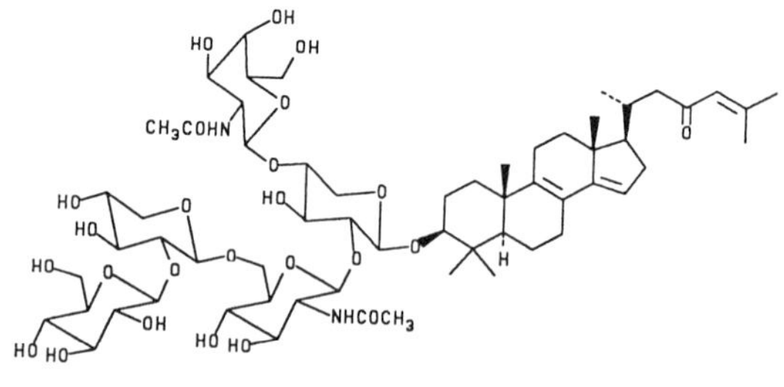

$C_{61}H_{98}N_2O_{25}$ **Sarasinoside B_1**

Mol. Wt.: 1260
Bioactivity: Inhibition of growth of starfish eggs: LD_{50} 0.71 μg/ml; LD_{100} 10 μg/ml
Ichthyotoxicity
Melting Point: 197–199°C
$[\alpha]_D^{20}$: −16 Solvent: Me
Spectral Data: UV, CMR, x-ray c.s.; IR, PMR of the aglycone
Organism: *Asteropus sarasinosum* (Porifera)
Location: Palau
Reference: 567, 568

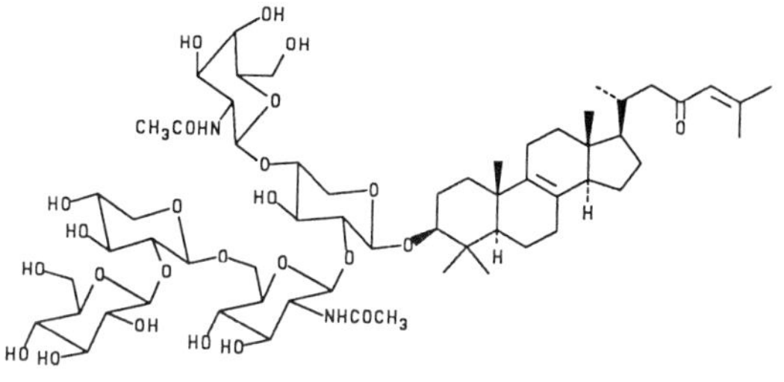

$C_{62}H_{98}N_2O_{26}$ **Sarasinoside A_2**

Mol. Wt: 1288
Spectral Data: UV, CMR; PMR of the aglycone
Organism: *Asteropus sarasinosum* (Porifera)
Location: Palau
Reference: 567

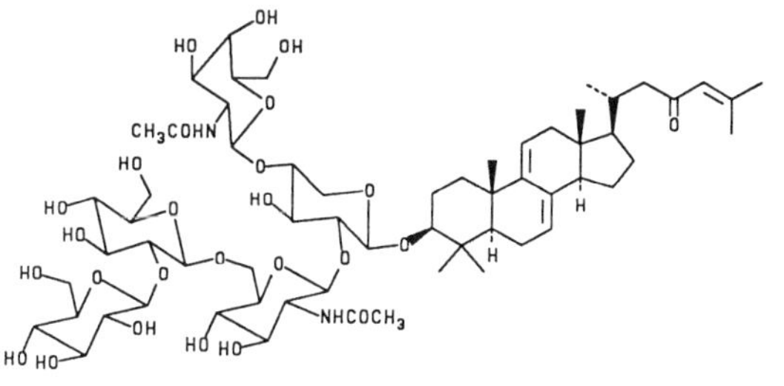

$C_{62}H_{98}N_2O_{26}$ **Sarasinoside A_3**

Mol. Wt.: 1288
Spectral Data: UV, CMR; PMR of the aglycone
Organism: *Asteropus sarasinosum* (Porifera)
Location: Palau
Reference: 567

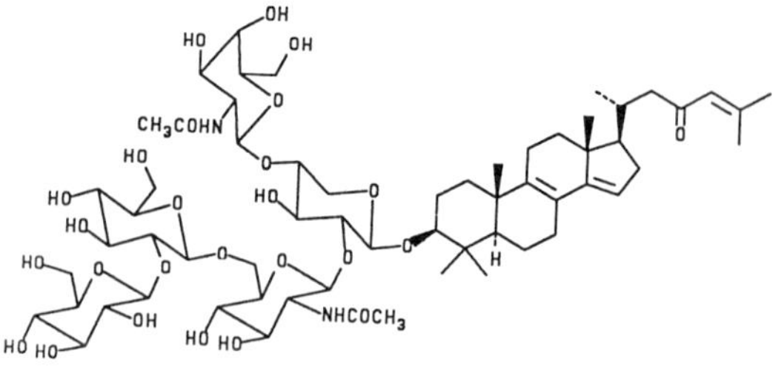

$C_{62}H_{101}NaO_{33}S$ **Pectinioside F**

Mol. Wt.: 1430
Melting Point: 225–230°C (dec.)
$[\alpha]_D^{25}$: −5.8 Solvent: Aq
Spectral Data: IR, CMR, PMR, Mass Spec.
Organism: *Asterina pectinifera* Müller et Troschel (Echinodermata)
Location: Fukuoka, Japan
Reference: 247

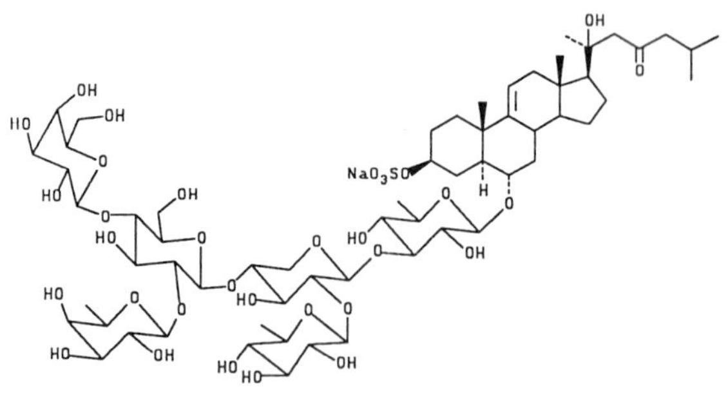

$C_{63}H_{103}NaO_{32}S$ **Acanthaglycoside F**

Mol. Wt.: 1428
Bioactivity: Sea urchin assay: ED_{50} 5 μg/ml; LD_{99} 2 μg/ml;
Starfish assay: ED_{50} 100 μg/ml
Hemolytic activity
Melting Point: 223–228°C (dec.)
$[\alpha]_D$" +11.3 Solvent: Aq
Spectral Data: CD, IR, CMR, Mass Spec.
Organism: *Acanthaster planci* (Echinodermata)
Location: Okinawa, Japan
Reference: 331, 434, 478

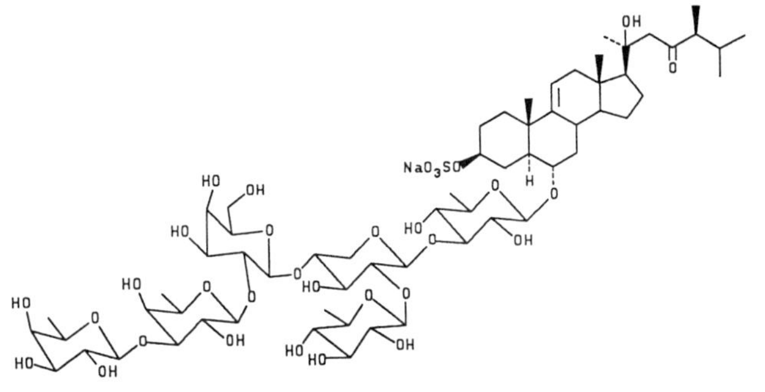

$C_{63}H_{103}NaO_{33}S$ **Pectinioside B**

Mol. Wt.: 1444
Melting Point: >300°C (dec.)
$[\alpha]_D$: +5.5 Solvent: Aq
Spectral Data: IR, CMR, Mass Spec.
Organism: *Asterina pectinifera* Müller et Troschel (Echinodermata)
Location: Fukuoka, Japan
Reference: 822

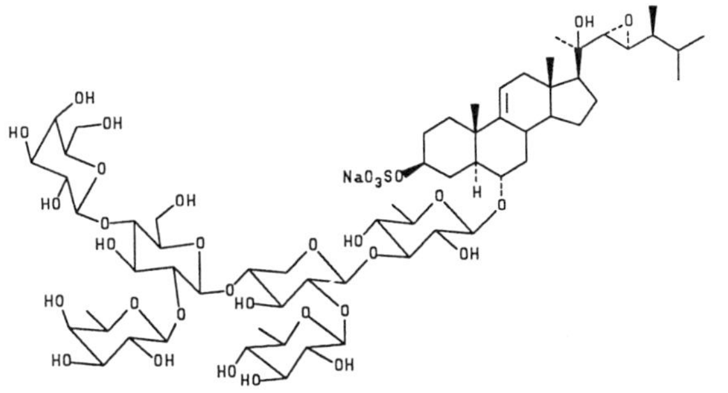

$C_{63}H_{103}NaO_{33}S$	**Versicoside B**
Mol. Wt.:	1444
Bioactivity:	Sea urchin assay: ED_{50} 10 μg/ml; LD_{99} 5 μg/ml; Starfish assay: ED_{50} 200 μg/ml; Hemolytic activity
Melting Point:	206.5–208.0°C
$[\alpha]_D$:	+8.4 Solvent: Aq
Spectral Data:	CD, IR, CMR, Mass Spec.
Organism:	*Asterias amurensis* [cf.] *versicolor* Sladen (Echinodermata)
Location:	Nagasaki, Japan
Reference:	331, 434, 477

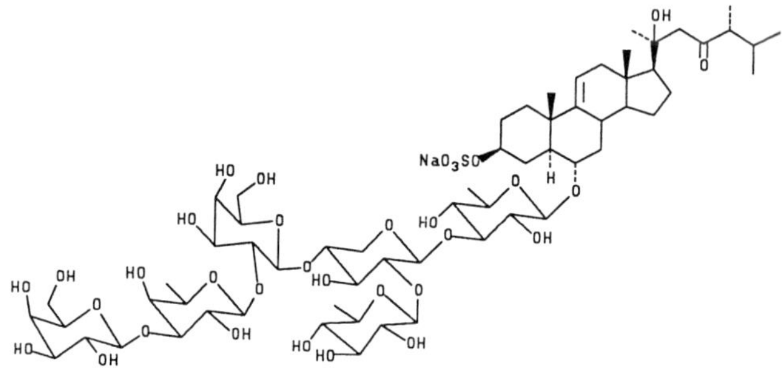

Chapter 16 FURANS, PYRANS, AND POLYETHERS

$C_7H_8O_4$ **2-Oxo-2,5-dihydrofuran-5-acetic acid methyl ester**

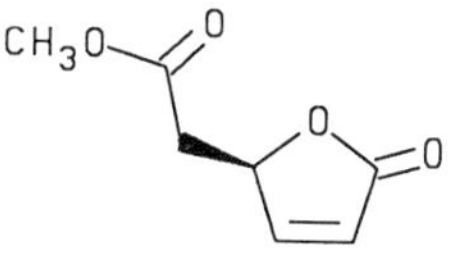

Mol. Wt.: 156
Melting Point: Oil
$[\alpha]_D^{20}$: +80.3 Solvent: Chf
Spectral Data: UV, CD, IR, CMR, PMR, Mass Spec.
Organism: *Xestospongia* sp. (Porifera)
Location: Fiji
Reference: 910

$C_9H_{14}O_5$ **Bissetone**

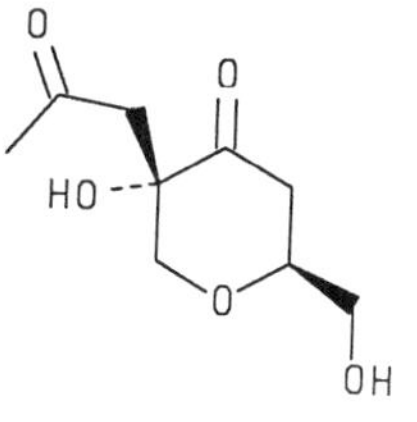

Mol. Wt.: 202
Bioactivity: Antimicrobial activity (gram-negative bacteria)
Melting Point: Oil
$[\alpha]_D$: -43.6 Solvent: Alc
Spectral Data: IR, CMR, PMR, Mass Spec., x-ray c.s.
Organism: *Briareum polyanthes* (Coelenterata)
Location: Bermuda
Reference: 147

$C_{11}H_{12}O_4$ **Didemnenone A**
Didemnenone B
(mixture)

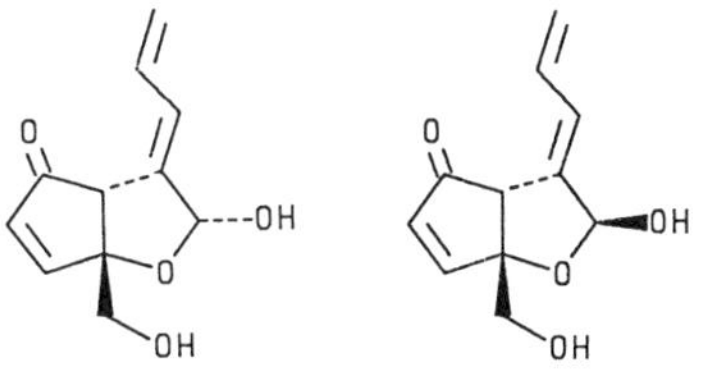

Didemnenone A Didemnenone B

Mol. Wt.: 208
Bioactivity: Antibacterial and antifungal activity
$[\alpha]_D$: +576.1 Solvent: DMSO
Spectral Data: UV, IR, CMR, PMR, Mass Spec.
Organism: *Trididemnum* cf. *cyanophorum* (Chordata/Tunicata)
Location: Bahamas
Reference: 661

$C_{15}H_{18}O$ **Tubipofuran**

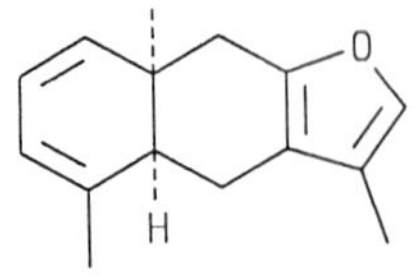

Mol. Wt.: 214
Bioactivity: Ichthyotoxic at 15 μg/ml
Melting Point: Oil
$[\alpha]_D$: +5.7 Solvent: Chf
Spectral Data: UV, CD, IR, CMR, PMR, Mass Spec.
Organism: *Tubipora musica* Linnaeus (Coelenterata)
Location: Okinawa, Japan
Reference: 453

$C_{15}H_{20}O$ **8,9-Z-Dehydrodendrolasin**

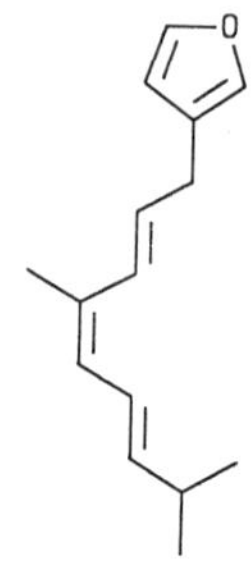

Mol. Wt.: 216
Melting Point: Oil
Spectral Data: CMR, PMR, Mass Spec.
Organism: *Ceratosoma brevicaudatum* (Mollusca)
Location: Adelaide, Australia
Reference: 616

$C_{15}H_{20}OS$ **Thiofurodysinin**

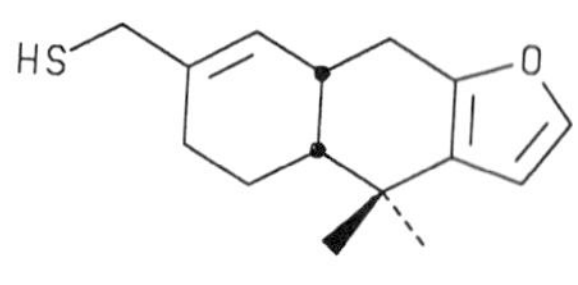

Mol. Wt.: 248
$[\alpha]_D$: +49.3 Solvent: Chf
Spectral Data: CMR, PMR, Mass Spec.
Organism: *Dysidea avara* Schmidt (Porifera)
Location: New South Wales, Australia
Reference: 143

$C_{15}H_{20}O_2$ **Pallescensone**

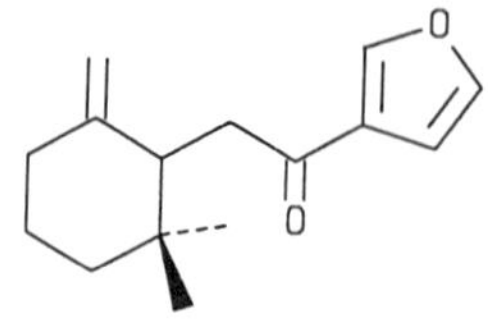

Mol. Wt.: 232
Melting Point: 42.5-43°C
$[\alpha]_D^{20}$: +36 Solvent: Chf
Spectral Data: UV, IR, CMR, PMR, Mass Spec.
Organism: *Dictyodendrilla cavernosa* Lendenfield (Porifera)
Location: Leigh, New Zealand
Reference: 133

$C_{16}H_{22}OS$ **(Methylthio)furodysinin**

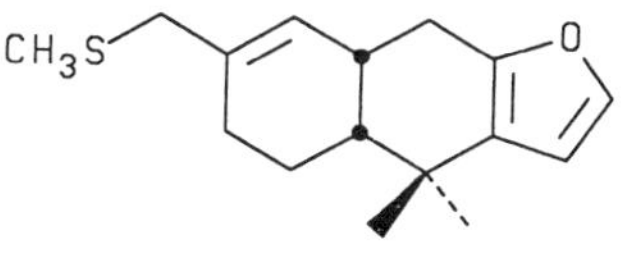

Mol. Wt.: 262
Melting Point: Oil
Spectral Data: CMR, PMR, Mass Spec.
Organism: *Ceratosoma brevicaudatum* (Mollusca)
Location: Adelaide, Australia
Reference: 616

$C_{19}H_{30}O_2$ **Gracilin F**

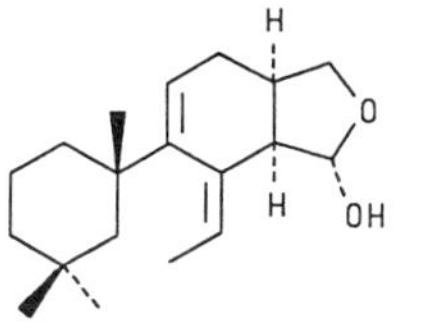

Mol. Wt.: 290
Melting Point: Oil
$[\alpha]_D$: +0.5 Solvent: Chf
Spectral Data: UV, IR, CMR, PMR, Mass Spec.
Organism: *Spongionella gracilis* (Porifera)
Location: Naples, Italy
Reference: 718

$C_{20}H_{24}O_3$ **Kallolide B**

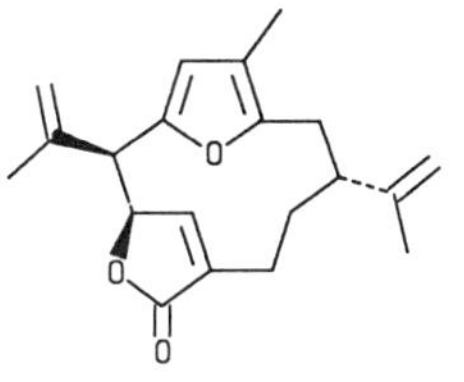

Mol. Wt.: 312
Melting Point: Oil
$[\alpha]_D^{20}$: +123 Solvent: Chf
Spectral Data: UV, IR, CMR, PMR, Mass Spec.
Organism: *Pseudopterogorgia kallos* (Coelenterata)
Location: Bahamas
Reference: 293, 669

$C_{20}H_{24}O_3$ **Rubifolide**

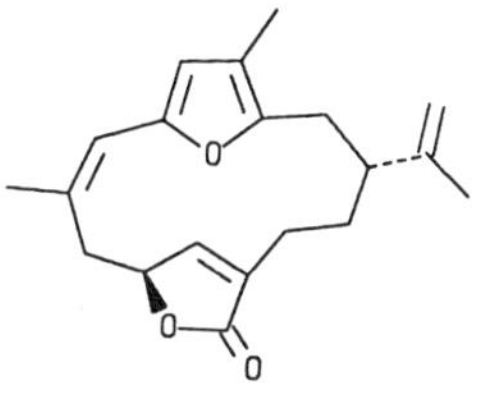

Mol. Wt.: 312
Melting Point: 159-160°C
$[\alpha]_D^{25}$: +31.7 Solvent: Dcm
Spectral Data: UV, IR, CMR, PMR, Mass Spec.
Organism: *Gersemia rubiformis* (Coelenterata)
Tochuina tetraquetra (Mollusca)
Location: British Columbia, Canada
Reference: 1179, 1181

$C_{20}H_{24}O_4$ **Kallolide A**

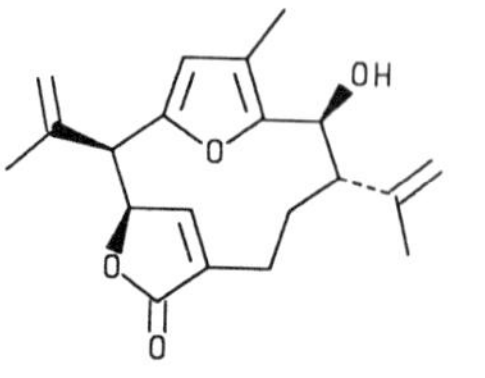

Mol. Wt.: 328
Bioactivity: Antiinflammatory activity
$[\alpha]_D^{20}$: +145 Solvent: Chf
Spectral Data: UV, IR, CMR, PMR, Mass Spec.
Organism: *Pseudopterogorgia kallos* (Coelenterata)
Location: Bahamas
Reference: 293, 669

$C_{20}H_{24}O_6$ **Kallolide C**

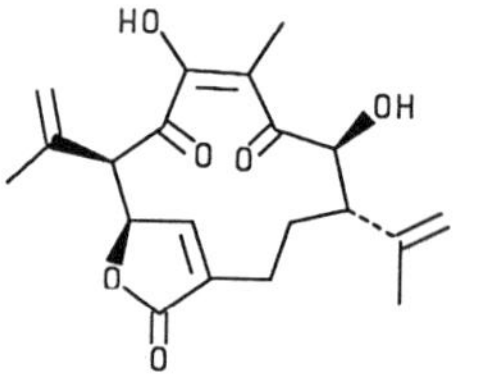

Mol. Wt.: 360
$[\alpha]_D^{20}$: -14 Solvent: Chf
Spectral Data: UV, IR, CMR, PMR, Mass Spec.
Organism: *Pseudopterogorgia kallos* (Coelenterata)
Location: Bahamas
Reference: 293, 669

$C_{20}H_{26}O_5$ **Spongialactone A**

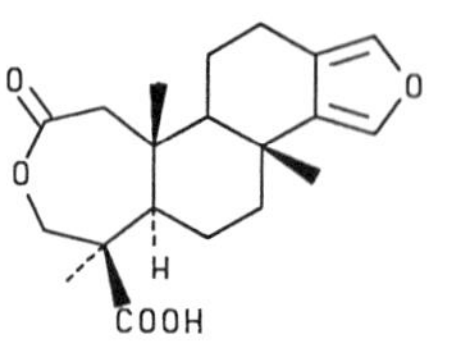

Mol. Wt.: 346
$[\alpha]_D^{25}$: +15 Solvent: Chf
Spectral Data: IR, PMR, CMR, Mass Spec.
Organism: *Spongia arabica* (*S. officinalis* var. *arabica*, Vacelet) (Porifera)
Location: Red Sea
Reference: 426

$C_{20}H_{28}O_3$ **19-Hydroxyspongia-13(16),14-dien-3-one**

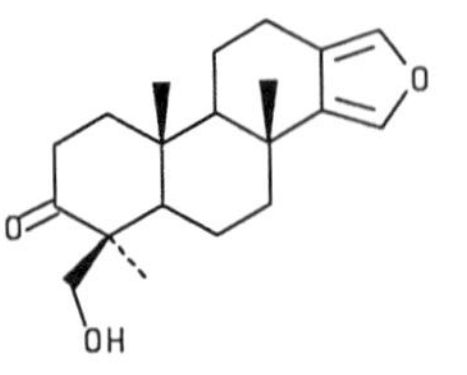

Mol. Wt.: 316
Melting Point: 143-144°C
$[\alpha]_D^{21}$: +18.8 Solvent: Chf
Spectral Data: UV, IR, CMR, PMR, Mass Spec.
Organism: *Hyatella intestinalis* (Lamarck) (Porifera)
Location: Darwin, Australia
Reference: 135

$C_{20}H_{28}O_3$ **Marginatafuran**

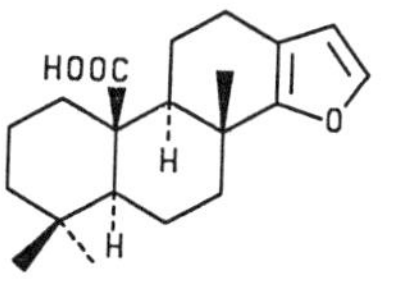

Mol. Wt.: 316
Melting Point: 208°C
$[\alpha]_D$: -102 Solvent: Chf
Spectral Data: IR, PMR, Mass Spec., x-ray c.s.
Organism: *Cadlina luteomarginata* (Mollusca)
Location: British Columbia, Canada
Reference: 380

$C_{20}H_{28}O_4$ **2α,19-Dihydroxyspongian-13(16),-14-dien-3-one**

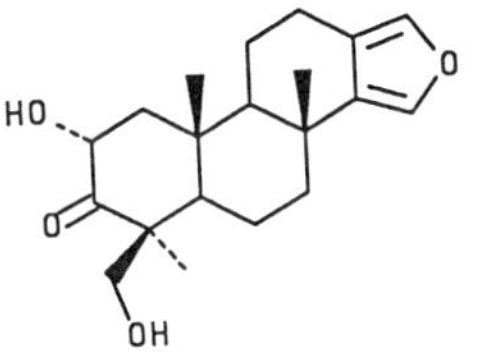

Mol. Wt.: 332
Melting Point: 180-182°C
$[\alpha]_D$: -48 Solvent: Chf
Spectral Data: UV, IR, CMR, PMR, Mass Spec.
Organism: *Hyatella intestinalis* (Lamarck) (Porifera)
Lacation: Darwin, Australia
Reference: 135

$C_{20}H_{30}O$ **Ambliofuran**

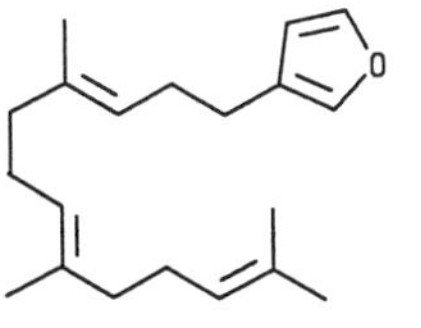

Mol. Wt.: 286
Melting Point: Oil
$[\alpha]_D^{25}$: 0 Solvent: Chf
Spectral Data: UV, IR, CMR, PMR, Mass Spec.
Organism: *Aplysilla* sp.
Aplysilla rosea Barrois
Darwinella sp.
Dendrilla rosea
(Porifera)
Location: Sydney, Australia;
Leigh, New Zealand
Reference: 513, 516, 753, 1149

$C_{20}H_{36}O$ **Hexahydroambliofuran**

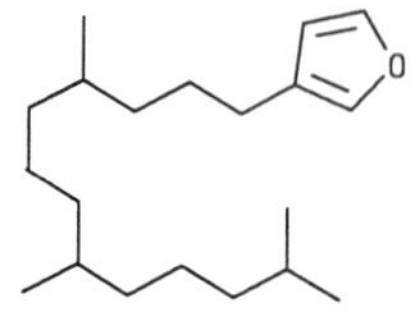

Mol. Wt.: 292
Melting Point: Oil
$[\alpha]_D^{25}$: 0 Solvent: Chf
Spectral Data: PMR, Mass Spec.
Organism: *Aplysilla rosea* Barrois (Porifera)
Location: Sydney, Australia
Reference: 516

$C_{21}H_{22}O_4$ **Kurospongin**

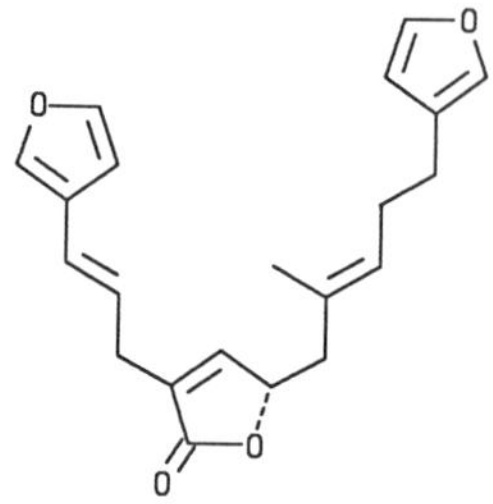

Mol. Wt.: 338
Bioactivity: Ichthyotoxic to goldfish at 5 μg/ml
Antifeedant activity towards *Tilapia mosambica*
Melting Point: Oil
$[\alpha]_D$: -16.8 Solvent: Chf
Spectral Data: UV, IR, CMR, PMR, Mass Spec.
Organism: *Spongia* sp. (Porifera)
Location: Okinawa, Japan
Reference: 1079

$C_{21}H_{26}O_5$ **Macfarlandin A**

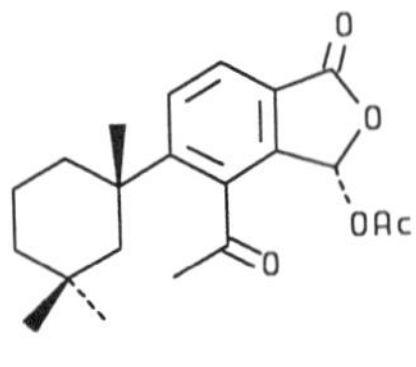

Mol. Wt.: 358
Bioactivity: Growth inhibition of *Bacillus subtilis*
Melting Point: 183-184°C
$[\alpha]_D$: +189 Solvent: Chf
Spectral Data: UV, CD, IR, CMR, PMR, Mass Spec.
Organism: *Chromodoris macfarlandi* (Mollusca)
Location: La Jolla, California
Reference: 754

$C_{21}H_{26}O_5$ **Macfarlandin B**

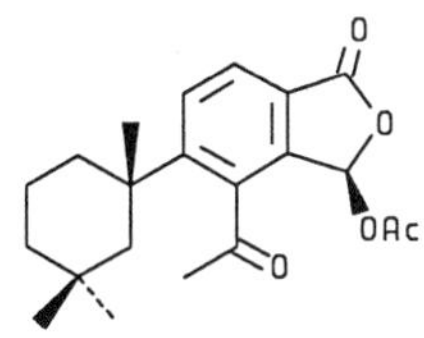

Mol. Wt.: 358
Bioactivity: Growth inhibition of *Bacillus subtilis* and *Staphylococcus aureus*
Melting Point: Glass
$[\alpha]_D$: -128 Solvent: Chf
Spectral Data: UV, CD, IR, CMR, PMR, Mass Spec.
Organism: *Chromodoris macfarlandi* (Mollusca)
Location: La Jolla, California
Reference: 754

$C_{21}H_{28}O_3$ **12,13-Didehydrofurospongin-1**

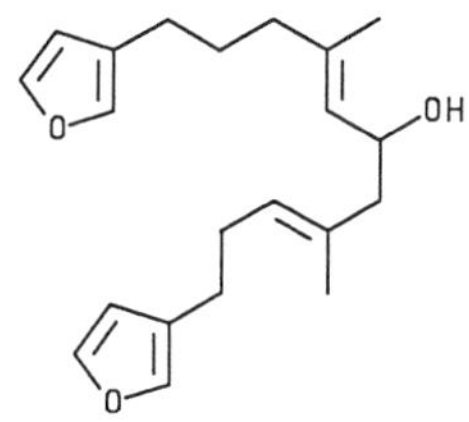

Mol. Wt.: 328
Spectral Data: IR, CMR, PMR, Mass Spec.
Organism: *Carteriospongia flabellifera* (syn. *Phyllospongia flabellifera*) (Porifera)
Location: Great Barrier Reef, Australia
Reference: 983

$C_{21}H_{30}O_5$ **Spongionellin**

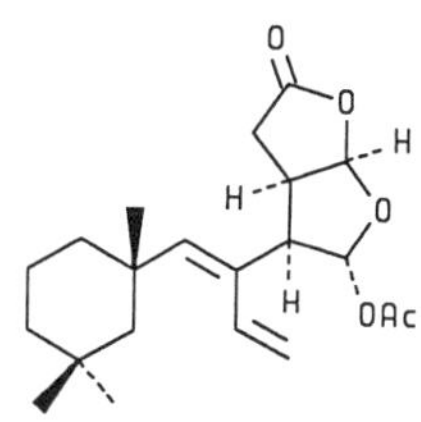

Mol. Wt.: 362
$[\alpha]_D$: +1.2 Solvent: Chf
Spectral Data: UV, IR, CMR, PMR, Mass Spec.
Organism: *Spongionella gracilis* (Porifera)
Location: Naples, Italy
Reference: 718

$C_{21}H_{32}O_3$ **Gracilin E**

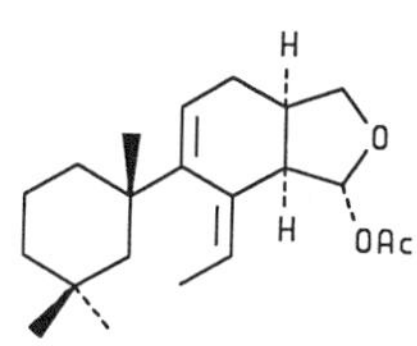

Mol. Wt.: 332
$[\alpha]_D$: -55.6 Solvent: Chf
Spectral Data: UV, IR, CMR, PMR, Mass Spec.
Organism: *Spongionella gracilis* (Porifera)
Location: Naples, Italy
Reference: 718

$C_{22}H_{26}O_5$ **Kallolide A acetate**

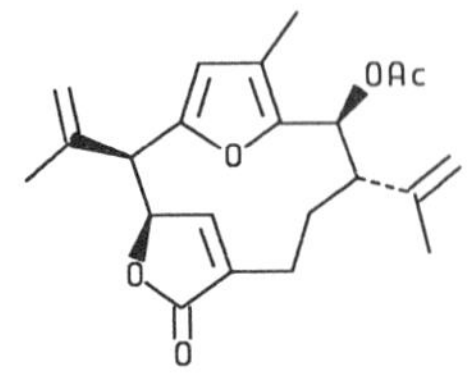

Mol. Wt.: 370
Melting Point: 198-199.5°C
$[\alpha]_D^{20}$: +55 Solvent: Chf
Spectral Data: UV, IR, CMR, PMR, Mass Spec., x-ray c.s.
Organism: *Pseudopterogorgia kallos* (Coelenterata)
Location: Bahamas
Reference: 669

$C_{22}H_{28}O_4$ **Verecynarmin A**

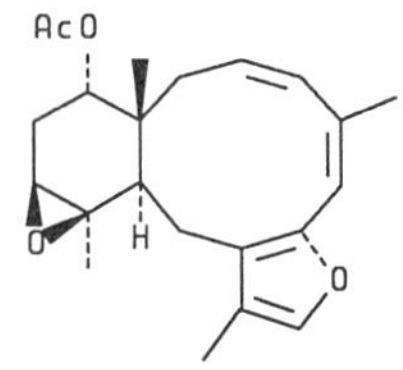

Mol. Wt.: 356
Melting Point: 127-135°C
$[\alpha]_D^{20}$: -255.7 Solvent: Alc
Spectral Data: UV, IR, CMR, PMR, Mass Spec.
Organism: *Armina maculata* Rafinesque (Mollusca)
Veretillum cynomorium Pallas (Coelenterata)
Location: Northeast Mediterranean
Reference: 374

$C_{22}H_{28}O_8$ **Gracilin C**

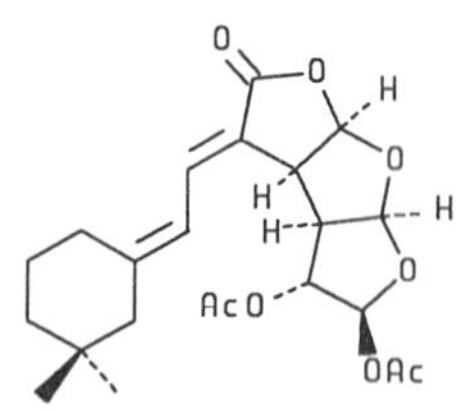

Mol. Wt.: 420
Melting Point: 240-241°C
$[\alpha]_D^{25}$: +273.3 Solvent: Chf
Spectral Data: UV, IR, CMR, PMR, Mass Spec.
Organism: *Spongionella gracilis* Vosmaer (Porifera)
Location: Naples, Italy
Reference: 717

$C_{22}H_{30}O_5$ **3β-Acetoxy-19-hydroxy-spongia-13(16),14-dien-2-one**

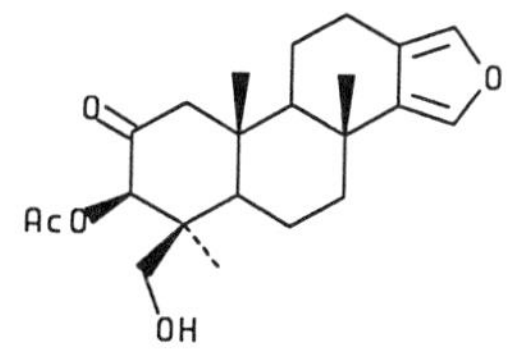

Mol. Wt.: 374
Melting Point: 216-218°C
$[\alpha]_D$: +34.0 Solvent: Chf
Spectral Data: UV, IR, CMR, PMR, Mass Spec.
Organism: *Hyatella intestinalis* (Lamarck) (Porifera)
Location: Darwin, Australia
Reference: 135

$C_{22}H_{32}O_5$ **Aplyviolene**

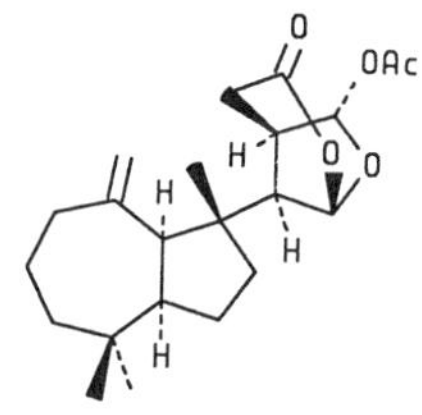

Mol. Wt.: 376
Melting Point: 163°C
$[\alpha]_D^{25}$: -29.5
Spectral Data: IR, CMR, PMR, x-ray c.s.
Organism: *Chelonaplysilla violacea* (Porifera)
Location: Eastern Australia
Reference: 391

$C_{22}H_{32}O_5$ **Macfarlandin C**

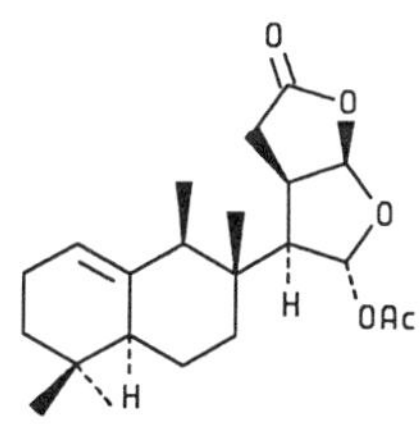

Mol. Wt.: 376
Melting Point: 195-196°C
$[\alpha]_D^{26}$: -29.1 Solvent: Chf
Spectral Data: IR, CMR, PMR, Mass Spec., x-ray c.s.
Organism: *Chromodoris macfarlandi* (Mollusca)
Location: La Jolla, California
Reference: 757

$C_{22}H_{32}O_5$ **Macfarlandin D**

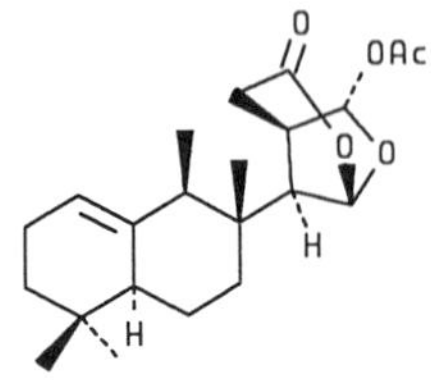

Mol. Wt.: 376
Bioactivity: Antimicrobial activity against *Bacillus subtilis*
Melting Point: 190-191°C
$[\alpha]_D^{26}$: -169 Solvent: Chf
Spectral Data: IR, CMR, PMR, Mass Spec.
Organism: *Chromodoris macfarlandi* (Mollusca)
Location: La Jolla, California
Reference: 757

$C_{23}H_{30}O_8$ **Gracilin D**

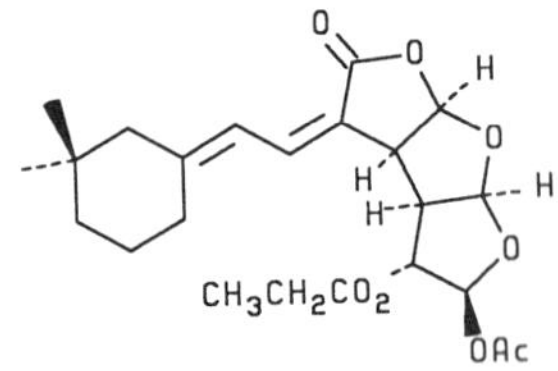

Mol. Wt.: 434
Melting Point: Oil
$[\alpha]_D^{25}$: +130.10 Solvent: Chf
Spectral Data: UV, IR, CMR, PMR, Mass Spec.
Organism: *Spongionella gracilis* Vosmaer (Porifera)
Location: Naples, Italy
Reference: 717

$C_{23}H_{36}O_5$ **9,11-Dihydrogracilin A**

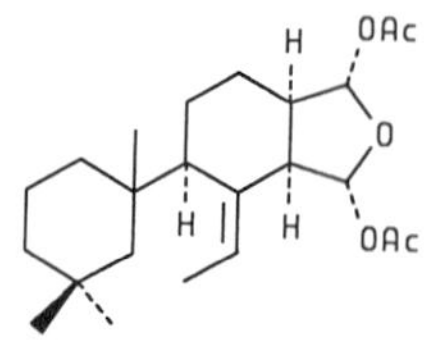

Mol. Wt.: 392
Bioactivity: Antibacterial activity *Bacillus subtilis:* growth inhibition at 100 μg/disk
Melting Point: Oil
$[\alpha]_D$: -11 Solvent: Chf
Spectral Data: IR, CMR, PMR, Mass Spec.
Organism: *Dendrilla membranosa* (Porifera)
Location: McMurdo Sound, Antarctica
Reference: 755

$C_{23}H_{38}O_5$ **Muamvatin**

Mol. Wt.: 394
Melting Point: Oil
$[\alpha]_D^{25}$: +61.1 Solvent: Dcm
Spectral Data: UV, IR, CMR, PMR, Mass Spec.
Organism: *Siphonaria normalis* (Mollusca)
Location: Muamvatu, Fiji
Reference: 942

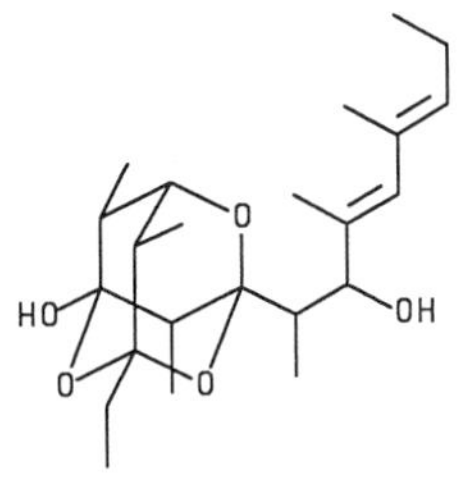

$C_{24}H_{34}O_7$ **Aplyviolacene**
(Macfarlandin E)
(previously known)

Mol. Wt.: 434
Bioactivity: Antimicrobial activity against *Vibrio anguillarum* and *Beneckea harveyi*
Melting Point: Glass
$[\alpha]_D$: -34 Solvent: Chf
Spectral Data: IR, CMR, PMR, Mass Spec.
Organism: *Chromodoris macfarlandi* (Mollusca)
Dysidea sp.
Chelonaplysilla violacea (Porifera)
Location: La Jolla, California; Red Sea; Eastern Australia
Reference: 150, 391, 431, 757

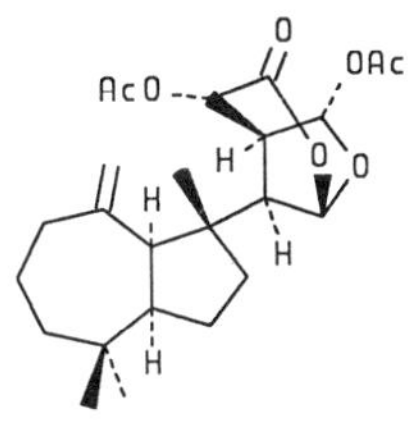

$C_{25}H_{32}O_4$ **Hippospongin**

Mol. Wt.: 396
Bioactivity: Antibacterial activity against *Bacillus subtilis*
Antispasmodic activity
Melting Point: Oil
$[\alpha]_D^{25}$: +15 Solvent: Chf
Spectral Data: UV, IR, CMR, PMR, Mass Spec.
Organism: *Hippospongia* sp. (Porifera)
Location: Okinawa, Japan
Reference: 584

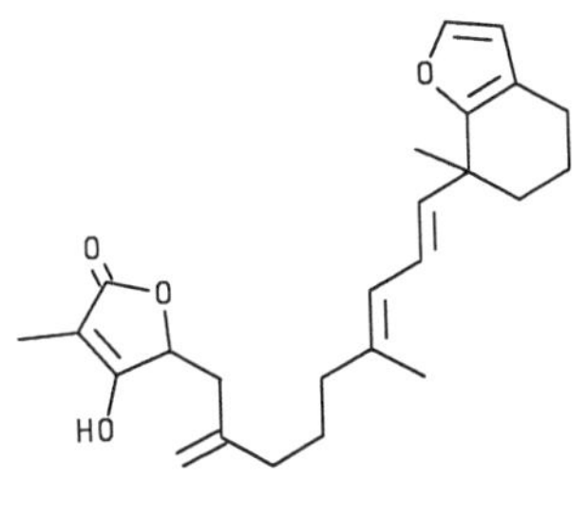

$C_{25}H_{32}O_4$ **Okinonellin A**

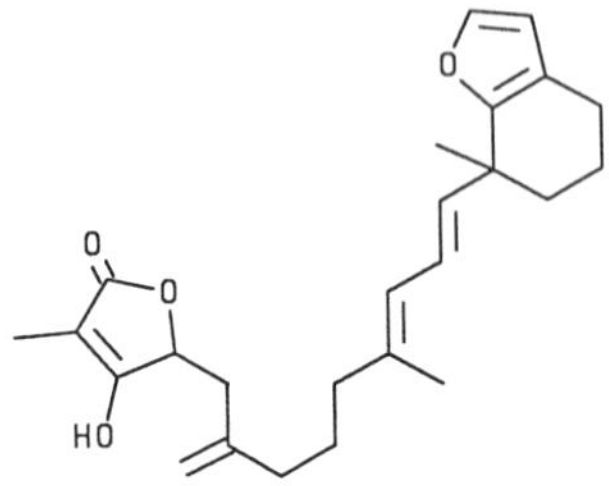

Mol. Wt.:	396
Bioactivity:	Fertilized starfish egg assay: activity at 5 μg/ml
Melting Point:	Oil
$[\alpha]_D^{20}$:	+42.5 Solvent: Alc
Spectral Data:	UV, IR, CMR, PMR, Mass Spec.
Organism:	*Spongionella* sp. (Porifera)
Location:	Japan
Reference:	524

$C_{25}H_{34}O_4$ **7E,12E,20E-Variabilin**

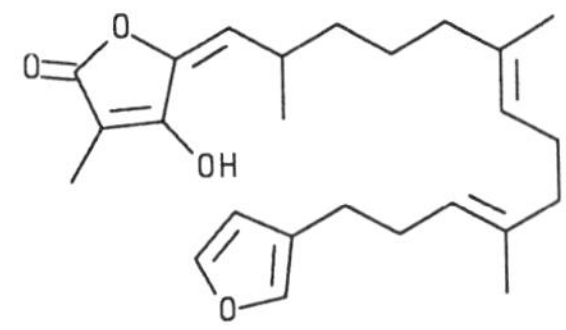

Mol. Wt.:	398
Bioactivity:	Cytotoxicity
Spectral Data:	UV, IR, CMR, PMR, Mass Spec.
Organism:	*Sarcotragus* sp. (Porifera)
Location:	New Zealand
Reference:	51

$C_{25}H_{34}O_4$ **7E,13Z,20Z-Variabilin**

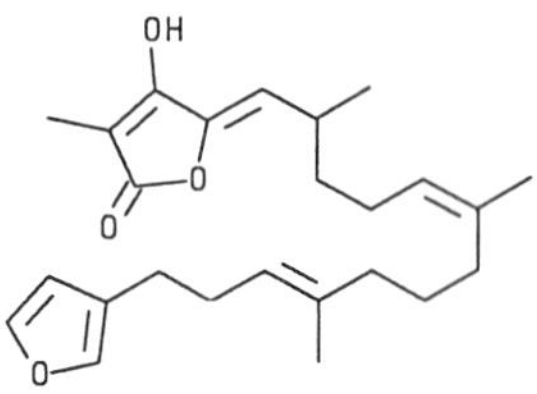

Mol. Wt.:	398
Bioactivity:	Cytotoxicity
Melting Point:	Oil
$[\alpha]_D$:	-4.4 Solvent: Chf
Spectral Data:	UV, IR, CMR, PMR, Mass Spec.
Organism:	*Sarcotragus* sp. (Porifera)
Location:	New Zealand
Reference:	51

$C_{25}H_{34}O_5$

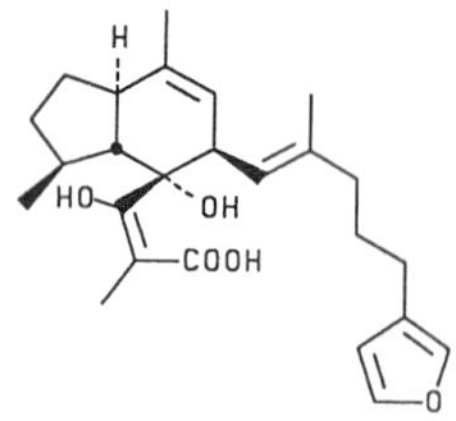

Mol. Wt.:	414
Bioactivity:	Antimicrobial activity; Coronary vasodilative activity (ED_{50} 11 μg/heart)
Organism:	*Ircinia wistarii* (Porifera)
Location:	Queensland, Australia
Reference:	270

$C_{25}H_{36}O_4$ **Cacospongionolide**

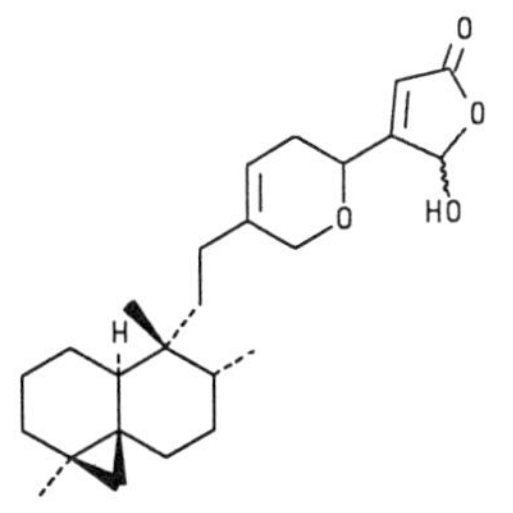

Mol. Wt.: 400
Bioactivity: Cytotoxicity in brine shrimp assay: LD_{50} 0.1 μg/ml
Ichthyotoxic at 1 ppm
75% Inhibition in crown-gall potato disc assay
Melting Point: 163-165°C
$[\alpha]_D$: +27 Solvent: Chf
Spectral Data: UV, IR, CMR, PMR, Mass Spec.
Organism: *Cacospongia mollior* (Porifera)
Location: Adriatic Sea
Reference: 235

$C_{25}H_{36}O_4$ **5-[13-(Furan-3-yl)-2,6,10-trimethyltrideca-6,8-dienyl]-4-hydroxy-3-methylfuran-2(5H)-one**

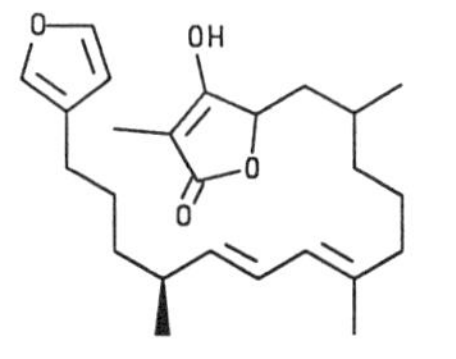

Mol. Wt.: 400
Bioactivity: Antimicrobial: inhibits growth of *Bacillus subtilis*
Melting Point: Oil
$[\alpha]_D$: +41 Solvent: Chf
Spectral Data: IR, CMR, PMR, Mass Spec.
Organism: *Ircinia* sp. (Porifera)
Location: New South Wales, Australia
Reference: 144

$C_{25}H_{36}O_4$ **Okinonellin B**

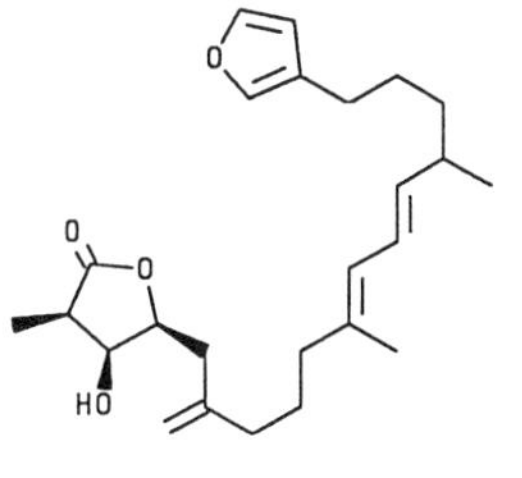

Mol. Wt.: 400
Bioactivity: Fertilized starfish egg assay: activity at 5 μg/ml
$[\alpha]_D^{20}$: +17.9 Solvent: Alc
Spectral Data: UV, IR, CMR, PMR, Mass Spec.
Organism: *Spongionella* sp. (Porifera)
Location: Japan
Reference: 524

$C_{25}H_{36}O_5$ **8-Hydroxy-12E,20Z-variabilin**

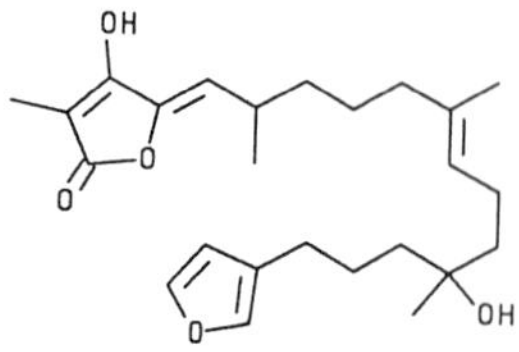

Mol. Wt.: 416
Bioactivity: Cytotoxicity
Melting Point: Oil
$[\alpha]_D$: -24.5 Solvent: Me
Spectral Data: UV, IR, CMR, PMR, Mass Spec.
Organism: *Sarcotragus* sp. (Porifera)
Location: New Zealand
Reference: 51

$C_{25}H_{36}O_5$ **Luffariellin A**

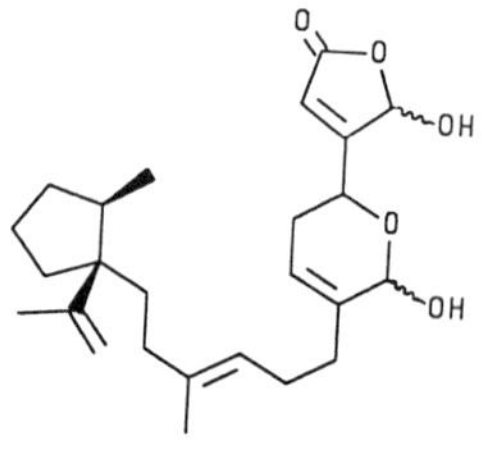

Mol. Wt.: 416
Bioactivity: Antiinflammatory activity
Melting Point: Oil
$[\alpha]_D$: +40.1 Solvent: Chf
Spectral Data: UV, IR, CMR, PMR, Mass Spec.
Organism: *Luffariella variabilis* (Porifera)
Location: Palau
Reference: 547

$C_{25}H_{36}O_5$ **Luffariellin B**

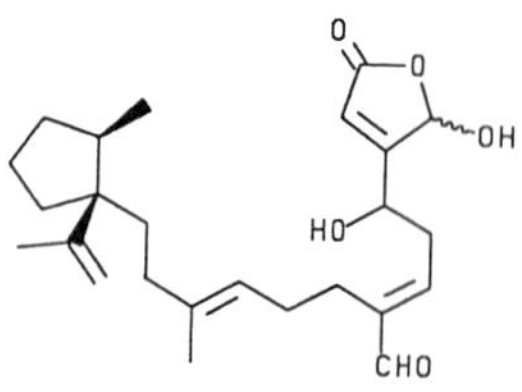

Mol. Wt.: 416
Bioactivity: Antiinflammatory activity
Melting Point: Oil
$[\alpha]_D$: -5.5 Solvent: Chf
Spectral Data: UV, IR, CMR, PMR, Mass Spec.
Organism: *Luffariella variabilis* (Porifera)
Location: Palau
Reference: 547

$C_{25}H_{39}NaO_5S$ **Halisulfate 2**

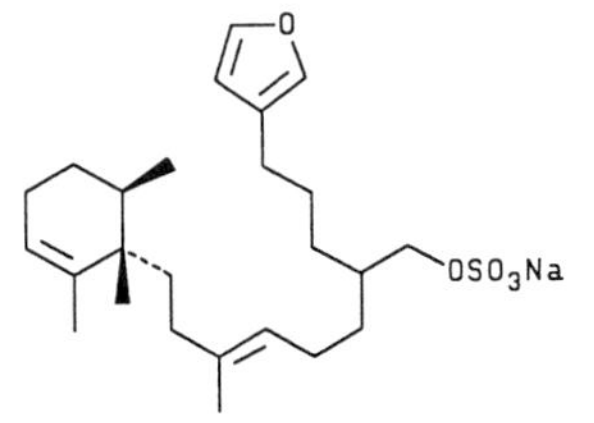

Mol. Wt.: 474
Bioactivity: Antiinflammatory and antimicrobial activities assayed in mixtures
Spectral Data: IR, CMR, PMR; IR, CMR, PMR, Mass Spec. of corresponding alcohol
Organism: *Halichondriidae* sp. (Porifera)
Location: La Jolla, California
Reference: 546

$C_{25}H_{39}NaO_5S$ **Halisulfates 3 and 4**

Mol. Wt.: 474
Bioactivity: Antiinflammatory activity (mixture of halisulfates 2, 3 and 4)
Antimicrobial activity (mixtures of halisulfates 2, 3, 4 and 5)
Spectral Data: IR, CMR, PMR of mixture;
IR, CMR, PMR, Mass Spec. of both corresponding alcohols
Organism: *Halichondriidae* sp. (Porifera)
Location: La Jolla, California
Reference: 546

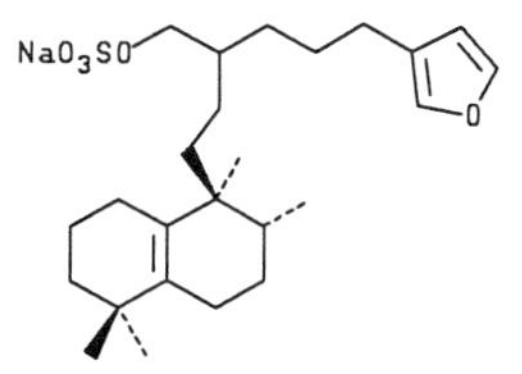

Halisulfate 3

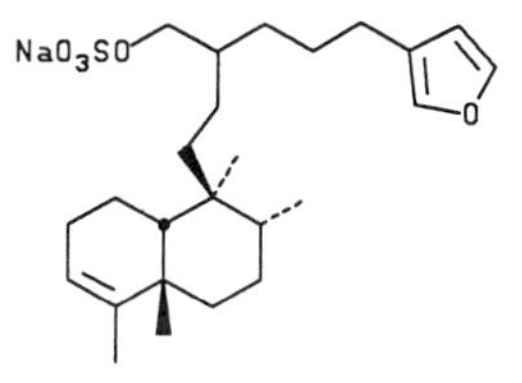

Halisulfate 4

$C_{25}H_{39}NaO_5S$ **Halisulfates 5 and 6**

Mol. Wt.: 474
Bioactivity: Antimicrobial activity (halisulfate 5 - assayed as part of mixtures)
Spectral Data: IR, CMR, PMR of mixture; IR, CMR, PMR, Mass Spec. of halisulfate 5's corresponding alcohol
Organism: *Halichondriidae* sp. (Porifera)
Location: La Jolla, California
Reference: 546

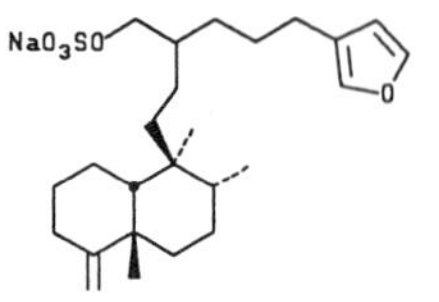

Halisulfate 5

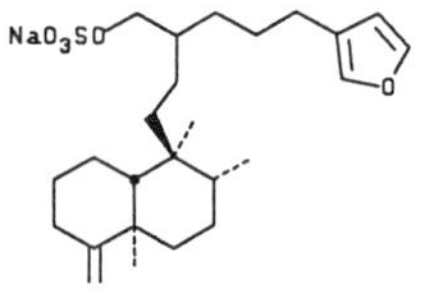

Halisulfate 6

$C_{30}H_{38}O_2S_2$ **Dithiofurodysinin disulfide**

Mol. Wt.: 494
Melting Point: Oil
Spectral Data: CMR, PMR, Mass Spec.
Organism: *Ceratosoma brevicaudatum* (Mollusca)
Location: Adelaide, Australia
Reference: 616

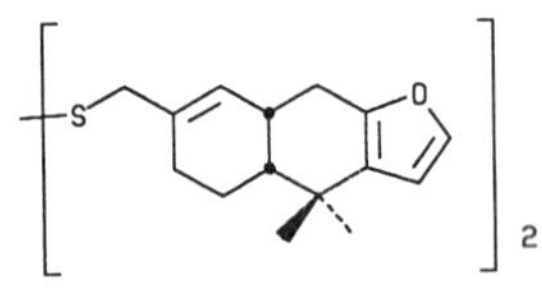

$C_{30}H_{42}O_7$ **Isolaulimalide**

Mol. Wt.: 514
Spectral Data: UV, IR, CMR, PMR, Mass Spec.
Organism: *Hyattella* sp. (Porifera)
Chromodoris lochi (Mollusca)
Location: Indonesia
Reference: 199

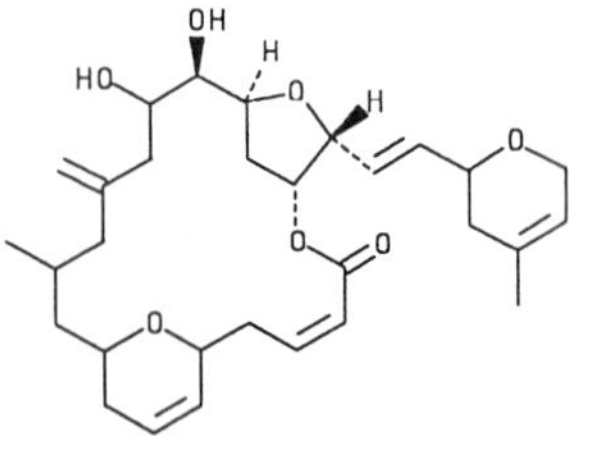

$C_{47}H_{68}O_{15}$ **Pectenotoxin-3 (PTX 3)**

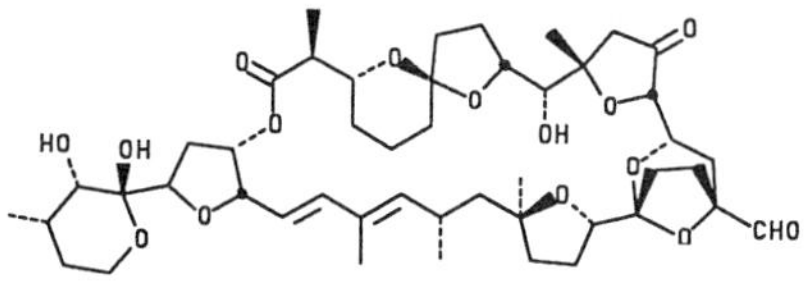

Mol. Wt.: 874
Bioactivity: Toxicity: minimum lethal dose 350 μg/kg of mouse (ip)
Melting Point: 159-160°C
$[\alpha]_D^{20}$: +2.22 Solvent: Me
Spectral Data: UV, IR, CMR, PMR, Mass Spec.
Organism: *Patinopecten yessoensis* (Mollusca)
Location: Aomori, Japan
Reference: 784

$C_{55}H_{80}Na_2O_{21}S_2$ **Yessotoxin (YTX)**

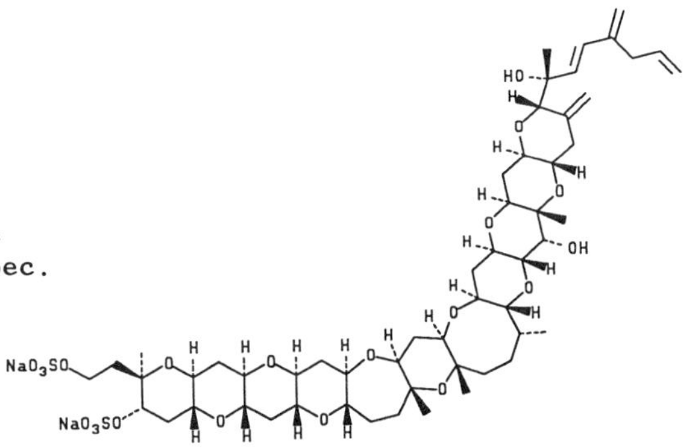

Mol. Wt.: 1188
Bioactivity: Diarrhetic toxin: toxic at 100 μg/kg in mice (i.p.)
$[\alpha]_D^{20}$: +3.01 Solvent: Me
Spectral Data: UV, IR, CMR, PMR, Mass Spec.
Organism: *Patinopecten yessoensis* (Mollusca)
Location: Japan
Reference: 620, 781

$C_{59}H_{82}O_{19}$ **Norhalichondrin B**

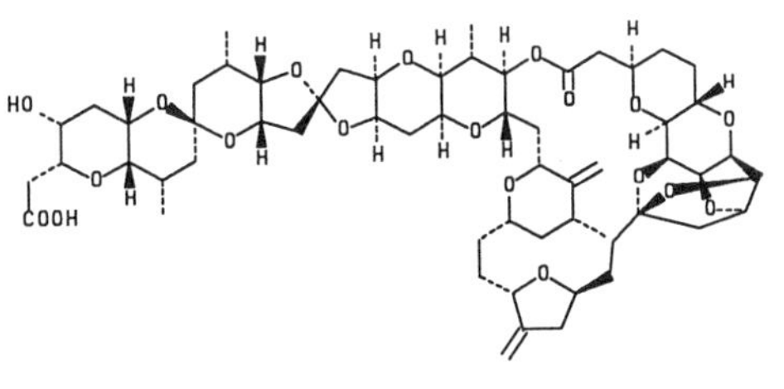

Mol. Wt.: 1096
Spectral Data: CMR, PMR, Mass Spec.
Organism: *Halichondria okadai* (Porifera)
Location: Japan
Reference: 423

$C_{59}H_{82}O_{20}$ **Norhalichondrin C**

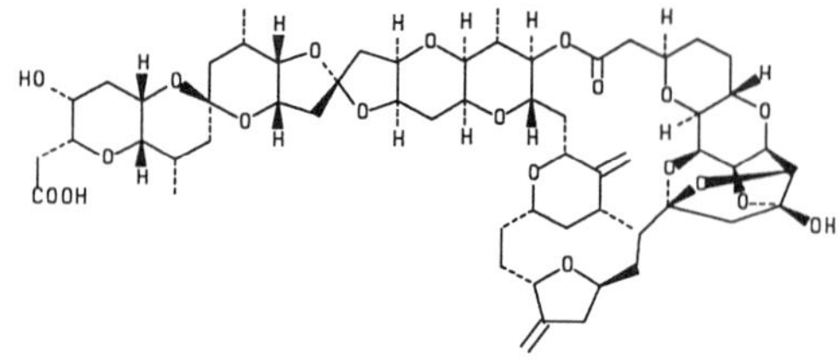

Mol. Wt.: 1112
Spectral Data: PMR, Mass Spec.
Organism: *Halichondria okadai* (Porifera)
Location: Japan
Reference: 423

$C_{61}H_{86}O_{20}$ **Homohalichondrin C**

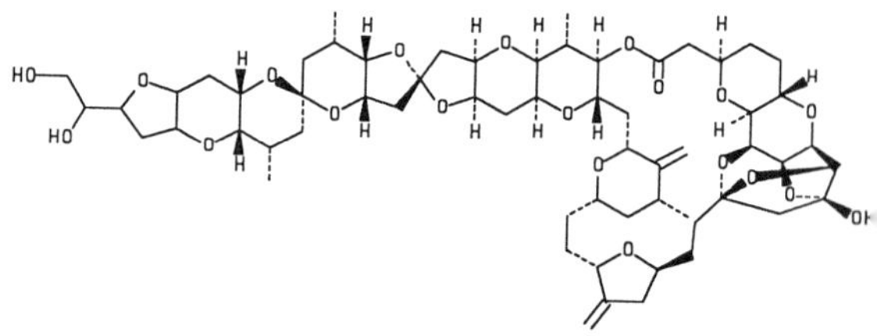

Mol. Wt.: 1140
Spectral Data: PMR, Mass Spec.
Organism: *Halichondria okadai* (Porifera)
Location: Japan
Reference: 423

$C_{61}H_{100}O_{14}$ **7-O-Palmitoyl DTX1**

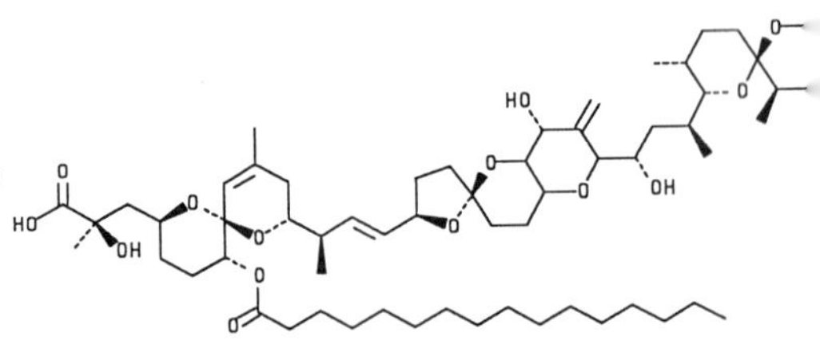

Mol. Wt.: 1058
Bioactivity: Diarrhetic shellfish toxin
Melting Point: 78°C
$[\alpha]_D^{20}$: +5.9 Solvent: $CDCl_3$
Spectral Data: PMR, Mass Spec.
Organism: *Patinopecten* sp. (Mollusca)
Location: Japan
Reference: 783

$C_{73}H_{126}O_{20}$ **Bistheonellide B**

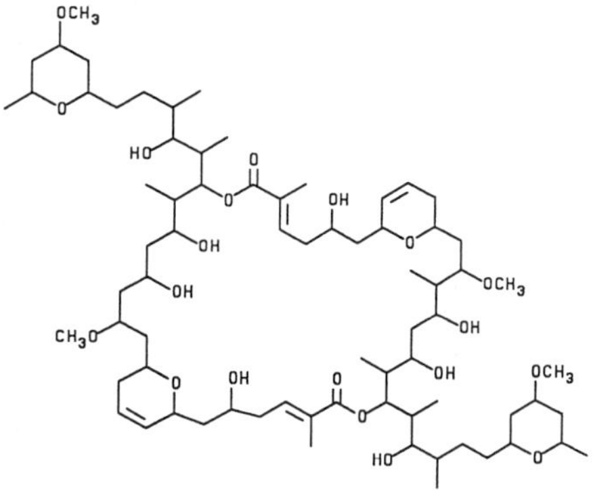

Mol. Wt.: 1324
Bioactivity: Growth inhibition of starfish eggs at 0.2 μg/ml
$[\alpha]_D^{20}$: -30 Solvent: Alc
Spectral Data: UV, IR, CMR, PMR, Mass Spec.
Organism: *Theonella* sp. (Porifera)
Location: Hachijo-jima, Japan
Reference: 528, 529

Chapter 17 PHENOLS, QUINONES, AND RELATED COMPOUNDS

$C_6H_4Br_2O$ **2,4-Dibromophenol**
(previously known)

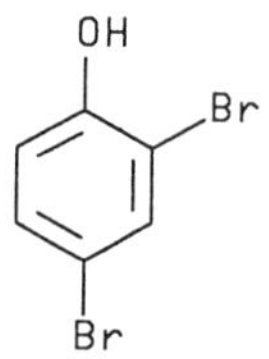

Mol. Wt.: 252
Melting Point: 33.5–34.5°C
Spectral Data: PMR
Organism: *Ptychodera* sp. (Hemichordata)
Location: Maui, Hawaii
Reference: 416, 418

$C_6H_4Br_2O_2$ **2,6-Dibromohydroquinone**
(previously known)

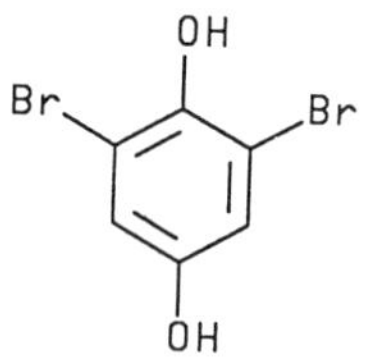

Mol. Wt.: 268
Melting Point: 168–169°C
Spectral Data: PMR
Organism: *Ptychodera* sp. (Hemichordata)
Location: Maui, Hawaii
Reference: 416, 418

$C_6H_4Br_2O_2$ **2,4-Dibromoresorcinol**
(previously known)

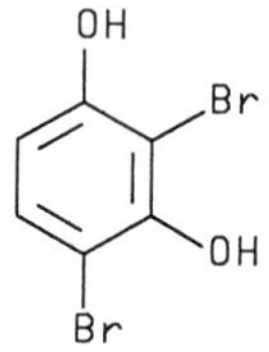

Mol. Wt.: 268
Spectral Data: PMR, Mass Spec.
Organism: *Ptychodera* sp. (Hemichordata)
Location: Maui, Hawaii
Reference: 418, 441

$C_6H_5BrO_3$ **(4S,5R,6R)-2-Bromo-5,6-epoxy-4-hydroxycyclohex-2-enone**

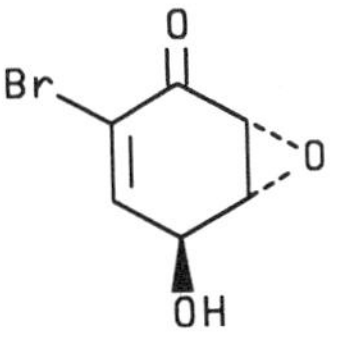

Mol. Wt.: 205
Melting Point: 123–127°C
$[\alpha]_D^{22}$: +220 Solvent: Chf
Spectral Data: PMR
Organism: *Ptychodera* sp. (Hemichordata)
Location: Maui, Hawaii
Reference: 418

$C_7H_7NO_4$ **3-Nitro-4-hydroxybenzyl alcohol**

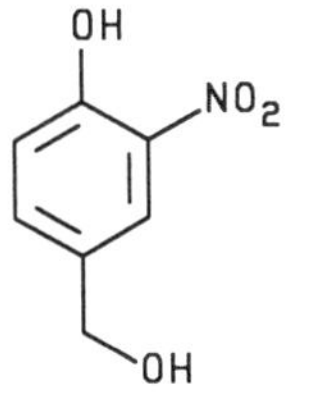

Mol. Wt.: 169
Bioactivity: Antibacterial, antifungal and antialgal activity
Spectral Data: PMR, Mass Spec.
Organism: *Phidolopora pacifica*
Diaperoecia californica
Heteropora alaskensis
Hippodiplosia insculpta
(Bryozoa)
Location: British Columbia, Canada
Reference: 1093

$C_8H_8Br_2O_4$ **(4S,5R,6R)-4-Acetoxy-2,6-dibromo-5-hydroxycyclohex-2-enone**

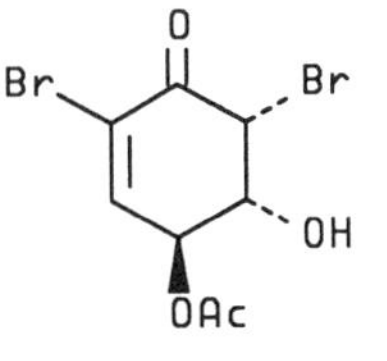

Mol. Wt.: 328
Bioactivity: Antifeedant
$[\alpha]_D^{23}$: +130 Solvent: Dcm
Spectral Data: UV, IR, CMR, PMR, Mass Spec.
Organism: *Ptychodera* sp. (Hemichordata)
Location: Maui, Hawaii
Reference: 418

$C_{10}H_7NO_5$ **4,5,8-Trihydroxyquinoline-2-carboxylic acid**

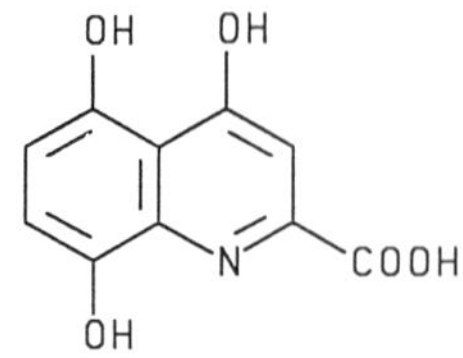

Mol. Wt.: 221
Bioactivity: Antibacterial activity
Melting Point: 295–300°C
Spectral Data: UV, IR, CMR, PMR, Mass Spec.
Organism: *Dendrilla membranosa* (Porifera)
Location: Antarctic
Reference: 756

$C_{12}H_8Br_2O_3$ **Aplysinadiene**

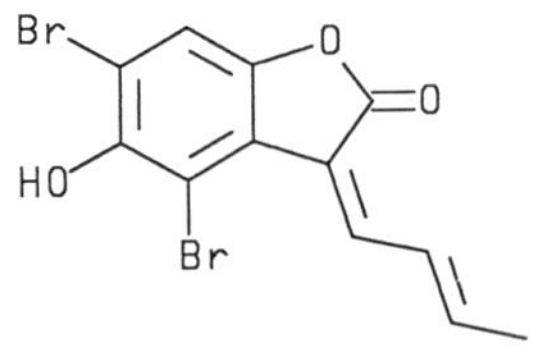

Mol. Wt.: 360
Melting Point: 218–220°C
Spectral Data: UV, IR, CMR, PMR, Mass Spec.
Organism: *Aplysina aerophoba* (Porifera)
Location: Canary Islands
Reference: 827, 828

$C_{15}H_{19}BrO$ **9-((Z)-Bromomethylidene)-1,2,5-trimethylspiro[5.5]undeca-1,7-dien-3-one**

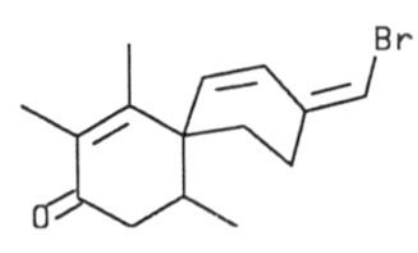

Mol. Wt.: 295
Melting Point: 97–99.5°C
$[\alpha]_D^{20}$: +33.5 Solvent: Chf
Spectral Data: UV, IR, CMR, PMR, Mass Spec.
Organism: *Aplysia dactylomela* (Mollusca)
Location: Okinawa, Japan
Reference: 962

$C_{15}H_{20}BrClO$ **8-Bromo-9-chloro-5,5,9-trimethyl-1-methylidenespiro[5.5]undec-3-en-2-one**

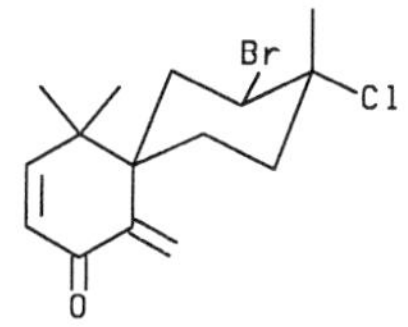

Mol. Wt.: 331
Melting Point: 98–100°C
$[\alpha]_D$: +19.6 Solvent: Chf
Spectral Data: UV, IR, CMR, PMR, Mass Spec., x-ray c.s.
Organism: *Aplysia dactylomela* (Mollusca)
Location: Okinawa, Japan
Reference: 962

$C_{15}H_{20}O$ **8,9-Dehydrocurcuphenol**

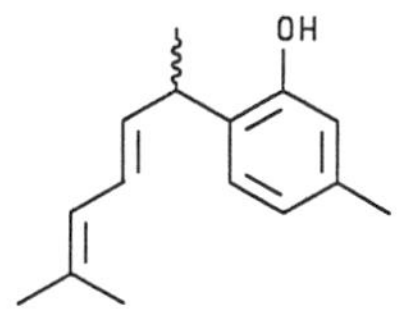

Mol. Wt.: 216
Bioactivity: Inhibition of gastric H,K–ATPase: IC_{50} $2.3x10^{-5}M$
Inhibition of gastric acid secretion
Melting Point: Oil
$[\alpha]_D^{23}$: −1.2 Solvent: Chf
Spectral Data: UV, PMR, Mass Spec.
Organism: *Epipolasis* sp. (Porifera)
Location: Izu Archipelago
Reference: 334

$C_{15}H_{20}O_2$ **7-Hydroxycalamenen-3-one**

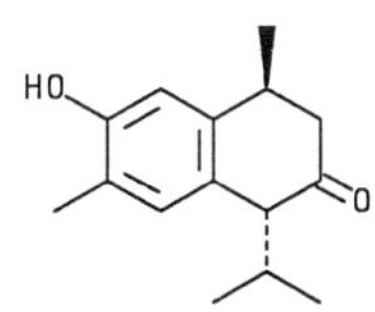

Mol. Wt.: 232
Melting Point: 121–123°C
$[\alpha]_D$: +178.1 Solvent: Chf
Spectral Data: UV, IR, CMR, PMR, Mass Spec.; x-ray c.s. of derivative
Organism: *Lemnalia cervicornis* (Coelenterata)
Location: Great Barrier Reef, Australia
Reference: 99

$C_{15}H_{22}O_2$ **Calamenene-3,7-diol**

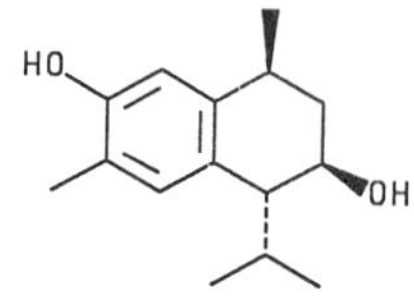

Mol. Wt.:	234
Melting Point:	Oil
$[\alpha]_D$:	+23.3 Solvent: Chf
Spectral Data:	UV, IR, CMR, PMR, Mass Spec.
Organism:	*Lemnalia cervicornis* (Coelenterata)
Location:	Great Barrier Reef, Australia
Reference:	99

$C_{15}H_{22}O_3$ **(4R)-Calamenene-3,4,7-triol**

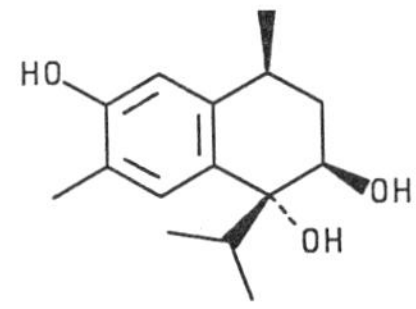

Mol. Wt.:	250
Melting Point:	160–162°C
$[\alpha]_D$:	+21.6 Solvent: Me
Spectral Data:	UV, IR, CMR, PMR, Mass Spec.
Organism:	*Lemnalia cervicornis* (Coelenterata)
Location:	Great Barrier Reef, Australia
Reference:	99

$C_{15}H_{22}O_3$ **(4S)-Calamenene-3,4,7-triol**

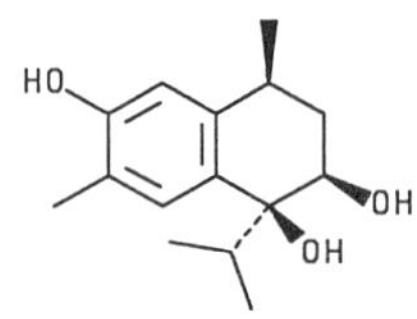

Mol. Wt.:	250
Melting Point:	162–164°C
$[\alpha]_D$:	+89.3 Solvent: Me
Spectral Data:	UV, IR, CMR, PMR, Mass Spec.
Organism:	*Lemnalia cervicornis* (Coelenterata)
Location:	Great Barrier Reef, Australia
Reference:	99

$C_{15}H_{24}O_2$ **(+)-Curcudiol**

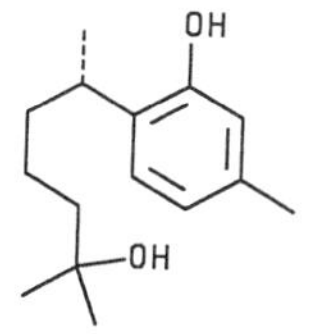

Mol. Wt.: 236
Bioactivity: Antifungal activity against *Candida albicans*
Melting Point: Oil
$[\alpha]_D^{22}$: +9.2 Solvent: Chf
Spectral Data: UV, IR, CMR, PMR, Mass Spec.
Organism: *Didiscus flavus* Van Soest (Porifera)
Location: Bahamas; Belize
Reference: 1189

$C_{16}H_{22}O$ **7-Methoxy-1,2-dihydrocadalene**

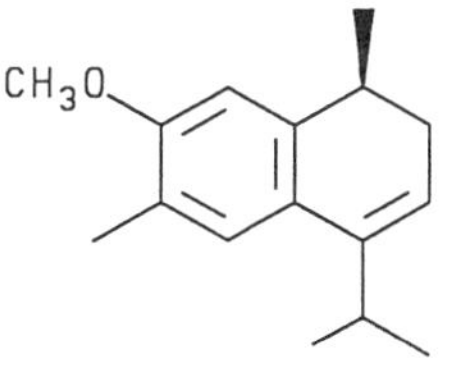

Mol. Wt.: 230
Melting Point: Oil
$[\alpha]_D$: -54.9 Solvent: Chf
Spectral Data: UV, IR, CMR, PMR, Mass Spec.
Organism: *Lemnalia cervicornis* (Coelenterata)
Location: Great Barrier Reef, Australia
Reference: 99

$C_{16}H_{22}O_2$ **7-Methoxycalamenen-3-one**

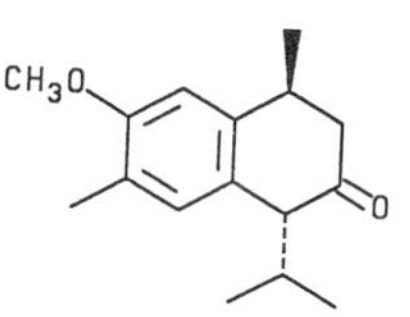

Mol. Wt.: 246
$[\alpha]_D$: +136.6 Solvent: Chf
Spectral Data: UV, IR, CMR, PMR, Mass Spec.
Organism: *Lemnalia cervicornis* (Coelenterata)
Location: Great Barrier Reef, Australia
Reference: 99

$C_{16}H_{24}O_2$ **7-Methoxycalamenen-3-ol**

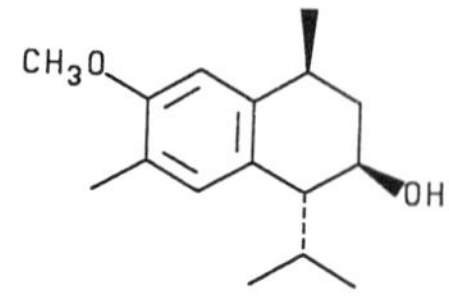

Mol. Wt.:	248
Melting Point:	Oil
$[\alpha]_D$:	+22 Solvent: Chf
Spectral Data:	UV, IR, CMR, PMR, Mass Spec.
Organism:	*Lemnalia cervicornis* (Coelenterata)
Location:	Great Barrier Reef, Australia
Reference:	99

$C_{16}H_{24}O_2$ **(4R)-7-Methoxycalamenen-4-ol**

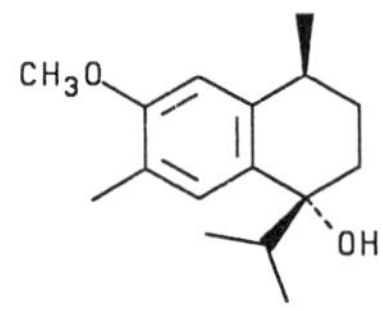

Mol. Wt.:	248
Melting Point:	Oil
$[\alpha]_D$:	−1.2 Solvent: Chf
Spectral Data:	UV, IR, CMR, PMR, Mass Spec.
Organism:	*Lemnalia cervicornis* (Coelenterata)
Location:	Great Barrier Reef, Australia
Reference:	99

$C_{16}H_{24}O_2$ **(4S)-7-Methoxycalamenen-4-ol**

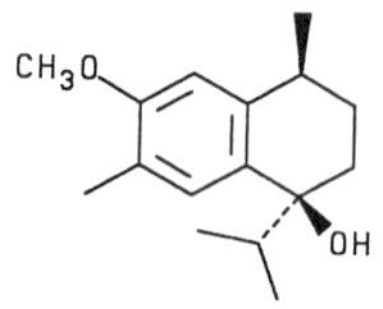

Mol. Wt.:	248
Melting Point:	Oil
$[\alpha]_D$:	+33.5 Solvent: Chf
Spectral Data:	UV, IR, CMR, PMR, Mass Spec.
Organism:	*Lemnalia cervicornis* (Coelenterata)
Location:	Great Barrier Reef, Australia
Reference:	99

$C_{16}H_{28}O_3$ **Maurenone**

Mol. Wt.: 268
Melting Point: Oil
Spectral Data: UV, IR, CMR, PMR, Mass Spec.
Organism: *Siphonaria maura* (Mollusca)
Location: Costa Rica
Reference: 697

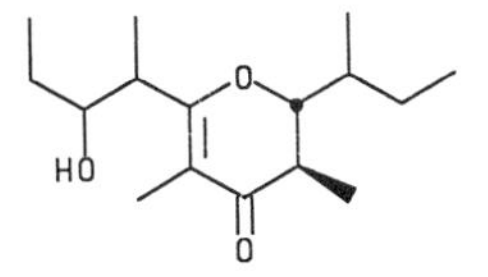

$C_{17}H_{22}BrClO_3$ **4-Bromo-3-chloro-3,7,7-trimethyl-11-methylidene-10-oxospiro[5.5]undec-8-en-1-yl acetate**

Mol. Wt.: 389
Melting Point: 105–106°C
$[\alpha]_D^{20}$: −27.8 Solvent: Chf
Spectral Data: UV, IR, CMR, PMR, Mass Spec.; x-ray c.s. of derivative
Organism: *Aplysia dactylomela* (Mollusca)
Location: Okinawa, Japan
Reference: 962

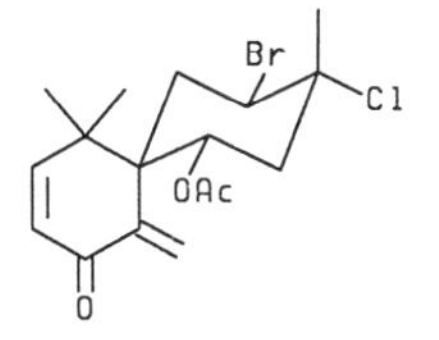

$C_{17}H_{22}O_3$ **7-Acetoxycalamenen-3-one**

Mol. Wt.: 274
Melting Point: Oil
$[\alpha]_D$: +173.6 Solvent: Chf
Spectral Data: UV, IR, CMR, PMR, Mass Spec.
Organism: *Lemnalia cervicornis* (Coelenterata)
Location: Great Barrier Reef, Australia
Reference: 99

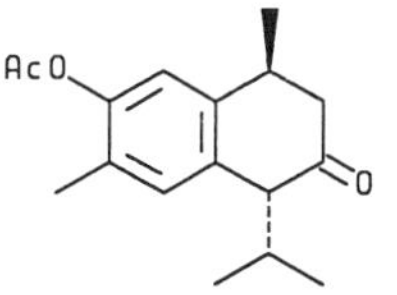

$C_{17}H_{22}O_3$ **Verapliquinone A**

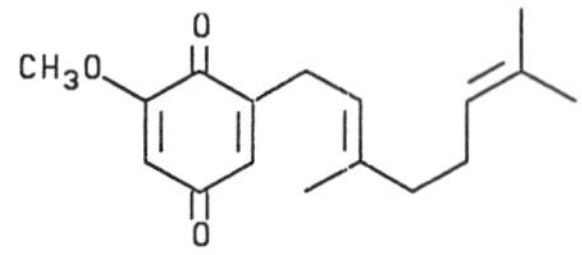

Mol. Wt.: 274
Melting Point: Oil
Spectral Data: UV, IR, CMR, PMR, Mass Spec.
Organism: *Aplidium* sp. (Chordata/Tunicata)
Location: Brittany, France
Reference: 369

$C_{17}H_{22}O_3$ **Verapliquinone B**

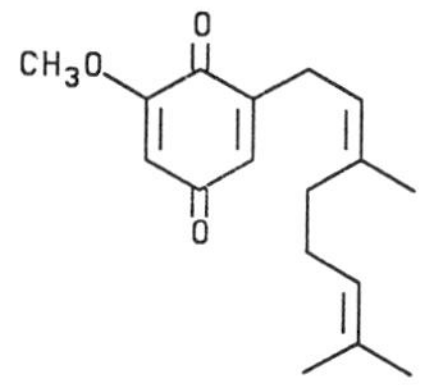

Mol. Wt.: 274
Melting Point: Oil
Spectral Data: UV, IR, CMR, PMR, Mass Spec.
Organism: *Aplidium* sp. (Chordata/Tunicata)
Location: Brittany, France
Reference: 369

$C_{17}H_{24}O_4$ **Verapliquinone C**

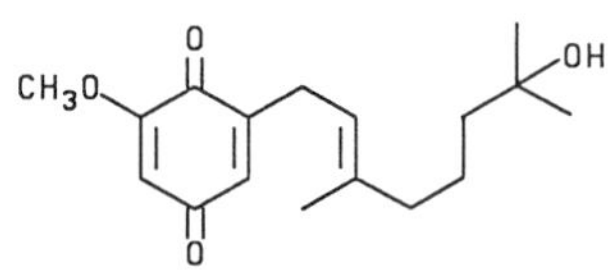

Mol. Wt.: 292
Melting Point: Oil
Spectral Data: UV, IR, CMR, PMR, Mass Spec.
Organism: *Aplidium* sp. (Chordata/Tunicata)
Location: Brittany, France
Reference: 369

$C_{17}H_{24}O_4$ **Verapliquinone D**

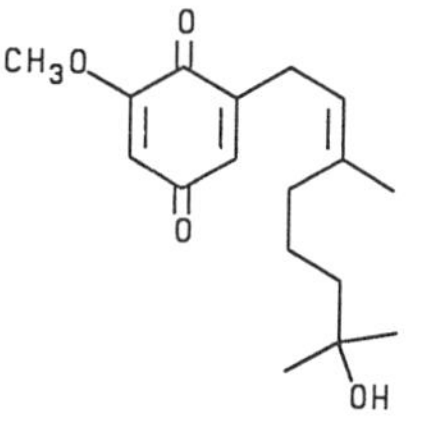

Mol. Wt.: 292
Melting Point: Oil
Spectral Data: UV, IR, CMR, PMR, Mass Spec.
Organism: *Aplidium* sp. (Chordata/Tunicata)
Location: Brittany, France
Reference: 369

$C_{18}H_{26}O_3$ **7-Methoxycalamenen-3-yl acetate**

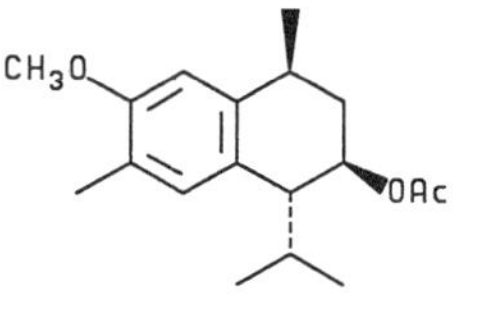

Mol. Wt.: 290
Melting Point: Oil
$[\alpha]_D$: +22.3 Solvent: Chf
Spectral Data: UV, IR, CMR, PMR, Mass Spec.
Organism: *Lemnalia cervicornis* (Coelenterata)
Location: Great Barrier Reef, Australia
Reference: 99

$C_{19}H_{20}O_7$ **Annulin A**

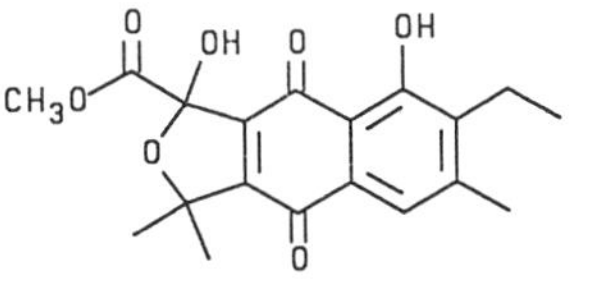

Mol. Wt.: 360
Bioactivity: Antibacterial activity
Melting Point: 174–176°C
Spectral Data: UV, IR, CMR, PMR, Mass Spec., x-ray c.s.
Organism: *Garveia annulata* (Coelenterata)
Location: British Columbia, Canada
Reference: 279

$C_{20}H_{20}O_4$ **13,14,15,16-Tetrahydroxestoquinol**

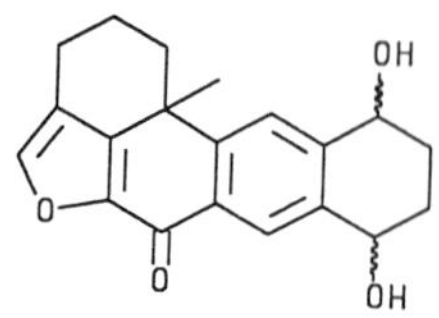

Mol. Wt.: 324
Melting Point: 224–229°C
Spectral Data: UV, IR, CMR, PMR, Mass Spec.
Organism: *Adocia* sp.
(Porifera)
Location: Truk
Reference: 982

$C_{20}H_{20}O_5$ **3,13-Dideoxo-1,2,14,15-tetrahydro-3,13-dihydroxyhalenaquinone**

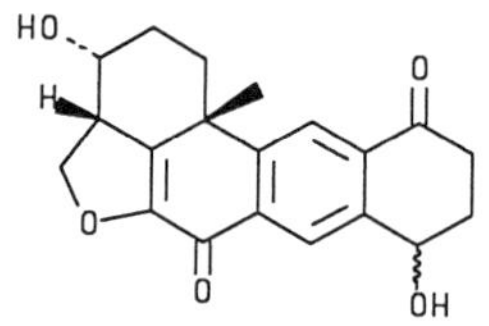

Mol. Wt.: 340
Melting Point: 235–245°C
Specral Data: UV, IR, CMR, PMR, Mass Spec.
Organism: *Adocia* sp.
(Porifera)
Location: Truk
Reference: 982

$C_{20}H_{22}O_4$ **Garveatin B**

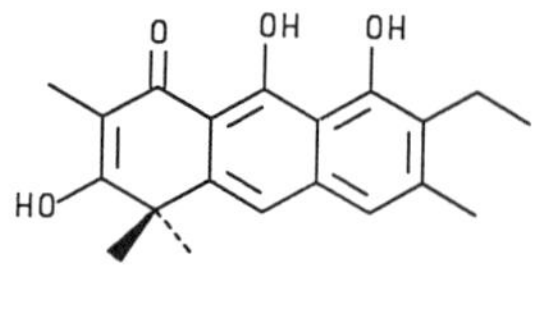

Mol. Wt.: 326
Bioactivity: Antimicrobial activity
Melting Point: Oil
Spectral Data: UV, IR, PMR, Mass Spec.
Organism: *Garveia annulata*
(Coelenterata)
Location: British Columbia, Canada
Reference: 278

$C_{20}H_{28}O_4$

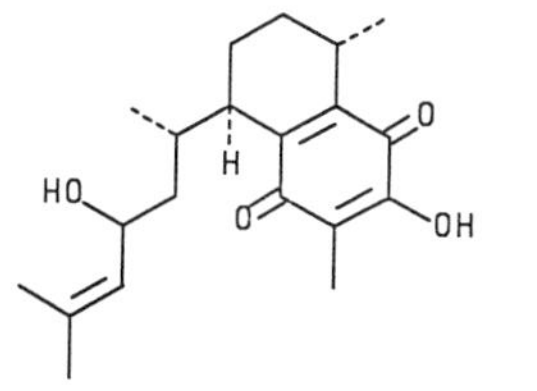

Mol. Wt.: 332
Melting Point: Oil
Spectral Data: UV, IR, CMR, PMR, Mass Spec.
Organism: *Pseudopterogorgia* sp. (Coelenterata)
Location: Bahamas
Reference: 401

$C_{21}H_{22}O_7$ **Annulin B**

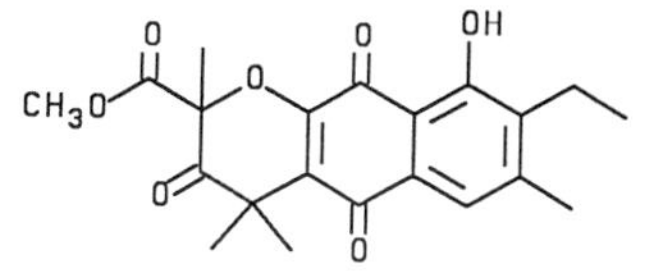

Mol. Wt.: 386
Bioactivity: Antibacterial activity
Melting Point: Oil
$[\alpha]_D$: +8.0 Solvent: Chf
Spectral Data: UV, IR, CMR, PMR, Mass Spec.
Organism: *Garveia annulata* (Coelenterata)
Location: British Columbia, Canada
Reference: 279

$C_{22}H_{24}O_5$ **Garveatin C**

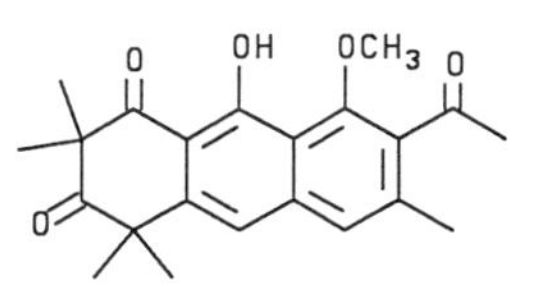

Mol. Wt.: 368
Bioactivity: Antimicrobial activity
Melting Point: 125°C
Spectral Data: UV, IR, CMR, PMR, Mass Spec.
Organism: *Garveia annulata* (Coelenterata)
Location: British Columbia, Canada
Reference: 278

$C_{22}H_{28}O_4$ **Tridachiapyrone-E**

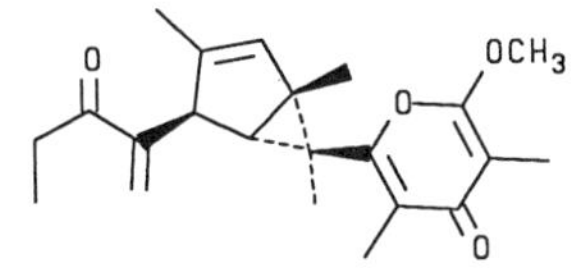

Mol. Wt.: 356
Melting Point: Oil
Spectral Data: UV, IR, PMR, Mass Spec.
Organism: *Tridachia crispata* (Mollusca)
Location: Jamaica
Reference: 613

$C_{22}H_{28}O_5$ **Tridachiapyrone-F**

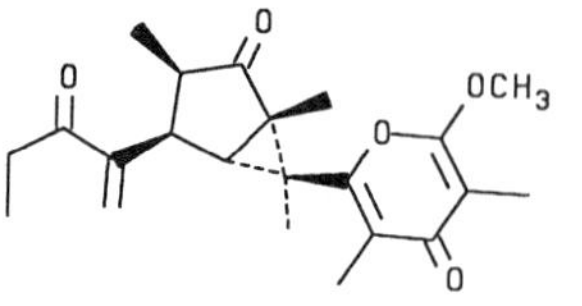

Mol. Wt.: 372
Spectral Data: UV, PMR, Mass Spec.
Organism: *Tridachia crispata* (Mollusca)
Location: Jamaica
Reference: 613

$C_{22}H_{29}NaO_7S$ **Siphonodictyal D**

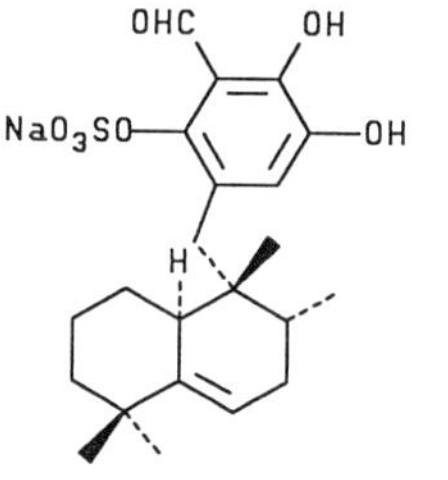

Mol. Wt.: 460
Bioactivity: Antimicrobial activity against *Staphylococcus aureus*, *Bacillus subtilis*, and *Vibrio anguillarum*
Melting Point: 131–132°C
$[\alpha]_{546}$: −67.65 Solvent: Me
$[\alpha]_{578}$: −56.54 Solvent: Me
Spectral Data: UV, IR, CMR, PMR, Mass spec., x-ray c.s.
Organism: *Siphonodictyon coralliphagum* Rützler (Porifera)
Location: Ponape, Pacific Ocean
Reference: 1044

$C_{22}H_{30}O_3$

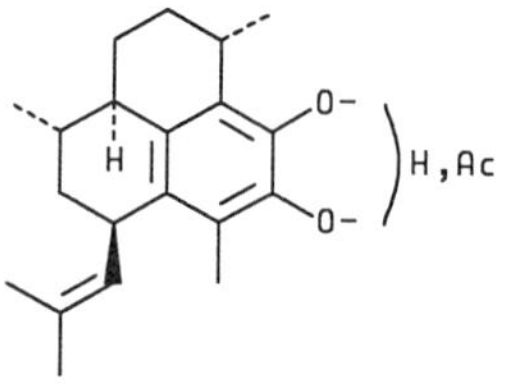

Mol. Wt.: 342 (mixture of monoacetates)
Melting Point: Oil
$[\alpha]_D$: −41.7 Solvent: Me (diacetate)
Spectral Data: UV, IR, CMR, PMR (diacetate)
Organism: *Pseudopterogorgia* sp. (Coelenterata)
Location: Bahamas
Reference: 401

$C_{22}H_{30}O_3$ **(+)-9,10-Deoxytridachione**

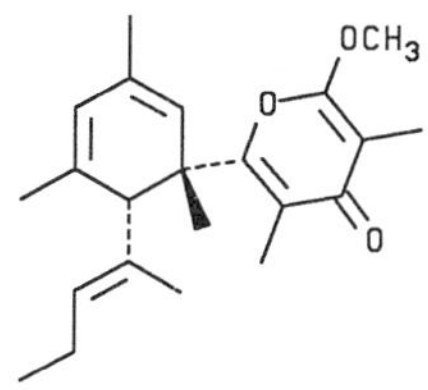

Mol. Wt.: 342
Bioactivity: Antibacterial activity against *Micrococcus luteus* and *Bacillus subtilis*
Melting Point: Oil
$[\alpha]_D$: +400° Solvent: Chf
Spectral Data: UV, CD, IR, CMR, PMR, Mass Spec.
Organism: *Elysia chlorotica* (Gould) (Mollusca)
Location: Nova Scotia, Canada
Reference: 223

$C_{22}H_{30}O_4$ **Siphonodictyal B**
(previously known)

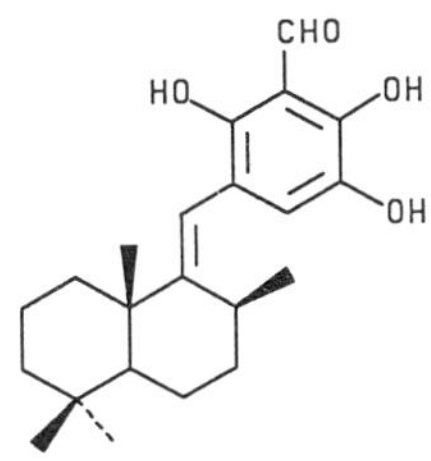

Mol. Wt.: 358
Bioactivity: Antimicrobial activity against *Staphylococcus aureus* and *Bacillus subtilis*
Melting Point: 145–147°C
Spectral Data: PMR (as dimethoxy derivative)
Organism: *Siphonodictyon coralliphagum* f. *typica* Rützler (Porifera)
Location: Bahamas; Belize
Reference: 1043, 1044

$C_{22}H_{30}O_4$ **Siphonodictyal C**

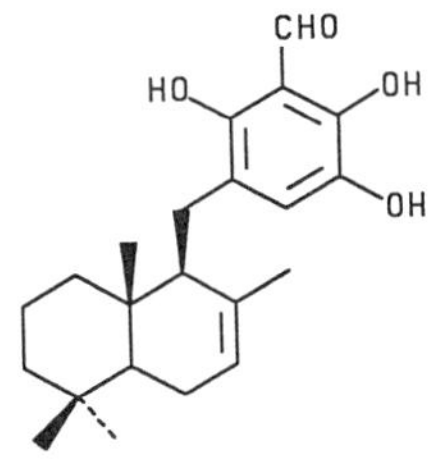

Mol. Wt.: 358
Bioactivity: Antimicrobial activity against *Staphylococcus aureus*, *Bacillus subtilis* and *Vibrio anguillarum*
$[\alpha]_{578}$: -23.60 Solvent: Me
$[\alpha]_{546}$: -30.47 Solvent: Me
Spectral Data: UV, IR, CMR, PMR, Mass Spec.
Organism: *Siphonodictyon coralliphagum* Rützler (Porifera)
Location: Ponape and Kwajalein, Pacific Ocean
Reference: 1044

$C_{22}H_{30}O_4$ **Siphonodictyoic acid**

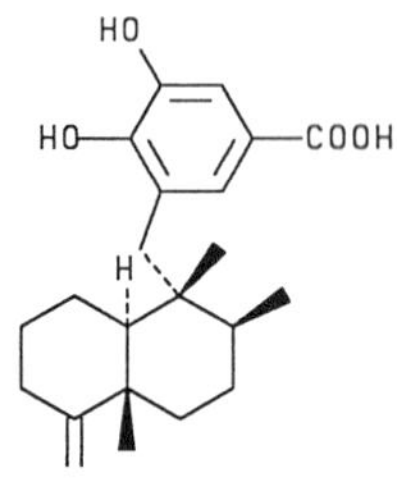

Mol. Wt.:	358
[α]$_{578}$:	−5.69 Solvent: Me
[α]$_{546}$:	−12.60 Solvent: Me
Spectral Data:	UV, IR, CMR, PMR, Mass Spec.
Organism:	*Siphonodictyon coralliphagum* f. *typica* Rützler (Porifera)
Location:	Belize
Reference:	1044

$C_{22}H_{30}O_5$

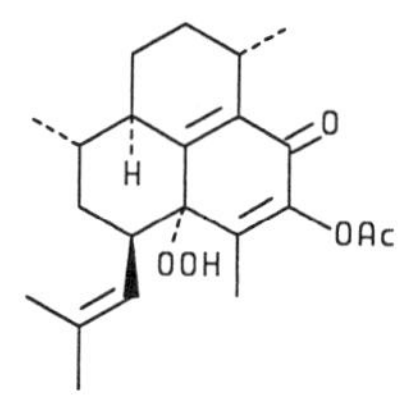

Mol. Wt.:	374
Melting Point:	Oil
[α]$_D$:	−11.3 Solvent: Me
Spectral Data:	UV, IR, CMR, PMR, Mass Spec.
Organism:	*Pseudopterogorgia* sp. (Coelenterata)
Location:	Bahamas
Reference:	401

$C_{22}H_{30}O_6$ **Siphonodictyal E**

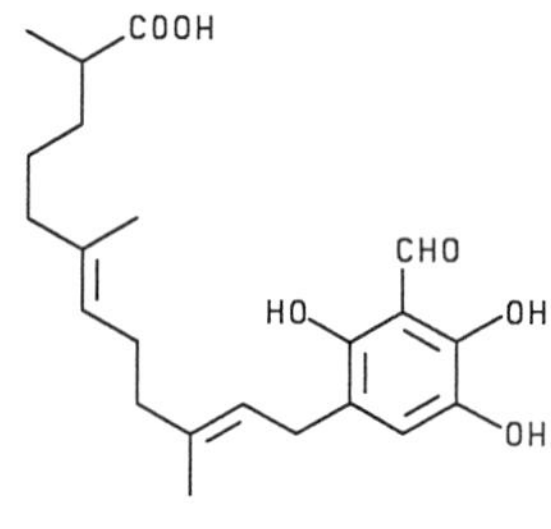

Mol. Wt.:	390
Spectral Data:	UV, IR, CMR, PMR, Mass Spec.
Organism:	*Siphonodictyon coralliphagum* f. *typica* Rützler *Siphonodictyon coralliphagum* f. *tubulosa* Rützler *Siphonodictyon coralliphagum* Rützler (Porifera)
Location:	Bahamas; Belize; Ponape and Kwajalein, Pacific Ocean
Reference:	1044

$C_{22}H_{31}NaO_6S$ **Siphonodictyol G**

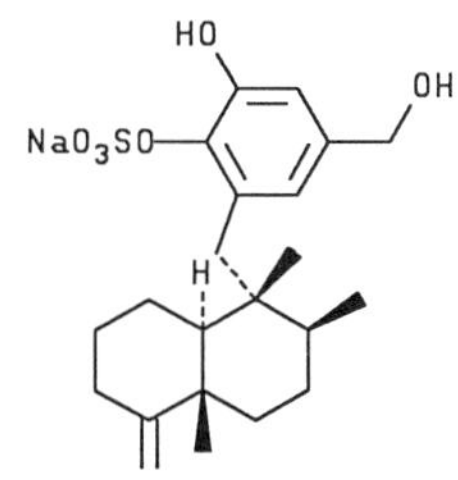

Mol. Wt.: 446
Bioactivity: Antimicrobial activity against *Staphylococcus aureus* and *Bacillus subtilis*
$[\alpha]_{578}$: −24.92 Solvent: Me
$[\alpha]_{546}$: −28.02 Solvent: Me
Spectral Data: UV, IR, CMR, PMR, Mass Spec.
Organism: *Siphonodictyon coralliphagum* f. *typica* Rützler
Siphonodictyon coralliphagum f. *tubulosa* Rützler
(Porifera)
Location: Bahamas; Belize
Reference: 1044

$C_{22}H_{31}NaO_6S$ **Siphonodictyol H**

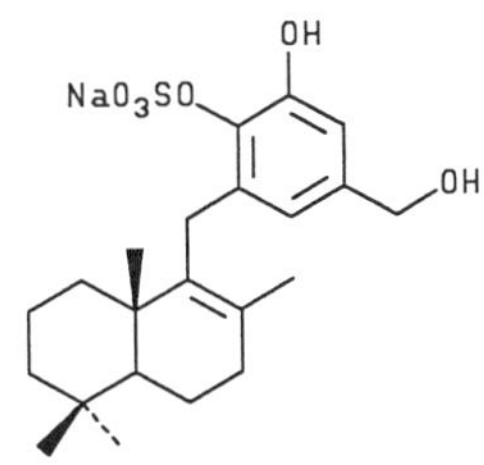

Mol. Wt.: 446
Bioactivity: Antimicrobial activity against *Staphylococcus aureus* and *Bacillus subtilis*
Spectral Data: UV, IR, CMR, PMR, Mass Spec.
Organism: *Siphonodictyon coralliphagum* Rützler
(Porifera)
Location: Ponape, Pacific Ocean
Reference: 1044

$C_{23}H_{24}O_7$ **Garvin A quinone**

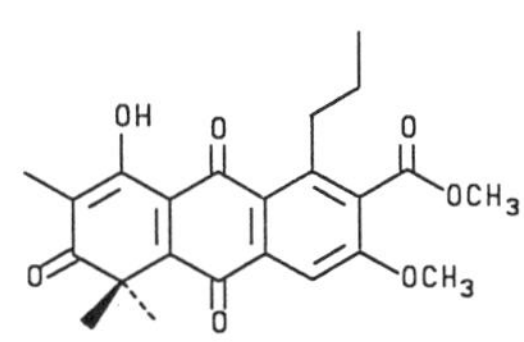

Mol. Wt.: 412
Bioactivity: Antimicrobial activity
Melting Point: Oil
Spectral Data: UV, PMR, Mass Spec., x-ray c.s.
Organism: *Garveia annulata*
(Coelenterata)
Location: British Columbia, Canada
Reference: 278

$C_{23}H_{26}O_7$ **2-Hydroxygarvin A**

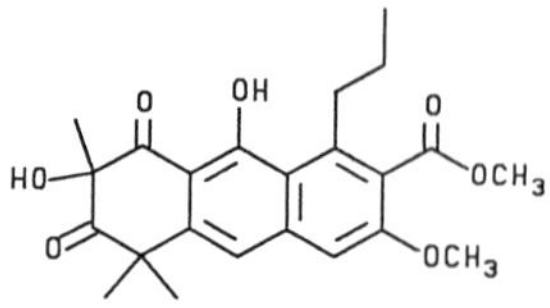

Mol. Wt.: 414
Melting Point: 195°C
$[\alpha]_D$: +5.5 Solvent: Chf
Spectral Data: UV, IR, CMR, PMR, Mass Spec.
Organism: *Garveia annulata* (Coelenterata)
Location: British Columbia, Canada
Reference: 278

$C_{23}H_{32}O_4$ **Dictyoceratin-A**

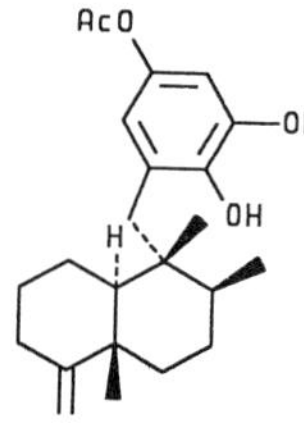

Mol. Wt.: 372
Bioactivity: Antimicrobial activity (against *Staphylococcus aureus* and *Bacillus subtilis*)
Melting Point: 180–181.5°C
$[\alpha]_D^{25}$: +5.8 Solvent: Chf
Spectral Data: UV, IR, CMR, PMR, Mass Spec.
Organism: *Hippospongia* sp. (Porifera)
Location: Okinawa, Japan
Reference: 796

$C_{23}H_{32}O_5$ **Dictyoceratin-B**

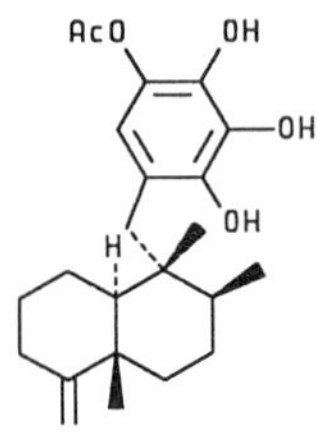

Mol. Wt.: 388
Bioactivity: Antimicrobial activity (against *Staphylococcus aureus* and *Bacillus subtilis*)
Melting Point: 154.5–155.5°C
$[\alpha]_D^{25}$: –1.22 Solvent: Chf
Spectral Data: UV, IR, CMR, PMR, Mass Spec.
Organism: *Hippospongia* sp. (Porifera)
Location: Okinawa, Japan
Reference: 796

$C_{25}H_{32}O_5$ **Isotridachiapyrone-B**

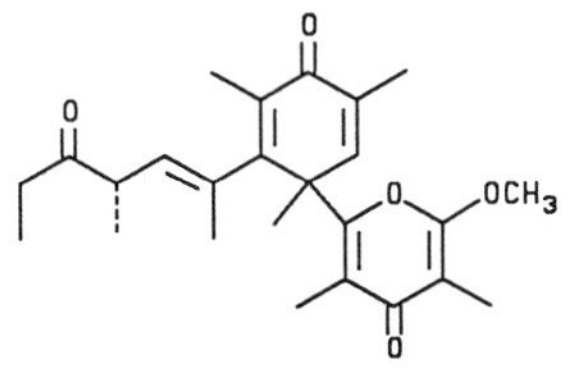

Mol. Wt.: 412
Melting Point: Oil
Spectral Data: UV, IR, CMR, PMR, Mass Spec.
Organism: *Tridachia crispata* (Mollusca)
Location: Jamaica
Reference: 613

$C_{25}H_{34}O_4$ **Elysione**

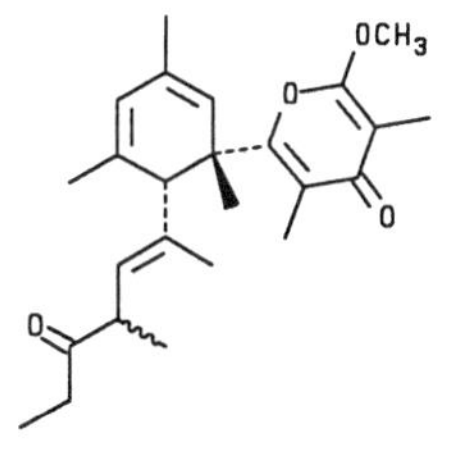

Mol. Wt.: 398
Bioactivity: Antibacterial activity (against *Micrococcus luteus*)
Melting Point: Oil
$[\alpha]_D$: +213 Solvent: Chf
Spectral Data: UV, CD, IR, CMR, PMR, Mass Spec.
Organism: *Elysia chlorotica* Gould (Mollusca)
Location: Nova Scotia, Canada
Reference: 223

$C_{25}H_{34}O_4$ **Isotridachiapyrone-A**

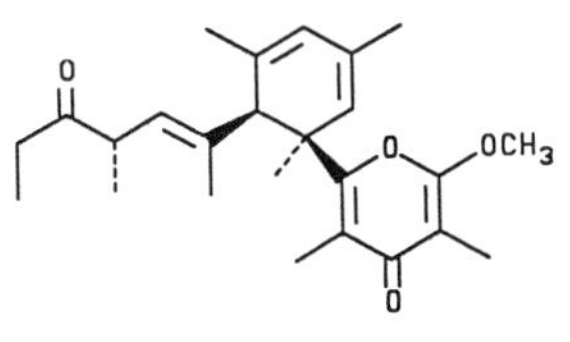

Mol. Wt.: 398
Melting Point: Oil
Spectral Data: UV, IR, CMR, PMR, Mass Spec.
Organism: *Tridachia crispata* (Mollusca)
Location: Jamaica
Reference: 613

$C_{25}H_{34}O_5$ **Maurapyrone C**

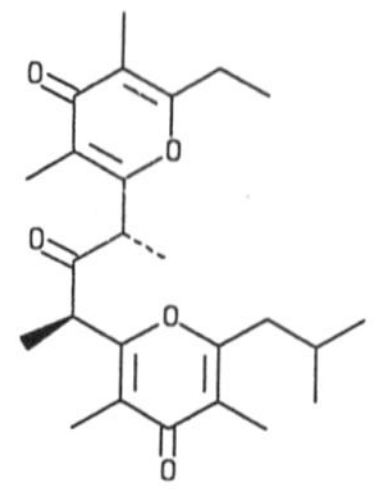

Mol. Wt.: 414
Bioactivity: Antimicrobial activity against *Vibrio anguillarum*
Melting Point: Wax
Spectral Data: UV, IR, PMR, Mass Spec.
Organism: *Siphonaria maura* (Mollusca)
Location: Costa Rica
Reference: 697

$C_{25}H_{34}O_5$ **Maurapyrone D**

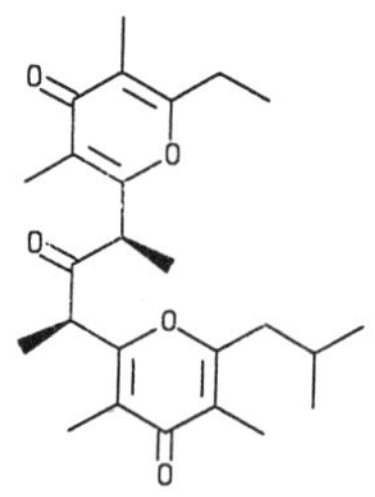

Mol. Wt.: 414
Bioactivity: Antimicrobial activity against *Vibrio anguillarum*
Melting Point: Oil
Spectral Data: UV, IR, PMR, Mass Spec.
Organism: *Siphonaria maura* (Mollusca)
Location: Costa Rica
Reference: 697

$C_{25}H_{34}O_5$ **Tridachiapyrone-C**

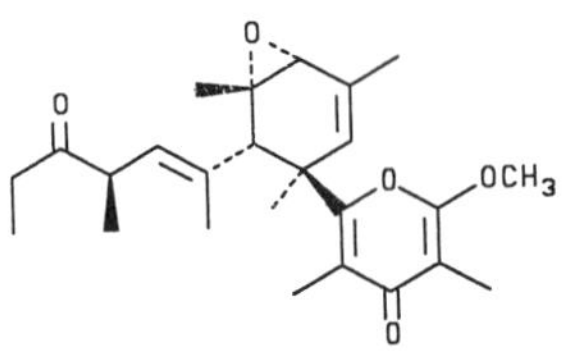

Mol. Wt.: 414
Melting Point: Oil
Spectral Data: UV, IR, PMR, Mass Spec.
Organism: *Tridachia crispata* (Mollusca)
Location: Jamaica
Reference: 613

$C_{25}H_{36}O_6$ **Pseudopterosin A**

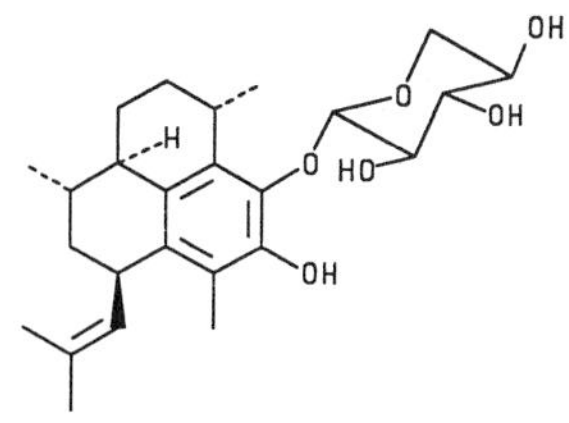

Mol. Wt.: 432
Bioactivity: Antiinflammatory and analgesic activities
$[\alpha]_D^{20}$: -85 Solvent: Chf
Spectral Data: UV, IR, CMR, PMR, Mass Spec.
Organism: *Pseudopterogorgia elisabethae* (Coelenterata)
Location: Bahamas
Reference: 293, 671, 672

$C_{25}H_{38}O_6$ **Seco-pseudopterosin A**

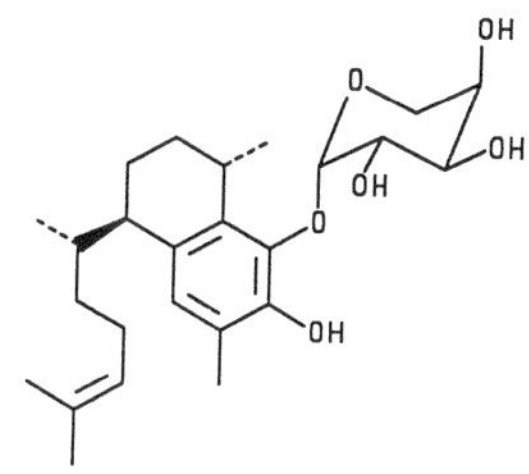

Mol. Wt.: 434
Bioactivity: Antimicrobial activity
Antiinflammatory and analgesic activities
$[\alpha]_D$: -118 Solvent: Chf
Spectral Data: UV, IR, CMR, PMR, Mass Spec.
Organism: *Pseudopterogorgia kallos* (tentative) (Coelenterata)
Location: Florida Keys
Reference: 293, 670

$C_{26}H_{36}O_5$ **Maurapyrone A**

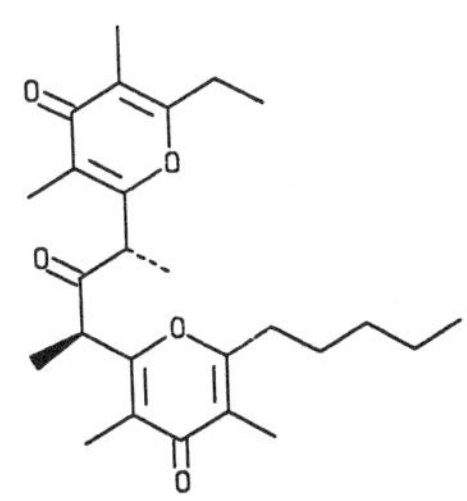

Mol. Wt.: 428
Bioactivity: Antimicrobial activity against *Vibrio anguillarum*
Melting Point: 110-112°C
Spectral Data: UV, IR, PMR, Mass Spec., x-ray c.s.
Organism: *Siphonaria maura* (Mollusca)
Location: Costa Rica
Reference: 697

$C_{26}H_{36}O_5$ **Maurapyrone B**

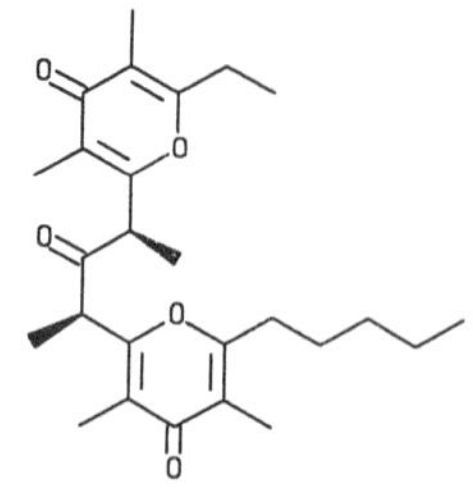

Mol. Wt.: 428
Bioactivity: Antimicrobial activity against *Vibrio anguillarum*
Melting Point: Wax
Spectral Data: UV, IR, PMR, Mass Spec.
Organism: *Siphonaria maura* (Mollusca)
Location: Costa Rica
Reference: 697

$C_{27}H_{38}O_7$ **Pseudopterosin B**

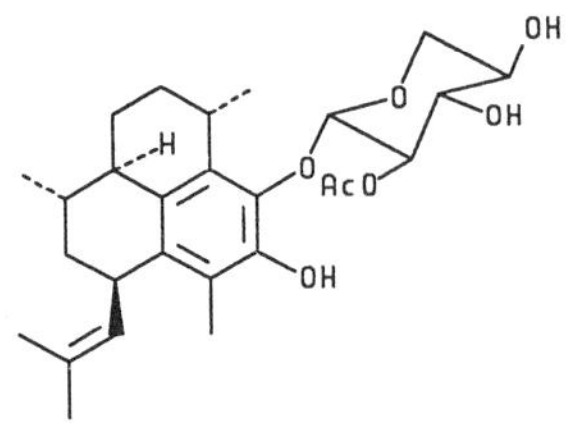

Mol. Wt.: 474
Bioactivity: Antiinflammatory and analgesic activities
Melting Point: Oil
$[\alpha]_D^{20}$: −55.2 Solvent: Chf
Spectral Data: UV, IR, CMR, PMR, Mass Spec.
Organism: *Pseudopterogorgia elisabethae* (Coelenterata)
Location: Bahamas
Reference: 293, 672

$C_{27}H_{38}O_7$ **Pseudopterosin C**

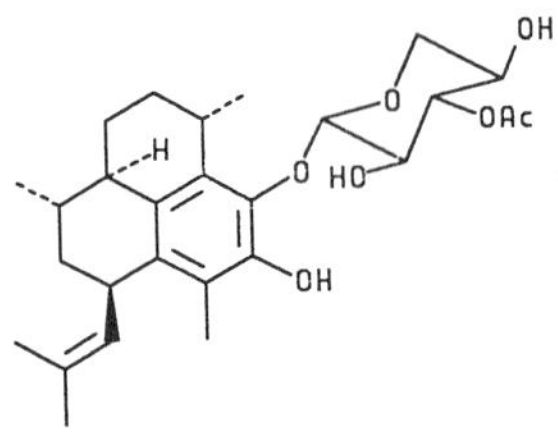

Mol. Wt.: 474
Bioactivity: Antiinflammatory and analgesic activities
Melting Point: 113.5–115°C
$[\alpha]_D^{20}$: −77 Solvent: Chf
Spectral Data: UV, IR, CMR, PMR, Mass Spec., x-ray c.s.
Organism: *Pseudopterogorgia elisabethae* (Coelenterata)
Location: Bahamas
Reference: 293, 672

$C_{27}H_{38}O_7$ **Pseudopterosin D**

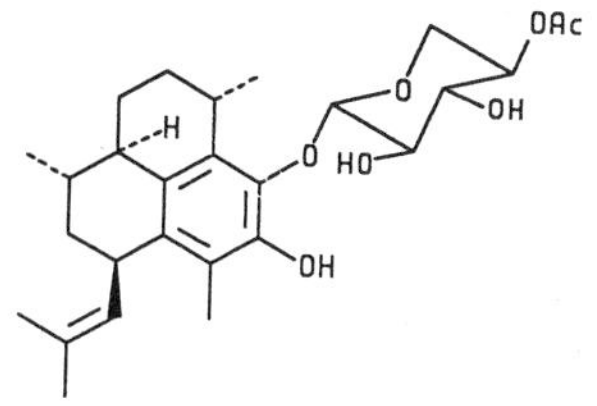

Mol. Wt.: 474
Bioactivity: Antiinflammatory and analgesic activities
Melting Point: Oil
$[\alpha]_D^{20}$: −107.3 Solvent: Chf
Spectral Data: UV, IR, CMR, PMR, Mass Spec.
Organism: *Pseudopterogorgia elisabethae* (Coelenterata)
Location: Bahamas
Reference: 293, 672

$C_{27}H_{40}O_7$ **Seco-pseudopterosin C**

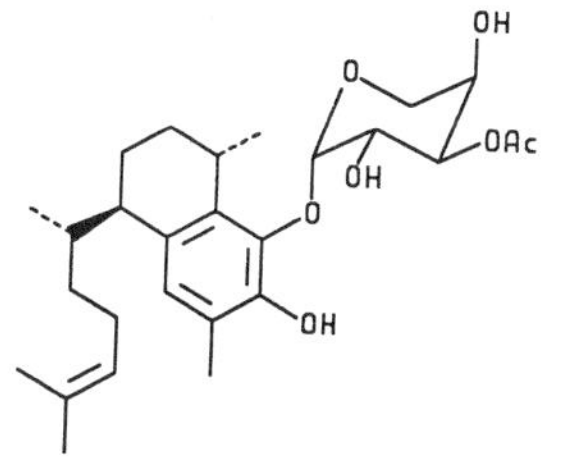

Mol. Wt.: 476
Bioactivity: Antimicrobial activity
Antiinflammatory and analgesic activities
$[\alpha]_D$: −89 Solvent: Chf
Spectral Data: UV, IR, CMR, PMR, Mass Spec.
Organism: *Pseudopterogorgia kallos* (tentative) (Coelenterata)
Location: Florida Keys
Reference: 293, 670

$C_{27}H_{40}O_7$ **Seco-pseudopterosin D**

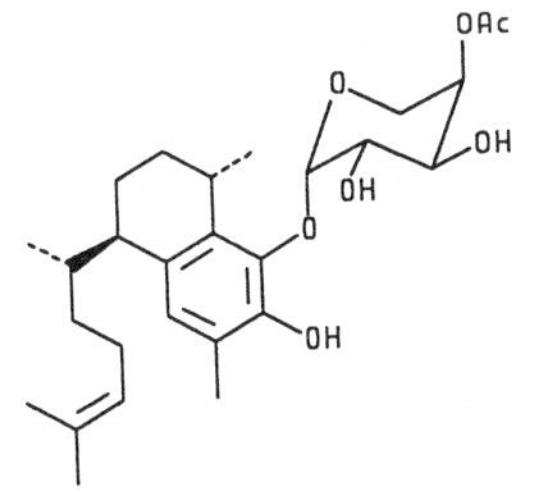

Mol. Wt.: 476
Bioactivity: Antimicrobial activity
Antiinflammatory and analgesic activities
$[\alpha]_D$: −139 Solvent: Chf
Spectral Data: UV, IR, CMR, PMR, Mass Spec.
Organism: *Pseudopterogorgia kallos* (tentative) (Coelenterata)
Location: Florida Keys
Reference: 293, 670

$C_{31}H_{47}NaO_6S$ **Halisulfate 1**

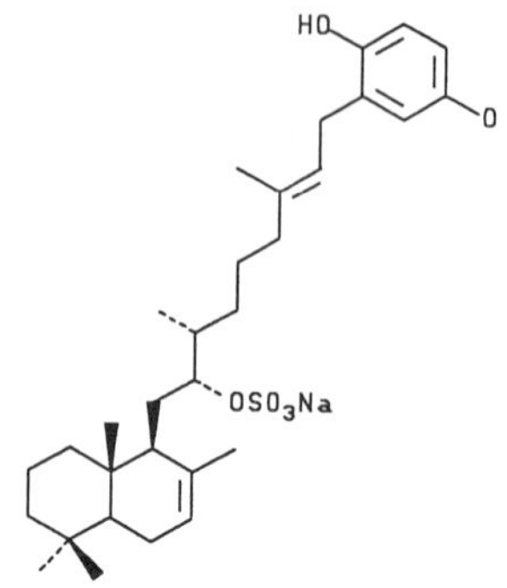

Mol. Wt.: 570
Bioactivity: Sea urchin egg assay:
70% inhibition at 8 μg/ml
100% Inhibition of phospholipase A_2 at 16 μg/ml
Antimicrobial activity
Melting Point: >300°C
$[\alpha]_D$: −27.3 Solvent: Me
Spectral Data: IR, CMR, PMR, Mass Spec.
Organism: *Halichondriidae* sp. (Porifera)
Location: La Jolla, California
Reference: 546

$C_{34}H_{48}O_{11}$ **Moritoside**

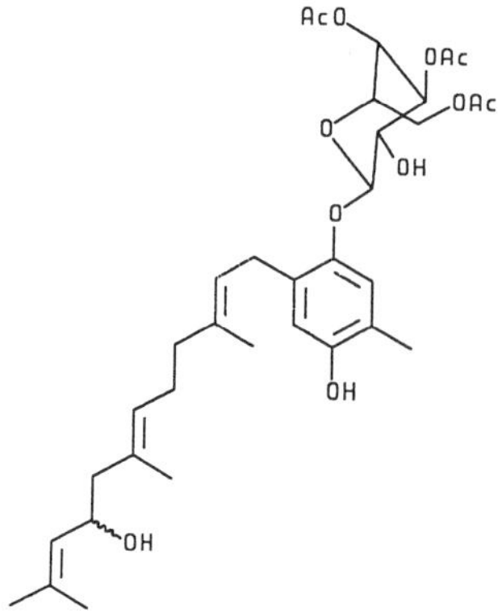

Mol. Wt.: 632
Bioactivity: Inhibition of cell division of fertilized starfish eggs at 1 μg/ml
Melting Point: Oil
$[\alpha]_D^{23}$: +22.6 Solvent: Chf
Spectral Data: UV, IR, CMR, PMR, Mass Spec.
Organism: *Euplexaura* sp. (Coelenterata)
Location: Japan
Reference: 337

$C_{36}H_{53}NaO_5S$ **Hexaprenylhydroquinone sulfate**

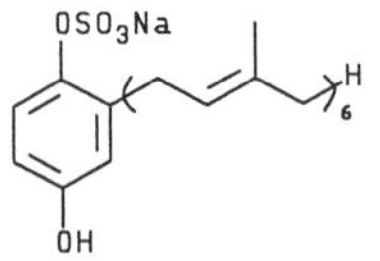

Mol. Wt.: 620
Bioactivity: Inhibition of H,K-ATPase:
IC_{50} $4.6x10^{-6}M$
Inhibition of gastric acid secretion
Inhibition of phospholipase A_2:
IC_{50} $1.8x10^{-6}M$
Melting Point: Gum
Spectral Data: UV, IR, CMR, PMR, Mass Spec.
Organism: *Dysidea* sp. (Porifera)
Location: Izu Archipelago
Reference; 336

$C_{40}H_{32}O_{15}$ **Kelletinin A**

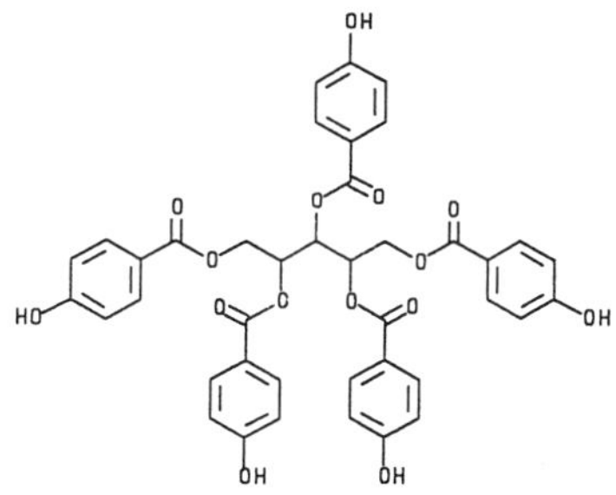

Mol. Wt.: 752
Spectral Data: UV, IR, CMR, PMR, Mass Spec.
Organism: *Buccinulum corneum* (Mollusca)
Location: Italy
Reference: 186

Chapter 18 AMINES AND NITROGEN HETEROCYCLIC COMPOUNDS

$C_6H_7N_5$ **3-Methyladenine**

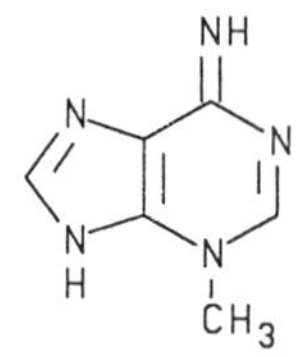

Mol. Wt.: 149
Melting Point: 302–305°C
Spectral Data: UV, CMR, PMR, Mass Spec.
Organism: *Topsentia genitrix* (Porifera)
Location: Mediterranean
Reference: 1036

$C_7H_9N_5O$ **1,9-Dimethyl-6-imino-8-oxopurine**

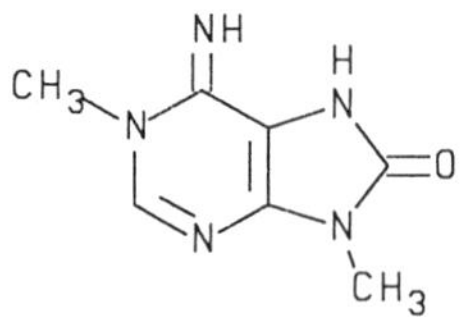

Mol. Wt.: 179
Melting Point: 245–246°C (acetate)
Spectral Data: UV, IR, PMR, Mass Spec., x-ray c.s. (acetate)
Organism: *Hymeniacidon sanguinea* (Porifera)
Location: English Channel
Reference: 183

$C_8H_4Br_3N$ **3,4,6-Tribromoindole** (previously known)

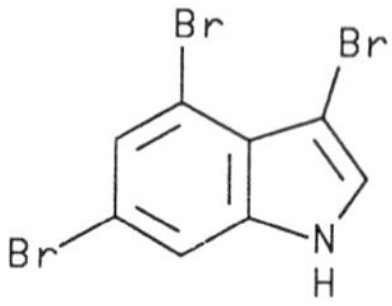

Mol. Wt.: 354
Melting Point: 90°C (dec.)
Spectral Data: PMR
Organism: *Ptychodera* sp. (Hemichordata)
Location: Maui, Hawaii
Reference: 416, 418

$C_8H_5Br_2N$ **4,6-Dibromoindole**

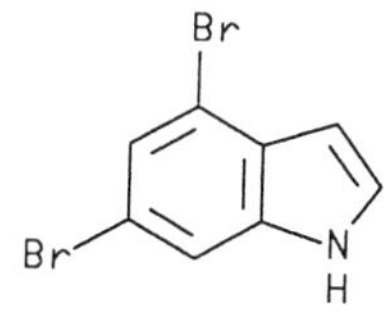

Mol. Wt.: 275
Spectral Data: PMR, Mass Spec.
Organism: *Glossobalanus* sp. (Hemichordata)
Location: Okinawa, Japan
Reference: 417

$C_8H_5BrN_2O_2$ **7-Bromo-2,4(1H,3H)-quinazolinedione**

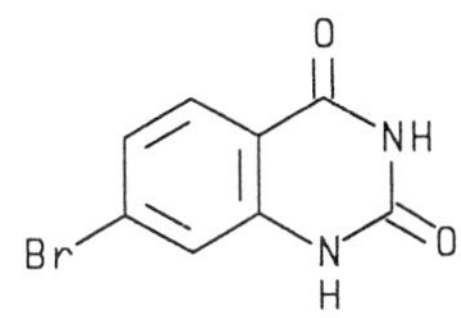

Mol. Wt.: 241
Melting Point: >330°C
Spectral Data: UV, IR, PMR, Mass Spec.
Organism: *Pyura sacciformis* (Chordata/Tunicata)
Location: Japan
Reference: 821

$C_8H_{10}N_4O_2$ **Caffeine**

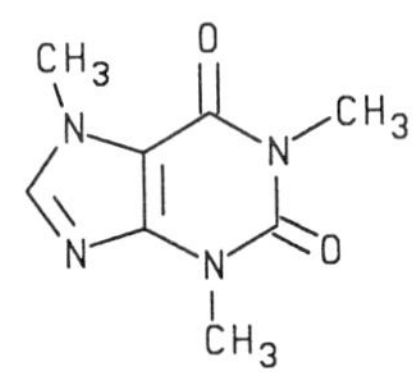

Mol. Wt.: 194
Organism: *Paramuricea chamaeleon* (Coelenterata)
Location: Sea of Marmara
Reference: 455

$C_8H_{12}ClN_5O$ **Caissarone hydrochloride**

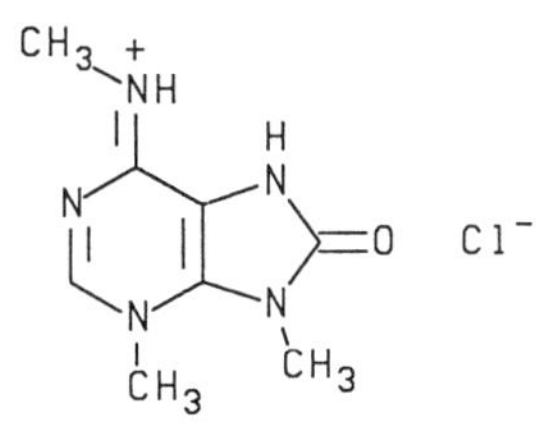

Mol. Wt.: 229
Melting Point: 285–290°C
Spectral Data: UV, IR, CMR, PMR, Mass Spec., x-ray c.s.
Organism: *Bunodosoma caissarum* (Coelenterata)
Location: São Sebastião, Brazil
Reference: 1220

$C_8H_{12}N_6$ **2-Iminomethyl-3-methyl-6-aminomethyl-9H-purine**

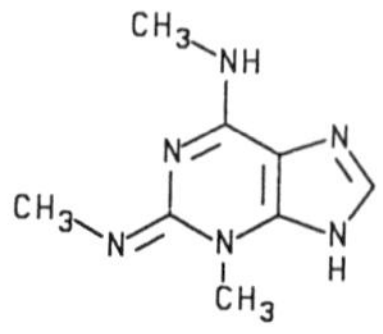

Mol. Wt.: 192
Melting Point: 226–227°C
Spectral Data: UV, PMR, Mass Spec., x-ray c.s.
Organism: *Sagartia troglodytes* Price (Coelenterata)
Location: Naples, Italy
Reference: 233

$C_9H_7Br_2N$ **4,6-Dibromo-2-methylindole**

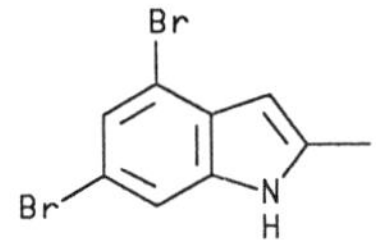

Mol. Wt.: 289
Melting Point: 96–96.5°C
Spectral Data: PMR, Mass Spec.
Organism: *Glossobalanus* sp. (Hemichordata)
Location: Okinawa, Japan
Reference: 417

$C_9H_{10}N_2O_6$ **2'-Deoxyuridine-5'-carboxylic acid**

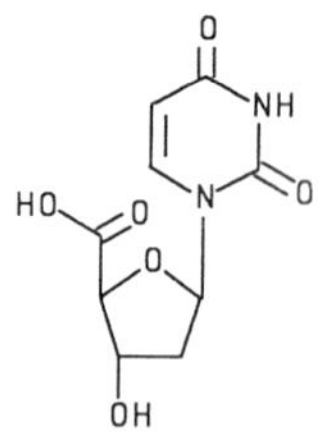

Mol. Wt.: 242
Melting Point: >210°C
$[\alpha]_{435}^{22}$: 20.4 Solvent: Aq
Spectral Data: UV, CMR, PMR, Mass Spec.
Organism: *Aplidium (=Amaroucium) fuscum* (Chordata/Tunicata)
Location: Mediterranean
Reference: 230

$C_{10}H_{12}N_2O_6$ **Thymidine-5'-carboxylic acid**

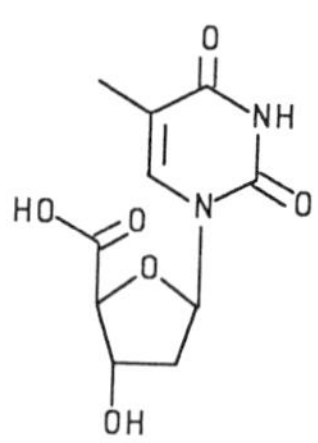

Mol. Wt.: 256
$[\alpha]_D^{22}$: +9.0 Solvent: Aq
Spectral Data: UV, CMR, PMR, Mass Spec.
Organism: *Aplidium (=Amaroucium) fuscum* (Chordata/Tunicata)
Location: Mediterranean
Reference: 230

$C_{10}H_{14}ClNO_2$ **1,1-Dimethyl-5,6-dihydroxy-indolinium chloride**

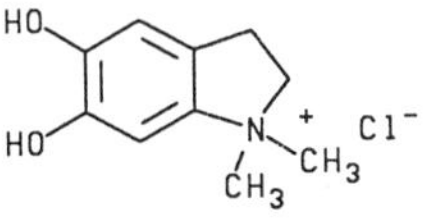

Mol. Wt.: 215
Melting Point: 244°C
Spectral Data: UV, IR, CMR, PMR, Mass Spec.
Organism: *Dercitus* sp. Gray (Porifera)
Location: Bahamas
Reference: 593

$C_{10}H_{15}N_3O_7$ **11-norTetrodotoxin-6(R)-ol [11-norTTX-6(R)-ol]**

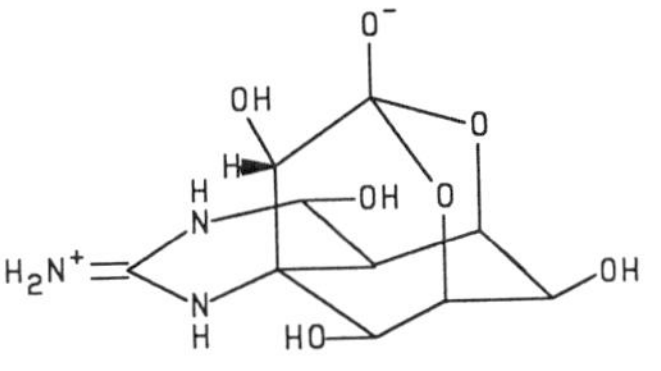

Mol. Wt.: 289
Bioactivity: Toxicity: LD_{99} 70 μg/kg (acetate)
Spectral Data: PMR, Mass Spec.
Organism: *Fugu niphobles*, *F. pardalis* *F. poecilonotus* (Chordata/Pisces)
Location: Japan
Reference: 268, 869

$C_{11}H_7BrN_2O$ **Eudistomin J**

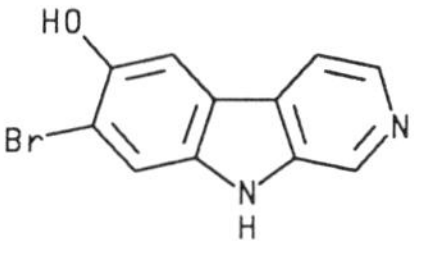

Mol. Wt.: 263
Spectral Data: UV, IR, PMR, Mass Spec. (diacetate)
Organism: *Eudistoma olivaceum* (Chordata/Tunicata)
Location: Caribbean
Reference: 935

$C_{11}H_{10}N_2O_3$

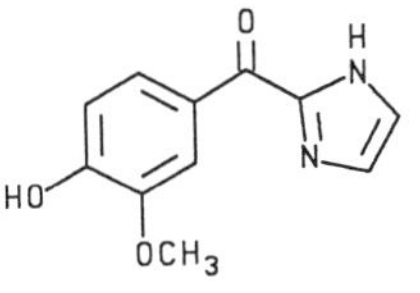

Mol. Wt.: 218
Melting Point: 226°C
Spectral Data: PMR, Mass Spec.
Organism: *Aplidium pliciferum* (Chordata/Tunicata)
Location: South Australia
Reference: 33

$C_{11}H_{11}Br_2N_5O$ **Dibromocantharelline**

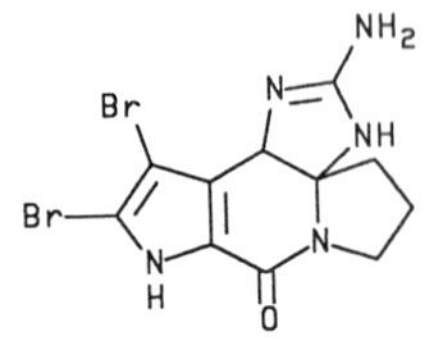

Mol. Wt.: 389
Melting Point: 260°C
$[\alpha]_D$: +95 Solvent: Me
Spectral Data: UV, CD, IR, CMR, PMR, Mass Spec., x-ray c.s.
Organism: *Pseudaxinyssa cantharella* (Porifera)
Location: New Caledonia
Reference: 232

$C_{11}H_{11}Br_2N_5O$ **Oroidin**

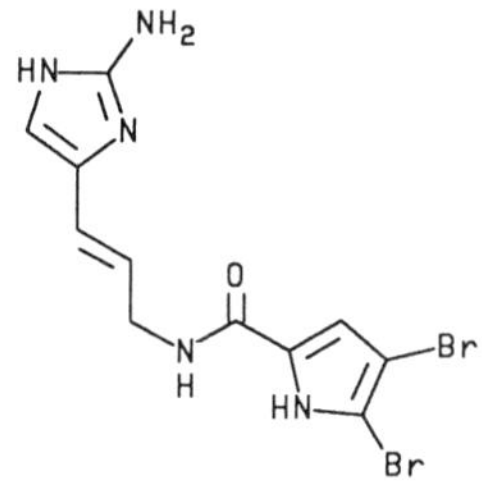

Mol. Wt.: 389
Bioactivity: Antimicrobial activity
Spectral Data: UV, IR, PMR
Organism: *Agelas oroides* (Porifera)
Location: Naples, Italy
Reference: 302, 340

$C_{11}H_{12}Br_2ClN_5O$ **Dibromoisophakellin**

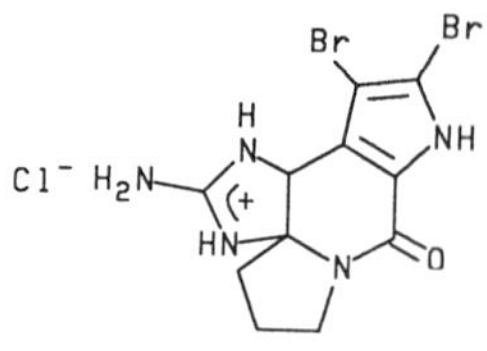

Mol. Wt.: 425
Melting Point: 275–277°C
$[\alpha]_D^{20}$: −101 Solvent: Me
Spectral Data: UV, CD, IR, CMR, PMR, Mass Spec., x-ray c.s.
Organism: *Acanthella carteri* (Porifera)
Location: Madagascar
Reference: 290

$C_{11}H_{15}N_3O_6$ **4,9-Anhydro-11-deoxyTTX**

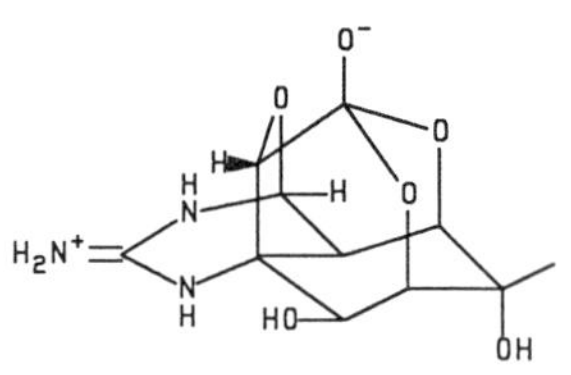

Mol. Wt.: 285
Spectral Data: PMR, Mass Spec.
Organism: *Cynops ensicauda* (Chordata/Vertebrata)
Location: Okinawa, Japan
Reference: 1207

$C_{11}H_{15}N_3O_7$ **4,9-Anhydro-6-epiTTX**

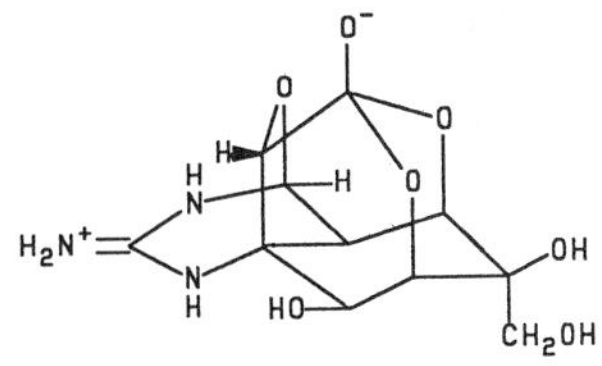

Mol. Wt.: 301
$[\alpha]_D^{25}$: +10 Solvent: 0.05N Ac
Spectral Data: PMR, Mass Spec.
Organism: *Cynops ensicauda* (Chordata/Vertebrata)
Location: Okinawa, Japan
Reference: 1207

$C_{11}H_{17}N_3O_7$ **11-Deoxy-4-epiTTX**

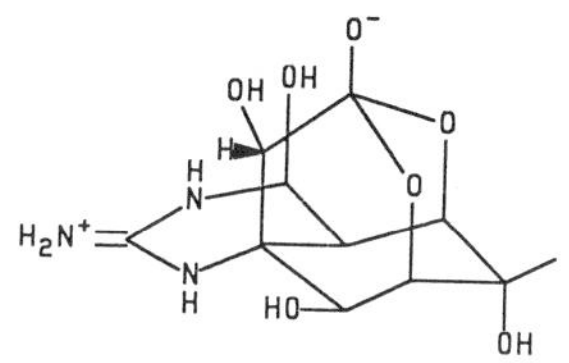

Mol. Wt.: 303
Spectral Data: PMR, Mass Spec.
Organism: *Cynops ensicauda* (Chordata/Vertebrata)
Location: Okinawa, Japan
Reference: 1207

$C_{11}H_{17}N_3O_7$ **11-Deoxytetrodotoxin (11-DeoxyTTX)**

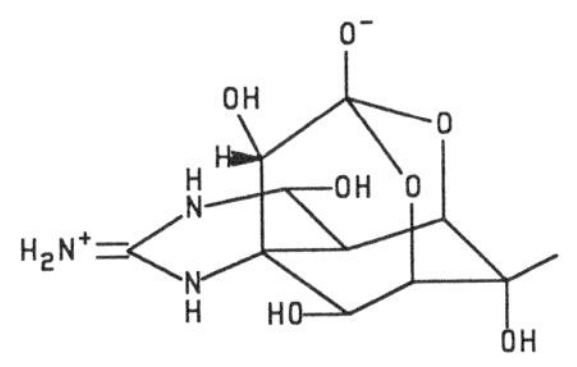

Mol. Wt.: 303
Bioactivity: Toxicity: mice: LD_{50} 71 μg/kg
Melting Point: 202°C (dec.)
$[\alpha]_D^{25}$: +5.37 Solvent: 0.05N Ac
Spectral Data: CMR, PMR, Mass Spec.
Organism: *Cynops ensicauda* (Chordata/Vertebrata)
Fugu niphobles (Chordata/Pisces)
Location: Okinawa, Japan
Reference: 268, 1207, 1213

$C_{11}H_{17}N_3O_8$ **6-*epi*Tetrodotoxin (6-*epi*TTX)**

Mol. Wt.: 319
Bioactivity: Toxicity: mice: LD_{50} 60 μg/kg
$[\alpha]_D^{25}$: -4.8 Solvent: 0.05N Ac
Spectral Data: CMR, PMR, Mass Spec.
Organism: *Cynops ensicauda* (Chordata/Vertebrata) *Fugu niphobles* (Chordata/Pisces)
Location: Okinawa, Japan
Reference: 268, 1207, 1213

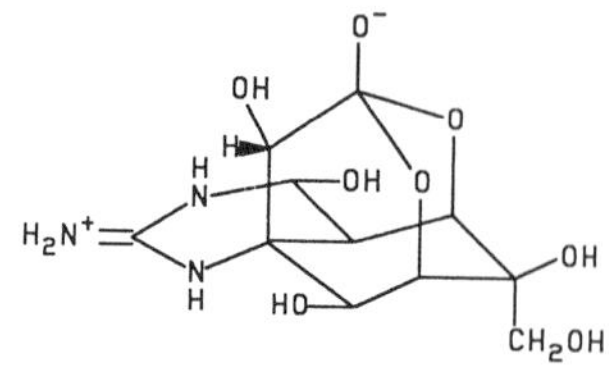

$C_{11}H_{17}N_3O_8$ **Tetrodotoxin (TTX)**

Mol. Wt.: 319
Spectral Data: Mass Spec.
Organism: *Lineus fuscoviridis* *Tubulanus punctatus* (Nemertinea)
Location: Hiroshima and Ehime, Japan
Reference: 749

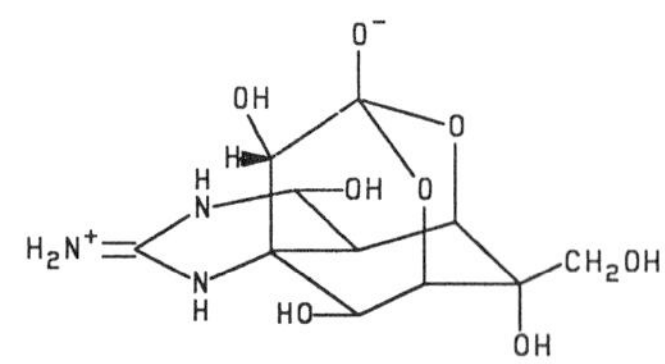

$C_{12}H_9BrN_2$ **6-Bromo-1-methyl-β-carboline**

Mol. Wt.: 261
Spectral Data: UV, CMR, PMR, Mass Spec.
Organism: *Aglaophenia pluma* Linnaeus (Coelenterata)
Location: Italy
Reference: 9

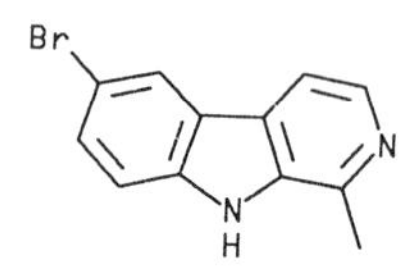

$C_{12}H_{10}N_2$ **Harman**
(1-Methyl-β-carboline)
(previously known)

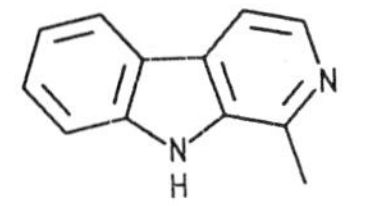

Mol. Wt.: 182
Bioactivity: Sedative and antidepressive properties
Organism: *Costaticella hastata* Busk (Bryozoa)
Location: Tasmania, Australia
Reference: 12, 75

$C_{13}H_{10}Br_2N_2$ **6,8-Dibromo-1-ethyl-β-carboline**

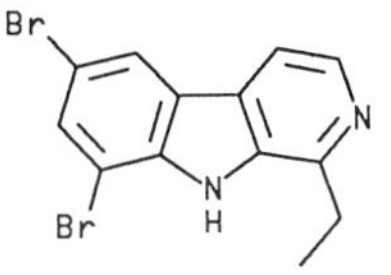

Mol. Wt.: 354
Spectral Data: UV, CMR, PMR, Mass Spec.
Organism: *Aglaophenia pluma* Linnaeus (Coelenterata)
Location: Italy
Reference: 9

$C_{13}H_{10}N_2$ **Pavettine**
(previously known)

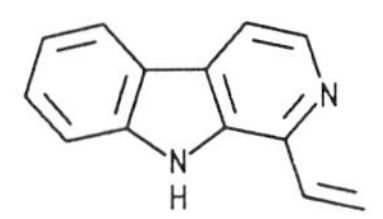

Mol. Wt.: 194
Spectral Data: UV, PMR
Organism: *Costaticella hastata* Busk (Bryozoa)
Soulamea fraxinifolia (Simaroubaceae)
Location: Tasmania, Australia; New Caledonia
Reference: 12, 75, 166, 502

$C_{13}H_{11}BrN_2$ **6-Bromo-1-ethyl-β-carboline**

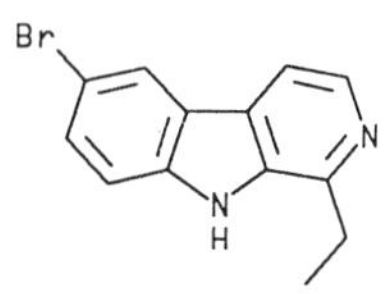

Mol. Wt.: 275
Spectral Data: UV, CMR, PMR, Mass Spec.
Organism: *Aglaophenia pluma* Linnaeus (Coelenterata)
Location: Italy
Reference: 9

$C_{13}H_{11}N_5O_5$ **Desmethyl phidolopin**

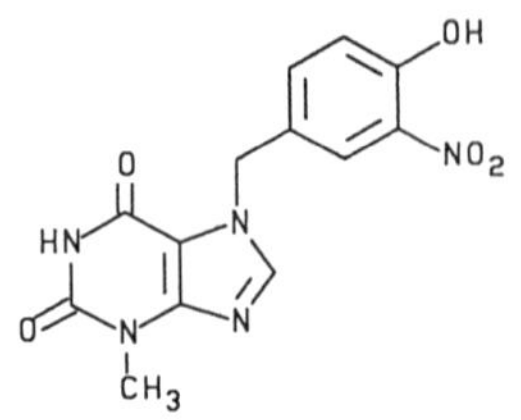

Mol. Wt.: 317
Bioactivity: Antibacterial, antifungal and antialgal activity
Spectral Data: PMR, Mass Spec.
Organism: *Phidolopora pacifica* *Diaperoecia californica* (Bryozoa)
Location: British Columbia, Canada
Reference: 1093

$C_{13}H_{12}N_2$ **1-Ethyl-β-carboline** (previously known)

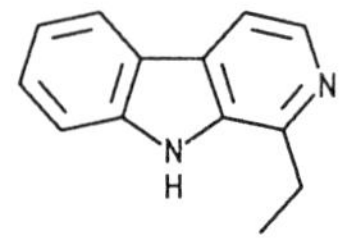

Mol. Wt.: 196
Spectral Data: UV, IR, PMR, Mass Spec.
Organism: *Costaticella hastata* Busk (Bryozoa) *Hannoa klaineana* (Simaroubaceae)
Location: Tasmania, Australia; Zaire
Reference: 75, 679

$C_{13}H_{12}N_2O$ **(S)-1-(1′-Hydroxyethyl)-β-carboline**

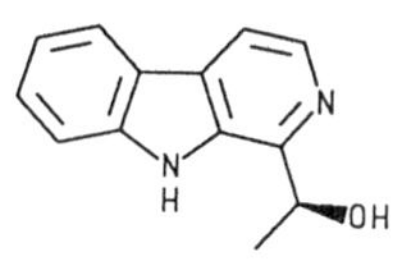

Mol. Wt.: 212
Melting Point: 163–169°C
$[\alpha]_D^{25}$: −11.4 Solvent: Me
Spectral Data: UV, IR, PMR, Mass Spec.
Organism: *Costaticella hastata* Busk (Bryozoa)
Location: Tasmania, Australia
Reference: 75

$C_{13}H_{12}Br_2N_2O_5$ **(R,R)-5-[3,5-Dibromo-4-(2-oxo-5-oxazolidinyl)methoxyphenyl]-2-oxazolidinone**

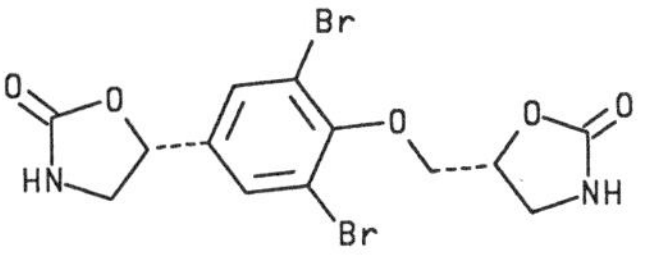

Mol. Wt.: 436
Melting Point: 220–222°C
$[\alpha]_D$: −33 Solvent: Me
Spectral Data: UV, IR, CMR, PMR, Mass Spec., x-ray c.s.
Organism: *Aplysina aerophoba* (Porifera)
Location: Canary Islands
Reference: 828

$C_{13}H_{12}N_4O_4$ **Mycalisine B**

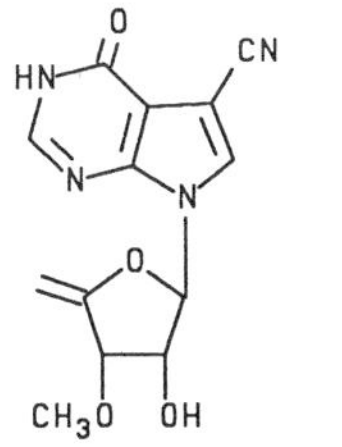

Mol. Wt.: 288
Bioactivity: Fertilized starfish egg assay: activity at 200 μg/ml
Melting Point: Oil
$[\alpha]_D^{21}$: −75.9 Solvent: Alc
Spectral Data: UV, IR, CMR, PMR, Mass Spec.
Organism: *Mycale* sp. (Porifera)
Location: Gulf of Sagami, Japan
Reference: 523

$C_{13}H_{13}NO_3$ **4-Hydroxy-5-(indole-3-yl)-5-oxo-pentan-2-one**

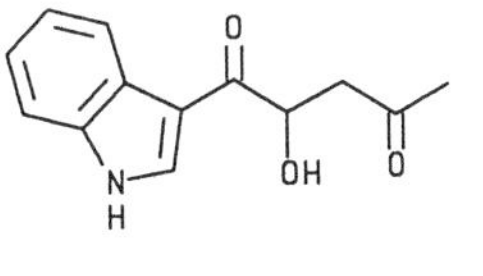

Mol. Wt. 231
Bioactivity: Plant growth promotion
Spectral Data: IR, PMR, Mass Spec.
Organism: *Dysidea etheria* de Laubenfels
Ulosa ruetzleri Wiedenmayer
(Porifera)
Location: Bermuda
Reference: 148

$C_{13}H_{13}N_5O_3$ **Mycalisine A**

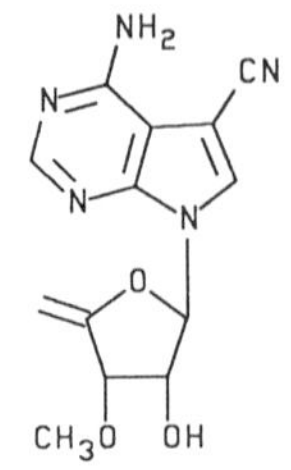

Mol. Wt.: 287
Bioactivity: Fertilized starfish egg assay: activity at 0.5 μg/ml
Melting Point: Oil
$[\alpha]_D^{21}$: −88.0 Solvent: Alc
Spectral Data: UV, IR, CMR, PMR, Mass Spec.
Organism: *Mycale* sp. (Porifera)
Location: Gulf of Sagami, Japan
Reference: 523

$C_{13}H_{16}N_2O_4$ **(-)-Bursatellin**

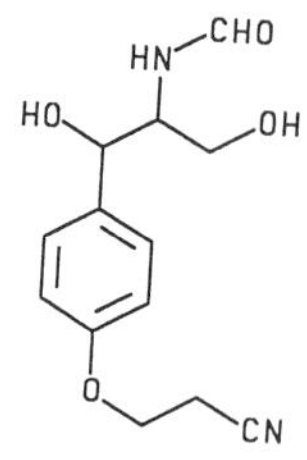

Mol. Wt.: 264
$[\alpha]_D$: −8.8 Solvent: Me
Spectral Data: IR, CMR, PMR
Organism: *Bursatella leachii leachii*
B. leachii savignyana
(Mollusca)
Location: Naples and Taranto, Italy
Reference: 188

$C_{14}H_{13}BrN_4O$ **6-Bromoaplysinopsin**

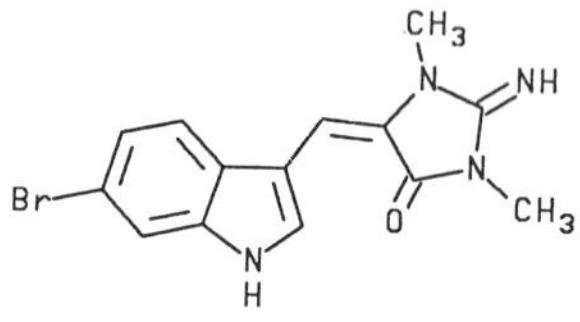

Mol. Wt.: 333
Melting Point: 283–285°C
Spectral Data: UV, CMR, PMR, Mass Spec.
Organism: *Astroides calycularis* Pallas (Coelenterata)
Location: Naples, Italy
Reference: 286

$C_{15}H_{10}BrN_3O$ **Eudistomin A**

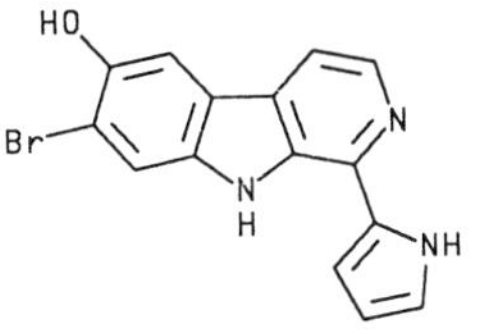

Mol. Wt.: 328
Melting Point: Oil
Spectral Data: UV, IR, CMR, PMR, Mass Spec.
Organism: *Eudistoma olivaceum* (Chordata/Tunicata)
Location: Caribbean
Reference: 935

$C_{15}H_{11}N_3O$ **Eudistomin M**

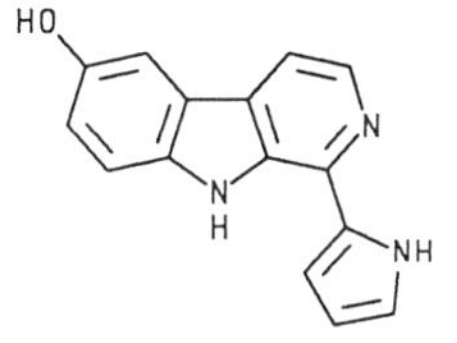

Mol. Wt.: 249
Melting Point: Oil
Spectral Data: UV, IR, PMR, Mass Spec. (acetate)
Organism: *Eudistoma olivaceum* (Chordata/Tunicata)
Location: Caribbean
Reference: 935

$C_{15}H_{12}BrN_3O$ **Eudistomidin A**

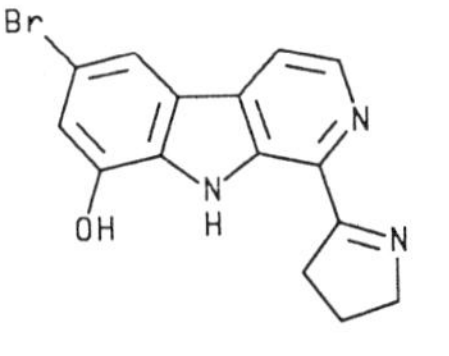

Mol. Wt.: 330
Bioactivity: Calmodulin antagonist
Melting Point: 225–230°C (dec.)
Spectral Data: UV, IR, CMR, PMR, Mass Spec.
Organism: *Eudistoma glaucus* (Chordata/Tunicata)
Location: Okinawa, Japan
Reference: 583

$C_{15}H_{17}Br_2N_5O_3$ **Ianthelline**

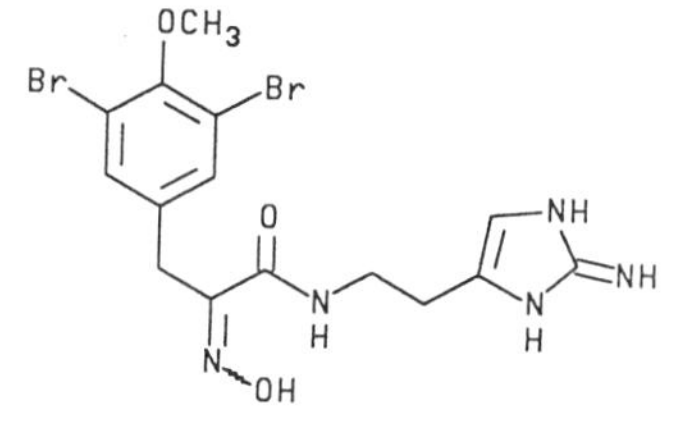

Mol. Wt.: 475
Bioactivity: Antibiotic activity against *Staphylococcus aureus*
Antifungal activity against *Candida albicans*
Melting Point: 113–115°C
Spectral Data: CMR, PMR, Mass Spec.
Organism: *Ianthella ardis* (syn. *Aiolochroia crassa* *Pseudoceratina crassa*) (Porifera)
Location: Bahamas
Reference: 666

$C_{15}H_{17}Br_3N_2O_2$ **Amathamide E**

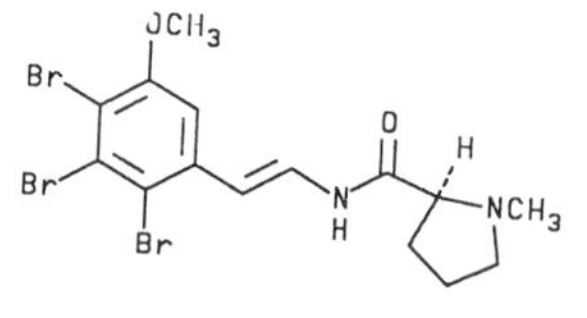

Mol. Wt.: 497
Melting Point: Oil
Spectral Data: IR, CMR, PMR, Mass Spec.
Organism: *Amathia wilsoni* Kirkpatrick (Bryozoa)
Location: Tasmania
Reference: 72

$C_{15}H_{17}Br_3N_2O_2$ **Amathamide F**

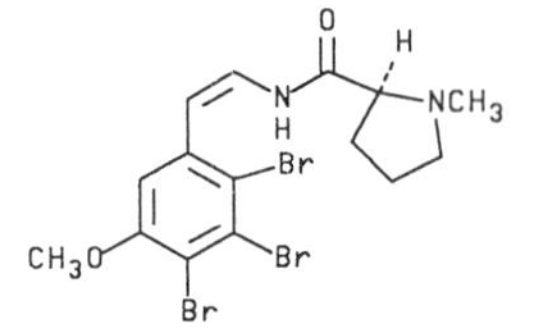

Mol. Wt.: 497
Melting Point: Oil
Spectral Data: IR, CMR, PMR
Organism: *Amathia wilsoni* Kirkpatrick (Bryozoa)
Location: Tasmania
Reference: 72

$C_{15}H_{18}Br_2N_2O_2$ **Amathamide A**

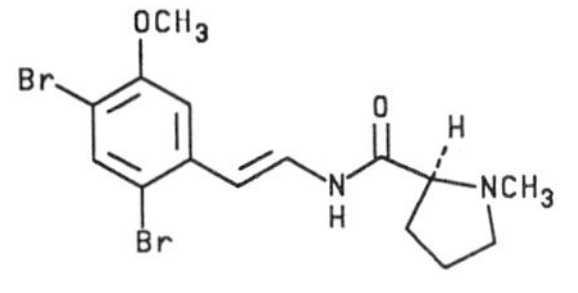

Mol. Wt.: 418
Melting Point: 189–190.5°C
Spectral Data: CD, IR, CMR, PMR, Mass Spec.
Organism: *Amathia wilsoni* Kirkpatrick (Bryozoa)
Location: Tasmania
Reference: 74

$C_{15}H_{18}Br_2N_2O_2$ **Amathamide B**

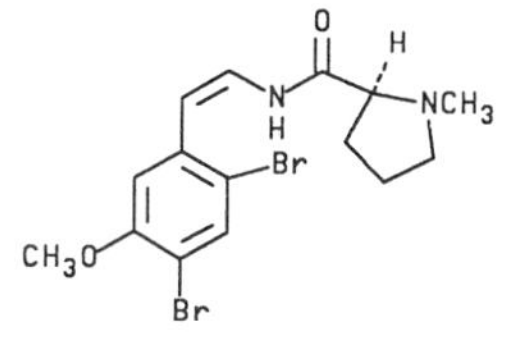

Mol. Wt.: 418
Melting Point: Oil
Spectral Data: IR, PMR, Mass Spec.
Organism: *Amathia wilsoni* Kirkpatrick (Bryozoa)
Location: Tasmania
Reference: 74

$C_{15}H_{19}N$ **cis-Trikentrin A**

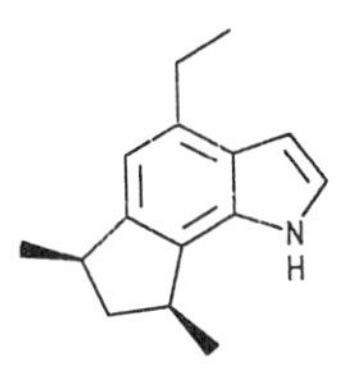

Mol. Wt.: 213
Bioactivity: Antimicrobial activity
Melting Point: Oil
$[\alpha]_D$: +48 Solvent: Chf
Spectral Data: UV, IR, CMR, PMR, Mass Spec.
Organism: *Trikentrion flabelliforme* (Porifera)
Location: Darwin, Australia
Reference: 145

$C_{15}H_{19}N$ **trans-Trikentrin A**

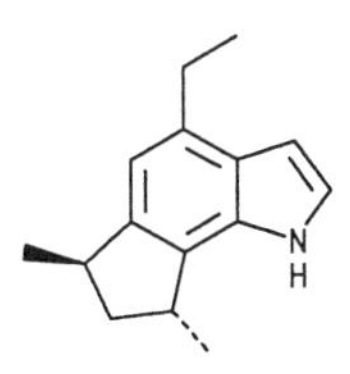

Mol. Wt.: 213
Bioactivity: Antimicrobial activity
Melting Point: Oil
$[\alpha]_D$: +23.3 Solvent: Chf
Spectral Data: UV, IR, CMR, PMR, Mass Spec.
Organism: *Trikentrion flabelliforme* (Porifera)
Location: Darwin, Australia
Reference: 145

$C_{15}H_{19}Br_3N_2O_2$ **Amathamide D**

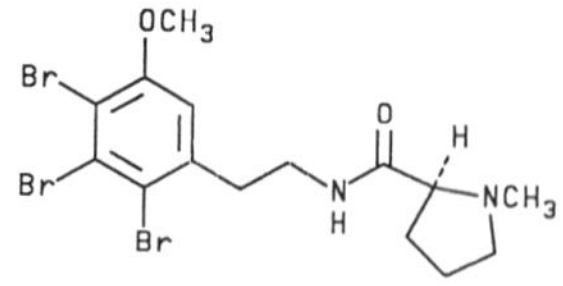

Mol. Wt.: 499
Melting Point: Oil
Spectral Data: IR, CMR, PMR, Mass Spec.
Organism: *Amathia wilsoni* Kirkpatrick (Bryozoa)
Location: Tasmania
Reference: 72

$C_{15}H_{21}Cl_6NO_3$ **Dysidamide**

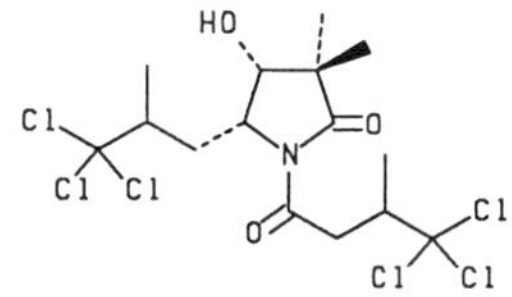

Mol. Wt.: 476
Melting Point: 123–124°C
$[\alpha]_D^{21}$: −14.9 Solvent: Chf
Spectral Data: IR, CMR, PMR, Mass Spec.
Organism: *Dysidea* sp. (Porifera)
Location: Red Sea
Reference: 345

$C_{15}H_{27}NO$ **Aminobisabolenol**

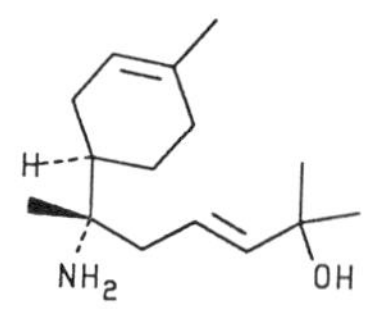

Mol. Wt.: 237
Melting Point: Oil
$[\alpha]_D^{16}$: +29 Solvent: Me
Spectral Data: IR, CMR, PMR
Organism: *Theonella* sp. (Porifera)
Location: Okinawa, Japan
Reference: 565, 569

$C_{15}H_{27}NO$ **Isoaminobisabolenol-a**

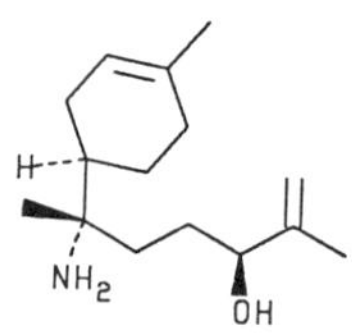

Mol. Wt.: 237
Melting Point: Oil
$[\alpha]_D$: +34 Solvent: Me
Spectral Data: IR, CMR, PMR
Organism: *Theonella* sp. (Porifera)
Location: Okinawa, Japan
Reference: 565, 569

$C_{15}H_{27}NO$ **Isoaminobisabolenol-b**

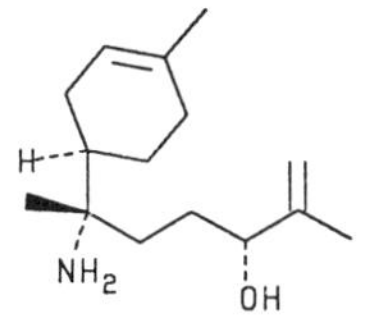

Mol. Wt.: 237
Melting Point: Oil
$[\alpha]_D$: +40 Solvent: Me
Spectral Data: IR, CMR, PMR
Organism: *Theonella* sp. (Porifera)
Location: Okinawa, Japan
Reference: 565, 569

$C_{15}H_{28}NCl$ **(6R,7S)-7-Amino-7,8-dihydro-α-bisabolene hydrochloride**

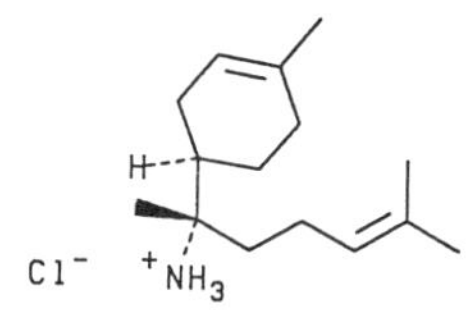

Mol. Wt.: 257
Bioactivity: Antimicrobial activity
$[\alpha]_D^{20}$: +64.1 Solvent: Chf
Spectral Data: IR, CMR, PMR, Mass Spec.
Organism: *Halichondria* sp. (Porifera)
Location: Ponape, Marshall Islands
Reference: 1045

$C_{15}H_{28}NCl$ **7-Ammonio-7,8-dihydro-α-bisabolene chloride**

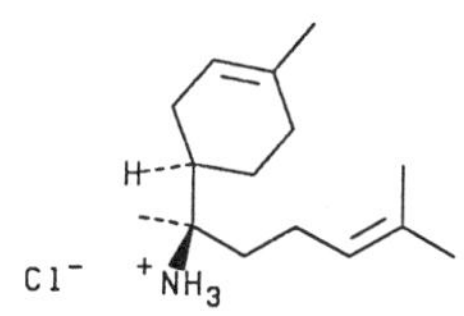

Mol. Wt.: 257
Bioactivity: Growth inhibition of *Bacillus subtilis*
Melting Point: Oil
$[\alpha]_D^{23}$: -8.3 Solvent: Me
Spectral Data: IR, PMR, Mass Spec.
Organism: *Ciocalypta* sp. (Porifera)
Location: O'ahu, Hawaii
Reference: 377

$C_{16}H_{14}BrN_3O_2$ **Barettin**

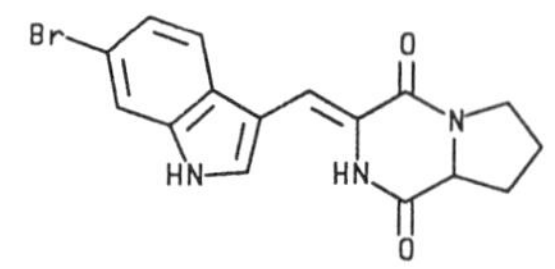

Mol. Wt.: 360
Bioactivity: Inhibits contractions of guinea-pig ileum
Melting Point: 207–210°C
$[\alpha]_D$: −25 Solvent: Me
Spectral Data: UV, IR, CMR, PMR, Mass Spec.
Organism: *Geodia baretti* (Bowerbank) Lamarck (Porifera)
Location: Northern Swedish West Coast
Reference: 655

$C_{16}H_{18}BrN_3O_4S$ **Eudistomin F**

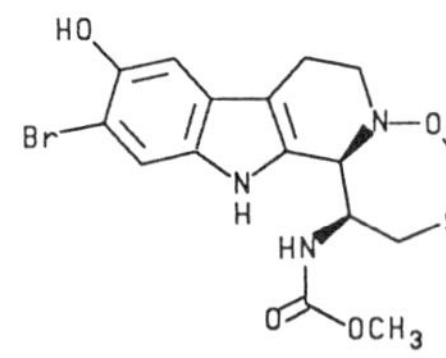

Mol. Wt.: 428
Spectral Data: UV, IR, PMR, Mass Spec.
Organism: *Eudistoma olivaceum* (Chordata/Tunicata)
Location: Caribbean
Reference: 935

$C_{16}H_{19}Br_3N_2O_2$ **Amathamide C**

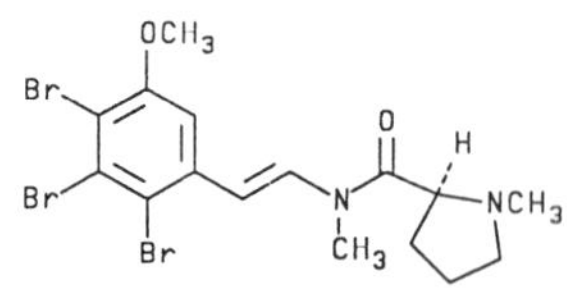

Mol. Wt.: 511
Melting Point: Oil
Spectral Data: IR, CMR, PMR, Mass Spec.
Organism: *Amathia wilsoni* Kirkpatrick (Bryozoa)
Location: Tasmania
Reference: 72

$C_{16}H_{21}BrN_2O$ **Dihydroflustramine C** **N-oxide**

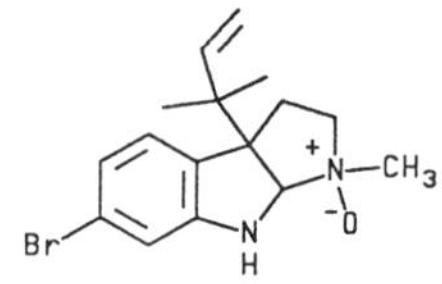

Mol. Wt.: 337
Bioactivity: Antibacterial activity
Melting Point: Oil
$[\alpha]_D^{25}$: −67.1 Solvent: Dcm
Spectral Data: UV, IR, CMR, PMR, Mass Spec.
Organism: *Flustra foliacea* (Bryozoa)
Location: Eastern Canada
Reference: 638

$C_{16}H_{26}N_3O_3$ **Amphikuemin**

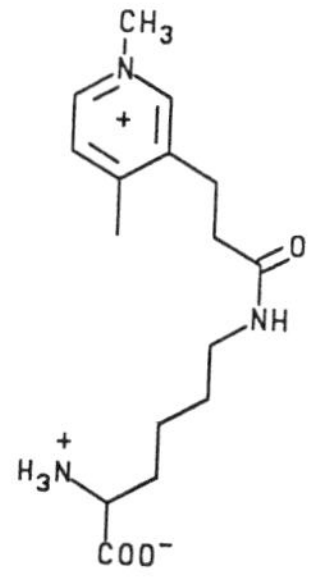

Mol. Wt.: 308
Bioactivity: Fish attractant
Spectral Data: UV, PMR, Mass Spec.
Organism: *Radianthus kuekenthali* (Coelenterata)
Location: Okinawa, Japan
Reference: 782

$C_{16}H_{27}NO$

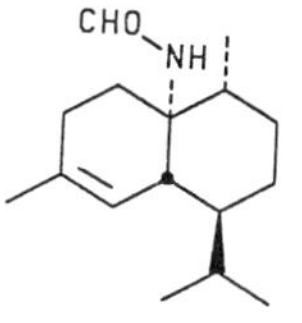

Mol. Wt.: 249
Melting Point: Oil
Spectral Data: IR, PMR, Mass Spec.
Organism: *Axinella cannabina* (Porifera)
Location: Taranto, Italy
Reference: 179

$C_{16}H_{27}NO$ **6α-Formamido-5αH,7αH,10α-eudesm-4(14)-ene**

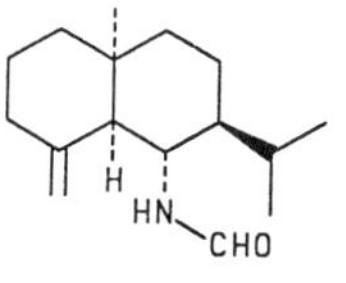

Mol. Wt.: 249
Spectral Data: IR, PMR, Mass Spec.
Organism: *Axinella cannabina* Esper (Porifera)
Location: Taranto, Italy
Reference: 180

$C_{17}H_{17}BrN_4O_2$ **6-Bromo-N-propionylaplysinopsin**

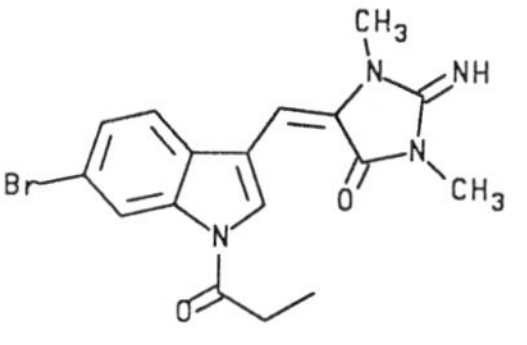

Mol. Wt.: 389
Melting Point: >300°C
Spectral Data: PMR, Mass Spec.
Organism: *Astroides calycularis* Pallas (Coelenterata)
Location: Naples, Italy
Reference: 286

$C_{17}H_{18}N_4O_2$ **N-Propionylaplysinopsin**

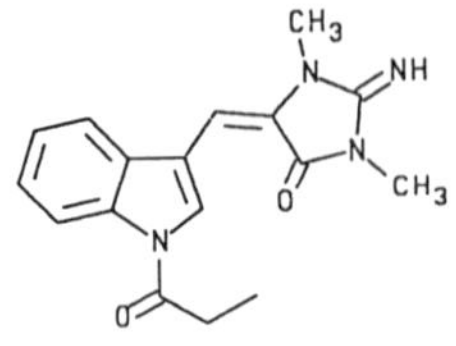

Mol. Wt.: 310
Melting Point: >300°C
Spectral Data: PMR, Mass Spec.
Organism: *Astroides calycularis* Pallas (Coelenterata)
Location: Naples, Italy
Reference: 286

$C_{17}H_{21}N$ **cis-Trikentrin B**
iso-trans-Trikentrin B
(mixture)

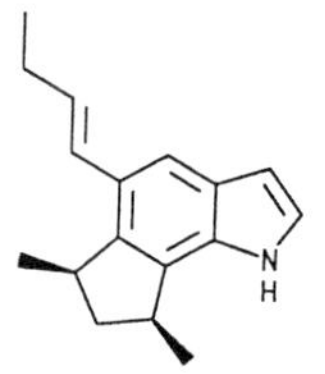

cis-Trikentrin B

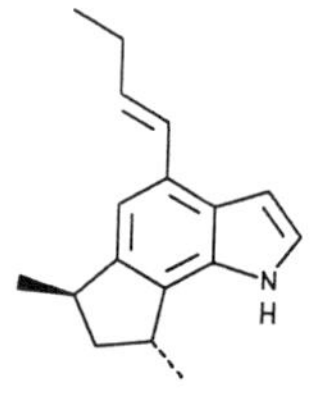

iso-trans-Trikentrin B

Mol. Wt.: 239
Bioactivity: Antimicrobial activity
Melting Point: Oil
Spectral Data: UV, IR, CMR, PMR, Mass Spec.
Organism: *Trikentrion flabelliforme* (Porifera)
Location: Darwin, Australia
Reference: 145

$C_{17}H_{21}N$ **trans-Trikentrin B**

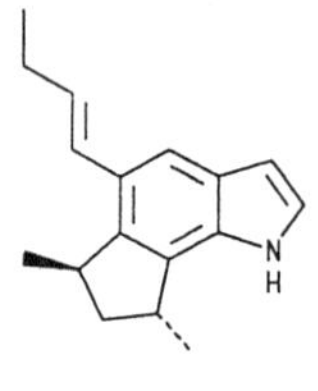

Mol. Wt.: 239
Bioactivity: Antimicrobial activity
Melting Point: Oil
$[\alpha]_D$: −13 Solvent: Chf
Spectral Data: UV, IR, CMR, PMR, Mass Spec.
Organism: *Trikentrion flabelliforme* (Porifera)
Location: Darwin, Australia
Reference: 145

$C_{18}H_{14}N_2O_3$ **Norsegoline**

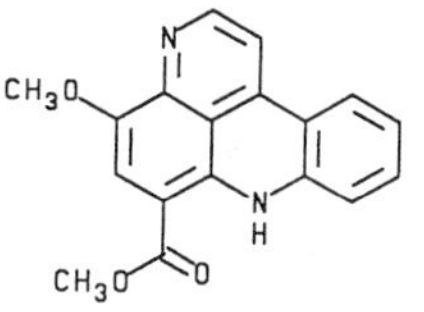

Mol. Wt.: 306
Spectral Data: UV, IR, CMR, PMR, Mass Spec.
Organism: *Eudistoma* sp. (Chordata/Tunicata)
Location: Gulf of Suez
Reference: 954

$C_{18}H_{14}N_4O_2$ **Calliactine** (revised formula)

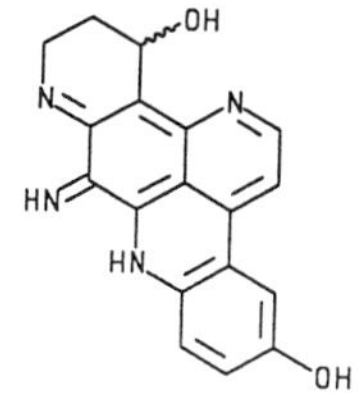

(other structures possible)

Mol. Wt.: 318
Spectral Data: UV, CMR, PMR, Mass Spec.
Organism: *Calliactis parasitica* (Coelenterata)
Location: Naples, Italy
Reference: 181

$C_{19}H_{13}BrN_2O$ **Eudistomin R**

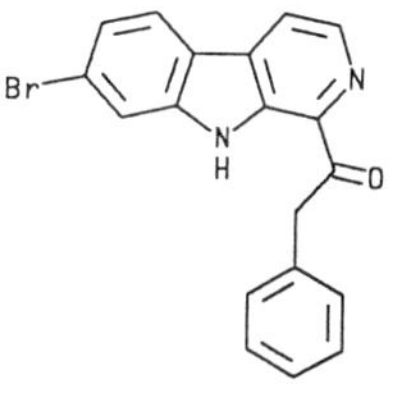

Mol. Wt.: 365
Spectral Data: UV, IR, PMR, Mass Spec.
Organism: *Eudistoma olivaceum* (Chordata/Tunicata)
Location: Bermuda
Reference: 561

$C_{19}H_{13}BrN_2O$ **Eudistomin S**

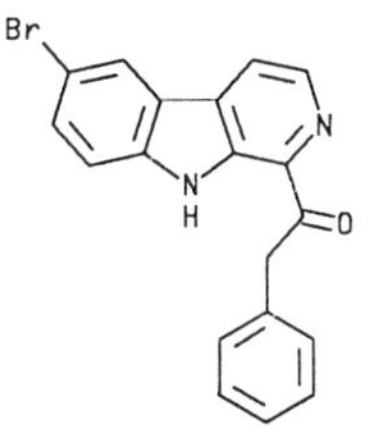

Mol. Wt.: 365
Spectral Data: UV, IR, PMR, Mass Spec.
Organism: *Eudistoma olivaceum* (Chordata/Tunicata)
Location: Bermuda
Reference: 561

$C_{19}H_{14}N_2O$ **Eudistomin T**

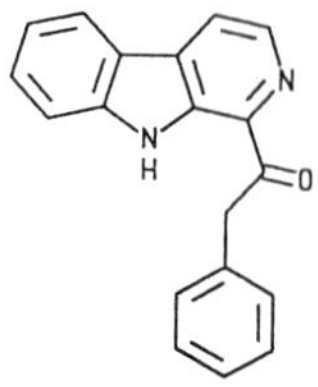

Mol. Wt.: 286
Spectral Data: IR, PMR, Mass Spec.
Organism: *Eudistoma olivaceum* (Chordata/Tunicata)
Location: Bermuda
Reference: 561

$C_{19}H_{14}Br_3N_3O$ **Hinckdentine-A**

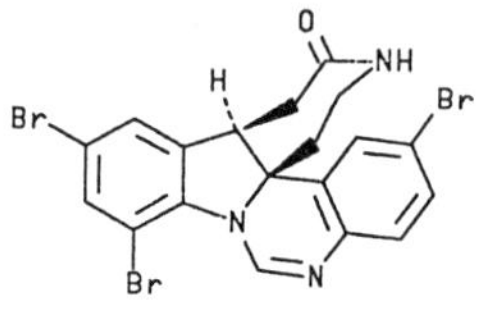

Mol. Wt.: 540
Melting Point: 196–197°C
$[\alpha]_D^{25}$: +274
Spectral Data: UV, IR, PMR, Mass Spec., x-ray c.s.
Organism: *Hincksinoflustra denticulata* (Bryozoa)
Location: Tasmania
Reference: 73

$C_{19}H_{19}N_3O_6$ **Mm-1**

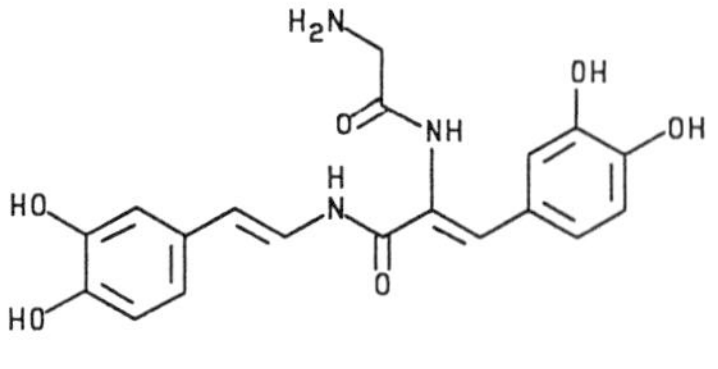

Mol. Wt.: 385
Bioactivity: Blood reducing pigment
Spectral Data: UV, PMR, Mass Spec. (acetate)
Organism: *Molgula manhattensis* (Chordata/Tunicata)
Location: Cape Cod Canal
Reference: 852

$C_{19}H_{19}ClN_4O_2$

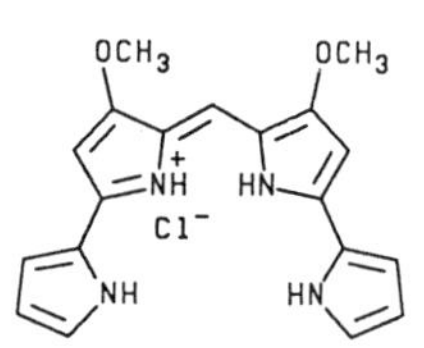

Mol. Wt.: 370
Bioactivity: Antimicrobial activity
Spectral Data: UV, CMR, PMR, Mass Spec.
Organism: *Bugula dentata* (Bryozoa)
Location: Japan
Reference: 712

$C_{19}H_{33}N_3O_5$ **Janolusimide**

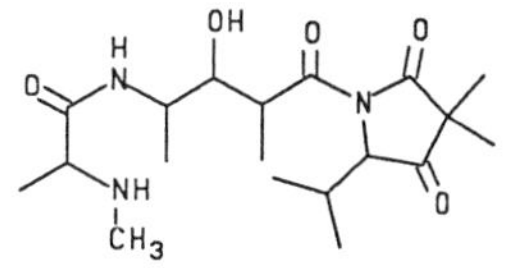

Mol. Wt.: 383
Bioactivity: Toxic to mice at 5mg/kg
$[\alpha]_D^{25}$: -10.3 Solvent: Chf
Spectral Data: IR, CMR, PMR, Mass Spec.
Organism: *Janolus cristatus* Delle Chiaje (Mollusca)
Location: Naples, Italy
Reference: 184, 1026

$C_{20}H_{11}Br_5N_4O_2$ **Chartellamide B**

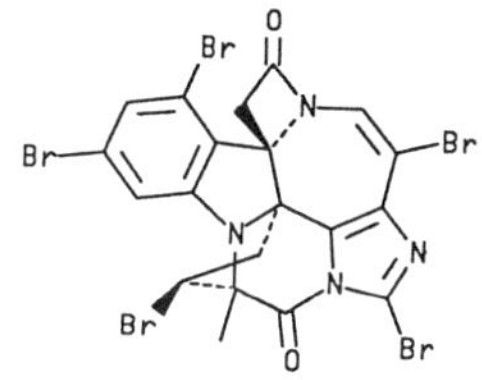

Mol. Wt.: 739
Spectral Data: UV, CD, IR, CMR, PMR, Mass Spec.
Organism: *Chartella papyracea* (Ellis and Solander) (syn. *Flustra papyracea*) (Bryozoa)
Location: Brittany, France
Reference: 28

$C_{20}H_{12}Br_4N_4O_2$ **Chartellamide A**

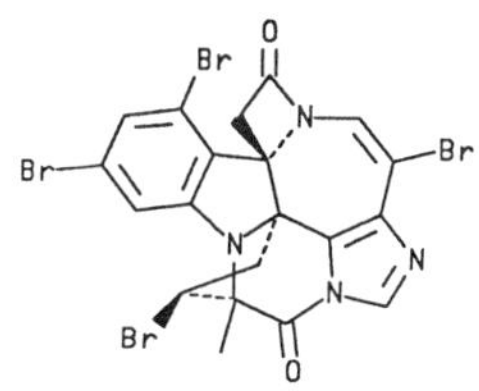

Mol. Wt.: 660
Spectral Data: UV, CD, IR, CMR, PMR, Mass Spec.
Organism: *Chartella papyracea* (Ellis and Solander) (syn. *Flustra papyracea*) (Bryozoa)
Location: Brittany, France
Reference: 28

$C_{20}H_{14}Br_3ClN_4O$ **Chartelline B**

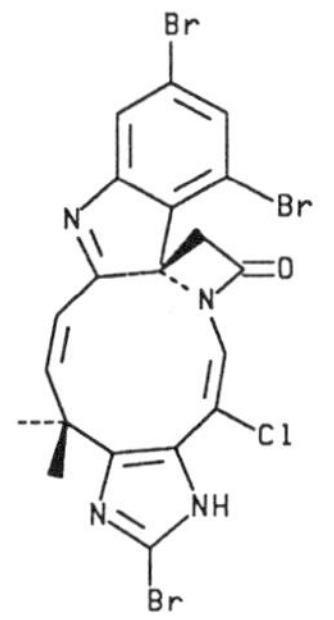

Mol. Wt.: 601
$[\alpha]_D^{20}$: -339.1 Solvent: Alc
Spectral Data: UV, CD, IR, CMR, PMR, Mass Spec.
Organism: *Chartella papyracea* (Ellis and Solander) (syn. *Flustra papyracea*) (Bryozoa)
Location: Brittany, France
Reference: 29

$C_{20}H_{15}Br_2ClN_4O$ **Chartelline C**

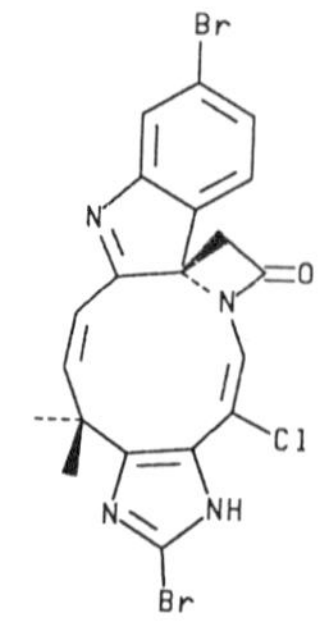

Mol. Wt.: 522
$[\alpha]_D^{20}$: −217.4 Solvent: Alc
Spectral Data: UV, CD, IR, PMR, Mass Spec.
Organism: *Chartella papyracea* (Ellis and Solander)
(syn. *Flustra papyracea*)
(Bryozoa)
Location: Brittany, France
Reference: 29

$C_{21}H_{17}BrClN_3O_2$ **Petrosamine**

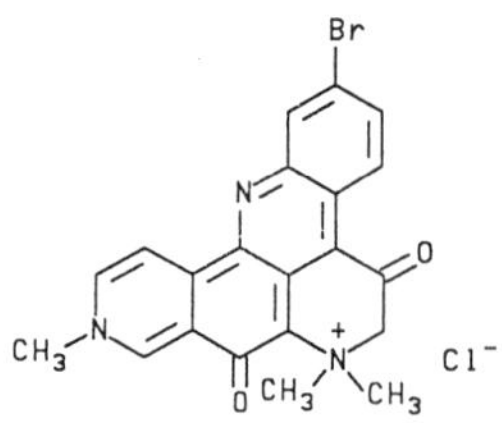

Mol. Wt.: 458
Melting Point: >330°C
Spectral Data: UV, IR, CMR, PMR, Mass Spec.,
x-ray c.s.
Organism: *Petrosia* sp.
(Porifera)
Location: Belize
Reference: 752

$C_{21}H_{17}BrN_4O_2S$ **Shermilamine A**

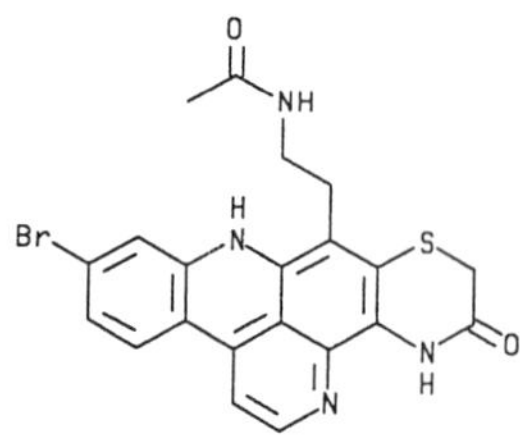

Mol. Wt.: 469
Melting Point: 135°C
Spectral Data: UV, IR, CMR, PMR, Mass Spec.,
x-ray c.s.
Organism: *Trididemnum* sp.
(Chordata/Tunicata)
Location: Guam
Reference: 196

$C_{21}H_{24}N_2O_4$ **Isopteropodine**
(Previously known)

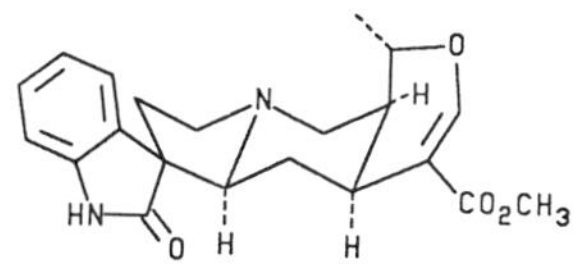

Mol. Wt.: 368
Melting Point: 205–206°C
$[\alpha]_D^{20}$: −109
Spectral Data: UV, IR, CMR, PMR, Mass Spec.
Organism: *Nerita albicilla* L.
(Mollusca)
Location: Queensland, Australia
Reference: 91, 704, 834

$C_{21}H_{27}BrN_2O$ **Flustramide B**

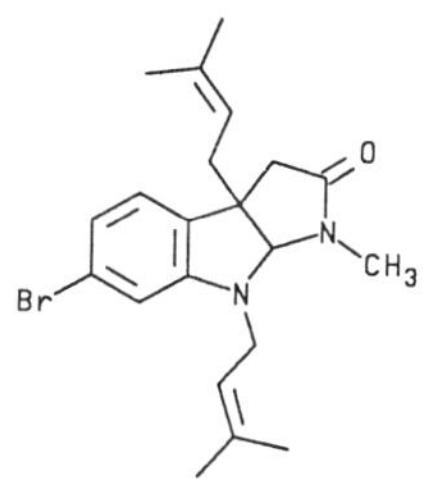

Mol. Wt.: 403
Melting Point: Oil
$[\alpha]_D^{20}$: −53.79 Solvent: Alc
Spectral Data: UV, IR, PMR, Mass Spec.
Organism: *Flustra foliaceae*
(Bryozoa)
Location: North Sea
Reference: 539

$C_{21}H_{29}BrN_2$ **Flustramine D**

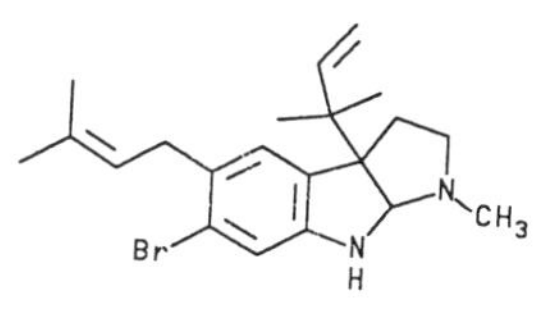

Mol. Wt.: 389
Bioactivity: Antibacterial activity
Melting Point: Oil
$[\alpha]_D^{25}$: −86.5 Solvent: Dcm
Spectral Data: UV, IR, CMR, PMR, Mass Spec.
Organism: *Flustra foliacea*
(Bryozoa)
Location: Eastern Canada
Reference: 638

$C_{21}H_{29}BrN_2$ **Isoflustramine D**
(isolated as part of mixture)

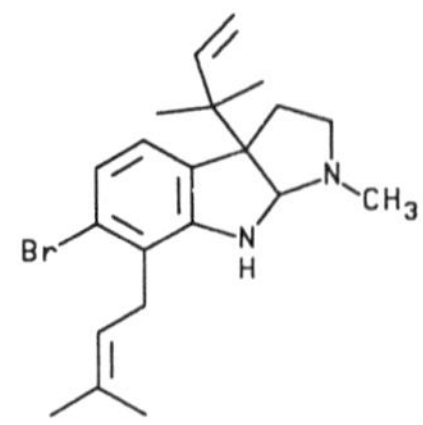

Mol. Wt.: 389
Bioactivity: Antibacterial activity
Spectral Data: UV, IR, PMR, Mass Spec.
Organism: *Flustra foliacea* (Bryozoa)
Location: Eastern Canada
Reference: 638

$C_{21}H_{29}BrN_2O$ **Flustramine D N-oxide**

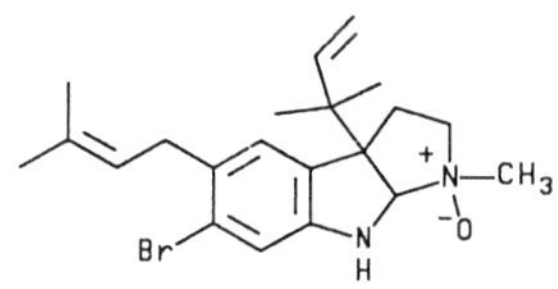

Mol. Wt.: 405
Bioactivity: Antibacterial activity
Melting Point: Oil
Spectral Data: UV, IR, CMR, PMR, Mass Spec.
Organism: *Flustra foliacea* (Bryozoa)
Location: Eastern Canada
Reference: 638

$C_{21}H_{29}BrN_2O$ **Flustrarine B**

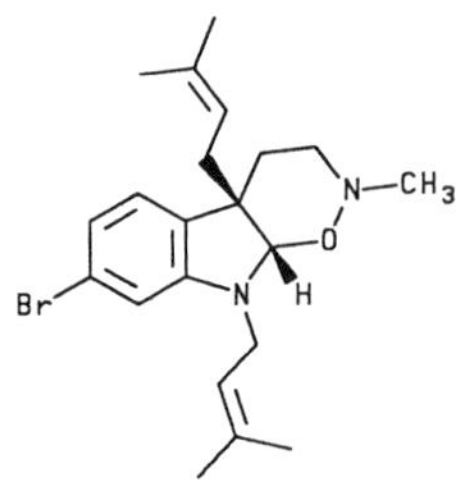

Mol. Wt.: 405
$[\alpha]_D^{20}$: −180 Solvent: Alc
Spectral Data: UV, IR, CMR, PMR, Mass Spec.
Organism: *Flustra foliaceae* (Bryozoa)
Location: North Sea
Reference: 539

$C_{21}H_{44}NO_6P$ **1-(1-Hexadecenyl)-sn-glycerol-3-phosphorylethanolamine**

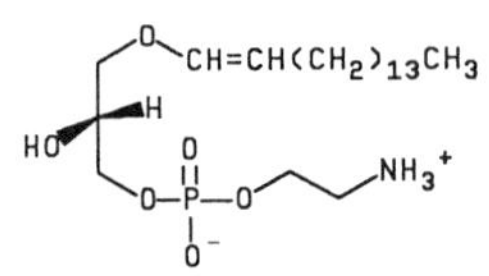

Mol. Wt.: 437
Bioactivity: Hemolytic activity
Melting Point: 187°C (dec.)
$[\alpha]_D^{23}$: −2.9 Solvent: Chf
Spectral Data: IR, CMR, PMR, Mass Spec.
Organism: *Solanderia secunda* (Coelenterata)
Location: Japan
Reference: 338

$C_{22}H_{15}NO_7S$ **3-Ketoadociaquinone A**

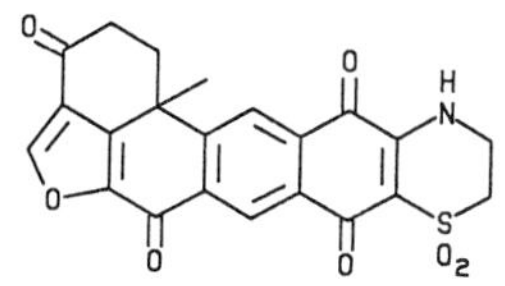

Mol. Wt.: 437
Melting Point: >300°C (dec.)
$[\alpha]_D$: +65.4
Spectral Data: UV, IR, CMR, PMR, Mass Spec.
Organism: *Adocia* sp. (Porifera)
Location: Truk
Reference: 982

$C_{22}H_{17}NO_6S$ **Adociaquinone A**

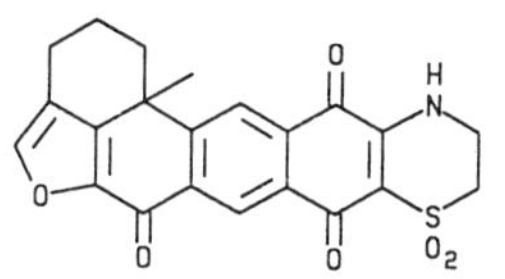

Mol. Wt.: 423
Melting Point: >300°C (dec.)
$[\alpha]_D$: +25
Spectral Data: UV, IR, CMR, PMR, Mass Spec.
Organism: *Adocia* sp. (Porifera)
Location: Truk
Reference: 982

$C_{22}H_{24}Br_2N_4O_6S_2$ **(E,E)-N,N'-Bis[3-(3'-bromo-4'-hydroxyphenyl)-2-oximidopropionyl]cystamine**

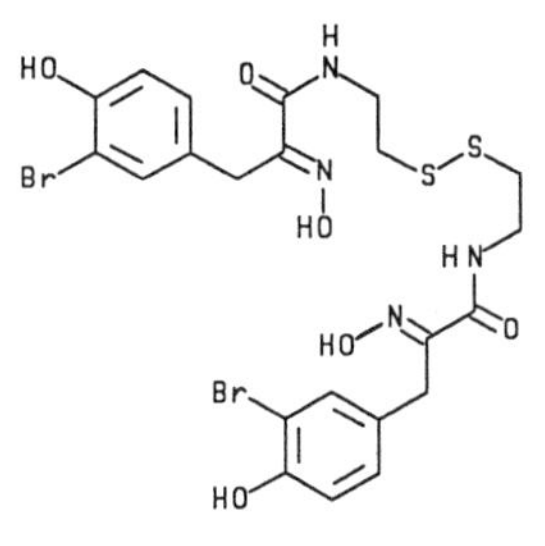

Mol. Wt.: 664
Melting Point: 172–174°C
Spectral Data: UV, IR, CMR, PMR, Mass Spec.
Organism: Unknown sp. (Porifera)
Location: Guam
Reference: 32

$C_{22}H_{24}Br_2N_4O_6S_2$ **(E,Z)-N,N'-Bis[3-(3'-bromo-4'-hydroxyphenyl)-2-oximidopropionyl] cystamine**

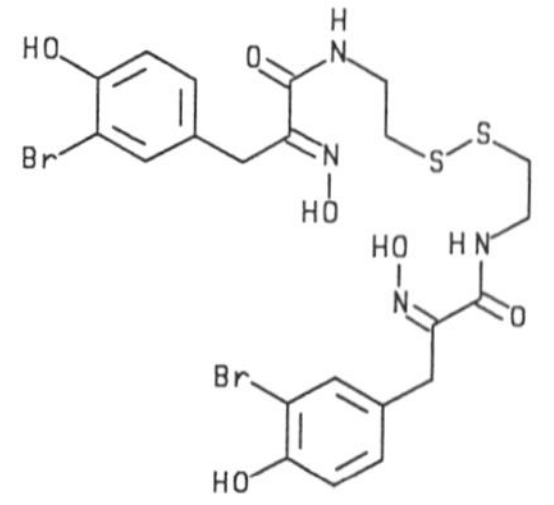

Mol. Wt.: 664
Spectral Data: IR, CMR, PMR
Organism: Unknown sp. (Porifera)
Location: Guam
Reference: 32

$C_{22}H_{36}N_2O$ **Niphatyne B**

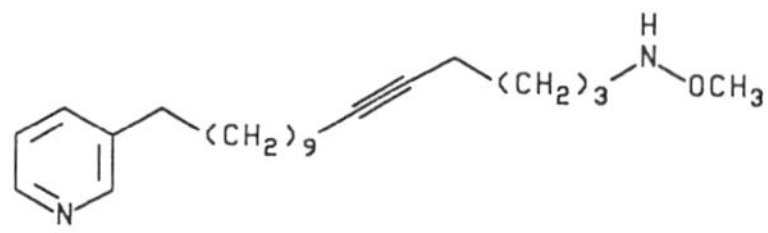

Mol. Wt.: 344
Spectral Data: UV, IR, CMR, PMR, Mass Spec.
Organism: *Niphates* sp. (Porifera)
Location: Vitu Levu, Fiji
Reference: 906

$C_{22}H_{48}NO_6P$ **1-Tetradecyl-sn-glycerol-3-phosphorylcholine**

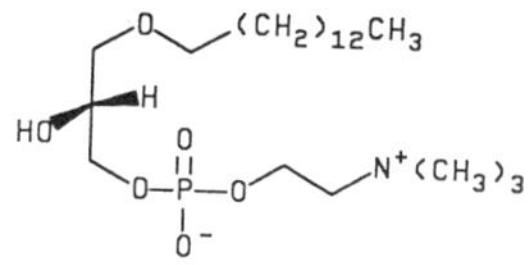

Mol. Wt.: 453
Bioactivity: 155°C (dec.)
$[\alpha]_D^{23}$: −2.4 Solvent: Chf
Spectral Data: IR, CMR, PMR, Mass Spec.
Organism: *Solanderia secunda* (Coelenterata)
Location: Japan
Reference: 338

$C_{23}H_{19}N_3O_3$ **Isosegoline A**

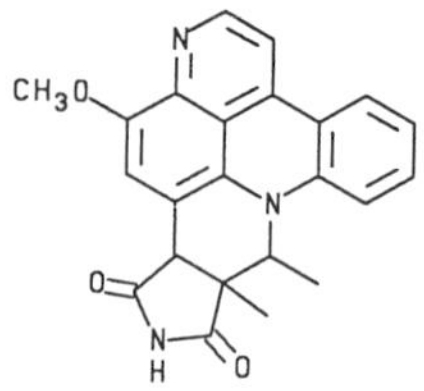

Mol. Wt.: 385
Spectral Data: UV, IR, CMR, PMR
Organism: *Eudistoma* sp. (Chordata/Tunicata)
Location: Gulf of Suez
Reference: 954

$C_{23}H_{19}N_3O_3$ **Segoline A**

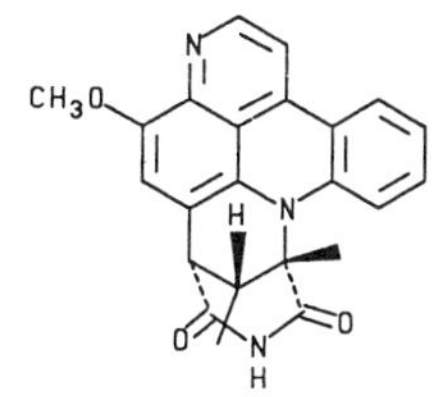

Mol. Wt.: 385
Melting Point: >300°C
$[\alpha]_D^{25}$: −322
Spectral Data: UV, IR, PMR, x-ray c.s.
Organism: *Eudistoma* sp. (Chordata/Tunicata)
Location: Gulf of Suez
Reference: 954

$C_{23}H_{27}N_3O_6$ **Mm-2**

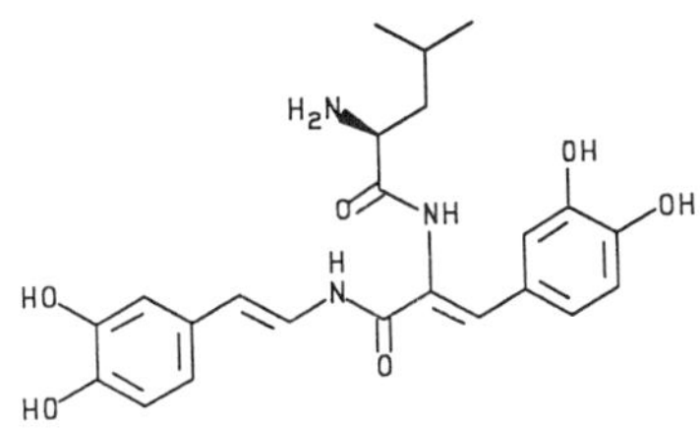

Mol. Wt.: 441
Bioactivity: Blood reducing pigment
Spectral Data: UV, CD, PMR, Mass Spec. (acetate)
Organism: *Molgula manhattensis* (Chordata/Tunicata)
Location: Cape Cod Canal
Reference: 852

$C_{24}H_{52}NO_6P$ **1-Hexadecyl-sn-glycerol-3-phosphorylcholine**

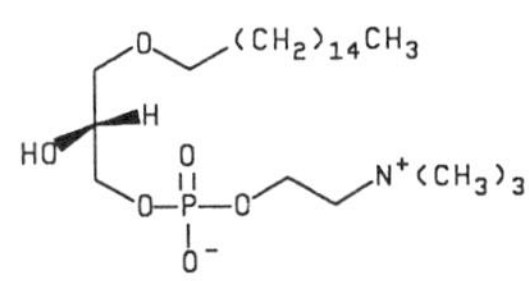

Mol. Wt.: 481
Bioactivity: Hemolytic activity
Melting Point: 155°C (dec.)
$[\alpha]_D^{23}$: −2.4 Solvent: Chf
Spectral Data: IR, CMR, PMR, Mass Spec.
Organism: *Solanderia secunda* (Coelenterata)
Location: Japan
Reference: 338

$C_{25}H_{15}NO_8$ **Lamellarin H**

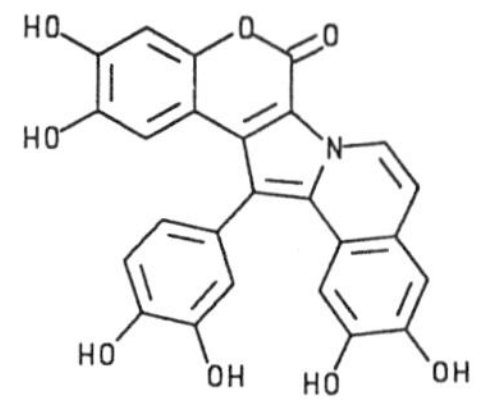

Mol. Wt.: 457
Spectral Data: UV, CMR, PMR, Mass Spec.
Organism: *Didemnum chartaceum* (Chordata/Tunicata)
Location: Seychelles
Reference: 662

$C_{25}H_{40}N_2$ **Haliclonadiamine** (also isolated as the hydrochloride salt)

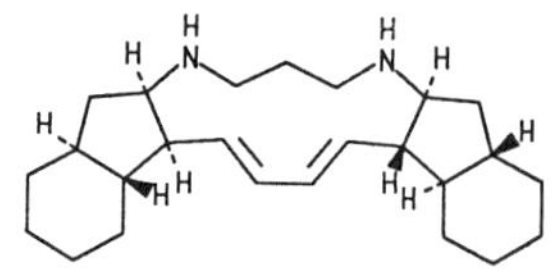

Mol. Wt.: 368
Bioactivity: Antimicrobial activity towards *Candida albicans*, *Bacillus subtilis* and *Staphylococcus aureus*
Melting Point: 115–117°C (hydrochloride)
$[\alpha]_D$: −18.2
Spectral Data: UV, IR, CMR, PMR, x-ray c.s. (of the diacetate)
Organism: *Haliclona* sp. (Porifera)
Location: Palau
Reference: 280

$C_{25}H_{40}N_2$ **Papuamine** (also isolated as the dihydrochloride)

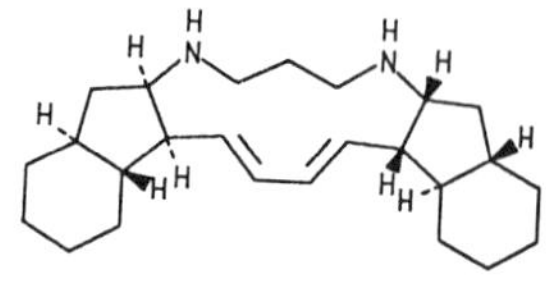

Mol. Wt.: 368
Bioactivity: Antifungal: inhibits growth of *Trichophyton mentagrophytes* Antimicrobial: inhibits growth of *Candida albicans*, *Bacillus subtilis*, and *Straphyloccus aureus*
Melting Point: 167.5–169°C
$[\alpha]_D$: −150 Solvent: Me
Spectral Data: IR, CMR, PMR, Mass Spec.
Organism: *Haliclona* sp. (Porifera)
Location: Papua New Guinea; Palau
Reference: 47, 280

$C_{26}H_{25}N_3O_9$ **An-3**

Mol. Wt.: 523
Bioactivity: Blood reducing pigment
Spectral Data: UV, CD, IR, CMR, PMR, Mass Spec. (acetate)
Organism: *Ascidia nigra* (Chordata/Tunicata)
Location: Florida
Reference: 852

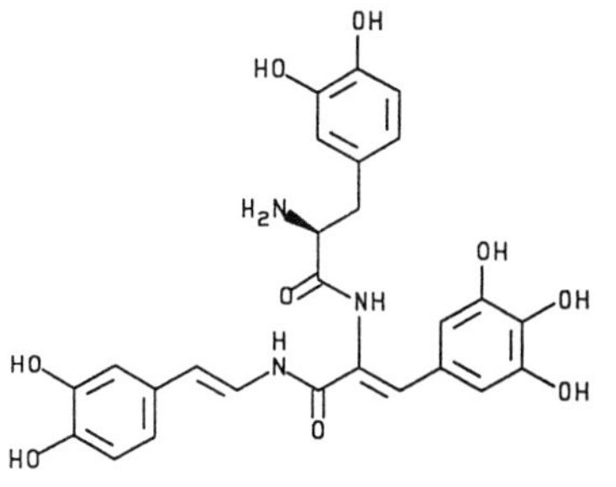

$C_{26}H_{25}N_3O_{10}$ **An-2**

Mol. Wt.: 539
Bioactivity: Reducing blood pigment
Spectral Data: UV, CD, IR, CMR, PMR, Mass Spec. (acetate)
Organism: *Ascidia nigra* (Chordata/Tunicata)
Location: Florida
Reference: 852

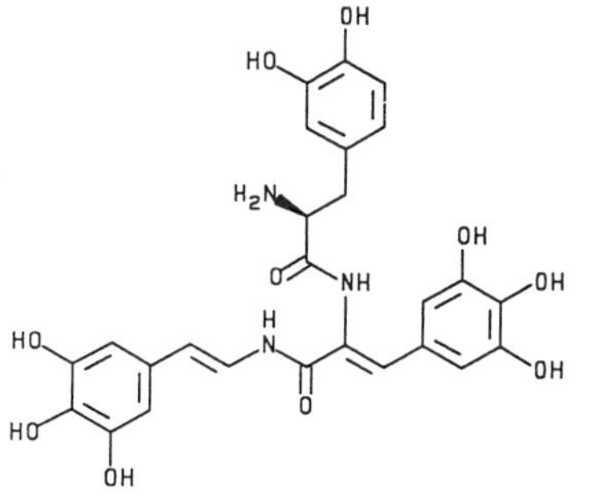

$C_{26}H_{25}N_3O_{11}$ **An-1 (Tunichrome B-1)**

Mol. Wt.: 555
Bioactivity: Reducing blood pigment
Spectral Data: UV, IR, CD, CMR, PMR, Mass Spec.
Organism: *Ascidia nigra* L.
A. ceratodes
Perophora viridis
(Chordata/Tunicata)
Location: Florida
Reference: 113, 114, 852

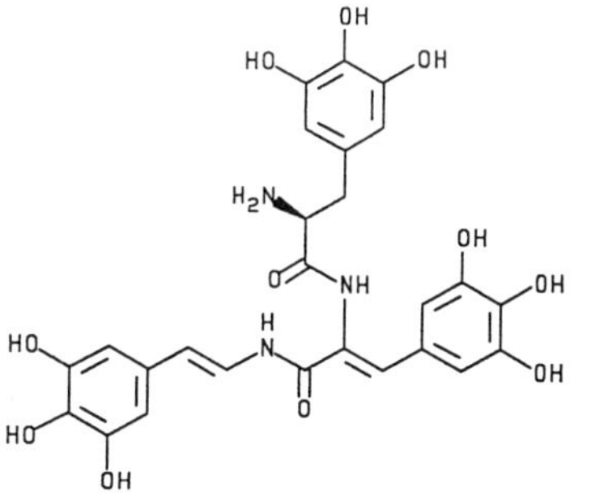

$C_{26}H_{40}ClN_5$ **Agelasine-A**

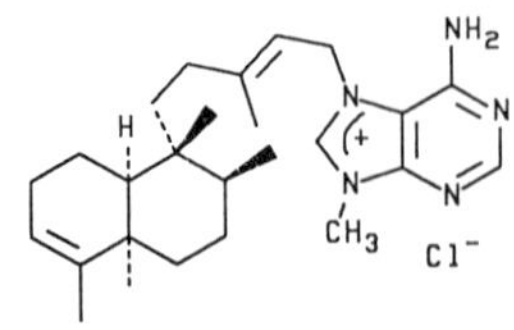

Mol. Wt.: 457
Melting Point: 173–174°C
$[\alpha]_D$: −31.3 Solvent: Me
Spectral Data: UV, IR, CMR, PMR, Mass Spec., CD of derivative
Organism: *Agelas nakamurai* (Porifera)
Location: Okinawa, Japan
Reference: 1190

$C_{26}H_{40}ClN_5$ **Agelasine-B**

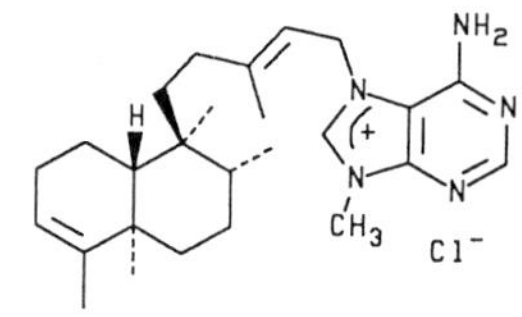

Mol. Wt.: 457
Melting Point: 167–170°C
$[\alpha]_D$: −21.5 Solvent: Me
Spectral Data: UV, IR, CMR, PMR, Mass Spec.
Organism: *Agelas nakamurai* (Porifera)
Location: Okinawa, Japan
Reference: 1190

$C_{26}H_{40}ClN_5$ **Agelasine-C**

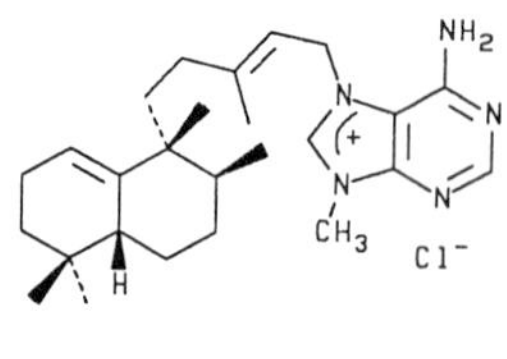

Mol. Wt.: 457
Melting Point: 176–179°C
$[\alpha]_D$: −55.1 Solvent: Me
Spectral Data: UV, IR, PMR, Mass Spec.; CD of derivative
Organism: *Agelas nakamurai* (Porifera)
Location: Okinawa, Japan
Reference: 1190

$C_{26}H_{40}ClN_5$ **Agelasine-D**

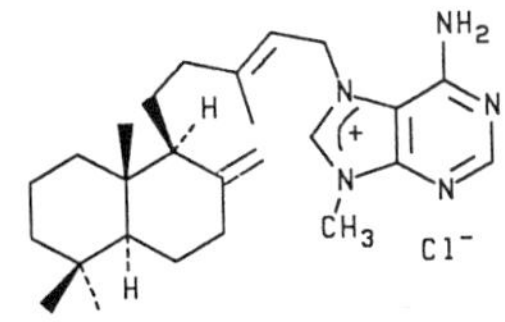

Mol. Wt.: 457
Melting Point: 175–176°C
$[\alpha]_D$: +10.4 Solvent: Me
Spectral Data: UV, IR, CMR, PMR, Mass Spec.
Organism: *Agelas nakamurai* (Porifera)
Location: Okinawa, Japan
Reference: 1190

$C_{26}H_{40}ClN_5$ **Agelasine-E**

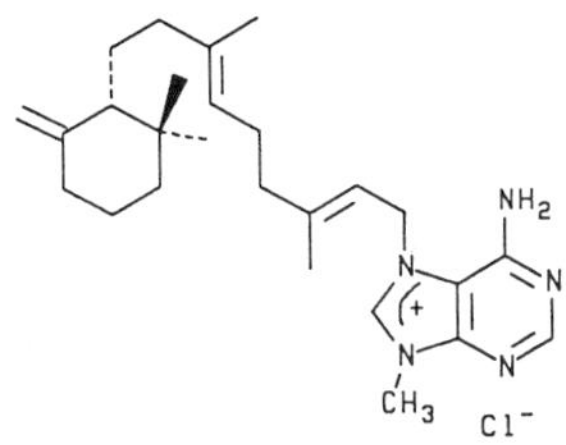

Mol. Wt.: 457
Melting Point: 180–182°C
$[\alpha]_D$: −17.1 Solvent: Me
Spectral Data: UV, IR, CMR, PMR, Mass Spec.; CD of derivative
Organism: *Agelas nakamurai* (Porifera)
Location: Okinawa, Japan
Reference: 1190

$C_{27}H_{44}N_2O_8$ **Bengazole A**

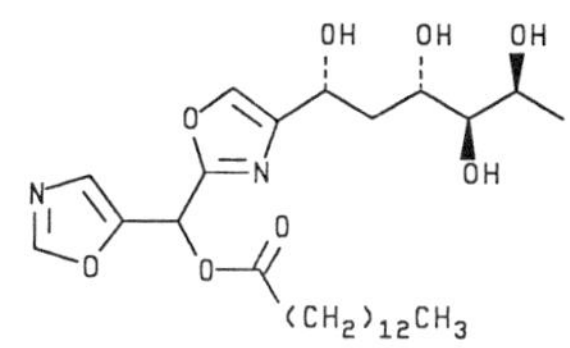

Mol. Wt.: 524
Bioactivity: Anthelminthic activity
Melting Point: Oil
$[\alpha]_D^{20}$: +5.0 Solvent: Me
Spectral Data: UV, IR, CMR, PMR, Mass Spec.
Organism: *Jaspidae* sp. (Porifera)
Location: Fiji
Reference: 4

$C_{28}H_{23}NO_8$ **Lamellarin G**

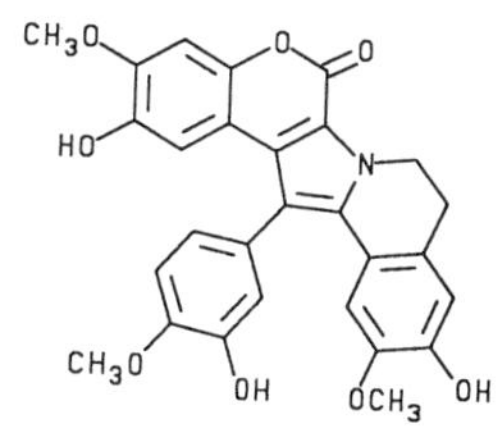

Mol. Wt.: 501
Melting Point: 263–265°C (dec.)
Spectral Data: UV, IR, CMR, PMR, Mass Spec.
Organism: *Didemnum chartaceum* (Chordata/Tunicata)
Location: Seychelles
Reference: 662

$C_{28}H_{36}N_2O_6$ **Sarcodictyin A**

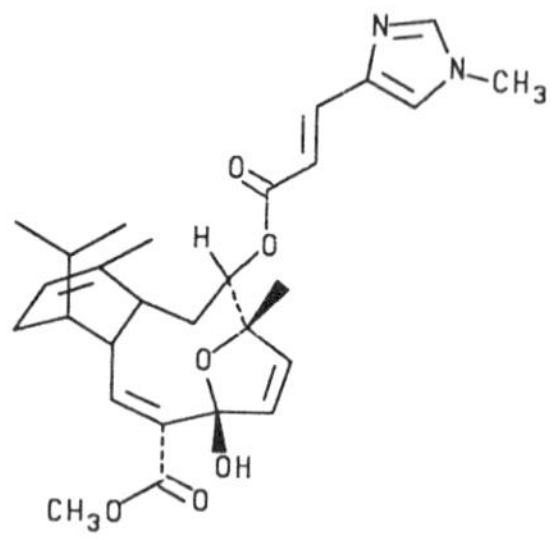

Mol. Wt.: 496
Melting Point: 219–222°C
$[\alpha]_D^{20}$: –15.2 Solvent: Alc
Spectral Data: UV, IR, CMR, PMR, Mass Spec.; CD of derivative
Organism: *Sarcodictyon roseum* (=*Rolandia rosea*) (Coelenterata)
Location: Northwest Mediterranean
Reference: 215

$C_{28}H_{36}N_2O_7$ **Sarcodictyin C**

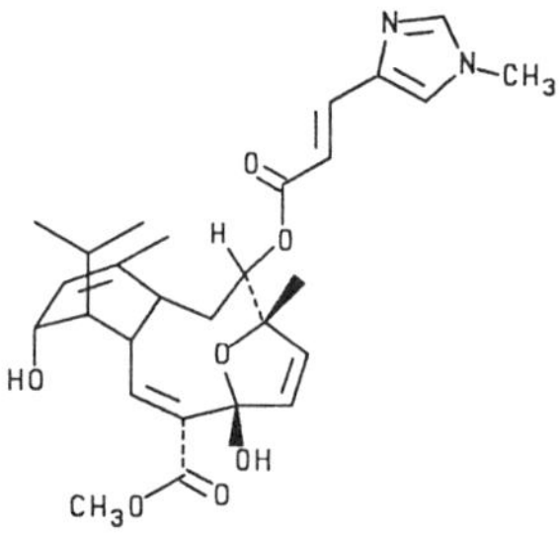

Mol. Wt.: 512
Melting Point: 225–227°C
$[\alpha]_D^{20}$: –16.5 Solvent: Alc
Spectral Data: UV, IR, CMR, PMR, Mass Spec.
Organism: *Sarcodictyon roseum* (Coelenterata)
Location: Northwest Mediterranean
Reference: 216

$C_{28}H_{36}N_2O_7$ **Sarcodictyin E**

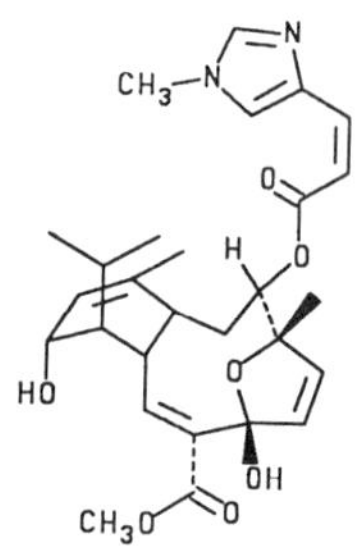

Mol. Wt.: 512
Melting Point: 212–214°C
$[\alpha]_D^{20}$: +15.6 Solvent: Me
Spectral Data: UV, CMR, PMR
Organism: *Sarcodictyon roseum* (Coelenterata)
Location: Northwest Mediterranean
Reference: 216

$C_{28}H_{36}N_2O_7$ **Sarcodictyin F**

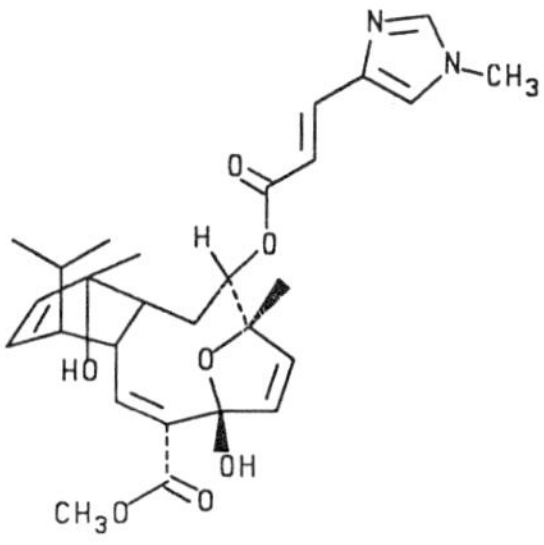

Mol. Wt.: 512
Melting Point: 228–229°
$[\alpha]_D^{20}$: +2.7 Solvent: Me
Spectral Data: PMR, CMR, Mass Spec.
Organism: *Sarcodictyon roseum* (Coelenterata)
Location: Northwest Mediterranean
Reference: 216

$C_{28}H_{40}BrN_3O_6$ **Geodiamolide B**

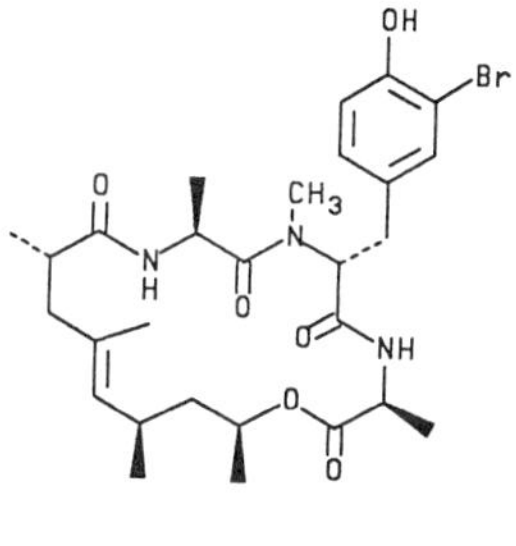

Mol. Wt.: 594
Bioactivity: Antifungal activity against *Candida albicans*
Melting Point: 203–204°C
$[\alpha]_D^{22}$: +101 Solvent: Chf
Spectral Data: UV, IR, CMR, PMR, Mass Spec., x-ray c.s.
Organism: *Geodia* sp. (Porifera)
Location: Trinidad and Tobago, West Indies
Reference: 162

$C_{28}H_{40}IN_3O_6$ **Geodiamolide A**

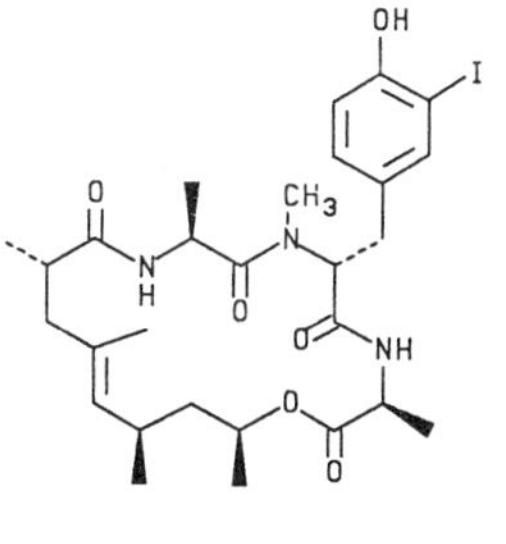

Mol. Wt.: 641
Bioactivity: Antifungal activity against *Candida albicans*
Melting Point: 217–218°C
$[\alpha]_D^{25}$: +53 Solvent: Chf
Spectral Data: UV, IR, CMR, PMR, Mass Spec., x-ray c.s.
Organism: *Geodia* sp. (Porifera)
Location: Trinidad and Tobago, West Indies
Reference: 162

$C_{28}H_{46}N_2O_8$ **Bengazole B**

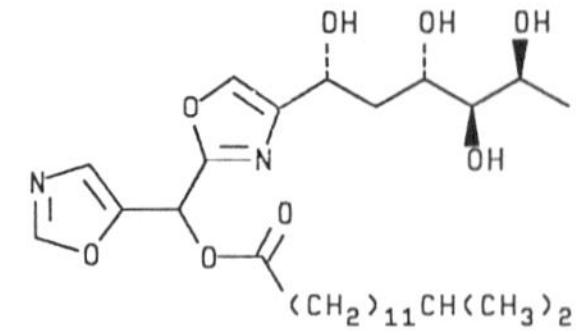

Mol. Wt.: 538
Bioactivity: Anthelmintic activity
Melting Point: Oil
$[\alpha]_D^{20}$: +4.7 Solvent: Me
Spectral Data: UV, IR, CMR, PMR, Mass Spec.
Organism: *Jaspidae* sp. (Porifera)
Location: Fiji
Reference: 4

$C_{29}H_{25}NO_9$ **Lamellarin E**

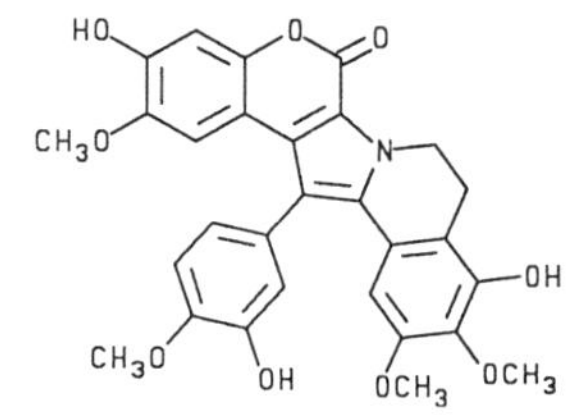

Mol. Wt.: 531
Melting Point: 228–232°C
Spectral Data: UV, IR, CMR, PMR, Mass Spec., x-ray c.s.
Organism: *Didemnum chartaceum* (Chordata/Tunicata)
Location: Seychelles
Reference: 662

$C_{29}H_{38}N_2O_6$ **Sarcodictyin B**

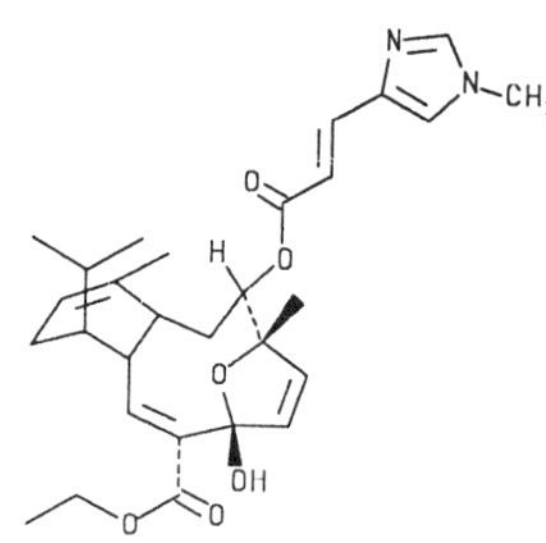

Mol. Wt.: 510
$[\alpha]_D^{20}$: −4.36 Solvent: Alc
Spectral Data: CMR, PMR
Organism: *Sarcodictyon roseum* (=*Rolandia rosea*) (Coelenterata)
Location: Northwest Mediterranean
Reference: 215

$C_{30}H_{27}NO_9$ **Lamellarin F**

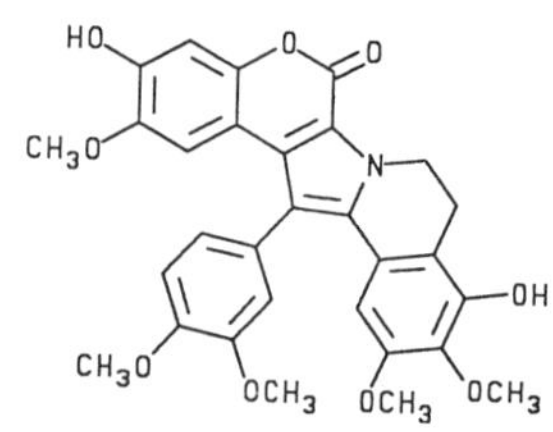

Mol. Wt.: 545
Melting Point: 273–276°C (dec.)
Spectral Data: UV, IR, CMR, PMR, Mass Spec.
Organism: *Didemnum chartaceum* (Chordata/Tunicata)
Location: Seychelles
Reference: 662

$C_{30}H_{38}N_2O_8$ **Sarcodictyin D**

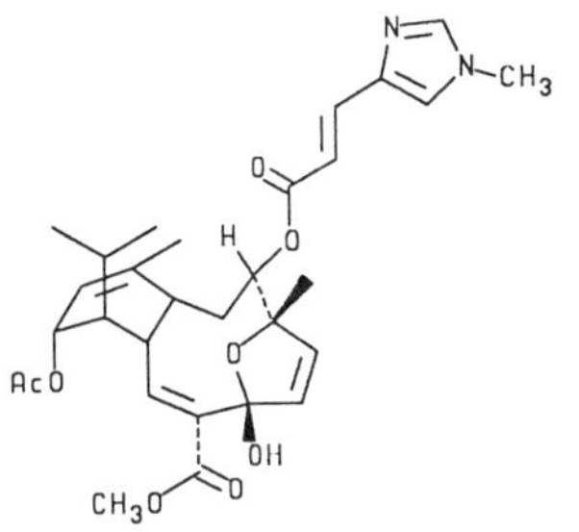

Mol. Wt.: 554
Melting Point: 130–132°
$[\alpha]_D^{20}$: −27.2 Solvent: Me
Spectral Data: CMR, PMR
Organism: *Sarcodictyon roseum* (Coelenterata)
Location: Northwest Mediterranean
Reference: 216

$C_{31}H_{49}Br_2ClN_6O_4$ **Lipopurealin-A**

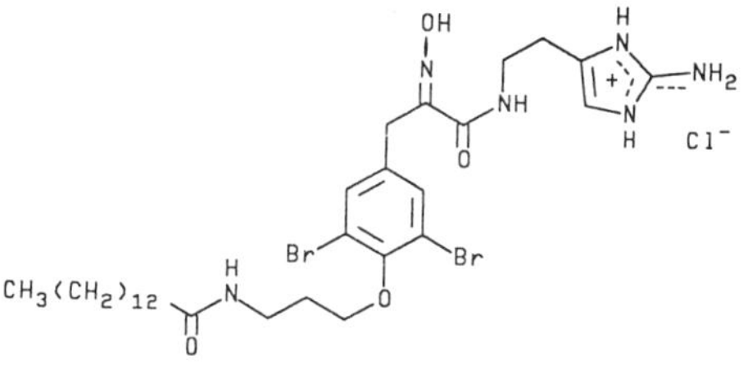

Mol. Wt.: 764
Bioactivity: ATPase inhibition
Melting Point: 94–95°C
Spectral Data: UV, IR, PMR, Mass Spec.
Organism: *Psammaplysilla purea* (Porifera)
Location: Okinawa, Japan
Reference: 1191

$C_{31}H_{56}N_2O_8$ **Bengamide A**

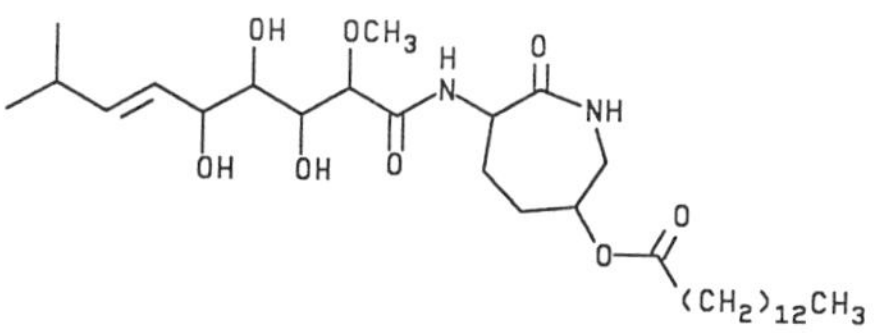

Mol. Wt.: 584
Bioactivity: Anthelmintic activity (against *Nippostrongylus braziliensis*)
Antimicrobial activity
Melting Point: 114–115°C
$[\alpha]_D^{20}$: +30.3 Solvent: Me
Spectral Data: IR, CMR, PMR, Mass Spec.
Organism: Unknown sp. (Porifera)
Location: Fiji Islands
Reference: 905

$C_{32}H_{32}N_4NiO_4$ **Tunichlorin (Nickel(II) 2-devinyl-2-hydroxymethylpyropheophorbide)**

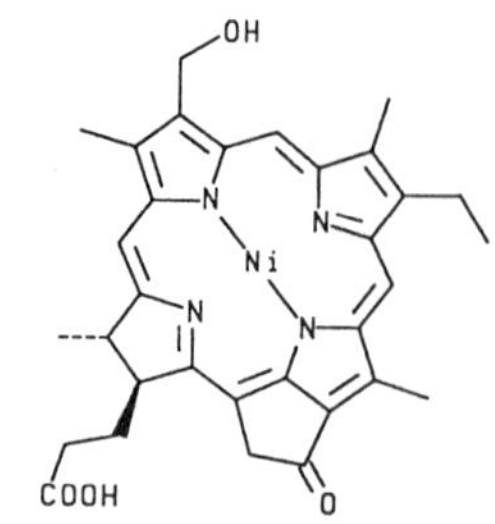

Mol. Wt.: 595
Spectral Data: UV, Mass Spec.; CD, ORD, IR, PMR, Mass Spec. of dimethyl derivative
Organism: *Trididemnum solidum* (Chordata/Tunicata)
Location: Belize
Reference: 66

$C_{32}H_{51}Br_2ClN_6O_4$ **Lipopurealin-B**

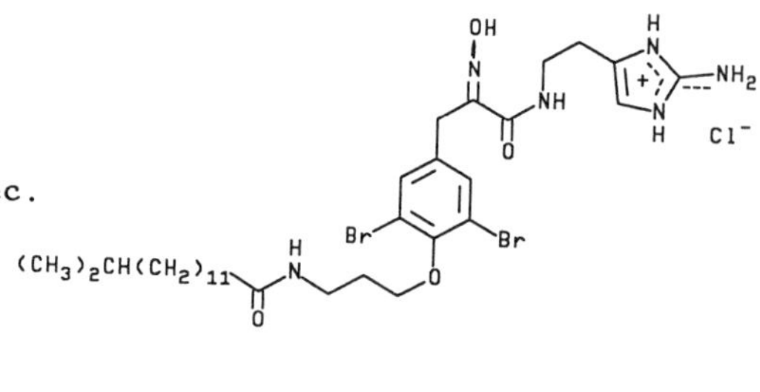

Mol. Wt.: 778
Bioactivity: ATPase inhibition
Melting Point: 93–95°C
Spectral Data: UV, IR, CMR, PMR, Mass Spec.
Organism: *Psammaplysilla purea* (Porifera)
Location: Okinawa, Japan
Reference: 1191

$C_{32}H_{58}N_2O_8$ **Bengamide B**

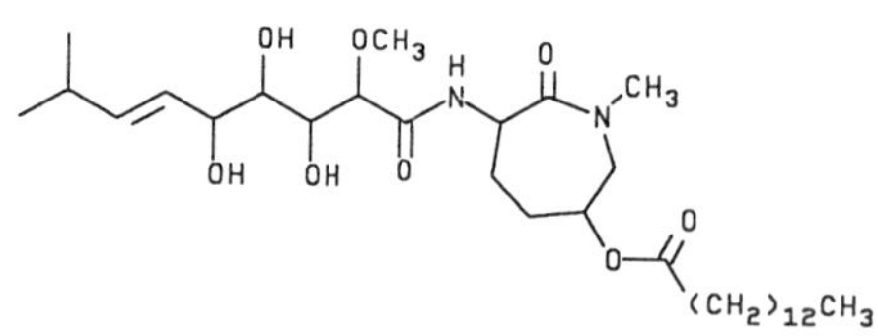

Mol. Wt.: 598
Bioactivity: Anthelmintic activity (against *Nippostrongylus braziliensis*)
Antimicrobial activity
Melting Point: Oil
$[\alpha]_D^{20}$: +34.6 Solvent: Me
Spectral Data: IR, CMR, PMR, Mass Spec.
Organism: Unknown sp. (Porifera)
Location: Fiji Islands
Reference: 905

$C_{33}H_{32}N_4O_2$ **13^2,17^3-Cyclopheophorbide enol**

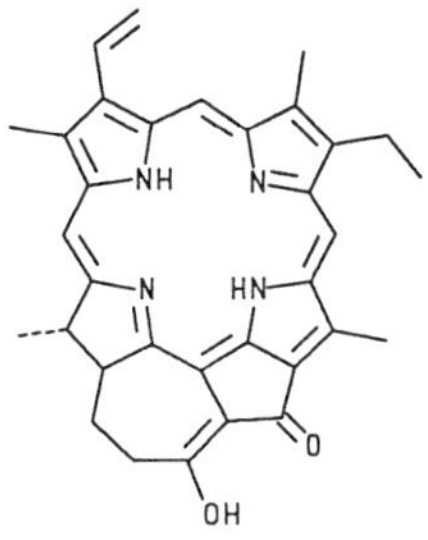

Mol. Wt.: 516
Melting Point: >360°C
Spectral Data: UV, IR, Mass Spec., x-ray c.s.
Organism: *Darwinella oxeata* (Berquist) (Porifera)
Reference: 512

$C_{33}H_{53}Br_2ClN_6O_4$ **Lipopurealin-C**

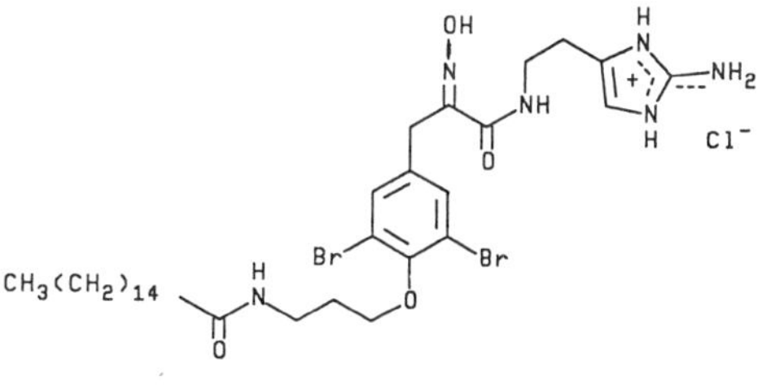

Mol. Wt.: 792
Bioactivity: ATPase inhibition
Melting Point: 108–110°C
Spectral Data: UV, IR, PMR, Mass Spec.
Organism: *Psammaplysilla purea* (Porifera)
Location: Okinawa, Japan
Reference: 1191

$C_{34}H_{65}NO_3$

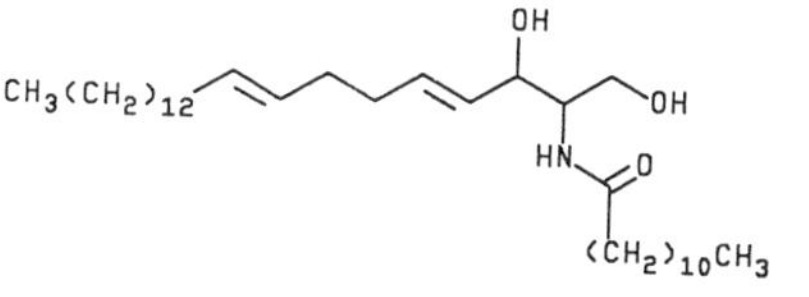

Mol. Wt.: 536
Melting Point: 297–298°C
$[\alpha]_D$: +2.94 Solvent: Chf
Spectral Data: IR, CMR, PMR, Mass Spec.
Organism: *Anemonia sulcata* (Coelenterata)
Location: Tunisia
Reference: 167

$C_{42}H_{57}N_3O_{13}$

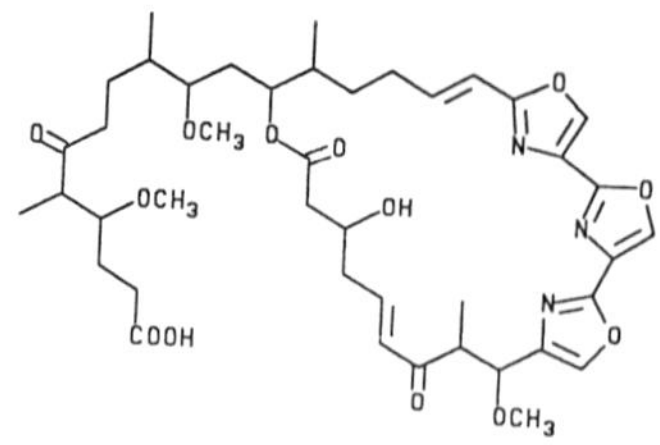

Mol. Wt.: 811
Bioactivity: Antifungal activity
Melting Point: Oil
Spectral Data: UV, IR, CMR, PMR, Mass Spec.
Organism: *Halichondria* sp. (Porifera)
Location: Marshall Islands
Reference: 548

$C_{43}H_{60}N_4O_{13}$

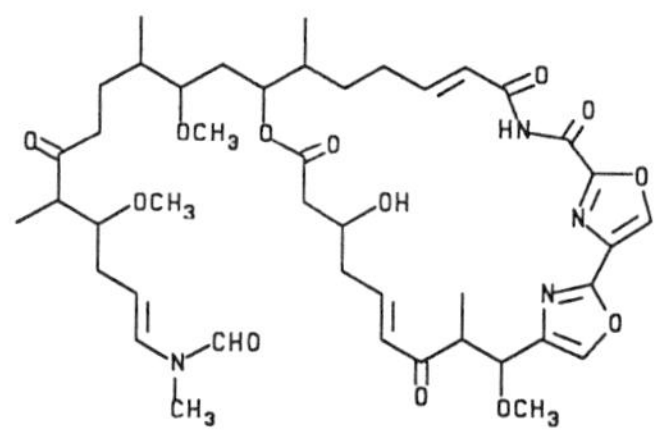

Mol. Wt.: 840
Melting Point: Oil
Spectral Data: UV, IR, CMR, PMR, Mass Spec.
Organism: *Halichondria* sp. (Porifera)
Location: Marshall Islands
Reference: 548

$C_{44}H_{46}Br_4N_8O_{12}S_4$ **Bisaprasin**

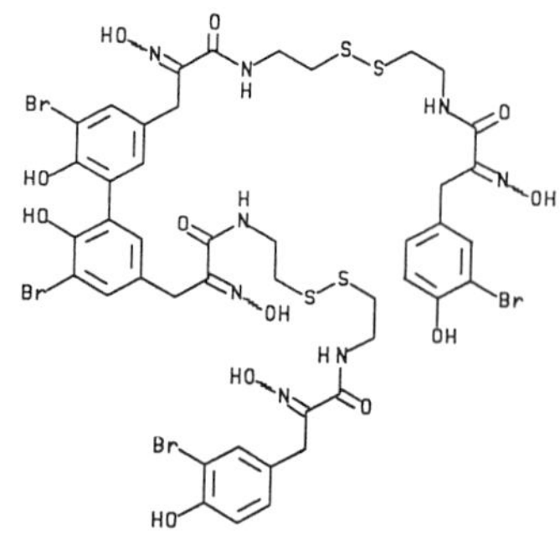

Mol. Wt.: 1326
Bioactivity: Antimicrobial activity
Melting Point: Foam
Spectral Data: UV, IR, CMR, PMR, Mass Spec.
Organism: *Thorectopsamma xana* (Porifera)
Location: Guam
Reference: 940

$C_{44}H_{60}N_4O_{12}$ **Halichondramide**

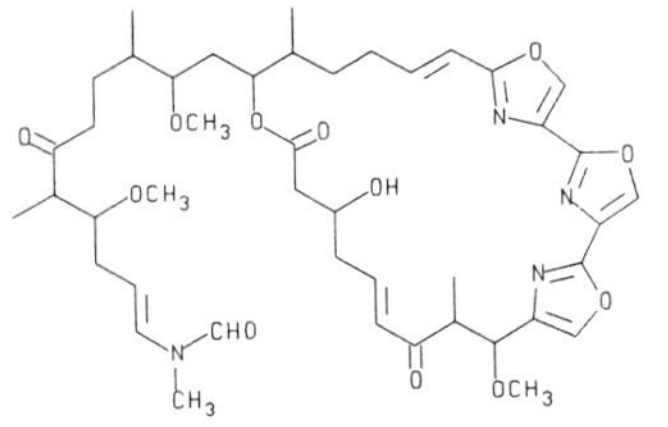

Mol. Wt.: 836
Bioactivity: Inhibition of growth of sea urchin eggs at 4 μg/ml
Antifungal activity
Toxic to mice at 1.4 mg/kg
Melting Point: 66–68°C
$[\alpha]_D$: −100.7 Solvent: Me
Spectral Data: UV, IR, CMR, PMR, Mass Spec.
Organism: *Halichondria* sp.
(Porifera)
Location: Marshall Islands
Reference: 548

$C_{44}H_{60}N_4O_{12}$ **Isohalichondramide**

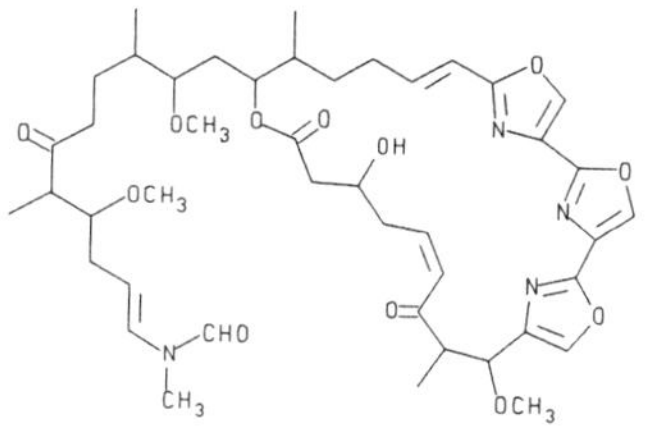

Mol. Wt.: 836
Bioactivity: Inhibition of growth of sea urchin eggs at 4 μg/ml
Antifungal activity
Melting Point: Oil
Spectral Data: CMR, PMR, Mass Spec.
Organism: *Halichondria* sp.
(Porifera)
Location: Marshall Islands
Reference: 548

$C_{44}H_{62}N_4O_{12}$ **Dihydrohalichondramide**

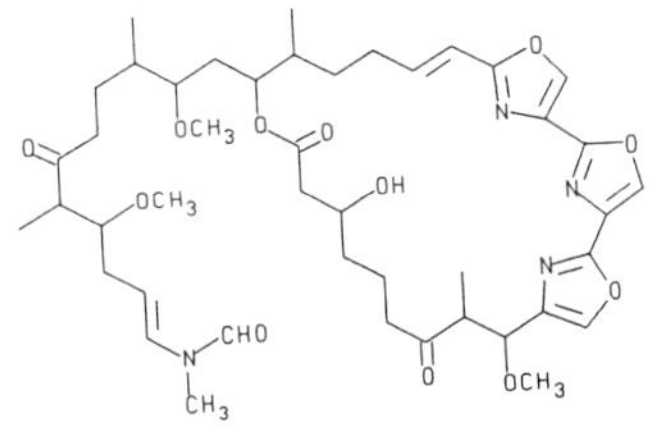

Mol. Wt.: 838
Bioactivity: Inhibition of growth of sea urchin eggs at 1 μg/ml
Antifungal activity
Melting Point: Glass
$[\alpha]_D$: −69.7 Solvent: Me
Spectral Data: UV, IR, CMR, PMR, Mass Spec.
Organism: *Halichondria* sp.
(Porifera)
Hexabranchus sanguineus
(Mollusca)
Location: Marshall Islands
Reference: 548

$C_{44}H_{64}N_4O_{12}$ **Tetrahydrohalichondramide**

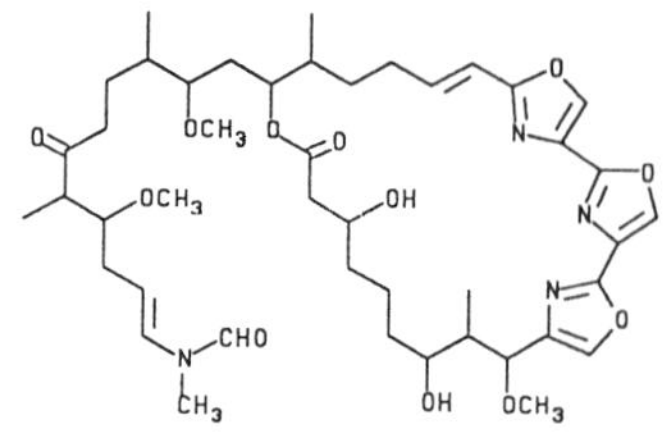

Mol. Wt.: 841
Bioactivity: Inhibition of growth of sea urchin eggs at 1 μg/ml
Antifungal activity
Melting Point: Glass
Spectral Data: UV, IR, PMR, Mass Spec.
Organism: *Hexabranchus sanguineus* (Mollusca)
Location: Marshall Islands
Reference: 548

$C_{44}H_{85}NO_{10}$ **Acanthacerebroside C**

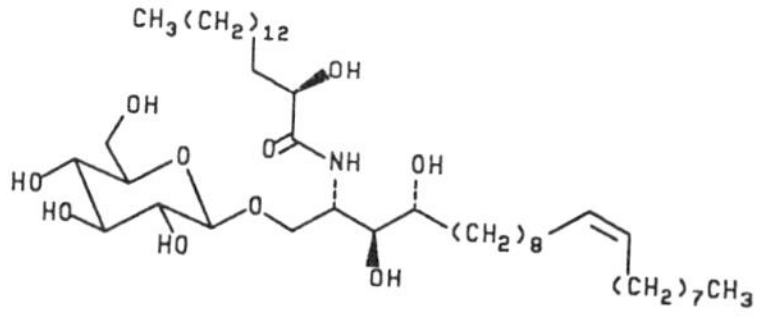

Mol. Wt.: 788
Melting Point: 203–204°C
$[\alpha]_D$: +18.3 Solvent: Pr
Spectral Data: IR, CMR, PMR, Mass Spec.
Organism: *Acanthaster planci* (Echinodermata)
Location: Japan
Reference: 534

$C_{44}H_{87}NO_{10}$ **Acanthacerebroside B**

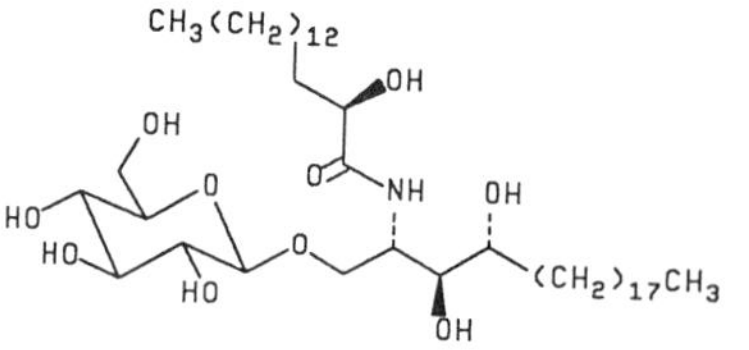

Mol. Wt.: 790
Melting Point: 218–219°C
$[\alpha]_D$: +7.8 Solvent: Pr
Spectral Data: IR, CMR, PMR, Mass Spec.
Organism: *Acanthaster planci* (Echinodermata)
Location: Japan
Reference: 534

$C_{46}H_{87}NO_9$ **Acanthacerebroside D**

Mol. Wt.: 799
Melting Point: 198–199°C
$[\alpha]_D$: +1.1 Solvent: Pr
Spectral Data: IR, CMR, PMR, Mass Spec.
Organism: *Acanthaster planci* (Echinodermata)
Location: Japan
Reference: 534

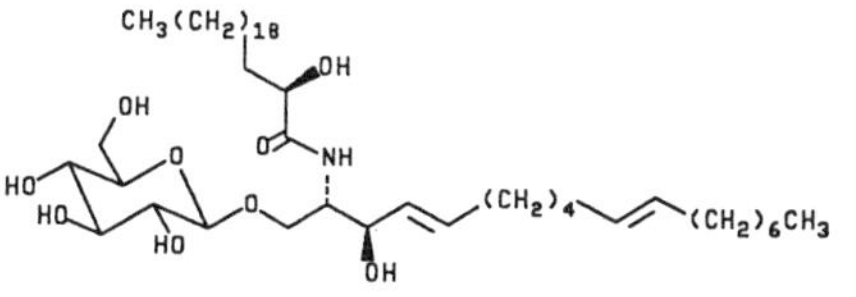

$C_{46}H_{91}NO_{10}$ **Acanthacerebroside A**

Mol. Wt.: 819
Melting Point: 209–210°C
$[\alpha]_D$: +2.4 Solvent: Pr
Spectral Data: IR, CMR, PMR, Mass Spec.
Organism: *Acanthaster planci* (Echinodermata)
Location: Japan
Reference: 534

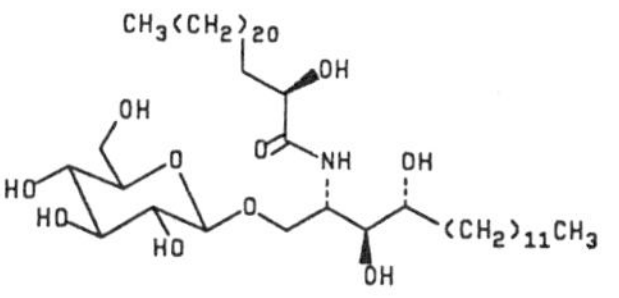

$C_{47}H_{89}NO_9$ **Acanthacerebroside E**

Mol. Wt.: 813
Melting Point: 194–195°C
$[\alpha]_D$: +1.0 Solvent: Pr
Spectral Data: IR, CMR, PMR, Mass Spec.
Organism: *Acanthaster planci* (Echinodermata)
Location: Japan
Reference: 534

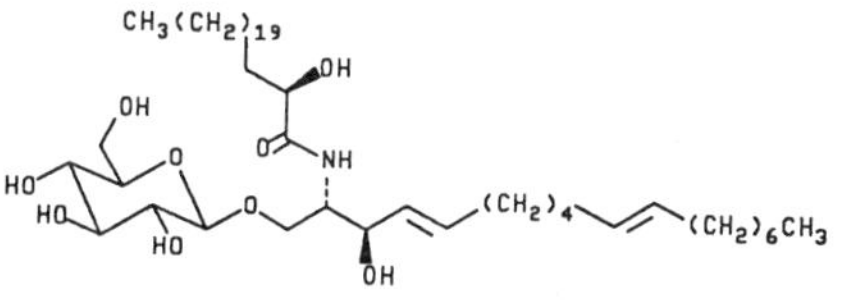

$C_{48}H_{71}N_5O_{14}$ **Kabiramide C**

Mol. Wt.: 943
Bioactivity: Antifungal activity
$[\alpha]_D^{23}$: +20 Solvent: Chf
Spectral Data: UV, IR, CMR, PMR, Mass Spec.
Organism: Unknown sp. (Mollusca)
Location: Japan
Reference: 713

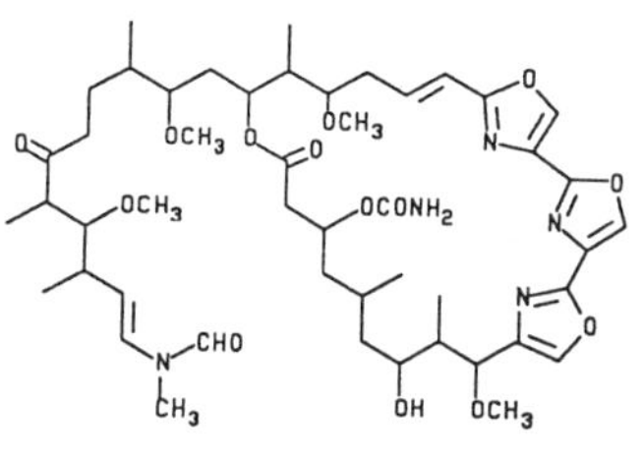

$C_{48}H_{91}NO_9$ **Acanthacerebroside F**

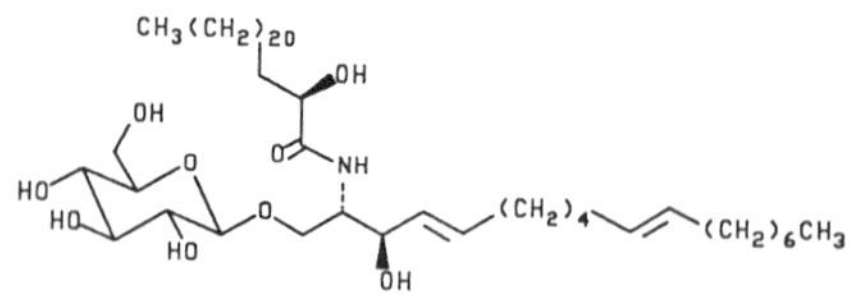

Mol. Wt.: 827
Melting Point: 193–194°C
$[\alpha]_D$: +1.2 Solvent: Pr
Spectral Data: IR, CMR, PMR, Mass Spec.
Organism: *Acanthaster planci* (Echinodermata)
Location: Japan
Reference: 534

$C_{48(49)}H_{93(95)}NO_{10}$ **Cerebrosides** (mixture)

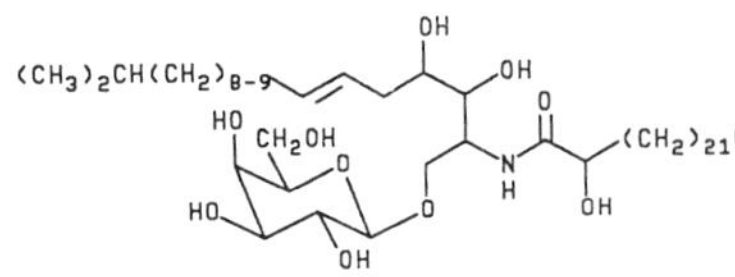

Mol. Wt.: 845 (859)
Bioactivity: Hypotensive activity
Inhibition of hystidine decarboxylase: IC_{50} $2.8x10^{-4}$ mg/ml
Spectral Data: IR, CMR, PMR
Organism: *Chondropsis* sp. (Porifera)
Location: Victoria, Australia
Reference: 270, 793

$C_{70}H_{125}N_{13}O_{16}$ **Theonellamine B (Theonellapeptolide Id)**

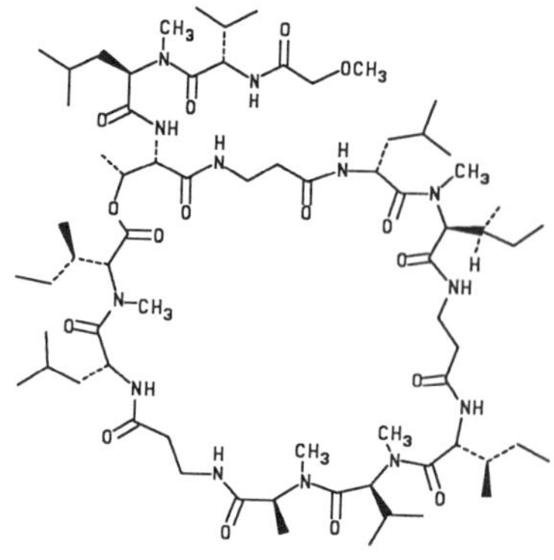

Mol. Wt.: 1405
Bioactivity: Inhibition of Na,K-ATPase
Fertilized sea urchin eggs assay: activity against *Hemicentrotus pulcherrimus* at 50 μg/ml
Melting Point: 168–169°C
$[\alpha]_D^{20}$: −68 Solvent: Me
Spectral Data: IR, CMR, PMR, Mass Spec.
Organism: *Theonella* sp. (Porifera)
Location: Okinawa, Japan
Reference: 565, 566, 800

$C_{75}H_{112}N_{20}O_{22}S$ **Discodermin D**

Mol. Wt.: 1678
Bioactivity: Antimicrobial activity
Fertilized starfish egg assay: activity at 50 μg/ml
Melting Point: 215–219°C
$[\alpha]_D^{23}$: –4.7 Solvent: Me
Spectral Data: UV, Mass Spec.
Organism: *Discodermia kiiensis* Hoshino (Porifera)
Location: Izu Archipelago, Japan
Reference: 716

HCO-D-Ala-L-Phe-L-Pro-D-Val-L-Val-D-Trp-L-Arg-D-Cys(O_3H)-L-Thr-L-MeGln-D-Leu-L-Asn-L-Thr-Sar

$C_{76}H_{114}N_{20}O_{22}S$ **Discodermin B**

Mol. Wt.: 1692
Bioactivity: Antimicrobial activity;
Melting Point: 217–219°C
$[\alpha]_D^{23}$: –3.2 Solvent: Me
Spectral Data: UV, Mass Spec.
Organism: *Discodermia kiiensis* Hoshino (Porifera)
Location: Izu Archipelago, Japan
Reference: 716

HCO-D-Ala-L-Phe-L-Pro-D-Val-L-t-Leu-D-Trp-L-Arg-D-Cys(O_3H)-L-Thr-L-MeGln-D-Leu-L-Asn-L-Thr-Sar

$C_{76}H_{114}N_{20}O_{22}S$ **Discodermin C**

Mol. Wt.: 1692
Bioactivity: Antimicrobial activity
Fertilized starfish egg assay: activity at 5 μg/ml
Melting Point: 222–224°C
$[\alpha]_D^{23}$: −6.6 Solvent: Me
Spectral Data: UV, Mass Spec.
Organism: *Discodermia kiiensis* Hoshino (Porifera)
Location: Izu Archipelago, Japan
Reference: 716

HCO-D-Ala-L-Phe-L-Pro-D-t-Leu-L-Val-D-Trp-L-Arg-D-Cys(O_3H)-L-Thr-L-MeGln-D-Leu-L-Asn-L-Thr-Sar

$C_{77}H_{116}N_{20}O_{22}S$ **Discodermin A**

Mol. Wt.: 1706
Bioactivity: Antimicrobial activity
Fertilized starfish egg assay: activity at 2 μg/ml
Melting Point: 226–228°C
$[\alpha]_D^{22}$: −6.3 Solvent: Me
Spectral Data: UV, IR, CMR, PMR, Mass Spec.
Organism: *Discodermia kiiensis* Hoshino (Porifera)
Location: Izu Archipelago, Japan
Reference: 714, 715, 716

HCO-D-Ala-L-Phe-L-Pro-D-t-Leu-L-t-Leu-D-Trp-L-Arg-D-Cys(O_3H)-L-Thr-L-MeGln-D-Leu-L-Asn-L-Thr-Sa

Chapter 19 ISONITRILES, ISOTHIOCYANATES, AND MISCELLANEOUS

$C_4H_{12}A_5I$ **Tetramethylarsonium iodide**

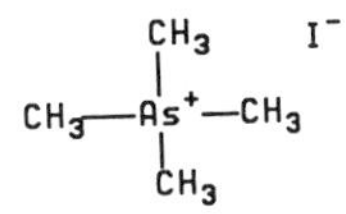

Mol. Wt.: 262
Spectral Data: Mass Spec.
Organism: *Parasicyonis actinostoloides*
(Coelenterata)
Aplysia kurodai
(Mollusca)
Location: Chiba, Japan
Reference: 1012

$C_{11}H_9NO_3S$

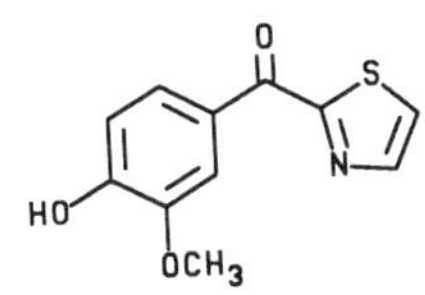

Mol. Wt.: 235
Melting Point: 104°C
Spectral Data: UV, IR, CMR, PMR, Mass Spec.
Organism: *Aplydium pliciferum*
(Chordata/Tunicata)
Location: South Australia
Reference: 33

$C_{11}H_{11}NO_3S$

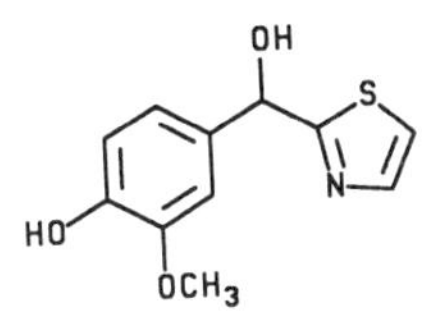

Mol. Wt.: 237
Spectral Data: PMR, Mass Spec.
Organism: *Aplydium pliciferum*
(Chordata/Tunicata)
Location: South Australia
Reference: 33

$C_{13}H_{20}N_2S_2$ **(Z)-1,11-Diisothiocyanoundec-1-ene**

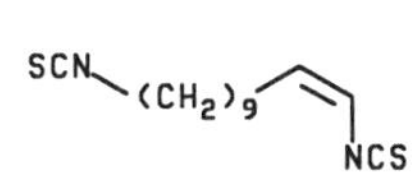

Mol. Wt.: 268
Organism: *Pseudaxinyssa* sp.
(Porifera)
Location: Fiji
Reference: 514

$C_{13}H_{21}NOS$ **12-Isothiocyanododec(Z)-11-enal**

Mol. Wt.: 239
Organism: *Pseudaxinyssa* sp. (Porifera)
Location: Fiji
Reference: 514

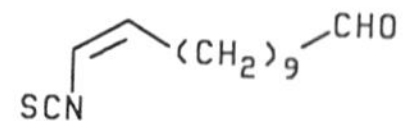

$C_{14}H_{20}N_2S_2$ **(Z,Z)-1,12-Diisothiocyanododeca-1,11-diene**

Mol. Wt.: 280
Organism: *Pseudaxinyssa* sp. (Poriera)
Location: Fiji
Reference: 514

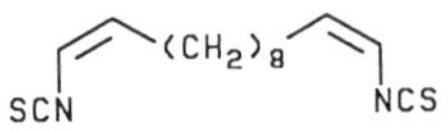

$C_{14}H_{22}N_2S_2$ **(Z)-1,12-Diisothiocyanododec-1-ene**

Mol. Wt.: 282
Organism: *Pseudaxinyssa* sp. (Porifera)
Location: Fiji
Reference: 514

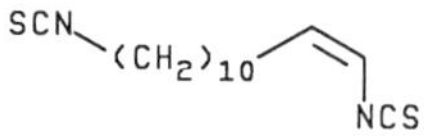

$C_{15}H_{22}N_2S_2$ **(Z,Z)-1,13-Diisothiocyanotrideca-1,12-diene**

Mol. Wt.: 294
Organism: *Pseudaxinyssa* sp. (Porifera)
Location: Fiji
Reference: 514

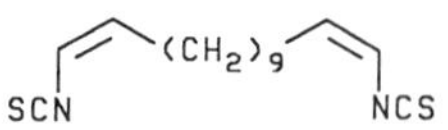

$C_{15}H_{24}N_2S_2$ **(Z)-1,13-Diisothiocyanotridec-1-ene**

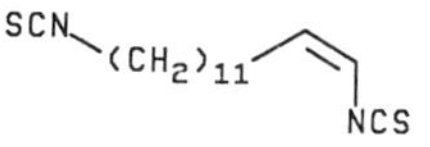

Mol. Wt.: 296
Organism: *Pseudaxinyssa* sp. (Porifera)
Location: Fiji
Reference: 514

$C_{16}H_{24}N_2S_2$ **(Z,Z)-1,14-Diisothiocyanotetradeca-1,13-diene**

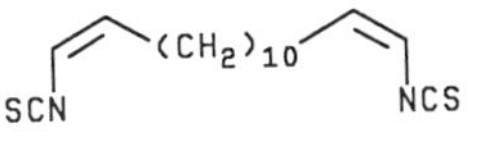

Mol. Wt.: 308
Organism: *Pseudaxinyssa* sp. (Porifera)
Location: Fiji
Reference: 514

$C_{16}H_{25}N$

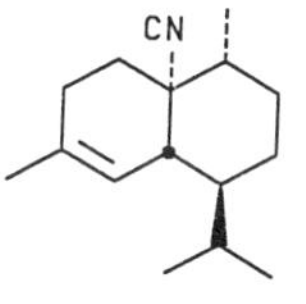

Mol. Wt.: 231
$[\alpha]_D$: -65.7 Solvent: Chf
Spectral Data: IR, CMR, PMR, Mass Spec.
Organism: *Axinella cannabina* (Porifera)
Location: Taranto, Italy
Reference: 179

$C_{16}H_{25}N$ **7-Isocyano-7,8-dihydro-α-bisabolene**

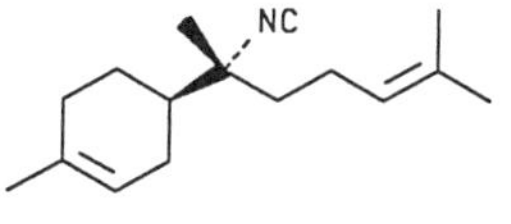

Mol. Wt.: 231
Melting Point: Oil
$[\alpha]_D^{22}$: -49.9 Solvent: He
Spectral Data: UV, IR, CMR, PMR, Mass Spec.
Organism: *Ciocalypta* sp. (Porifera)
Location: O'ahu, Hawaii
Reference: 377

$C_{16}H_{25}N$ **6α-Isocyano-5αH,7αH,10α-eudesm-4(14)-ene**

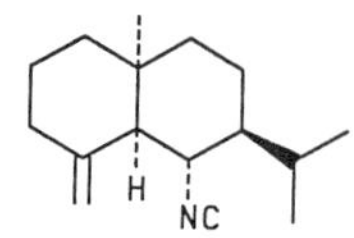

Mol. Wt.: 231
Melting Point: 78-79°C
$[\alpha]_D$: +92.9 Solvent: Chf
Spectral Data: IR, CMR, PMR, Mass Spec.
Organism: *Axinella cannabina* Esper
Acanthella acuta Schmitt
(Porifera)
Location: Taranto and Naples, Italy
Reference: 180

$C_{16}H_{25}N$ **3-Isocyanotheonellin**

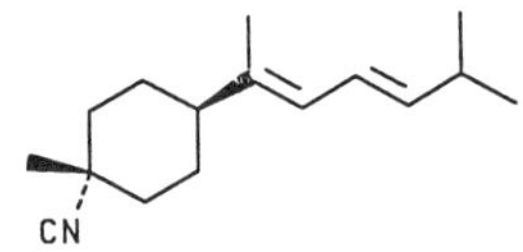

Mol. Wt.: 231
Bioactivity: Antibacterial activity (growth inhibition of *Bacillus subtilis*)
Melting Point: Oil
$[\alpha]_D^{25}$: 0 Solvent: Chf
Spectral Data: UV, IR, CMR, PMR, Mass Spec.
Organism: *Phyllidia* sp.
(Mollusca)
Location: Colombo, Sri Lanka
Reference: 377

$C_{16}H_{25}N$ **Stylotelline**

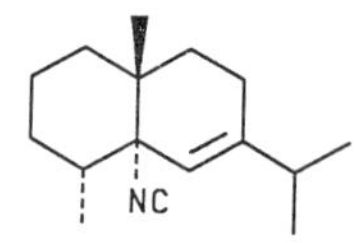

Mol. Wt.: 231
Melting Point: Oil
$[\alpha]_D$: -47 Solvent: Chf
Spectral Data: IR, CMR, PMR, Mass Spec.
Organism: *Stylotella* sp.
(Porifera)
Location: New Caledonia
Reference: 859

$C_{16}H_{25}NO$

7-Isocyanato-7,8-dihydro-α-bisabolene

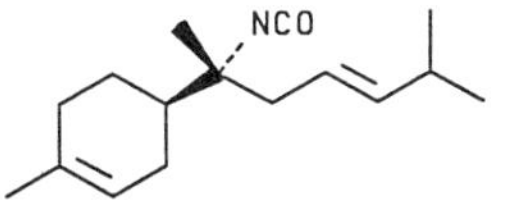

Mol. Wt.: 247
Melting Point: Oil
$[\alpha]_D^{25}$: -24.3 Solvent: He
Spectral Data: UV, IR, CMR, PMR, Mass Spec., x-ray c.s.
Organism: *Ciocalypta* sp. (Porifera)
Location: O'ahu, Hawaii
Reference: 377

$C_{16}H_{25}NS$

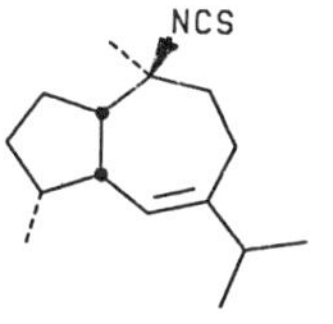

Mol. Wt.: 263
Spectral Data: IR, PMR, Mass Spec.
Organism: Unknown sp. (Porifera)
Location: Wakayama, Japan
Reference: 1068

$C_{16}H_{25}NS$

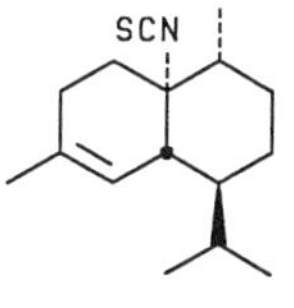

Mol. Wt.: 263
Melting Point: Oil
$[\alpha]_D$: -91.17
Spectral Data: IR, CMR, PMR, Mass Spec.
Organism: *Axinella cannabina* (Porifera)
Location: Taranto, Italy
Reference: 179

$C_{16}H_{25}NS$

6α-Isothiocyano-5αH,7αH,10α-eudesm-4(14)-ene

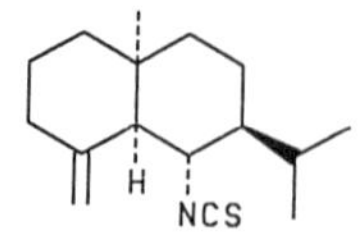

Mol. Wt.: 263
Melting Point: 52-53°C
$[\alpha]_D$: +88.4 Solvent: Chf
Spectral Data: IR, CMR, PMR, Mass Spec.
Organism: *Axinella cannabina* Esper
Acanthella acuta Schmitt
(Porifera)
Location: Taranto and Naples, Italy
Reference: 180

$C_{16}H_{25}NS$

7-Isothiocyanato-7,8-dihydro-α-bisabolene

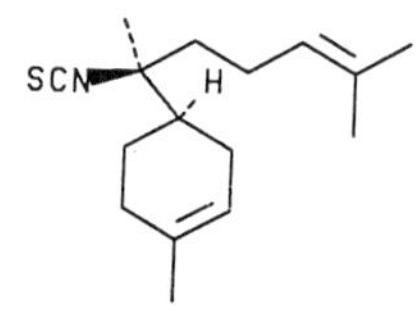

Mol. Wt.: 263
Melting Point: Oil
$[\alpha]_D^{20}$: +60.5 Solvent: Chf
Spectral Data: IR, CMR, PMR, Mass Spec.
Organism: *Halichondria* sp.
(Porifera)
Location: Ponape, Marshall Islands
Reference: 1045

$C_{16}H_{26}N_2S_2$

(Z)-1,14-Diisothiocyanotetradec-1-ene

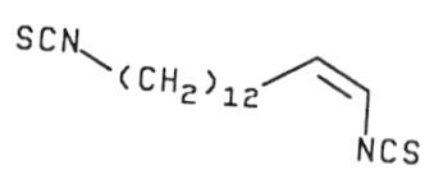

Mol. Wt.: 310
Organism: *Pseudaxinyssa* sp.
(Porifera)
Location: Fiji
Reference: 514

$C_{17}H_{26}N_2S_2$ **(Z,Z)-1,15-Diisothiocyanopentadeca-1,14-diene**

Mol. Wt.: 322
Organism: *Pseudaxinyssa* sp. (Porifera)
Location: Fiji
Reference: 514

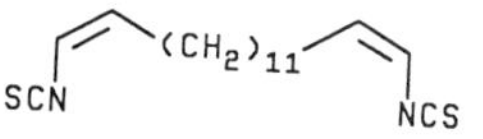

$C_{17}H_{28}N_2S_2$ **(Z)-1,15-Diisothiocyanopentadec-1-ene**

Mol. Wt.: 324
Organism: *Pseudaxinyssa* sp. (Porifera)
Location: Fiji
Reference: 514

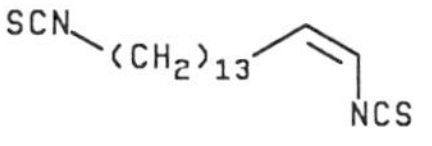

$C_{18}H_{28}N_2S_2$ **(Z,Z)-1,16-Diisothiocyanohexadeca-1,15-diene**

Mol. Wt.: 336
Organism: *Pseudaxinyssa* sp. (Porifera)
Location: Fiji
Reference: 514

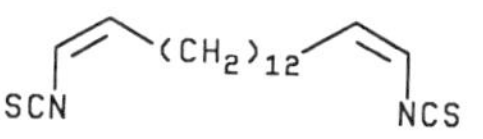

$C_{18}H_{30}N_2S_2$ **(Z)-1,16-Diisothiocyanohexadec-1-ene**

Mol. Wt.: 338
Organism: *Pseudaxinyssa* sp. (Porifera)
Location: Fiji
Reference: 514

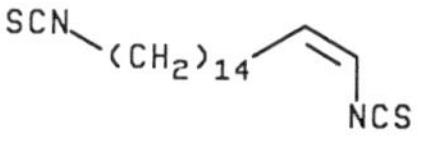

$C_{19}H_{30}N_2S_2$ **(Z,Z)-1,17-Diisothiocyanoheptadeca-1,16-diene**

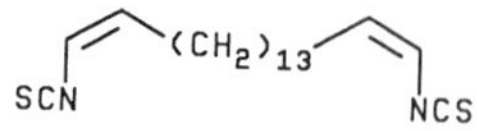

Mol. Wt.: 350
Organism: *Pseudaxinyssa* sp. (Porifera)
Location: Fiji
Reference: 514

$C_{19}H_{32}N_2S_2$ **(Z)-1,17-Diisothiocyanoheptadec-1-ene**

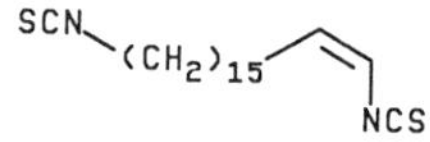

Mol. Wt.: 352
Organism: *Pseudaxinyssa* sp. (Porifera)
Location: Fiji
Reference: 514

$C_{19}H_{33}NOS$ **18-Isothiocyanooctadec(Z)-17-enal**

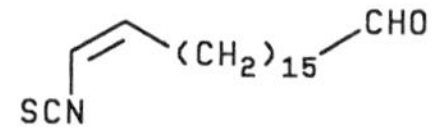

Mol. Wt.: 323
Spectral Data: UV, IR, CMR, PMR, Mass Spec.
Organism: *Pseudaxinyssa* sp. (Porifera)
Location: Fiji
Reference: 514

$C_{20}H_{32}N_2S_2$ **(Z,Z)-1,18-Diisothiocyanooctadeca-1,17-diene**

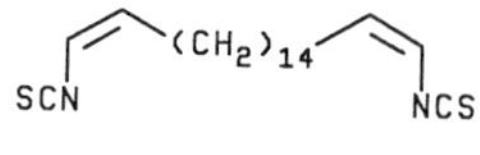

Mol. Wt.: 364
Melting Point: ~15°C
Spectral Data: UV, IR, CMR, PMR, Mass Spec.
Organism: *Pseudaxinyssa* sp. (Porifera)
Location: Fiji
Reference: 514

$C_{20}H_{34}N_2S_2$ **(Z)-1,18-Diisothiocyanooctadec-1-ene**

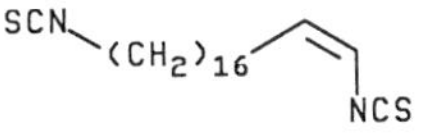

Mol. Wt.: 366
Spectral Data: UV, IR, CMR, PMR, Mass Spec.
Organism: *Pseudaxinyssa* sp. (Porifera)
Location: Fiji
Reference: 514

$C_{20}H_{35}NOS$ **19-Isothiocyanononadec(Z)-18-enal**

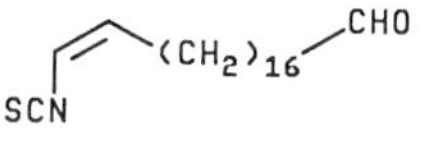

Mol. Wt.: 337
Organism: *Pseudaxinyssa* sp. (Porifera)
Location: Fiji
Reference: 514

$C_{21}H_{31}N$ **7-Isocyano-1-cycloamphilectene**

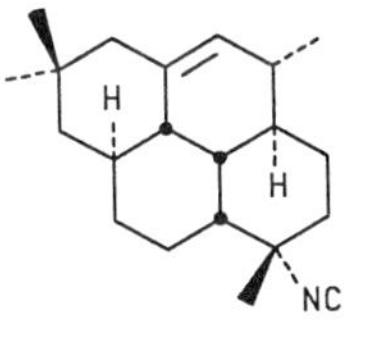

Mol. Wt.: 297
Melting Point: 182-183°C
$[\alpha]_D$: -14 Solvent: Chf
Spectral Data: IR, CMR, PMR, Mass Spec., x-ray c.s.
Organism: *Halichondria* sp. (Porifera)
Location: Palau
Reference: 758

$C_{21}H_{31}N$ **7-Isocyano-11-cycloamphilectene**

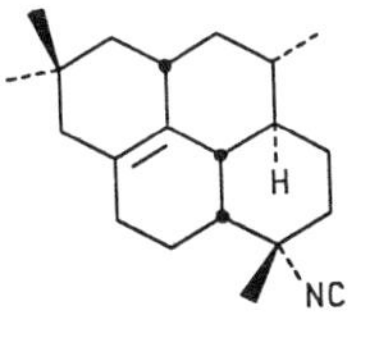

Mol. Wt.: 297
Melting Point: 134°C
Spectral Data: IR, PMR, Mass Spec., x-ray c.s.
Organism: *Halichondria* sp. (Porifera)
Location: Palau
Reference: 758

$C_{21}H_{31}N$ **8-Isocyano-1(12)-cycloamphilectene**
(previously known)
(revised structure)

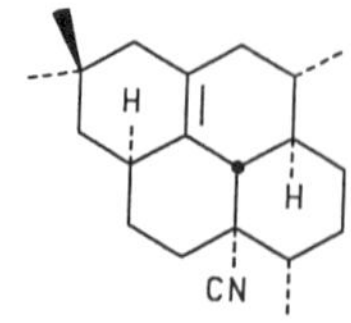

Mol. Wt.: 297
Bioactivity: Antibacterial activity against *Staphylococcus aureus* and *Bacillus subtilis*
Spectral Data: X-ray c.s.
Organism: *Halichondria* sp. (Porifera)
Location: Palau
Reference: 537, 758

$C_{21}H_{31}N$ **8-Isocyano-10,14-amphilectadiene**

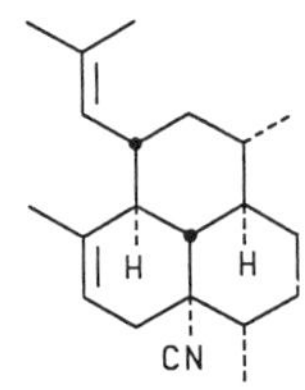

Mol. Wt.: 297
Bioactivity: Antibacterial activity against *Staphylococcus aureus* and *Bacillus subtilis*
Melting Point: Oil
$[\alpha]_D$: -79.8 Solvent: Chf
Spectral Data: IR, CMR, PMR, Mass Spec.
Organism: *Halichondria* sp. (Porifera)
Location: Palau
Reference: 758

$C_{21}H_{32}ClNO_2$ **Kalihinol Y**

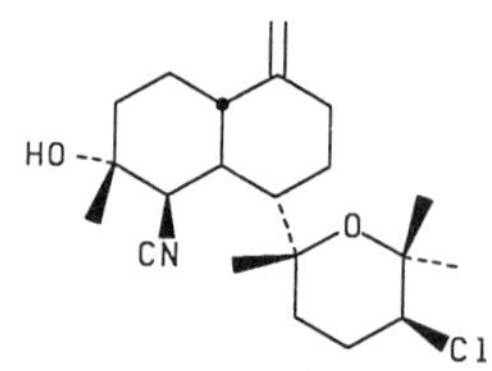

Mol. Wt.: 365
Bioactivity: Antimicrobial activity against *Bacillus subtilis*, *Staphylococcus aureus* and *Candida albicans*
Anthelmintic activity
Melting Point: 176-179°C
$[\alpha]_D$: -34 Solvent: Chf
Spectral Data: IR, CMR, PMR, Mass Spec.
Organism: *Acanthella* sp.
Acanthella carvenosa
(Porifera)
Location: Vita Levu, Fiji
Reference: 163, 853

$C_{21}H_{34}N_2S_2$

(Z,Z)-1,19-Diisothiocyanononadec-1,18-diene

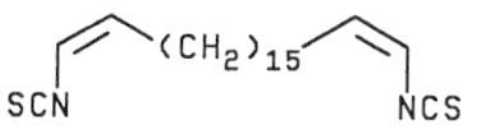

Mol. Wt.: 378
Organism: *Pseudaxinyssa* sp. (Porifera)
Location: Fiji
Reference: 514

$C_{21}H_{36}N_2S_2$

(Z)-1,19-Diisothiocyanononadec-1-ene

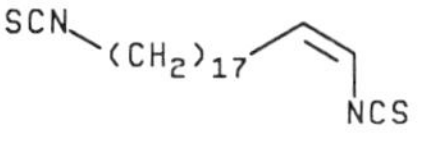

Mol. Wt.: 380
Organism: *Pseudaxinyssa* sp. (Porifera)
Location: Fiji
Reference: 514

$C_{22}H_{32}N_2$

Diisocyanoadociane
(previously known)
(revised structure)

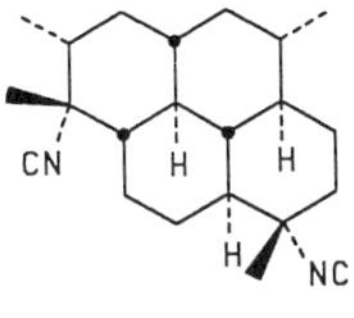

Mol. Wt.: 324
Bioactivity: Antimicrobial activity
Coronary vasodilative activity
Melting Point: 109-110°C
$[\alpha]_D^{22}$: +47.4 Solvent: Dcm
Spectral Data: IR, PMR, Mass Spec., x-ray c.s.
Organism: *Amphimedon* sp. (ex. *Adocia* sp.) (Porifera)
Location: Great Barrier Reef; Queensland, Australia
Reference: 48, 198, 270, 301, 537

$C_{22}H_{33}ClN_2O_2$	**Kalihinol A** (previously known) (revised structure)	
Mol. Wt.:	392	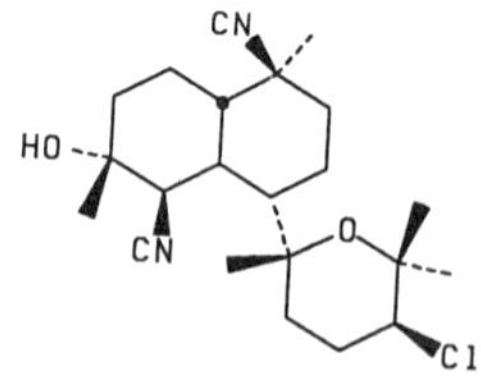
Bioactivity:	Antimicrobial activity against *Bacillus subtilis*, *Staphylococcus aureus*, and *Candida albicans* Anthelmintic activity	
Melting Point:	233°C	
$[\alpha]_D$:	+16 Solvent: Chf	
Spectral Data:	IR, CMR, PMR, Mass Spec., x-ray c.s.	
Organism:	*Acanthella* sp. *Acanthella carvenosa* (Porifera)	
Location:	Guam, Fiji	
Reference:	163, 164, 853	

$C_{22}H_{33}ClN_2O_2$	**Kalihinol D**	
Mol. Wt.:	392	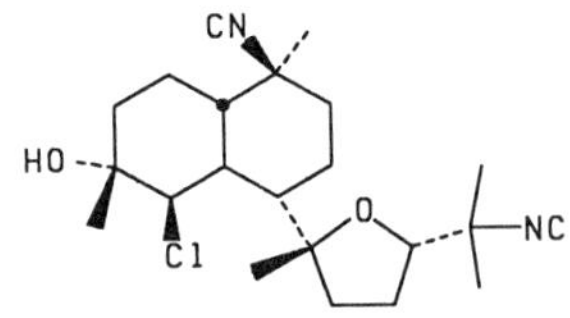
Bioactivity:	Antimicrobial activity against *Bacillus subtilis*, *Staphylococcus aureus*, and *Candida albicans*	
Melting Point:	183-184°C	
$[\alpha]_D$:	+8.0 Solvent: Chf	
Spectral Data:	IR, CMR, PMR, Mass Spec.	
Organism:	*Acanthella* sp. (Porifera)	
Location:	Guam	
Reference:	163	

$C_{22}H_{33}ClN_2O_2$ **Kalihinol E**
(previously known)
(revised structure)

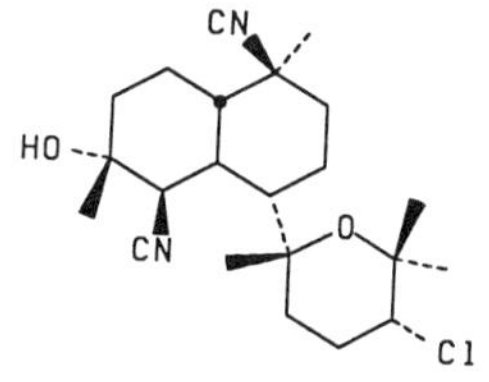

Mol. Wt.: 392
Bioactivity: Antimicrobial activity against *Bacillus subtilis*, *Staphylococcus aureus*, and *Candida albicans*
Melting Point: 197-199°C
[α]D: +4.0 Solvent: Chf
Spectral Data: IR, CMR, PMR, Mass Spec.
Organism: *Acanthella* sp.
(Porifera)
Location: Guam
Reference: 163, 866

$C_{22}H_{33}ClN_2O_2$ **Kalihinol Z**

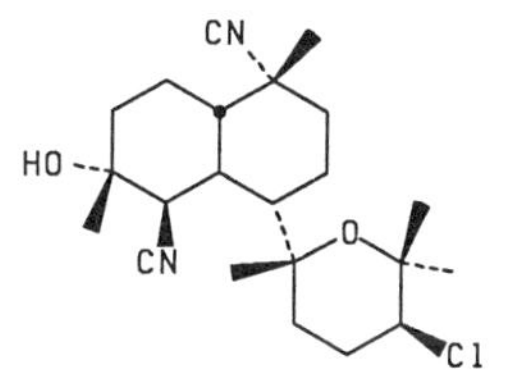

Mol. Wt.: 392
Bioactivity: Antimicrobial activity against *Bacillus subtilis*, *Staphylococcus aureus*, and *Candida albicans*
Anthelmintic activity
Melting Point: 228-230°C
[α]D: -10 Solvent: Chf
Spectral Data: IR, CMR, PMR, Mass Spec.
Organism: *Acanthella* sp.
Acanthella carvenosa
(Porifera)
Location: Vita Levu, Fiji
Reference: 163, 853

$C_{22}H_{33}ClN_2O_2S$ **Kalihinol X**

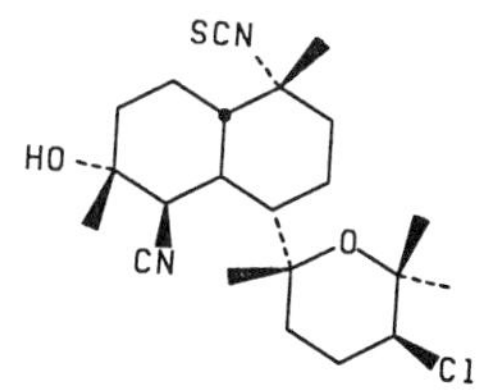

Mol. Wt.: 424
Bioactivity: Antimicrobial activity against *Bacillus subtilis*, *Staphylococcus aureus*, and *Candida albicans*
Anthelmintic activity
Melting Point: 199-200°C
[α]D: -22 Solvent: Chf
Spectral Data: UV, IR, CMR, PMR, Mass Spec.
Organism: *Acanthella* sp.
Acanthella carvenosa
(Porifera)
Location: Vita Levu, Fiji
Reference: 163, 853

$C_{22}H_{38}N_2S_2$ **(Z)-1,20-Diisothiocyanoeicos-1-ene**

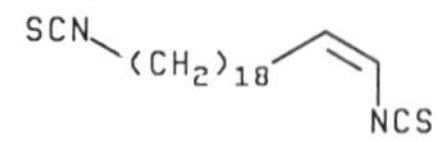

Mol. Wt.: 394
Organism: *Pseudaxinyssa* sp. (Porifera)
Location: Fiji
Reference: 514

$C_{23}H_{33}N_3O_2$ **Isokalihinol F**

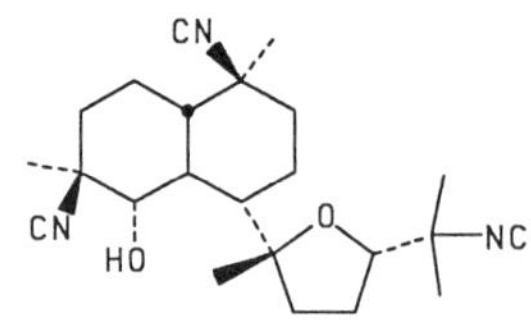

Mol. Wt.: 383
Melting Point: 180-182°C
$[\alpha]_D^{20}$: +13.6 Solvent: $CDCl_3$
Spectral Data: CMR, PMR, Mass Spec.
Organism: *Acanthella carvenosa* (Porifera)
Location: Fiji
Reference: 853

$C_{23}H_{33}N_3O_2S$ **Kalihinol G**

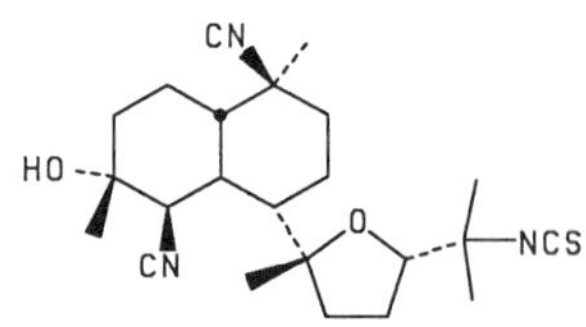

Mol. Wt.: 415
Bioactivity: Antimicrobial activity against *Bacillus subtilis*, *Staphylococcus aureus*, and *Candida albicans*
Melting Point: Oil
$[\alpha]_D$: -12 Solvent: Chf
Spectral Data: UV, IR, CMR, PMR, Mass Spec.
Organism: *Acanthella* sp. (Porifera)
Location: Guam
Reference: 163

$C_{23}H_{33}N_3O_2S$ **Kalihinol H**

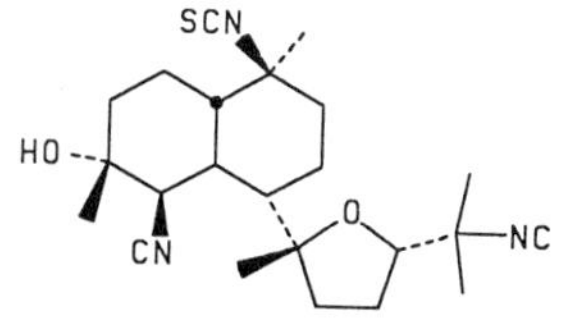

Mol. Wt.: 415
Bioactivity: Antimicrobial activity against *Bacillus subtilis*, *Staphylococcus aureus*, and *Candida albicans*
Melting Point: Oil
$[\alpha]_D$: +98 Solvent: Chf
Spectral Data: UV, IR, CMR, PMR, Mass Spec.
Organism: *Acanthella* sp. (Porifera)
Location: Guam
Reference: 163

$C_{30}H_{51}N_9O_{10}S_2$ **Sperm activating peptide**

Mol. Wt.: 762
Bioactivity: Stimulation of spermatozoan respiration rates
Elevation of cAMP and cGMP concentrations in spermatozoa at 10^{-10}M
Organism: *Glyptocidaris crenularis* (Echinodermata)
Location: Aomori, Japan
Reference: 1061

Leu-Cys-Pro-Gly-Gly-
Asn-Cys-Val

$C_{31}H_{53}N_9O_{10}S_2$ **Sperm activating peptide**

Mol. Wt.: 776
Bioactivity: Stimulation of spermatozoan respiration rates
Elevation of cAMP and cGMP concentrations in spermatozoa at 10^{-10}M
Organism: *Glyptocidaris crenularis* (Echinodermata)
Location: Aomori, Japan
Reference: 1061

Leu-Cys-Pro-Gly-Gly-
Gln-Cys-Val

$C_{36}H_{63}N_{11}O_{11}S_2$ **Sperm activating peptide (Alloresact)**

Mol. Wt.: 890
Bioactivity: Stimulation of spermatozoan respiration rates
Elevation of cAMP and cGMP concentrations in spermatozoa at 10^{-10}M
Organism: *Glyptocidaris crecularis* (Echinodermata)
Location: Aomori, Japan
Reference: 1061

Lys-Leu-Cys-Pro-Gly-Gly-Asn-Cys-Val

$C_{37}H_{65}N_{11}O_{11}S_2$ **Sperm activating peptide**

Mol. Wt.: 904
Bioactivity: Stimulation of spermatozoan respiration rates
Elevation of cAMP and cGMP concentrations in spermatozoa at 10^{-10}M
Organism: *Glyptocidaris crenularis* (Echinodermata)
Location: Aomori, Japan
Reference: 1061

Lys-Leu-Cys-Pro-Gly-Gly-Gln-Cys-Val

$C_{42}H_{73}N_{13}O_{14}S_2$ **Sperm activating peptide**

Mol. Wt.: 1048
Bioactivity: Stimulation of spermatozoan respiration rates
Elevation of cAMP and cGMP concentrations in spermatozoa at 10^{-10}M
Organism: *Glyptocidaris crenularis* (Echinodermata)
Location: Aomori, Japan
Reference: 1061

Ser-Ala-Lys-Leu-Cys-Pro-Gly-Gly-Asn-Cys-Val

$C_{49}H_{79}N_{13}O_{14}O_2$ **Sperm activating peptide**

Mol. Wt.: 1138
Bioactivity: Stimulation of spermatozoan respiration rates
Elevation of cAMP and cGMP concentrations in spermatozoa at $10^{-10}M$
Organism: *Glyptocidaris crenularis* (Echinodermata)
Location: Aomori, Japan
Reference: 1061

Ser-Phe-Lys-Leu-Cys-Pro-Gly-Gly-Gln-Cys-Val

Fibroblast growth inhibitory factor (FGIF)

Mol. Wt.: <2000
Bioactivity: Inhibition of DNA synthesis and cell proliferation
Organism: Chicken embryo fibroblasts (Chordata/Vertebrata)
Reference: 997

Pardaxin P-1

Mol. Wt.: ~2800
Bioactivity: Ichthyotoxic at 25 μg/ml
Organism: *Pardachirus pavoninus* (Chordata/Pisces)
Location: Ryukyu Archipelago, Japan
Reference: 1090

Gly-Phe-Phe-Ala-Leu-Ile-Pro-Lys-Ile-Ile-Ser-Ser-Pro-Leu-Phe-Lys-Thr-Leu-Leu-Ser-Ala-Val-Gly-Ser-Ala-Leu-Ser-Ser-Ser-Gly-Glu-Gln-Glu

Pardaxin P-2

Mol. Wt.: ~2800
Bioactivity: Ichthyotoxic at 25 μg/ml
Organism: *Pardachirus pavoninus* (Chordata/Pisces)
Location: Ryukyu Archipelago, Japan
Reference: 1090

Gly-Phe-Phe-Ala-Leu-Ile-Pro-Lys-Ile-Ile-Ser-Ser-Pro-Ile-Phe-Lys-Thr-Leu-Leu-Ser-Ala-Val-Gly-Ser-Ala-Leu-Ser-Ser-Ser-Gly-Gly-Gln-Glu

Pardaxin P-3

Mol. Wt.: ~2800
Organism: *Pardachirus pavoninus* (Chordata/Pisces)
Location: Ryukyu Archipelago, Japan
Reference: 1090

Gly-Phe-Phe-Ala-Phe-Ile-Pro-Lys-Ile-Ile-Ser-Ser-Pro-Leu-Phe-Lys-Thr-Leu-Leu-Ser-Ala-Val-Gly-Ser-Ala-Leu-Ser-Ser-Ser-(Gly)-(Glu)-Gln-Glu
(Residues in parentheses assumed)

Plasma antifreeze polypeptides (AFP)

Mol. Wt.: 3300-4500
Bioactivity: Antifreeze activity
Organism: *Pseudopleuronectes americanus* (Chordata/Pisces)
Location: Newfoundland, Nova Scotia, New Brunswick and Long Island
Reference: 305

Cytotoxin II

Mol. Wt.: 6646
Bioactivity: Cytotoxicity: FL 50% lysis at 10.6 μg/ml
Organism: *Naja naja siamensis* (Chordata/Reptilia)
Location: Thailand
Reference: 839

Cytotoxin I

Mol. Wt.: 6693
Bioactivity: Cytotoxicity: FL 50% lysis at 5.4 μg/ml
Organism: *Naja naja siamensis* (Chordata/Reptilia)
Location: Thailand
Reference: 839

Cytotoxin III

Mol. Wt.:	6709
Bioactivity:	Cytotoxicity: FL 50% lysis at 16.1 μg/ml
Organism:	*Naja naja siamensis* (Chordata/Reptilia)
Location:	Thailand
Reference:	839

Cytotoxin IV

Mol. Wt.:	6739
Bioactivity:	Cytotoxicity: FL 50% lysis at 12.6 μg/ml
Organism:	*Naja naja siamensis* (Chordata/Reptilia)
Location:	Thailand
Reference:	839

Tealiatoxin

Mol. Wt.:	~7800
Bioactivity:	Histaminolytic activity
Organism:	*Tealia felina* L. (Coelenterata)
Reference:	264

CTF-II
(Cytotoxic factor II)

Mol. Wt.:	13,905
Bioactivity:	Cytotoxicity: minimum cytotoxic dose (MCD) ~0.05 μg/ml Toxicity: LD_{50} >270 μg/mouse
Organism:	*Trimeresurus flavoviridis* (Chordata/Reptilia)
Location:	Okinawa, Japan
Reference:	854

CTF-I
(Cytotoxic factor I)

Mol. Wt.: 13,940
Bioactivity: Cytotoxicity: minimum cytotoxic dose (MCD) ~0.05 μg/ml
Toxicity: LD_{50} 270 μg/mouse
Organism: *Trimeresurus flavoviridis* (Chordata/Reptilia)
Location: Okinawa, Japan
Reference: 854

Parasitoxin

Mol. Wt.: ~17,200
Bioactivity: Toxic to mice: LD_{50} 65 μg/kg
Ichthyotoxic at 1.5 μg/ml
Hemolytic activity
Organism: *Parasicyonis actinostoloides* (Coelenterata)
Location: Chiba, Japan
Reference: 1013

Equinatoxin II
(EqT II)

Mol. Wt.: 17,770
Bioactivity: Toxicity: LD_{50} 35 μg/kg of mouse
Sheep erythrocyte lysis
Organism: *Actinia equina* L. (Coelenterata)
Location: Adriatic
Reference: 684

Equinatoxin I
(EqT I)

Mol. Wt.: 17,800
Bioactivity: Toxicity: LD_{50} 23 μg/kg of mouse
Sheep erythrocyte lysis
Organism: *Actinia equina* L (Coelenterata)
Location: Adriatic
Reference: 684

Equinatoxin III
(EqT III)

Mol. Wt.: 18,150
Bioactivity: Toxicity: LD_{50} 83 μg/kg of mouse
Sheep erythrocyte lysis
Organism: *Actinia equina* L.
(Coelenterata)
Location: Adriatic
Reference: 684

***Goniopora* toxin**

Mol. Wt.: 19,000
Bioactivity: Ca^{2+}-channel activator
Toxic to mice
Organism: *Goniopora* sp.
(Coelenterata)
Location: Red Sea, Japan
Reference: 904

Greenland cod trypsin (GCT)

Mol. Wt.: 23,500
Bioactivity: Catalysis
Spectral Data: CD
Organism: *Gadus ogac*
(Chordata/Pisces)
Location: Labrador
Reference: 1018

Hemagglutinin

Mol. Wt.: ~24,000
Bioactivity: Hemagglutinating activity
Organism: *Haliclona* sp.
(Porifera)
Location: Great Barrier Reef, Australia
Reference: 725

Fluorescent protein

Mol. Wt.: 30,000-32,000
Spectral Data: UV
Organism: *Malacosteus niger* (Chordata/Pisces)
Location: Eastern North Atlantic
Reference: 136

Fr.SM II
(Squid melanoprotein)

Mol. Wt.: ~39,000
Bioactivity: Gastric secretion inhibition in rats
Anti-ulcerogenic activity in rats
Antiinflammatory activity in rats
Organism: *Ommastrephes bartrami* Lesuel (Mollusca)
Reference: 736, 737, 738, 739

MAC (protein)

Mol. Wt.: 45,000-65,000
Bioactivity: Ichthyotoxic at 1 μg/g
Positive inotropic cardiotonic activity
Action on vas deferens - contractile response
Action on ileum - rhythmic contraction and relaxation
Organism: *Conus magus* Linné (Mollusca)
Location: Okinawa, Japan
Reference: 582

Toxin 2 (protein)

Mol. Wt.: ~150,000
Bioactivity: Myotoxic: elicits contractures of mammalian and crustacean musculature
Lethal to mice
Organism: *Chironex fleckeri* (Coelenterata)
Location: Queensland, Australia
Reference: 267

Toxin 1 (protein)

Mol. Wt.: ~600,000
Bioactivity: Myotoxic: elicits contractures of mammalian musculature
Lethal to mice
Organism: *Chironex fleckeri* (Coelenterata)
Location: Queensland, Australia
Reference: 267

Glycolipoproteins

Bioactivity: Vitellogenic substances
Spectral Data: PMR
Organism: *Asterias rubens* (Echinodermata)
Location: The Netherlands
Reference: 238

HvTX (Toxin)

Bioactivity: Blockage of resting potassium conductance in frog muscle fibers
Organism: *Haliclona viridis* (Porifera)
Location: Falcón State, Venezuela
Reference: 996

Neurotoxin II
(RTX II)

Bioactivity: Neurotoxicity
Organism: *Radianthus macrodactylus* (Coelenterata)
Reference: 1228

Section C

MARINE PLANT BIOSYNTHETIC PRODUCTS

Chapter 20 MARINE PLANT CONSTITUENTS

A. Hydrocarbons, Alcohols, and Esters

$C_{11}H_{16}$ **6-[(1E)-1-Butenyl]-cyclohepta-2,5-diene**

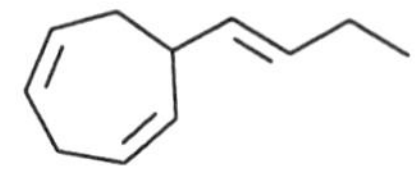

Mol. Wt.: 148
Spectral Data: PMR, Mass Spec.
Organism: *Dictyopteris membranacea* (Stackh.) Batt. (Phaeophyta)
Location: Mediterranean Coast, France
Reference: 87

$C_{11}H_{18}$ **4-[(1E)-1-Hexenyl]-cyclopentene**

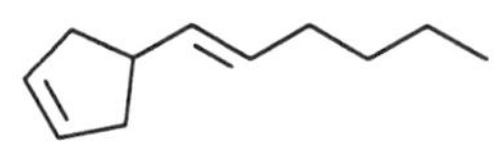

Mol. Wt.: 150
Spectral Data: PMR, Mass Spec.
Organism: *Dictyopteris membranacea* (Stackh.) Batt. (Phaeophyta)
Location: Mediterranean Coast, France
Reference: 87

$C_{20}H_{28}O_4$ **Ptilodene**

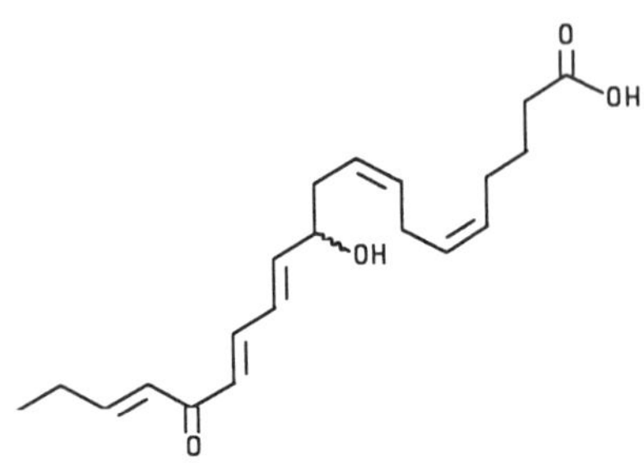

Mol. Wt.: 332
Bioactivity: Inhibition of arachidonic acid utilization by human polymorphonuclear leukocytes: IC_{50} 10^{-5}
Inhibition of growth of *E. coli* and *Bacillus subtilis*
Moderate inhibition of dog renal Na^+/K^+ ATPase
$[\alpha]_D$: 0 Solvent: Chf
Spectral Data: CMR, PMR, Mass Spec.; UV, IR, CMR, PMR, Mass Spec. (of acetate methyl ester)
Organism: *Ptilota fillicina* (Rhodophyta)
Location: Oregon
Reference: 673

$C_{20}H_{30}O_3$ **12(S)-Hydroxyeicosa-5(Z),8(Z),-10(E),14(Z),17(Z)-pentaenoic acid**
(Characterized as the 12-acetoxy methyl ester derivative)

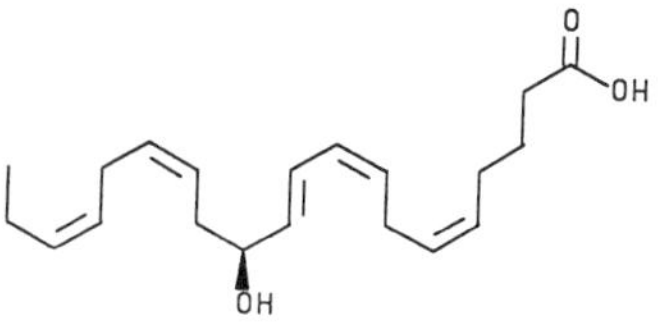

Mol. Wt.: 318
Bioactivity: Stimulates degranulation by neutrophils
$[\alpha]_D$: -11 Solvent: An
Spectral Data: UV, IR, CMR, PMR, Mass Spec.
Organism: *Murrayella periclados* (Rhodophyta)
Location: Caribbean
Reference: 63

$C_{30}H_{58}O$ **(E)-2-Tridecyl-2-heptadecenal**

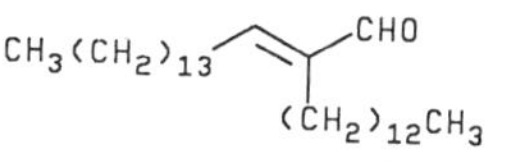

Mol. Wt.: 434
Spectral Data: UV, IR, CMR, PMR, Mass Spec.
Organism: *Laurencia undulata* Yamada (Rhodophyta)
Laurencia papillosa (Forsk.) Greville
Location: Ago Bay, Shirahama and Okinawa, Japan
Reference: 1058

$C_{52+x}H_{98+2x}O$ **Botryals 1**
(X=0,2,4,6,8,10,12)

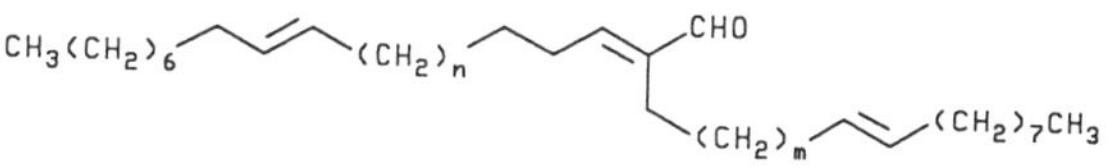

Mol. Wt.: 740–908
Melting Point: Oil
Spectral Data: IR, CMR, PMR, Mass Spec.
Organism: *Botryococcus braunii* (Chlorophyta)
Culture
Location: Austin
Reference: 731

$C_{52+x}H_{98+2x}O$ **Botryals 2**
(x=0,2,4,6,8,10,12)

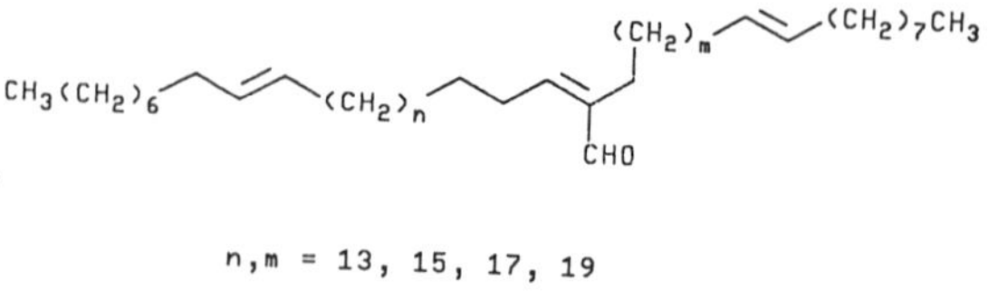

Mol. Wt.:	740–908
Melting Point:	Oil
Spectral Data:	IR, CMR, PMR, Mass Spec.
Organism:	*Botryococcus braunii* (Chlorophyta) Culture
Location:	Austin
Reference:	731

B. Sterols and Steroids

$C_{27}H_{44}O_2$ **5α-Cholestane-3,6-dione**

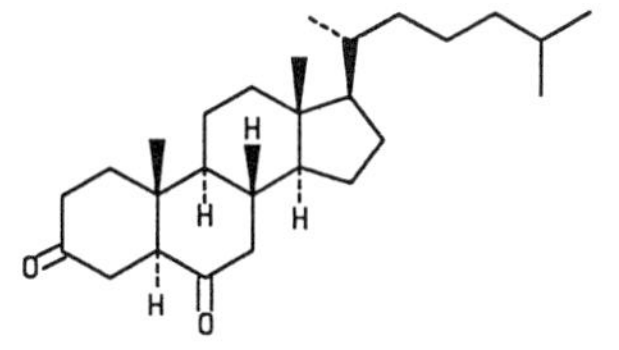

Mol. Wt.: 400
Melting Point: 168–170°C
Spectral Data: IR, CMR, PMR, Mass Spec.
Organism: *Acantophora spicifera* (Rhodophyta)
Location: Indian West Coast
Reference: 1145

$C_{27}H_{46}O$ **Cholest-8(9)-en-3β-ol**

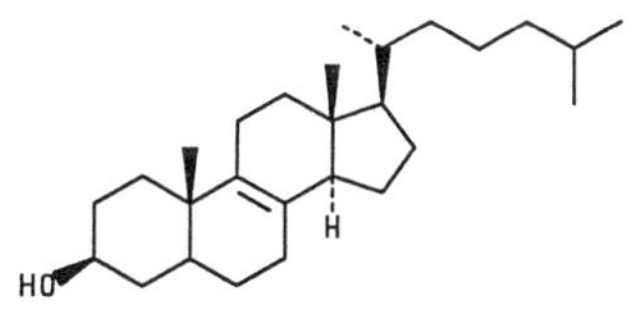

Mol. Wt.: 386
Organism: *Chattonella antiqua* (Raphidophyta) Culture
Location: Japan
Reference: 814

$C_{28}H_{48}O_5$ **24-Epicastasterone**

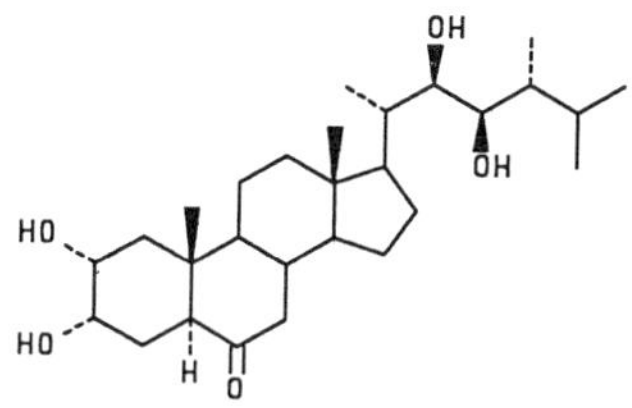

Mol. Wt.: 464
Bioactivity: Plant hormone
Organism: *Hydrodictyon reticulatum* (L.) Lagerheim (Chlorophyta)
Location: Japan
Reference: 1211

$C_{29}H_{50}O_5$ **(24S)-24-Ethylbrassinone**

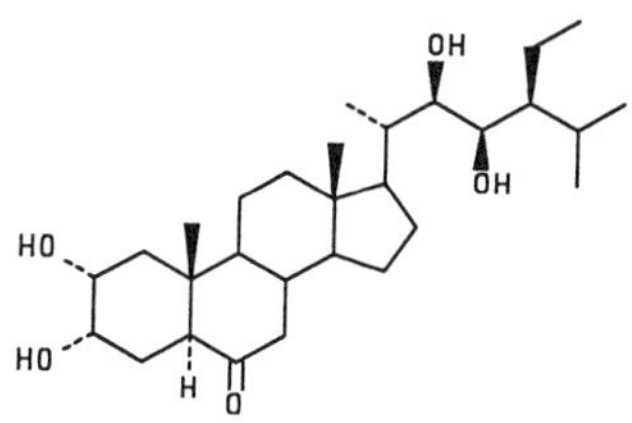

Mol. Wt.: 478
Bioactivity: Plant hormone
Spectral Data: Mass Spec. of derivative
Organism: *Hydrodictyon reticulatun* (L.) Lagerheim (Chlorophyta)
Location: Japan
Reference: 1211

$C_{29}H_{52}O$	**(23R,24R)-23,24-Dimethyl-5α-cholestan-3β-ol**
Mol. Wt.:	416
Spectral Data:	PMR
Organism:	*Orbulina universa* (Pyrrophyta)
Location:	Culture
Reference:	1223

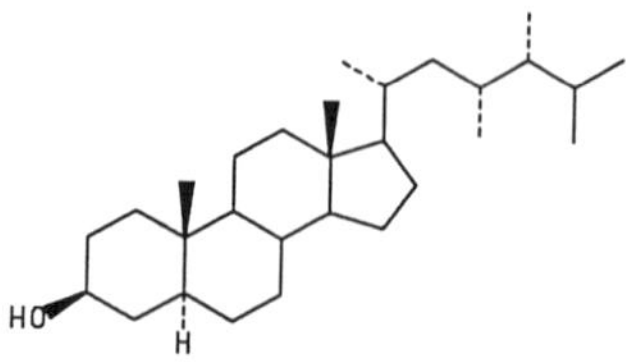

C. Terpenoids

$C_{10}H_{14}BrClO$ **(2R*,3(8)E,4S*,6R*)-6-Bromo-2-chloro-1,4-oxido-3(8)-ochtodene**

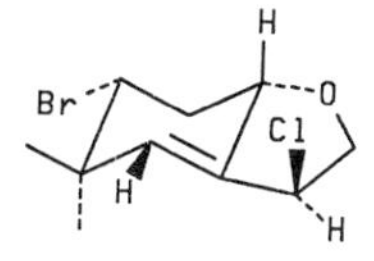

Mol. Wt.: 265
Melting Point: Oil
$[\alpha]_D$: +7.8 Solvent: Chf
Spectral Data: IR, CMR, PMR, Mass Spec.
Organism: *Chondrococcus hornemannii* (Rhodophyta)
Location: Great Barrier Reef, Australia
Reference: 191

$C_{10}H_{14}BrClO$ **(2S*,3(8)E,4S*,6R*)-6-Bromo-2-chloro-1,4-oxido-3(8)-ochtodene**

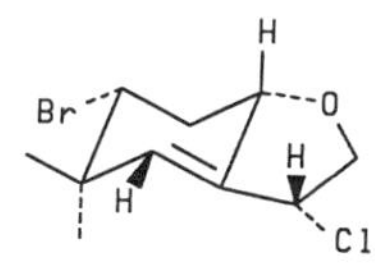

Mol. Wt.: 265
Melting Point: Oil
$[\alpha]_D$: -92.6 Solvent: Chf
Spectral Data: IR, CMR, PMR, Mass Spec.
Organism: *Chondrococcus hornemannii* (Rhodophyta)
Location: Great Barrier Reef, Australia
Reference: 191

$C_{10}H_{15}Br_2Cl$ **(E)-1,2-Dibromo-3-chloromethylene-7-methyloct-6-ene**

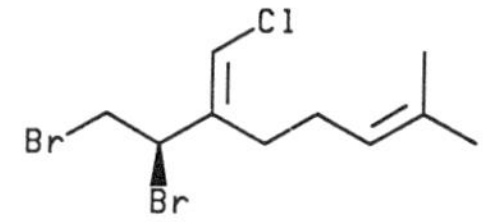

Mol. Wt.: 330
Melting Point: Oil
$[\alpha]_D$: +12.5 Solvent: Chf
Spectral Data: IR, CMR, PMR, Mass Spec.
Organism: *Chondrococcus hornemannii* (Rhodophyta)
Location: Great Barrier Reef, Australia
Reference: 191

$C_{10}H_{15}Cl_3$ **(<u>Z</u>)-1,6-Dichloro-3-chloromethyl-7-methylocta-2,7-diene**

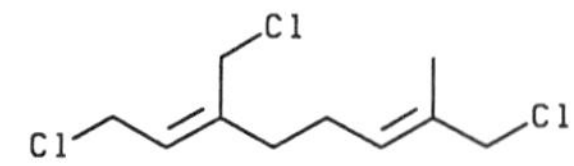

Mol. Wt.:	241
Melting Point:	Oil
$[\alpha]_D$:	−33.7 Solvent: Chf
Spectral Data:	IR, CMR, PMR, Mass Spec.
Organism:	*Chondrococcus hornemannii* (Rhodophyta)
Location:	Great Barrier Reef, Australia
Reference:	191

$C_{10}H_{15}Cl_3$ **(2<u>Z</u>,6<u>E</u>)-1,8-Dichloro-3-chloromethyl-7-methylocta-2,6-diene**

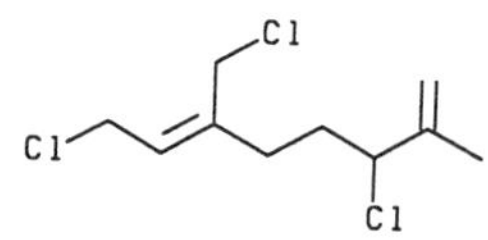

Mol. Wt.:	241
Melting Point:	Oil
Spectral Data:	IR, CMR, PMR, Mass Spec.
Organism:	*Chondrococcus hornemannii* (Rhodophyta)
Location:	Great Barrier Reef, Australia
Reference:	191

$C_{10}H_{16}Cl_2$ **(<u>Z</u>)-1-Chloro-3-chloromethyl-7-methylocta-2,6-diene**

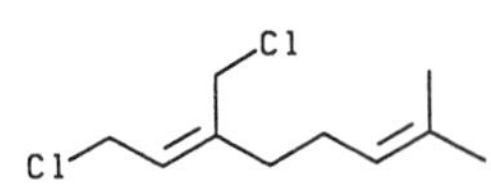

Mol. Wt.:	207
Melting Point:	Oil
Spectral Data:	IR, CMR, PMR, Mass Spec.
Organism:	*Chondrococcus hornemannii* (Rhodophyta)
Location:	Great Barrier Reef, Australia
Reference:	191

$C_{13}H_{22}O$ **Geranylacetone**

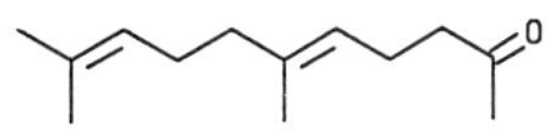

Mol. Wt.: 194
Bioactivity: Feeding deterrent
Melting Point: Oil
Spectral Data: IR, CMR, PMR, Mass Spec.
Organism: *Cystophora moniliformis* (Phaeophyta)
Location: South Australia
Reference: 1135

$C_{14}H_{18}O_2$ **Majusculone**

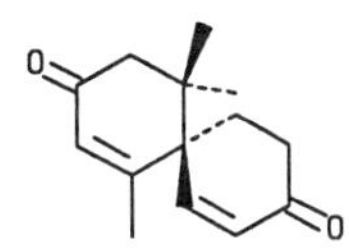

Mol. Wt.: 218
Melting Point: 91.1–92.0°C
$[\alpha]_D^{19}$: +145 Solvent: Chf
Spectral Data: UV, IR, CMR, PMR, Mass Spec.
Organism: *Laurencia majuscula* Harvey (Rhodophyta)
Location: Okino-Shima, Japan
Reference: 1059

$C_{15}H_{19}BrO$ **Isolaurenisol**

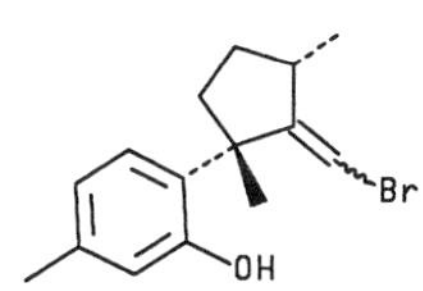

Mol. Wt.: 295
Melting Point: Oil
$[\alpha]_D^{25}$: −42 Solvent: Chf
Spectral Data: UV, IR, CMR, PMR, Mass Spec.
Organism: *Laurencia distichophylla* (Rhodophyta)
Location: Leigh, New Zealand
Reference: 82

$C_{15}H_{20}O$ (previously known)

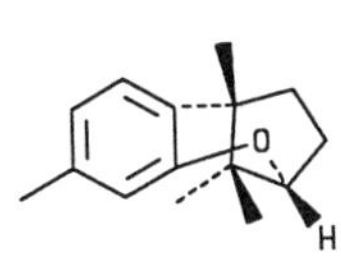

Mol. Wt.: 216
$[\alpha]_D$: −25
Organism: *Laurencia distichophylla* (Rhodophyta)
Location: Leigh, New Zealand
Reference: 82, 1055

$C_{15}H_{20}Br_2O_2$ **Dehydrochloroprepacifenol**

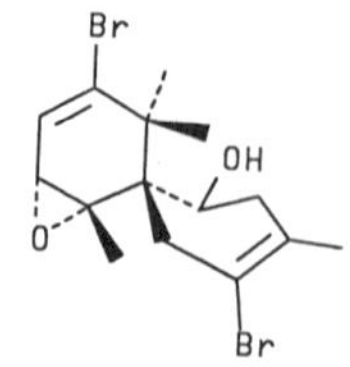

Mol. Wt.: 392
Melting Point: 124–125°C
$[\alpha]_D^{20}$: +51.7 Solvent: Alc
Spectral Data: IR, CMR, PMR, Mass Spec., x-ray c.s.
Organism: *Laurencia majuscula* (Rhodophyta)
Location: Sicily
Reference: 123

$C_{15}H_{20}O_4$ **Abscisic acid (ABA)**

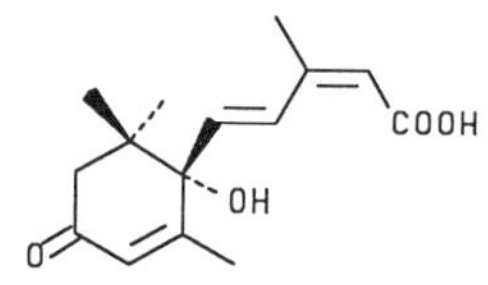

Mol. Wt.: 264
Bioactivity: Plant growth regulator
Spectral Data: Mass Spec. (methyl ester)
Organism: *Ascophyllum nodosum* (L.) Lejol (Phaeophyta)
Location: Maine and commercial extract (Nitrozyme™)
Reference: 107

$C_{15}H_{21}Br$ **α-Bromocuparene**
(previously known)

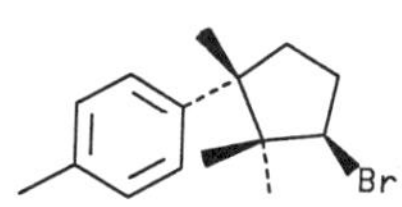

Mol. Wt.: 281
Melting Point: Oil
$[\alpha]_D$: +23.0 Solvent: Chf
Organism: *Laurencia distichophylla* (Rhodophyta)
Location: Leigh, New Zealand
Reference: 82, 1055, 1063

$C_{15}H_{21}BrO$ **Isoobtusadiene**

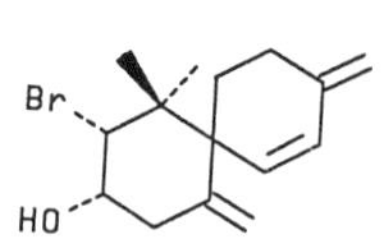

Mol. Wt.: 297
Melting Point: Oil
$[\alpha]_D^{25}$: -11.7 Solvent: Chf
Spectral Data: UV, IR, CMR, PMR, Mass Spec.
Organism: *Laurencia obtusa* (Hudson) Lamouroux (Rhodophyta)
Location: Puerto Rico, Tobago
Reference: 347

$C_{15}H_{21}BrO$ **Obtusadiene**

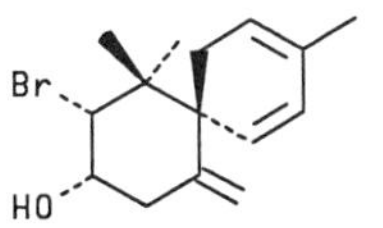

Mol. Wt.: 297
Melting Point: Oil
$[\alpha]_D^{25}$: -52.0 Solvent: Chf
Spectral Data: UV, CD, IR, CMR, PMR, Mass Spec.
Organism: *Laurencia obtusa* (Hudson) Lamouroux (Rhodophyta)
Location: Puerto Rico, Tobago
Reference: 347

$C_{15}H_{24}O_2$ **Humulenediol**

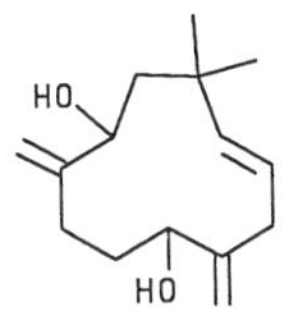

Mol. Wt.: 236
Melting Point: 104.5-107°C
$[\alpha]_D$: +0.8
Spectral Data: IR, CMR, PMR
Organism: *Laurencia obtusa* (Hud) Lamouroux (Rhodophyta)
Location: Hokkaido, Japan
Reference: 1065

$C_{15}H_{26}O$ **(1<u>R</u>,4<u>R</u>,10<u>R</u>)-1,4-Epoxycadinane**

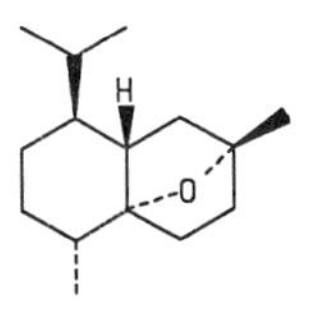

Mol. Wt.: 222
Melting Point: 54-55°C
$[\alpha]_D$: -46.6
Spectral Data: IR, CMR, PMR, Mass Spec.
Organism: *Dilophus fasciola* (Phaeophyta)
Location: Sicily
Reference: 287

$C_{15}H_{26}O$ **(5<u>S</u>,7<u>R</u>,10<u>R</u>)-Selin-4(14)-en-5α-ol**

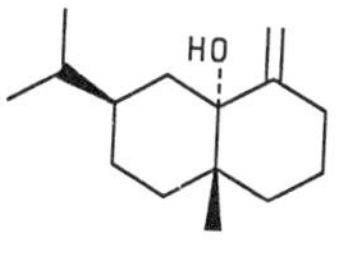

Mol. Wt.: 222
Melting Point: Oil
$[\alpha]_D^{20}$: +97.2 Solvent: Chf
Spectral Data: IR, CMR, PMR, Mass Spec.
Organism: *Laurencia nipponica* (Rhodophyta)
Location: Hokkaido, Japan
Reference: 1060

$C_{18}H_{29}Br$ **Norsphaerol**

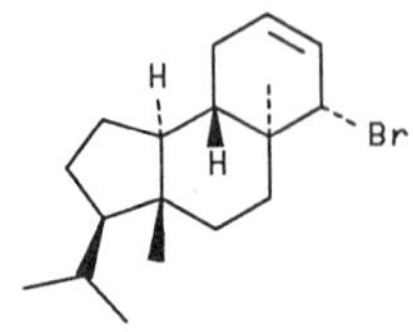

Mol. Wt.: 325
Melting Point: 107–109°C
$[\alpha]_D$: −39 Solvent: Chf
Spectral Data: CMR, PMR, Mass Spec., x–ray c.s.
Organism: *Sphaerococcus coronopifolius* (Rhodophyta)
Location: Naples, Italy
Reference: 55

$C_{18}H_{30}O_2$ **(5E,9E)-5,6-Epoxy-6,10,14-trimethylpentadeca-9,13-dien-2-one**

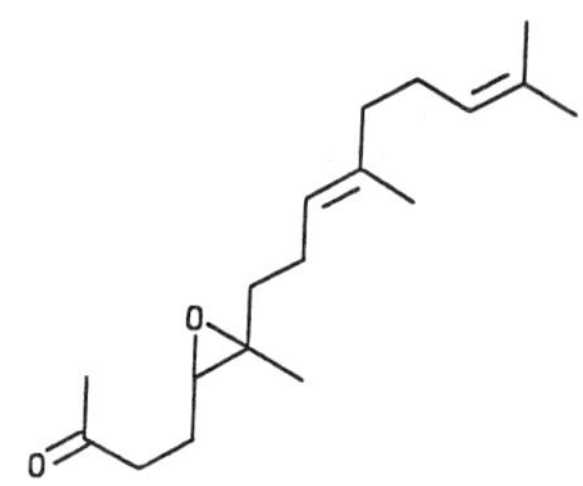

Mol. Wt.: 278
Melting Point: Oil
Spectral Data: IR, CMR, PMR, Mass Spec.
Organism: *Cystophora moniliformis* (Phaeophyta)
Location: South Australia
Reference: 1135

$C_{19}H_{34}O_3$ **(2S*,2'R*,5'S*,5E)-2-(5'-Methoxy-5'-methyltetrahydrofuran-2'-yl)-6,10-dimethylundeca-5,9-dien-2-ol**

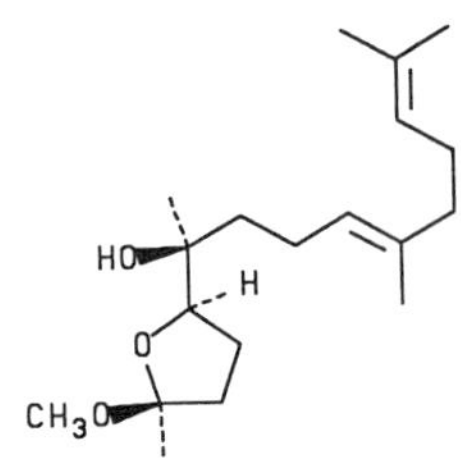

Mol. Wt.: 310
Melting Point: Oil
$[\alpha]_D$: +11 Solvent: Chf
Spectral Data: IR, CMR, PMR, Mass Spec.
Organism: *Cystophora moniliformis* (Phaeophyta)
Location: South Australia
Reference: 1135

$C_{20}H_{28}O$ **Fasciola-7,18-dien-17-al**

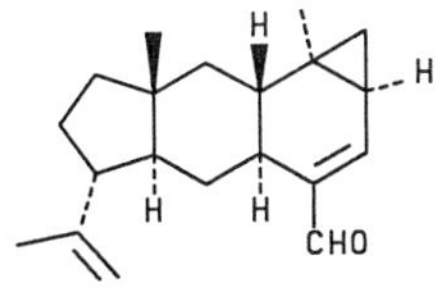

Mol. Wt.: 284
Melting Point: 103–104°C
$[\alpha]_D^{25}$: −150.9 Solvent: Alc
Spectral Data: UV, IR, CMR, PMR, Mass Spec.
Organism: *Dilophus fasciola* (Roth) Howe (Phaeophyta)
Location: Sicily
Reference: 1106

$C_{20}H_{30}O$ **Amijitrienol**

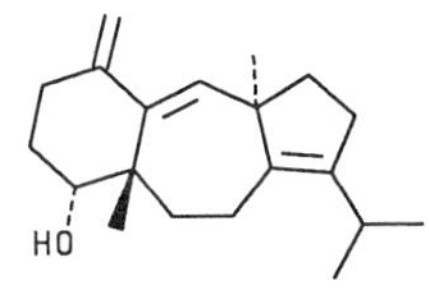

Mol. Wt.: 286
Bioactivity: Antimicrobial activity
Melting Point: 129–129.5°C
$[\alpha]_D^{18}$: +15.1 Solvent: Alc
Spectral Data: UV, IR, CMR, PMR, Mass Spec.
Organism: *Dictyota linearis* (Phaeophyta)
Location: Japan
Reference: 835

$C_{20}H_{30}O_2$ **(5S*,8S*,9S*,12S*,14R*)-9-Hydroxydolasta-1,3-dien-6-one**

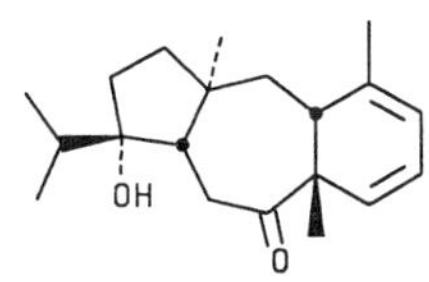

Mol. Wt.: 302
Melting Point: Oil
$[\alpha]_D^{23}$: +160 Solvent: Chf
Spectral Data: UV, IR, CMR, PMR, Mass Spec.
Organism: *Dictyota dichotoma* (Huds.) Lamouroux (Phaeophyta)
Location: Gulf of Mannar, India
Reference: 915

$C_{20}H_{31}BrO$ **Sphaeroxetane**

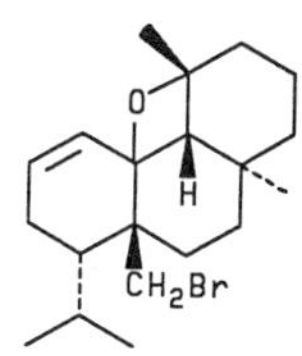

Mol. Wt.: 367
Melting Point: Oil
$[\alpha]_D$: −9.0 Solvent: Chf
Spectral Data: IR, CMR, PMR, Mass Spec.
Organism: *Sphaerococcus coronopifolius* (Rhodophyta)
Location: Yugoslavia
Reference: 234

$C_{20}H_{31}BrO_2$ **15-Bromo-7,16-dihydroxy-9(11)-parguerene**

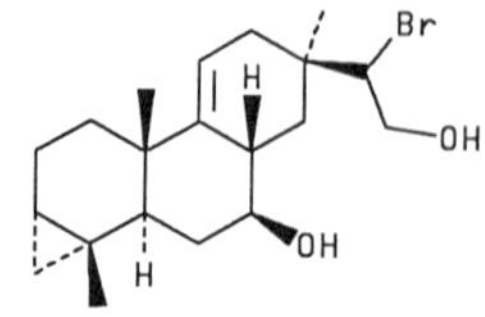

Mol. Wt.: 383
Melting Point: 87–90°C
$[\alpha]_D$: −17.8
Spectral Data: IR, CMR, PMR, Mass Spec.
Organism: *Laurencia obtusa* (Rhodophyta)
Location: Teuri Island, Japan
Reference: 1064

$C_{20}H_{32}$ **Isosphaerodiene-1**

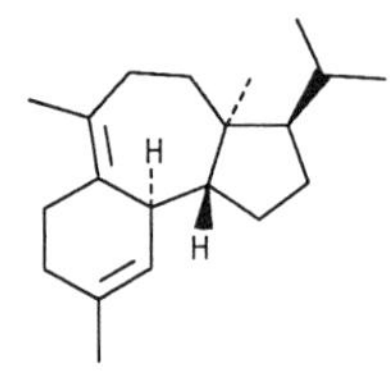

Mol. Wt.: 272
Melting Point: Oil
$[\alpha]_D$: +28 Solvent: Chf
Organism: *Sphaerococcus coronopifolius* (Rhodophyta)
Location: Naples, Italy
Reference: 125, 127

$C_{20}H_{32}$ **Isophaerodiene-2**

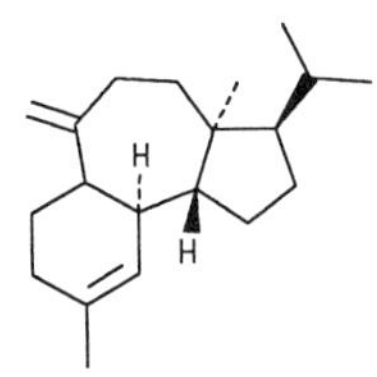

Mol. Wt.: 272
Melting Point: Oil
$[\alpha]_D$: +18 Solvent: Chf
Spectral Data: IR, PMR, Mass Spec.
Organism: *Sphaerococcus coronopifolius* (Rhodophyta)
Location: Naples, Italy
Reference: 125

$C_{20}H_{32}O$ **14-Deoxyisoamijiol**

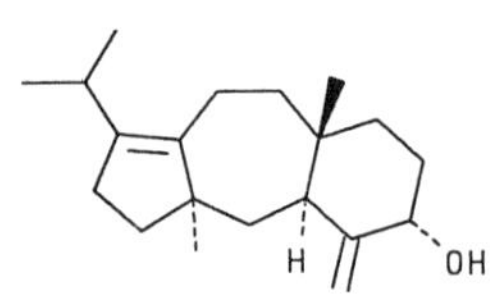

Mol. Wt.: 288
Bioactivity: Antimicrobial activity
Melting Point: 89–90°C
$[\alpha]_D^{18}$: −2.6 Solvent: Alc
Spectral Data: IR, CMR, PMR, Mass Spec.
Organism: *Dictyota linearis* (Phaeophyta)
Location: Japan
Reference: 835

$C_{20}H_{32}O$ **Dictymal**

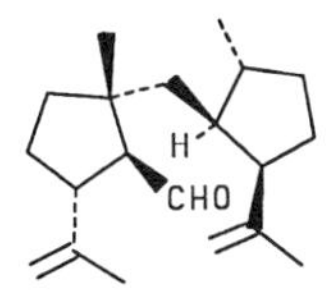

Mol. Wt.: 288
Melting Point: Oil
$[\alpha]_D^{18}$: +16.4 Solvent: Chf
Spectral Data: IR, CMR, PMR, Mass Spec.
Organism: *Dictyota dichotoma* (Phaeophyta)
Location: Hokkaido, Japan
Reference: 991

$C_{20}H_{32}O$ **Sphaeropyrane**

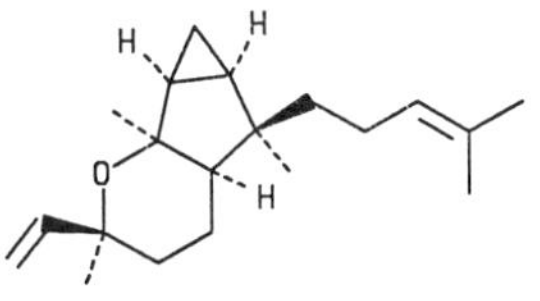

Mol. Wt.: 288
Melting Point: 136–138°C
$[\alpha]_D$: −43.9 Solvent: Chf
Spectral Data: IR, CMR, PMR, Mass Spec.
Organism: *Sphaerococcus coronopifolius* (Rhodophyta)
Location: Naples, Italy
Reference: 126

$C_{20}H_{32}Br_2O_2$ **12<u>R</u>-Hydroxybromosphaerol**

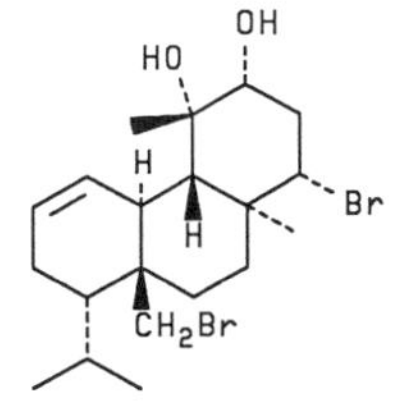

Mol. Wt.: 464
Melting Point: 89–92°C
$[\alpha]_D$: −34 Solvent: Chf
Spectral Data: IR, PMR, Mass Spec.
Organism: *Sphaerococcus coronopifolius* (Rhodophyta)
Location: Naples, Italy
Reference: 125

$C_{20}H_{32}O_2$ **Dictyol B**
(previously known)

Mol. Wt.: 304
Melting Point: 110–114°C
$[\alpha]_D$: +73.5
Spectral Data: CD, IR, CMR, PMR, Mass Spec.
Organism: *Dictyota* sp.
D. dichotoma var. *implexa*
(Phaeophyta)
Location: Canary Islands; Mediterranean
Reference: 288, 1140

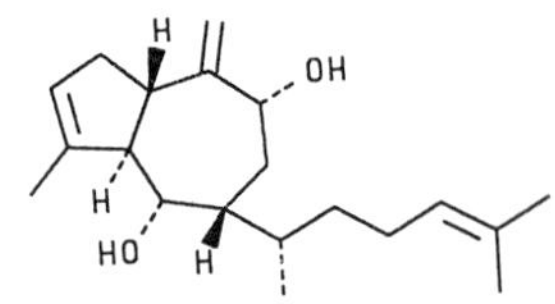

$C_{20}H_{32}O_2$ **Dictyotadiol**
(previously known)

Mol. Wt.: 304
Melting Point: 150–151°C
$[\alpha]_D$: +1.3 Solvent: Me
Spectral Data: UV, CD, PMR, Mass Spec. (derivative)
Organism: *Dictyota* sp.
D. dichotoma
(Phaeophyta)
Location: Canary Islands
Reference: 289, 1140

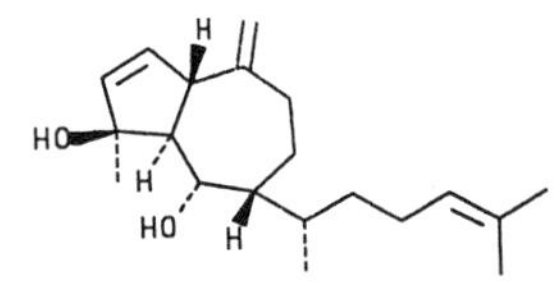

$C_{20}H_{32}O_2$ **Dilophic acid**

Mol. Wt.: 304
Bioactivity: Antibacterial activity against *Bacillus subtilis* at 100 μg/ml
Ichthyotoxic at 50 μg/ml
Melting Point: Oil
$[\alpha]_D^{25}$: −116 Solvent: Chf
Spectral Data: UV, IR, CMR, PMR, Mass Spec.
Organism: *Dilophus guineensis*
(Phaeophyta)
Location: Vega Baja, Puerto Rico
Reference: 979

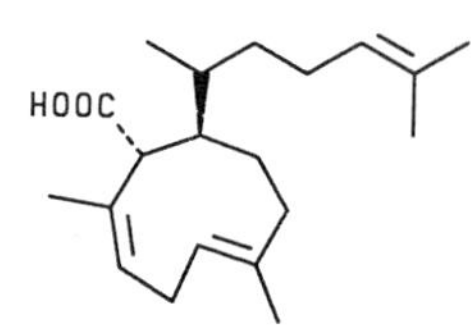

$C_{20}H_{32}O_2$

(2E,6E,10E)-14,15-Epoxy-3,7,11,15-tetramethylhexadeca-2,6,10-trienal

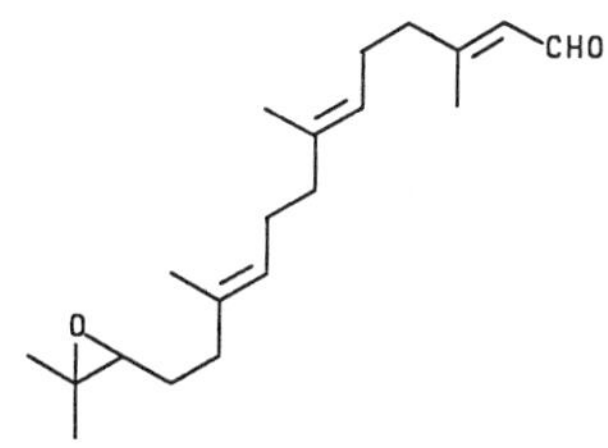

Mol. Wt.: 304
Melting Point: Oil
$[\alpha]_D$: -17 Solvent: Chf
Spectral Data: UV, IR, CMR, PMR, Mass Spec.
Organism: *Cystophora moniliformis* (Phaeophyta)
Location: South Australia
Reference: 1135

$C_{20}H_{32}O_2$

(2Z,6E,10E,)-14,15-Epoxy-3,7,11,15-tetramethylhexadeca-2,6,10-trienal

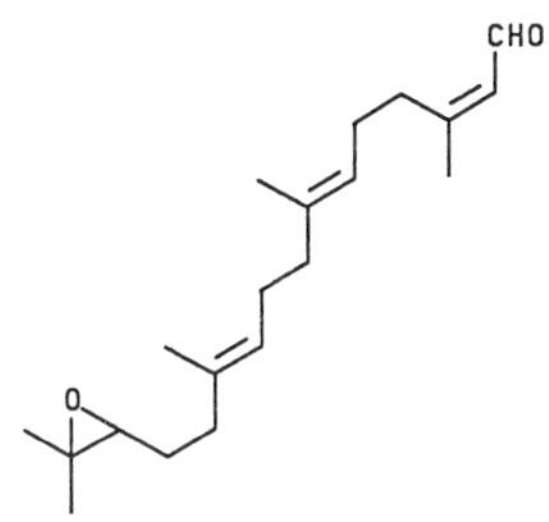

Mol. Wt.: 304
Melting Point: Oil
$[\alpha]_D$: -22 Solvent: Chf
Spectral Data: UV, IR, CMR, PMR, Mass Spec.
Organism: *Cystophora moniliformis* (Phaeophyta)
Location: South Australia
Reference: 1135

$C_{20}H_{32}O_2$

(1S*,3E,6Z,11S*,12S*)-12-Hydroxydolabella-3,6-dien-9-one
(two isomers)

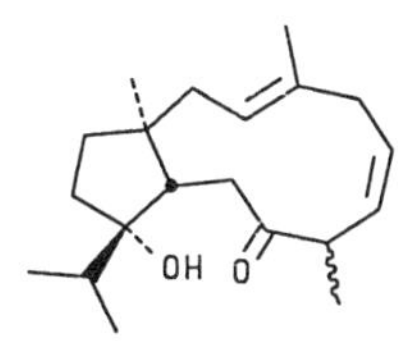

Mol. Wt.: 304
Melting Point: Oil
$[\alpha]_D^{23}$: +31.7 Solvent: Chf
+9.4 Solvent: Me
Spectral Data: UV, IR, CMR, PMR, Mass Spec.
Organism: *Dictyota dichotoma* (Huds.) Lamouroux (Phaeophyta)
Location: Gulf of Mannar, India
Reference: 915

$C_{20}H_{32}O_2$ **(1S*,3E,7E,11S*,12S*)-12-Hydroxydolabella-3,7-dien-9-one**

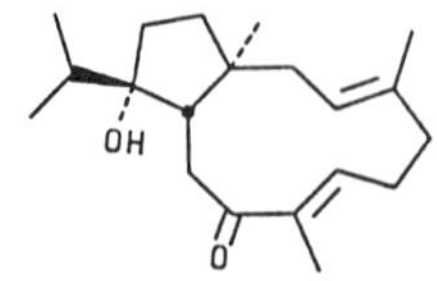

Mol. Wt.: 304
Melting Point: 93–95°C
$[\alpha]_D^{23}$: −53.3 Solvent: Chf
Spectral Data: UV, IR, CMR, PMR, Mass Spec.
Organism: *Dictyota dichotoma* (Huds.) Lamouroux (Phaeophyta)
Location: Gulf of Mannar, India
Reference: 915

$C_{20}H_{32}O_2$ **(1S*,3E,7Z,11S*,12S*)-12-Hydroxydolabella-3,7-dien-9-one**

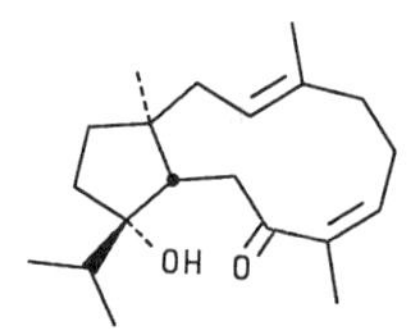

Mol. Wt.: 304
Melting Point: Oil
$[\alpha]_D^{23}$: +7.2 Solvent: Chf
Spectral Data: UV, IR, CMR, PMR, Mass Spec.
Organism: *Dictyota dichotoma* (Huds.) Lamouroux (Phaeophyta)
Location: Gulf of Mannar, India
Reference: 915

$C_{20}H_{32}Br_2O_3$ **12S-Hydroxybromosphaerodiol**

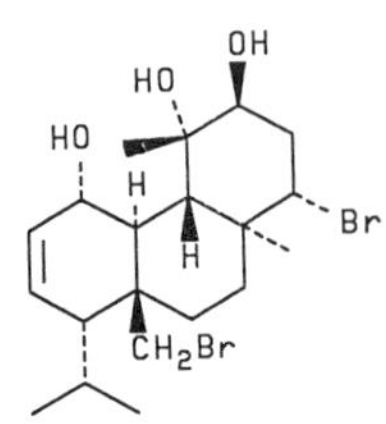

Mol. Wt.: 480
Melting Point: 88–90°C
$[\alpha]_D$: +39 Solvent: Chf
Spectral Data: IR, PMR, Mass Spec.
Organism: *Sphaerococcus coronopifolius* (Rhodophyta)
Location: Naples, Italy
Reference: 125

$C_{20}H_{32}O_3$ **Dictyotriol A**

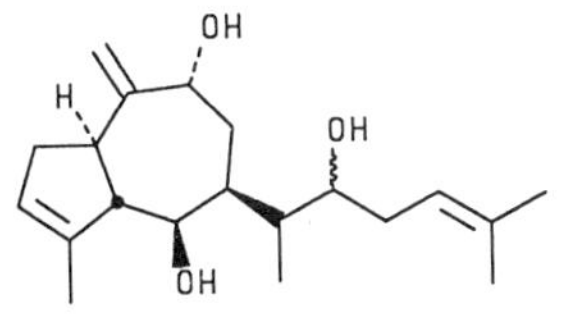

Mol. Wt.: 320
$[\alpha]_D^{25}$: +24.9 Solvent: Chf
Spectral Data: IR, CMR, PMR, Mass Spec.
Organism: *Glossophora kuntii* (C. Agardh) J. Agardh (Phaeophyta)
Location: V Región, Chile
Reference: 938

$C_{20}H_{32}O_3$ **Dictyotriol C**

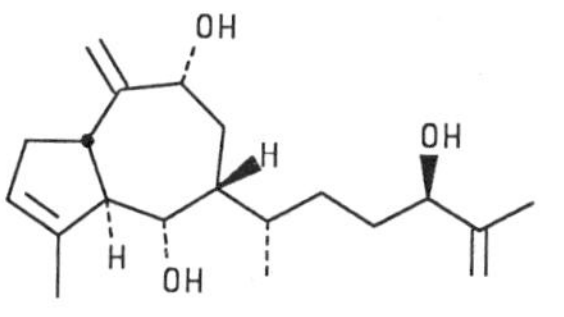

Mol. Wt.: 320
Melting Point: 165–167°C
$[\alpha]_D$: 77.4 Solvent: Chf
Spectral Data: IR, CMR, PMR, Mass Spec.; CD of derivative
Organism: *Dictyota* sp. (Phaeophyta)
Location: Canary Islands
Reference: 1140

$C_{20}H_{32}O_3$ **Dictyotriol D**

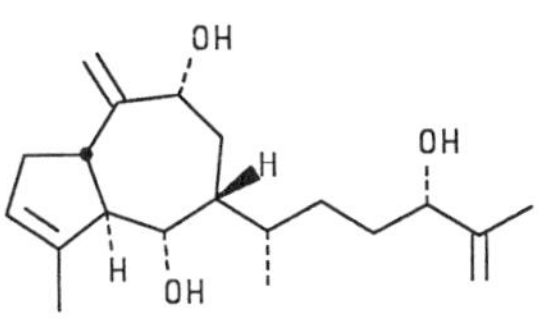

Mol. Wt.: 320
Melting Point: 164–166°C
$[\alpha]_D$: +72.4 Solvent: Chf
Spectral Data: IR, CMR, PMR, Mass Spec.; CD of derivative
Organism: *Dictyota* sp. (Phaeophyta)
Location: Canary Islands
Reference: 1140

$C_{20}H_{32}O_3$ **Dictyotriol E**

Mol. Wt.: 320
Melting Point: Oil
$[\alpha]_D$: +56.8 Solvent: Chf (acetate)
Spectral Data: IR, CMR, PMR, Mass Spec. (acetate); CD of derivative
Organism: *Dictyota* sp. (Phaeophyta)
Location: Canary Islands
Reference: 1140

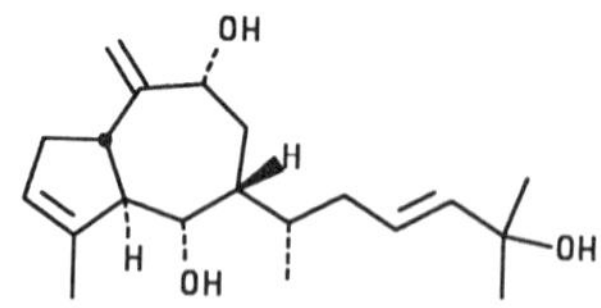

$C_{20}H_{32}O_3$ **Dictyoxetane**

Mol. Wt.: 320
Melting Point: 87–90°C
$[\alpha]_D$: +35 Solvent: Chf
Spectral Data: IR, CMR, PMR, Mass Spec., x–ray c.s.
Organism: *Dictyota dichotoma* (Phaeophyta)
Location: Gulf of Mannar, India
Reference: 902, 915

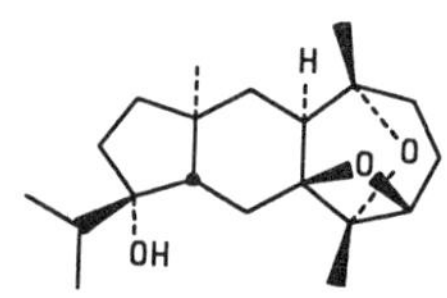

$C_{20}H_{32}O_3$ **(1S*,2E,4R*,6Z,11S*,12S*)-4,12-Dihydroxydolabella-2,6-dien-9-one** (two isomers)

Mol. Wt.: 320
Melting Point: Oil
$[\alpha]_D^{23}$: +13.3 Solvent: Chf
−52.3 Solvent: Chf
Spectral Data: UV, IR, CMR, PMR, Mass Spec.
Organism: *Dictyota dichotoma* (Huds.) Lamouroux (Phaeophyta)
Location: Gulf of Mannar, India
Reference: 915

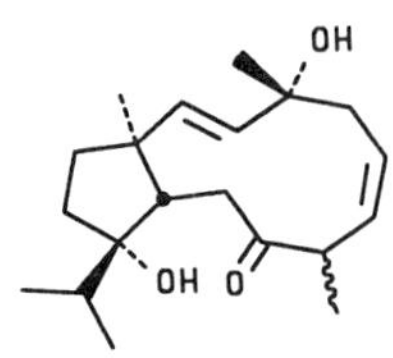

$C_{20}H_{32}O_3$

(1S*,2E,4R*,7E,11S*,12S*)-4,12-Dihydroxydolabella-2,7-dien-9-one

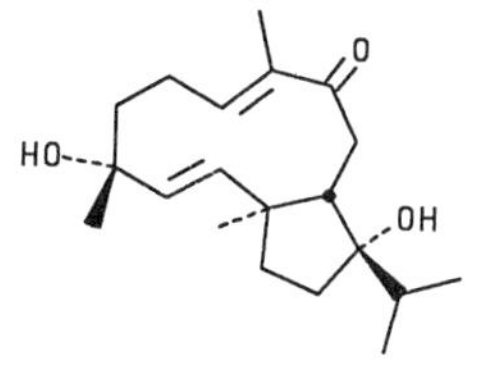

Mol. Wt.: 320
Melting Point: 212–213°C
$[\alpha]_D^{23}$: −6.5 Solvent: Me
Spectral Data: UV, IR, CMR, PMR, Mass Spec.
Organism: *Dictyota dichotoma* (Huds.) Lamouroux (Phaeophyta)
Location: Gulf of Mannar, India
Reference: 915

$C_{20}H_{32}O_3$

(1S*,2E,4R*,7Z,11S*,12S*)-4,12-Dihydroxydolabella-2,7-dien-9-one

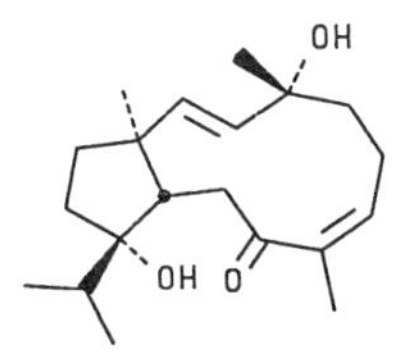

Mol. Wt.: 320
Melting Point: 153–155°C
$[\alpha]_D^{23}$: −99.3 Solvent: Chf
Spectral Data: UV, IR, CMR, PMR, Mass Spec., x–ray c.s.
Organism: *Dictyota dichotoma* (Huds.) Lamouroux (Phaeophyta)
Location: Gulf of Mannar, India
Reference: 915

$C_{20}H_{32}O_3$

(1S*,3E,7R*,8R*,11S*,12S*)-7,8-Epoxy-12-hydroxydolabella-3-en-9-one

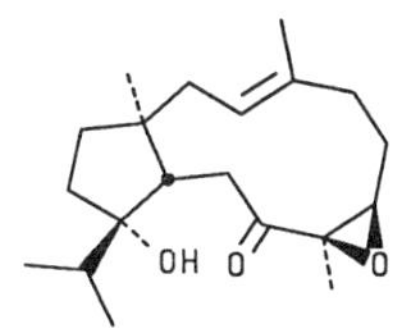

Mol. Wt.: 320
Melting Point: Oil
$[\alpha]_D^{23}$: −1.3 Solvent: Chf
Spectral Data: UV, IR, CMR, PMR, Mass Spec.
Organism: *Dictyota dichotoma* (Huds.) Lamouroux (Phaeophyta)
Location: Gulf of Mannar, India
Reference: 915

$C_{20}H_{32}O_3$ **(1S*,3S*,4R*,7E,11S*,12S*)-3,4-Epoxy-12-hydroxydolabella-7-en-9-one**

Mol. Wt.: 320
Melting Point: 113–115°C
$[\alpha]_D^{23}$: −32.7 Solvent: Chf
Spectral Data: UV, IR, CMR, PMR, Mass Spec.
Organism: *Dictyota dichotoma* (Huds.) Lamouroux (Phaeophyta)
Location: Gulf of Mannar, India
Reference: 915

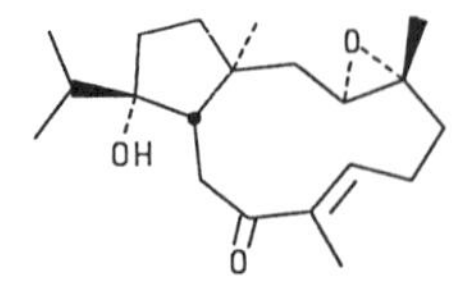

$C_{20}H_{32}O_4$ **Cervicol**

Mol. Wt.: 336
Melting Point: Gum
$[\alpha]_D^{25}$: −76.1 Solvent: Chf (acetate)
Spectral Data: IR, CMR, PMR, Mass Spec. (acetate)
Organism: *Dictyota cervicornis* (Phaeophyta)
Location: Rio de Janeiro, Brazil
Reference: 1087

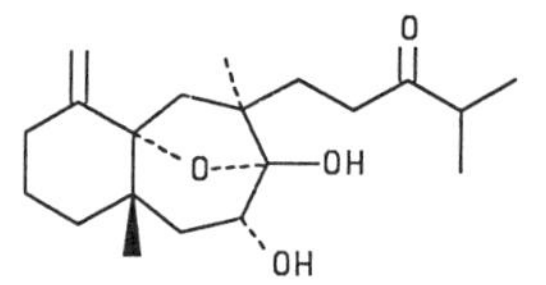

$C_{20}H_{32}O_4$ **Isolinearol**

Mol. Wt.: 336
Melting Point: Gum
$[\alpha]_D^{25}$: −52.1 Solvent: Chf
Spectral Data: IR, CMR, PMR, Mass Spec.
Organism: *Dictyota cervicornis* Kützing (Phaeophyta)
Location: Rio de Janiero, Brazil
Reference: 1086

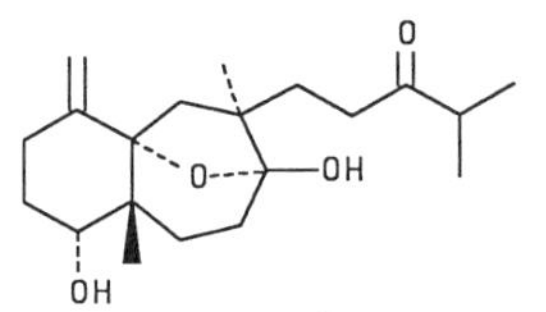

$C_{20}H_{33}BrO$ **Pinnatol B**

Mol. Wt.: 369
Melting Point: 106.5–107.5°C
$[a]_D$: −7.6 Solvent: Chf
Spectral Data: IR, PMR, Mass Spec.
Organism: *Laurencia pinnata* (Rhodophyta)
Location: Japan
Reference: 326

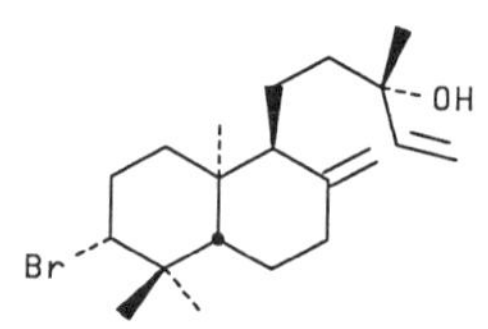

$C_{20}H_{33}BrO$ **Pinnatol C**

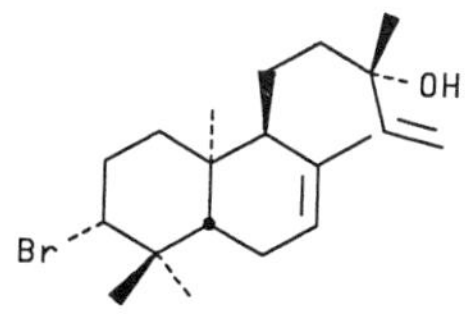

Mol. Wt.: 369
Melting Point: Oil
$[\alpha]_D$: +110.5 Solvent: Chf
Spectral Data: IR, PMR, Mass Spec.
Organism: *Laurencia pinnata* (Rhodophyta)
Location: Japan
Reference: 326

$C_{20}H_{33}BrO$ **Pinnatol D**

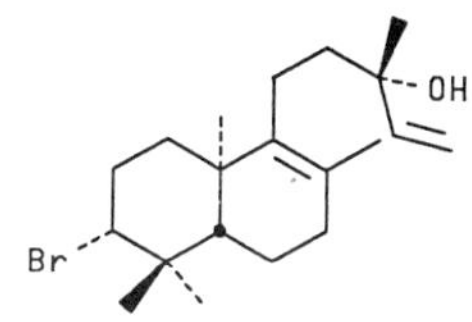

Mol. Wt.: 369
Melting Point: Oil
$[\alpha]_D$: −48.2 Solvent: Chf
Spectral Data: IR, PMR, Mass Spec.
Organism: *Laurencia pinnata* (Rhodophyta)
Location: Japan
Reference: 326

$C_{20}H_{33}BrO_2$ **Bromotetrasphaerol**

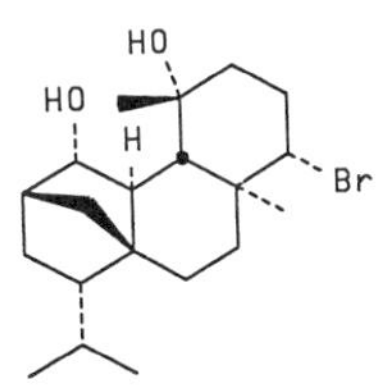

Mol. Wt.: 385
Melting Point: Oil
$[\alpha]_D$: −5.9 Solvent: Chf
Spectral Data: IR, CMR, PMR, Mass Spec.
Organism: *Sphaerococcus coronopifolius* (Rhodophyta)
Location: Naples, Italy
Reference: 129

$C_{20}H_{34}O_2$ **12-(S)-Hydroxygeranylgeraniol**

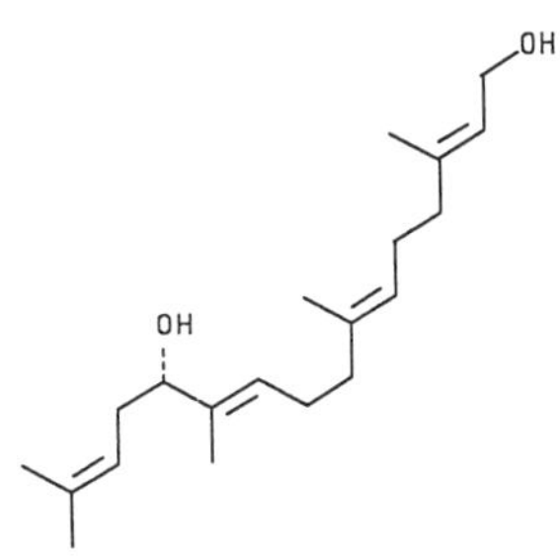

Mol. Wt.: 306
Melting Point: Oil
$[\alpha]_D$: −12.47 Solvent: Dcm
Spectral Data: IR, CMR, PMR, Mass Spec.
Organism: *Bifurcaria bifurcata* (Phaeophyta)
Location: Atlantic Coast, Morocco
Reference: 1134

$C_{20}H_{34}O_3$ **Isodictytriol**

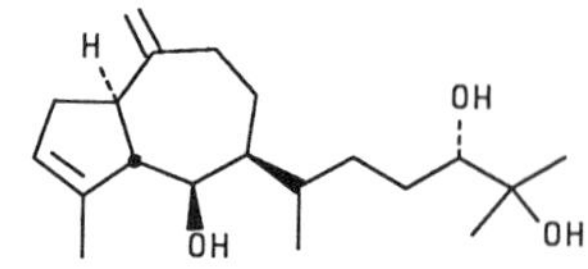

Mol. Wt.: 322
Melting Point: 125–126°C
Spectral Data: CD, IR, CMR, PMR, x-ray c.s.
Organism: *Dictyota dichotoma* (Phaeophyta)
Location: Okinawa, Japan
Reference: 627

$C_{20}H_{35}BrO_2$ **Pinnatol A**

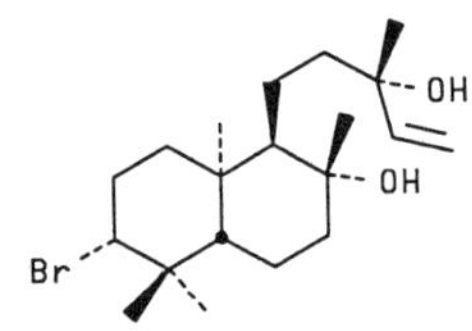

Mol. Wt.: 387
Melting Point: 49–51°C
$[\alpha]_D$: +24.5 Solvent: Chf
Spectral Data: IR, CMR, PMR, Mass Spec.; CD of derivative
Organism: *Laurencia pinnata* (Rhodophyta)
Location: Japan
Reference: 326

$C_{21}H_{28}O_5$ **Dendryphiellin A**

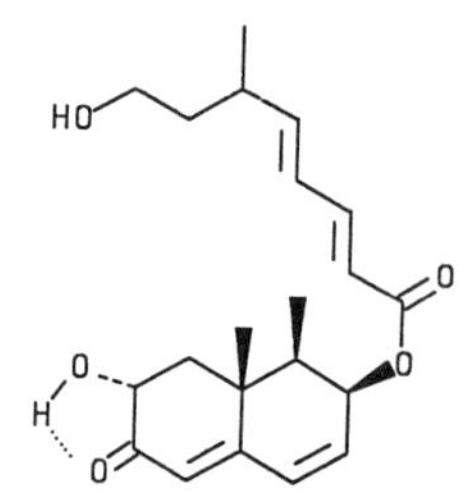

Mol. Wt.: 360
Melting Point: Oil
$[\alpha]_D^{20}$: +572.1 Solvent: Alc
Spectral Data: UV, CD, CMR, PMR, Mass Spec.
Organism: *Dendryphiella salina* (Dematiaceae) Culture
Reference: 373

$C_{22}H_{32}O_3$

(1R*,3E,7E,9S*,11S*)-9-Acetoxydolabella-3,7,12-trien-16-al

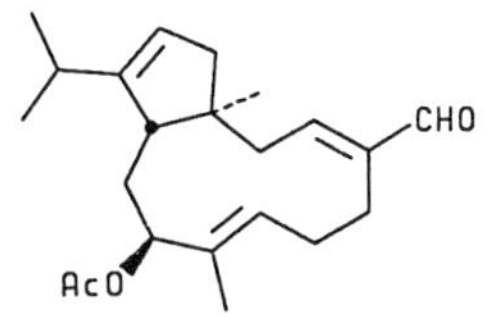

Mol. Wt.: 344
Melting Point: 163–165°C
$[\alpha]_D^{23}$: +10 Solvent: Chf
Spectral Data: UV, IR, CMR, PMR, Mass Spec., x-ray c.s.
Organism: *Dictyota dichotoma* (Huds.) Lamouroux (Phaeophyta)
Location: Gulf of Mannar, India
Reference: 915

$C_{22}H_{32}O_4$

(1R*,3E,7E,9S*,11S*)-9-Acetoxydolabella-3,7,12-trien-16-oic acid

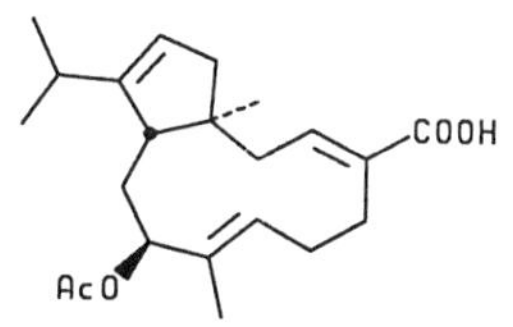

Mol. Wt.: 360
Melting Point: 152–154°C
$[\alpha]_D^{23}$: +60.2 Solvent: Chf
Spectral Data: UV, IR, CMR, PMR, Mass Spec.
Organism: *Dictyota dichotoma* (Huds.) Lamouroux (Phaeophyta)
Location: Gulf of Mannar, India
Reference: 915

$C_{22}H_{34}O_4$

(1R*,2R*,3E,7E,11S*,12S*)-2-Acetoxy-12-hydroxydolabella-3,7-dien-9-one

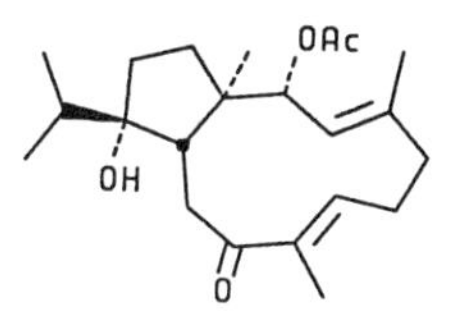

Mol. Wt.: 362
Melting Point: 173–174°C
$[\alpha]_D^{23}$: −73.2 Solvent: Chf
Spectral Data: UV, IR, CMR, PMR, Mass Spec.
Organism: *Dictyota dichotoma* (Huds.) Lamouroux (Phaeophyta)
Location: Gulf of Mannar, India
Reference: 915

$C_{22}H_{34}O_4$ **Dictyotriol A monoacetate**

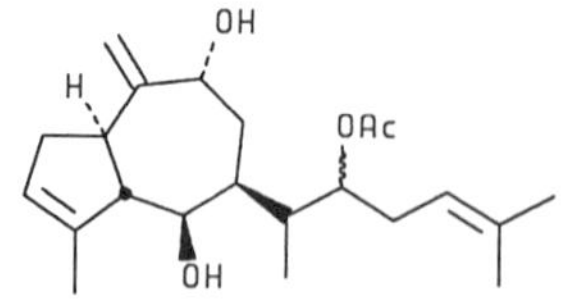

Mol. Wt.: 362
Melting Point: Oil
$[\alpha]_D^{25}$: +7.8 Solvent: Chf
Spectral Data: IR, CMR, PMR, Mass Spec.
Organism: *Glossophora kuntii* (C. Agardh) J. Agardh (Phaeophyta)
Location: V Región, Chile
Reference: 938

$C_{22}H_{34}O_5$ **Isolinearol acetate**

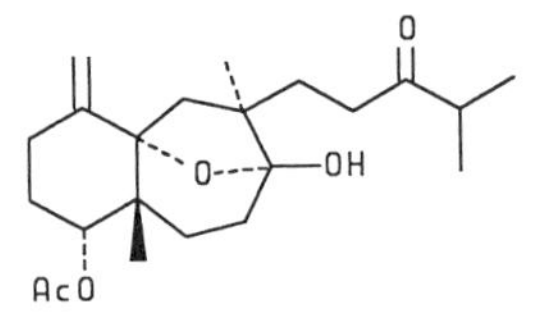

Mol. Wt.: 378
Melting Point: Gum
$[\alpha]_D^{25}$: -50.0 Solvent: Chf
Spectral Data: IR, CMR, PMR, Mass Spec.
Organism: *Dictyota cervicornis* Kützing (Phaeophyta)
Location: Rio de Janeiro, Brazil
Reference: 1086

$C_{22}H_{36}O_3$ **(1S*,3E,7E,11S*,12S*)-9-Acetoxydolabella-3,7-dien-12-ol**

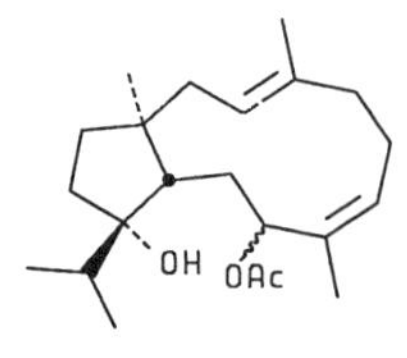

Mol. Wt.: 348
Melting Point: Oil
$[\alpha]_D^{23}$: +2.3 Solvent: Chf
Spectral Data: UV, IR, CMR, PMR, Mass Spec.
Organism: *Dictyota dichotoma* (Huds.) Lamouroux (Phaeophyta)
Location: Gulf of Mannar, India
Reference: 915

$C_{22}H_{36}O_3$ **Chromophycadiol monoacetate**

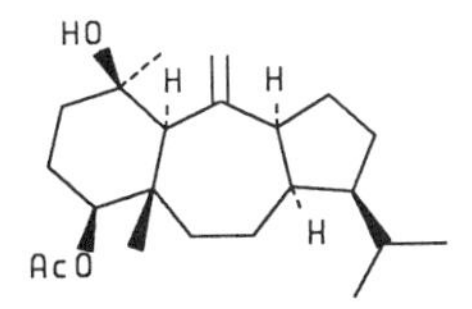

Mol. Wt.: 348
Melting Point: 137–139°C
$[\alpha]_D$: +26.5 Solvent: Chf
Spectral Data: IR, CMR, PMR, Mass Spec., x-ray c.s.
Organism: *Dictyota* sp. (Phaeophyta)
Location: Tenerife, Canary Islands
Reference: 189

$C_{22}H_{36}O_3$ **3-Hydroxyacetyldilophol**

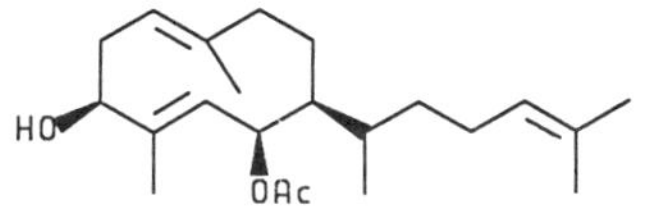

Mol. Wt.: 348
$[\alpha]_D$: −7.2 Solvent: Chf
Spectral Data: IR, PMR, Mass Spec.
Organism: *Pachydictyon coriaceum* (Phaeophyta)
Location: Japan
Reference: 472

$C_{22}H_{36}O_4$ **(1S*,3E,11S*,12S*)-9-Acetoxy-7,8-epoxydolabella-3-en-12-ol**

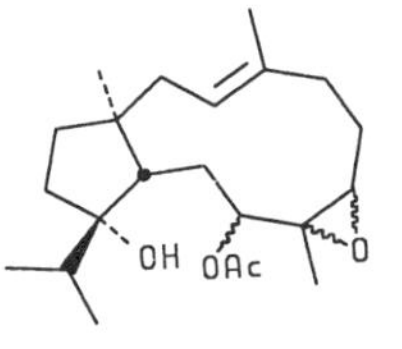

Mol. Wt.: 364
Melting Point: Oil
$[\alpha]_D^{23}$: −3.3 Solvent: Chf
Spectral Data: UV, IR, CMR, PMR, Mass Spec.
Organism: *Dictyota dichotoma* (Huds.) Lamouroux (Phaeophyta)
Location: Gulf of Mannar, India
Reference: 915

$C_{22}H_{36}O_4$ **Acetoxypachydiol**

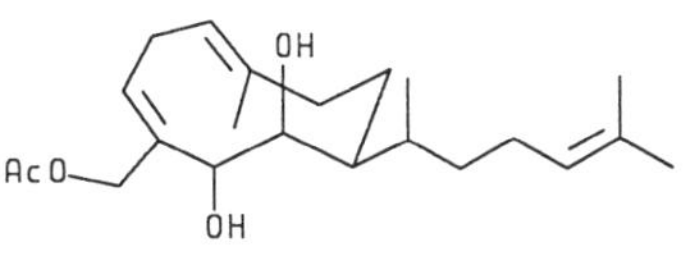

Mol. Wt.: 364
Melting Point: Oil
$[\alpha]_D$: −76.4 Solvent: Chf
Spectral Data: IR, CMR, PMR
Organism: *Pachydictyon coriaceum* (Phaeophyta)
Location: Japan
Reference: 472

$C_{22}H_{36}O_4$ **Crenulacetal A**

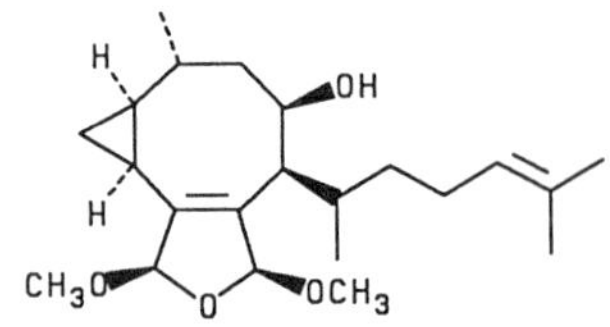

Mol. Wt.: 364
Melting Point: Oil
$[\alpha]_D$: +5.1 Solvent: Chf
Spectral Data: IR, CMR, PMR, Mass Spec.
Organism: *Dictyota dichotoma*, *D. spinulosa* (Phaeophyta)
Location: Okinawa, Japan
Reference: 626

$C_{22}H_{36}O_4$ **Crenulacetal B**

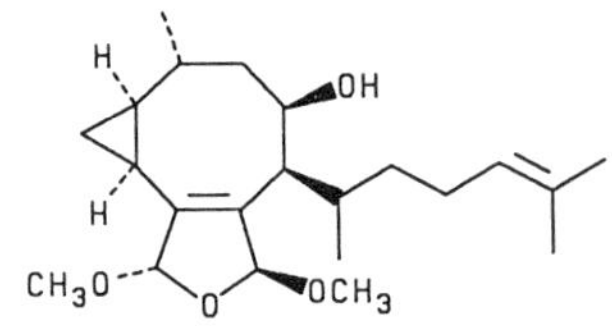

Mol. Wt.: 364
Melting Point: Oil
$[\alpha]_D$: +69.9 Solvent: Chf
Spectral Data: IR, CMR, PMR, Mass Spec.
Organism: *Dictyota spinulosa* (Phaeophyta)
Location: Okinawa, Japan
Reference: 626

$C_{24}H_{32}O_6$

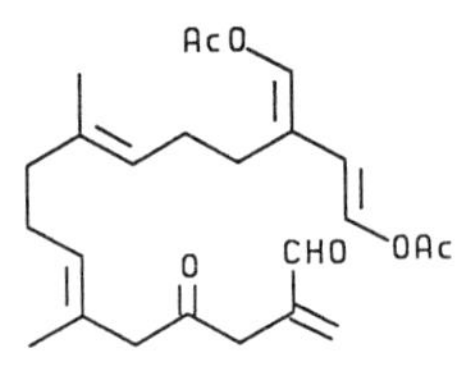

Mol. Wt.: 416
Bioactivity: Fertilized sea urchin egg assay: 100% inhibition of cell division at 8μg/ml
Antimicrobial activity
Melting Point: Oil
$[\alpha]_D^{25}$: 0 Solvent: Chf
Spectral Data: UV, IR, CMR, PMR, Mass Spec.
Organism: *Chlorodesmis fastigiata* (Chlorophyta)
Location: Guam
Reference: 868

$C_{24}H_{32}O_7$

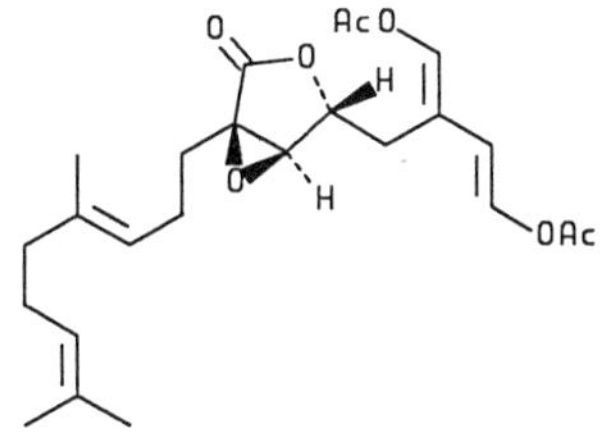

Mol. Wt.:	432
Bioactivity:	Fertilized sea urchin egg assay: 100% inhibition of cell division at 8 μg/ml Antimicrobial activity
$[\alpha]_D^{25}$:	+7.0 Solvent: Chf
Spectral Data:	UV, IR, CMR, PMR, Mass Spec.
Organism:	*Udotea argentea* (Chlorophyta)
Location:	Guam
Reference:	868

$C_{24}H_{32}O_7$

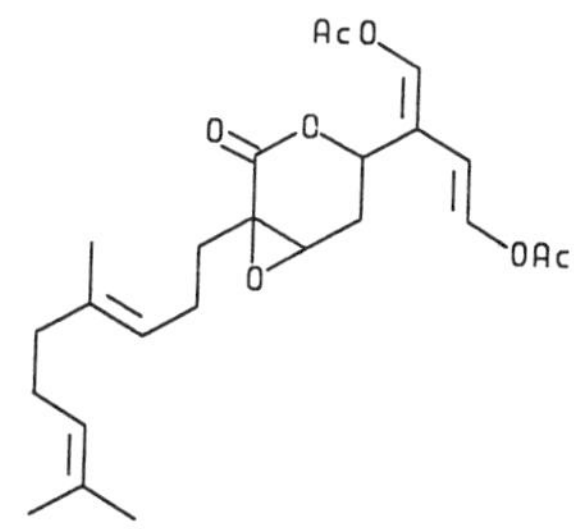

Mol. Wt.:	432
Bioactivity:	Feeding deterrent
$[\alpha]_D^{25}$:	+1.6 Solvent: Chf
Spectral Data:	UV, IR, CMR, PMR, Mass Spec.
Organism:	*Pseudochlorodesmis furcellata* (Chlorophyta)
Location:	Guam
Reference:	867

$C_{24}H_{38}O_5$

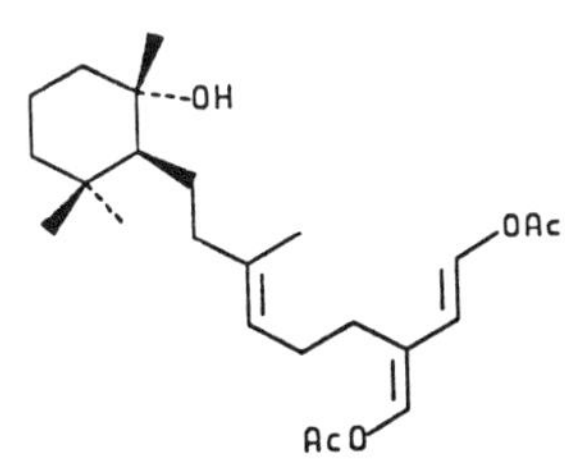

Mol. Wt.:	406
Bioactivity:	Fertilized sea urchin egg assay: 100% inhibition of cell division at 8 μg/ml Antimicrobial activity
Melting Point:	Oil
$[\alpha]_D^{25}$:	−0.5 Solvent: Chf
Spectral Data:	UV, IR, CMR, PMR, Mass Spec.
Organism:	*Caulerpa brownii* (Chlorophyta)
Location:	Melbourne, Australia
Reference:	868

$C_{24}H_{38}O_5$ **Crenulacetal C**

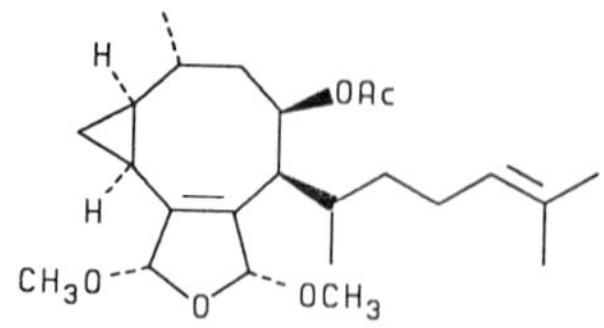

Mol. Wt.: 406
Melting Point: Oil
$[\alpha]_D$: −6.15 Solvent: Chf
Spectral Data: IR, CMR, PMR, Mass Spec.
Organism: Unknown sp. (Phaeophyta)
Location: Shimoda, Japan
Reference: 626

$C_{24}H_{38}O_5$ **Crenulacetal D**

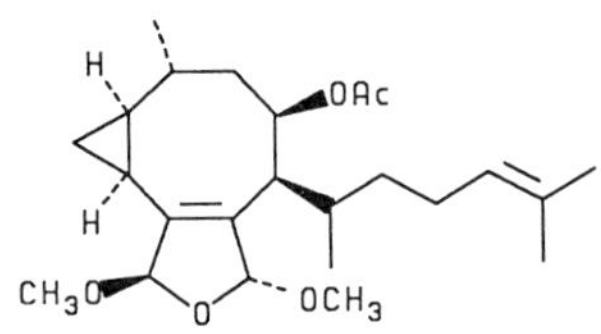

Mol. Wt.: 406
Melting Point: Oil
$[\alpha]_D$: +14.1 Solvent: Chf
Spectral Data: IR, PMR, Mass Spec.
Organism: Unknown sp. (Phaeophyta)
Location: Shimoda, Japan
Reference: 626

$C_{24}H_{42}O_4$

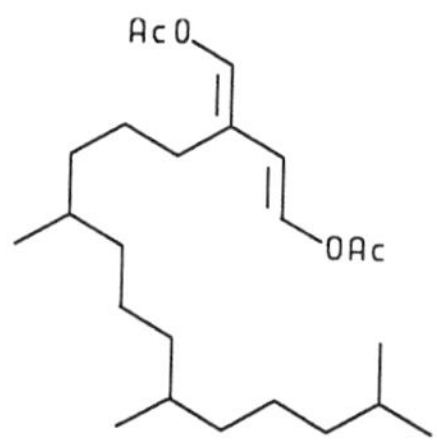

Mol. Wt.: 394
$[\alpha]_D^{25}$: +1.6
Spectral Data: UV, IR, CMR, PMR, Mass Spec.
Organism: *Pseudochlorodesmis furcellata* (Chlorophyta)
Location: Guam
Reference: 867

$C_{27}H_{38}O_5$ **Cystoseirol B**

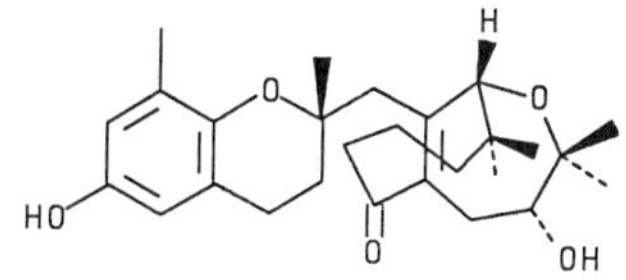

Mol. Wt.: 442
Melting Point: Oil
$[\alpha]_D$: +20 Solvent: Me
Spectral Data: UV, IR, CMR, PMR, Mass Spec.
Organism: *Cystoseira mediterranea*
C. tamariscifolia
C. stricta
(Phaeophyta)
Location: Banyuls-sur-Mer, Atlantic Coast, and Nice, France
Reference: 307

$C_{27}H_{38}O_5$ **Cystoseirol C**

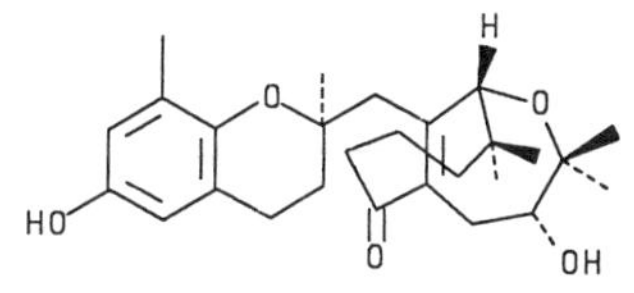

Mol. Wt.: 442
Melting Point: Oil
$[\alpha]_D$: +36 Solvent: Me
Spectral Data: UV, IR, PMR, Mass Spec.
Organism: *Cystoseira mediterranea*
C. tamariscifolia
C. stricta
(Phaeophyta)
Location: Banyuls-sur-Mer, Atlantic Coast, and Nice, France
Reference: 307

$C_{27}H_{38}O_5$ **Cystoseirol D**

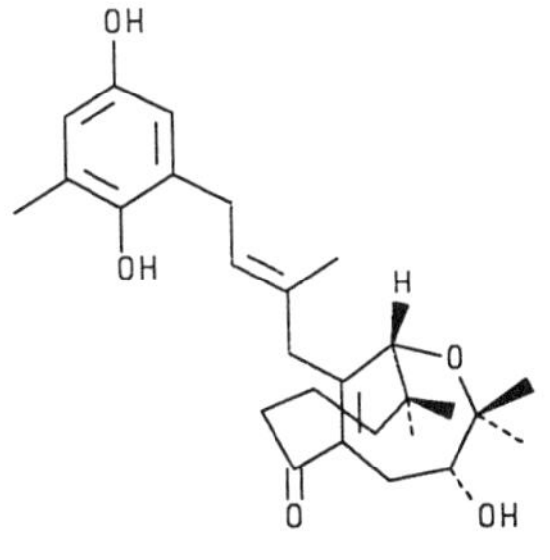

Mol. Wt.: 442
Melting Point: Oil
$[\alpha]_D$: −4.0 Solvent: Me
Spectral Data: UV, IR, CMR, PMR, Mass Spec.
Organism: *Cystoseira mediterranea*
C. tamariscifolia
C. stricta
(Phaeophyta)
Location: Banyuls-sur-Mer, Atlantic Coast, and Nice, France
Reference: 307

$C_{27}H_{38}O_5$ **Cystoseirol E**

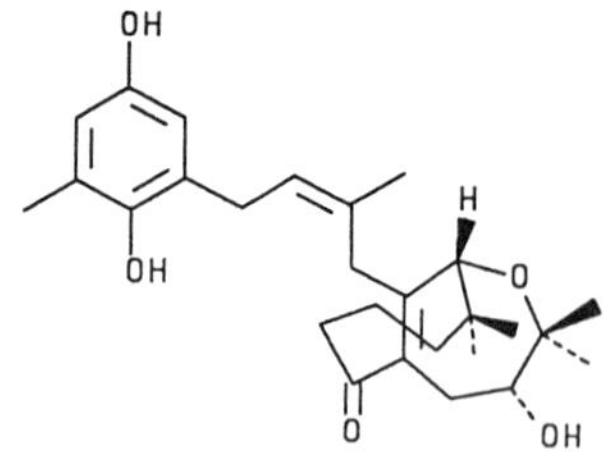

Mol. Wt.: 442
Melting Point: Oil
$[\alpha]_D$: +10 Solvent: Me
Spectral Data: UV, IR, PMR, Mass Spec.
Organism: *Cystoseira mediterranea*
C. tamariscifolia
C. stricta
(Phaeophyta)
Location: Banyuls-sur-Mer, Atlantic Coast, and Nice, France
Reference: 307

$C_{28}H_{38}O_9$ **4,9-Diacetoxyudoteal**

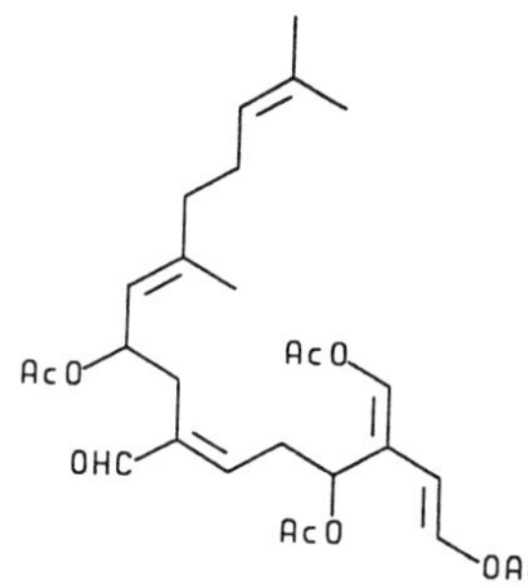

Mol. Wt.: 518
Melting Point: Oil
$[\alpha]_D$: −16.6 Solvent: Chf
Spectral Data: UV, IR, CMR, PMR, Mass Spec.
Organism: *Halimeda opuntia*
(Chlorophyta)
Location: La Parguera, Puerto Rico
Reference: 1092

$C_{28}H_{40}O_9$

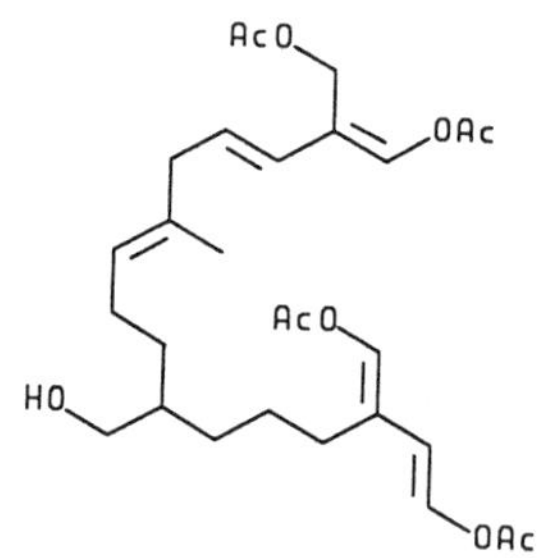

Mol. Wt.: 520
Bioactivity: Fertilized sea urchin egg assay: 100% inhibition of cell division at 8 μg/ml
Antimicrobrial activity
$[\alpha]_D^{25}$: −0.8 Solvent: Chf
Spectral Data: UV, IR, CMR, PMR, Mass Spec.
Organism: *Tydemania expeditionis*
(Chlorophyta)
Location: Guam
Reference: 868

$C_{30}H_{50}O$ **(10R,11R)-(+)-Squalene-10,11-epoxide**

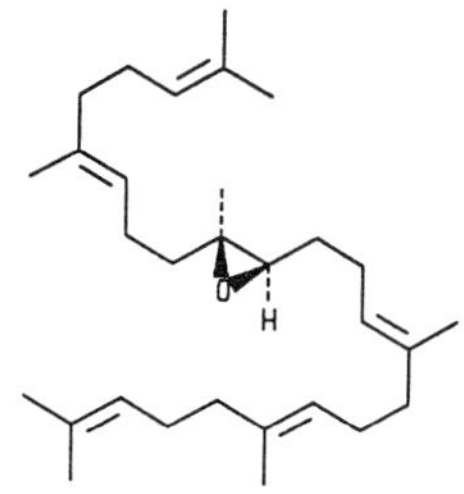

Mol. Wt.: 426
Melting Point: Oil
$[\alpha]_D^{25}$: +10.4 Solvent: Chf
Spectral Data: IR, CMR, PMR, Mass Spec.
Organism: *Laurencia okamurai* (Rhodophyta)
Location: Japan
Reference: 555, 556

$C_{30}H_{52}O_5$ **Teurilene**

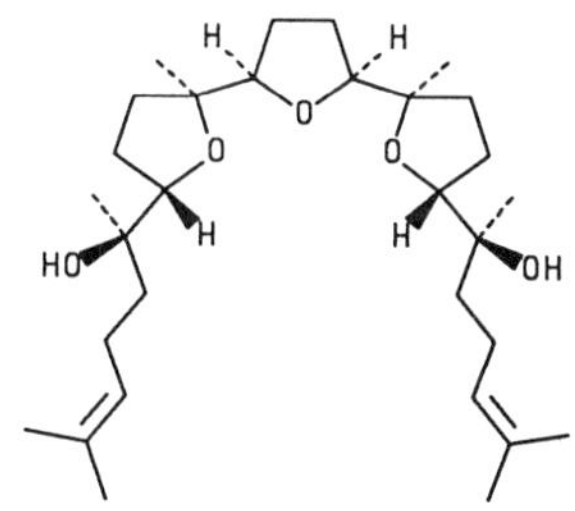

Mol. Wt.: 492
Melting Point: 84–85°C
$[\alpha]_D$: 0
Spectral Data: IR, CMR, PMR, Mass Spec., x-ray c.s.
Organism: *Laurencia obtusa* (Hud) Lamouroux (Rhodophyta)
Location: Hakkaido, Japan
Reference: 1065

$C_{40}H_{56}$ **β,β-Carotene**

Mol. Wt.: 536
Spectral Data: Mass Spec., visible spectrum
Organism: Algal clone Ω 48–23 (Chlorophyta)
Location: Northwest Atlantic
Reference: 303

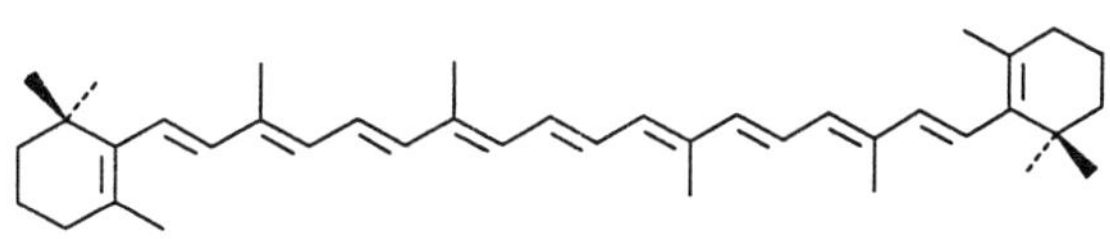

$C_{40}H_{56}$ **β,ϵ-Carotene**

Mol. Wt.: 536
Spectral Data: Visible spectrum
Organism: Algal clone Ω 48-23 (Chlorophyta)
Location: Northwest Atlantic
Reference: 303

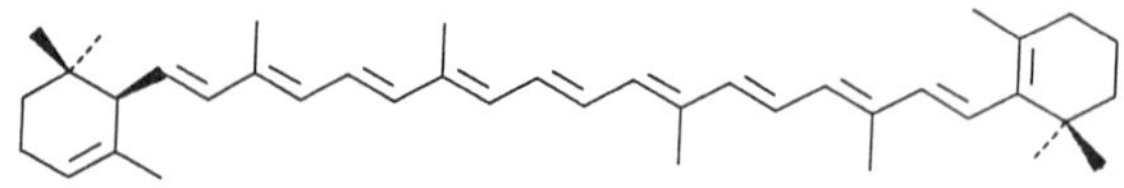

$C_{40}H_{56}O_4$ **Prasinoxanthin (Xanthophyll K)**

Mol. Wt.: 600
Spectral Data: IR, CMR, PMR, Mass Spec., visible spectrum
Organism: Algal clone Ω 48-23 (Chlorophyta)
Location: Northwest Atlantic
Reference: 303, 304

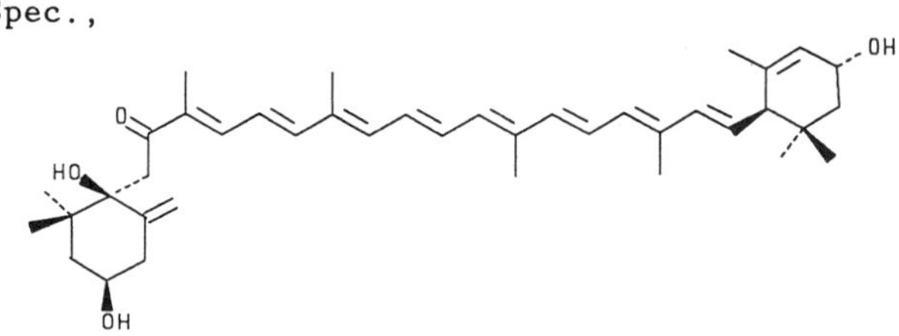

$C_{40}H_{78}$ **Lycopadiene**

Mol. Wt.: 558
Spectral Data: IR, CMR, PMR, Mass Spec.
Organism: *Botryococcus braunii* (Chlorophyta)
Location: Kossou and Yamoussoukro, Ivory Coast; Songkla Nakarin, Thailand
Reference: 730

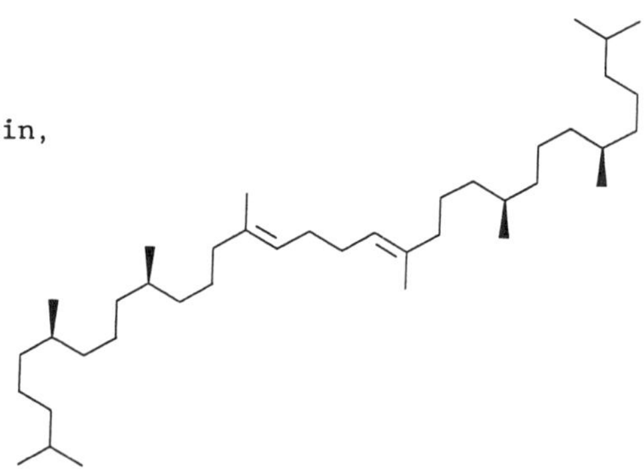

D. Pyrans and Polyethers

$C_{15}H_{18}Br_2O_2$

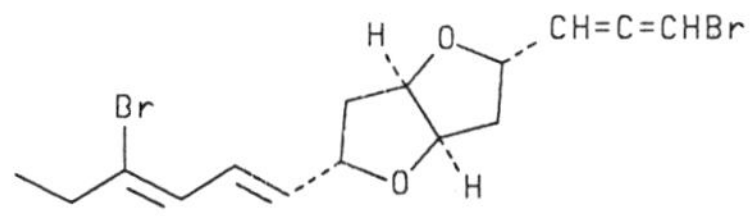

Mol. Wt.: 390
Melting Point: Oil
$[\alpha]_D^{23}$: -215 Solvent: Chf
Spectral Data: UV, IR, CMR, PMR, Mass Spec.
Organism: *Laurencia okamurai* (Rhodophyta)
Location: Japan
Reference: 1056

$C_{15}H_{19}Br_3O_3$ **Neoobtusin**

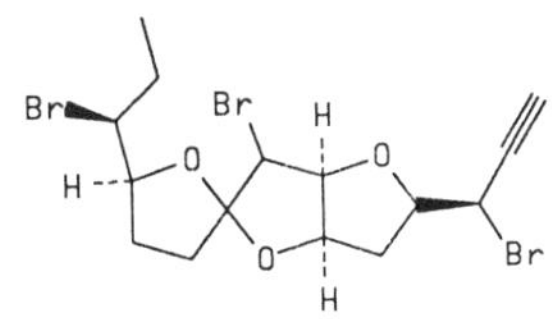

Mol. Wt.: 487
Melting Point: 107-108°C
Spectral Data: IR, CMR, PMR, Mass Spec.
Organism: *Laurencia obtusa* (Huds.) Lamour. (Rhodophyta)
Location: Syracuse, Sicily
Reference: 124

$C_{15}H_{20}Br_2O_2$ **Elatenyne**

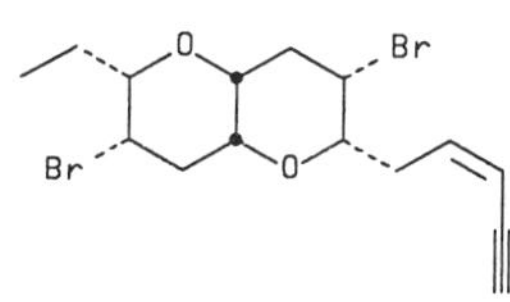

Mol. Wt.: 392
Melting Point: Oil
$[\alpha]_D^{25}$: +16.83 Solvent: Dcm
Spectral Data: UV, IR, CMR, PMR, Mass Spec.
Organism: *Laurencia elata* (Rhodophyta)
Location: Victoria, Australia
Reference: 386

$C_{15}H_{20}Br_2O_2$ **(3E)-Isolaureatin**

Mol. Wt.: 392
Melting Point: Oil
$[\alpha]_{D15}$: -8.73 Solvent: Chf
Spectral Data: UV, IR, CMR, PMR, Mass Spec.
Organism: *Laurencia nipponica* (Rhodophyta)
Location: Hokkaido and Honshu, Japan
Reference: 1057

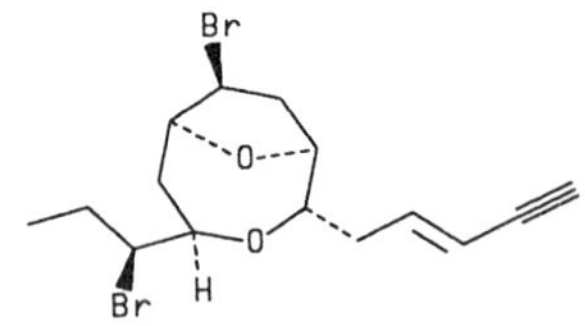

$C_{15}H_{20}Br_2O_2$ **(3E)-Laureatin**

Mol. Wt.: 392
Melting Point: 77-78°C
$[\alpha]_D^{18}$: +36.6 Solvent: Chf
Spectral Data: UV, IR, CMR, PMR, Mass Spec.
Organism: *Laurencia nipponica* (Rhodophyta)
Location: Hokkaido and Honshu, Japan
Reference: 1057

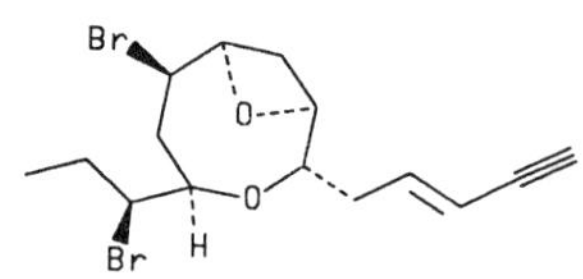

$C_{15}H_{20}O_8$

Mol. Wt.: 328
Melting Point: 182-185°C
Spectral Data: IR, PMR, Mass Spec., x-ray c.s.
Organism: *Laurencia chilensis* (Rhodophyta)
Location: Bahia de Concepcion, Chile
Reference: 70

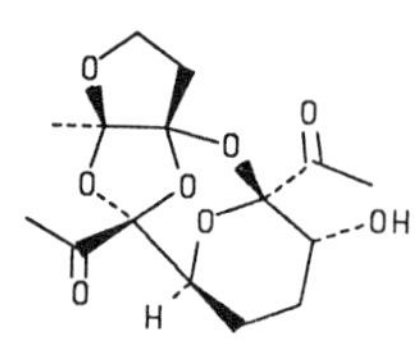

$C_{43}H_{60}O_{12}$ **Goniodomin A**

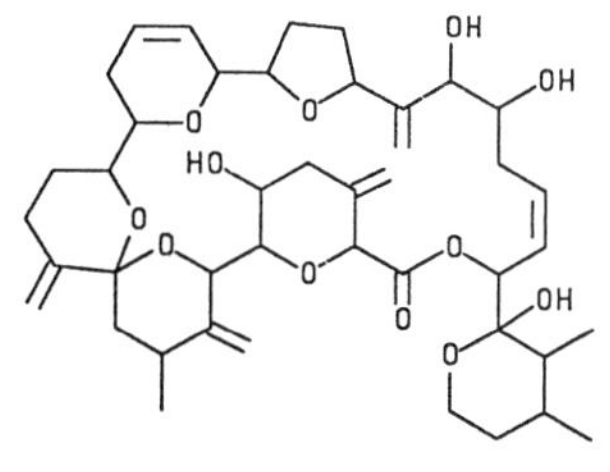

Mol. Wt.: 768
Bioactivity: Inhibition of growth of fertilized sea urchin eggs at 0.05 μg/ml
Antifungal activity
$[\alpha]_D^{20}$: +28 Solvent: Me
Spectral Data: IR, CMR, PMR, Mass Spec.
Organism: *Goniodoma pseudogoniaulax* (Pyrrophyta)
Location: Kanagawa, Japan
Reference: 779, 780

$C_{49}H_{70}O_{13}$ **Brevetoxin A (GB-1 toxin)**
(previously known)

Mol. Wt.: 868
Bioactivity: Neurotoxin
Ichthyotoxicity: *Brachydanio rerio*: LC_{50} 3 ng/ml; guppies: LC_{100} 4 ng/ml
Mouse toxicity: LD_{100} 0.3 mg/kg
Sodium channel binding
Melting Point: 197-199°C/218-220°C (double melting point)
Spectral Data: UV, CD, IR, CMR, PMR, Mass Spec., x-ray c.s.
Organism: *Gymnodinium breve* Davis (=*Ptychodiscus brevis* Davis) (Pyrrophyta)
Location: Cultured cells
Reference: 10, 177, 870, 1005

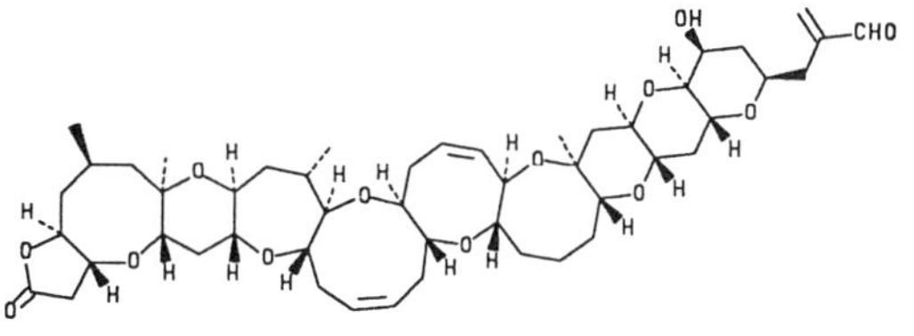

$C_{50}H_{70}O_{15}$ **GB-6 toxin (27S,28R-Epoxybrevetoxin B)**

Mol. Wt.: 912
Bioactivity: Ichthyotoxicity
Melting Point: 295-297°C
Spectral Data: CMR, PMR, x-ray c.s.
Organism: *Gymnodinium breve* Davis (=*Ptychodiscus brevis* Davis) (Pyrrophyta)
Location: Cultured cells
Reference: 177

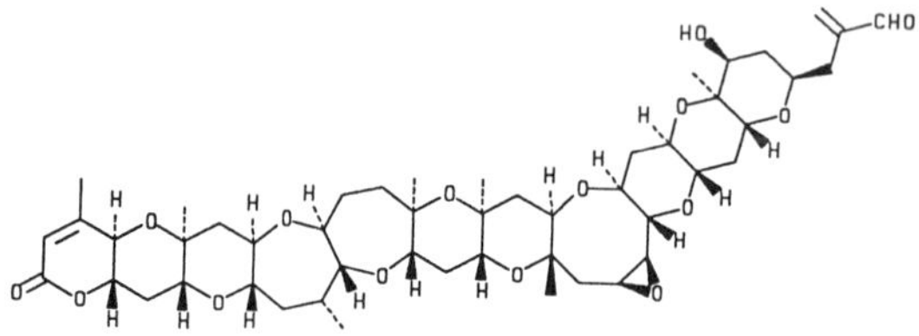

$C_{52}H_{72}O_{15}$ **GB-5 toxin (Brevetoxin B 37-O-acetate)**

Mol. Wt.: 938
Bioactivity: Ichthyotoxicity
Spectral Data: PMR
Organism: *Gymnodinium breve* Davis (=*Ptychodiscus brevis* Davis) (Pyrrophyta)
Location: Cultured cells
Reference: 177

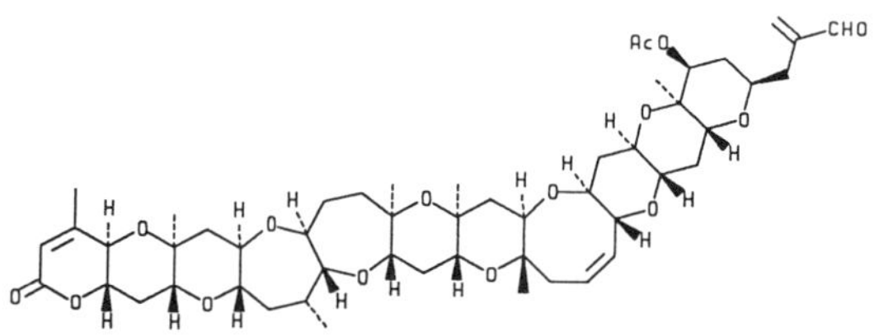

E. Carbohydrates

$C_{10}H_{21}AsO_7$ **(R)-2,3-Dihydroxypropyl-5-deoxy-5-(dimethylarsinoyl)-β-D-ribofuranoside**
(previously known)

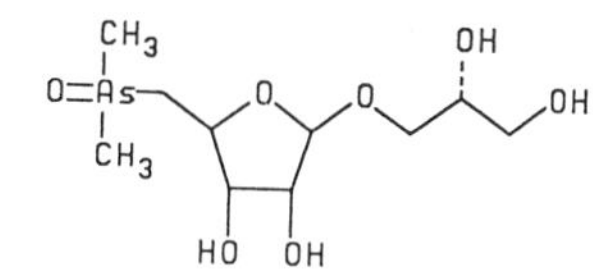

Mol. Wt.: 328
Spectral Data: CMR, PMR
Organism: *Sphaerotrichia divaricata*
Laminaria japonica
(Phaeophyta)
Location: Hokkaido, Japan
Reference: 253, 498, 1002

$C_{10}H_{21}AsO_9S$ **3-[5-Deoxy-5-(dimethylarsinoyl)-β-D-ribofuranosyloxy]-2-hydroxypropane-1-sulphonic acid**
(previously known)

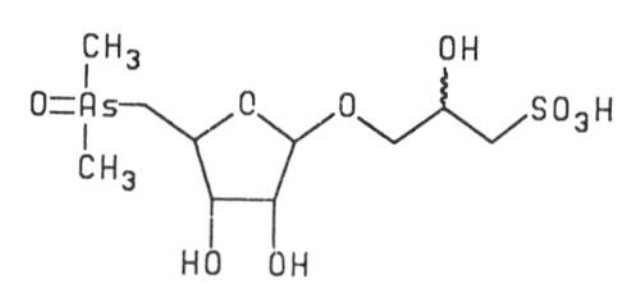

Mol. Wt.: 392
Melting Point: Syrup
Spectral Data: CMR, PMR
Organism: *Hizikia fusiforme* (Harvey) Okamura
Sphaerotrichia divaricata
Laminaria japonica
(Phaeophyta)
Location: Nakaminato and Hokkaido, Japan
Reference: 253, 254, 256, 498, 1002

$C_{10}H_{21}AsO_{10}S$ **(2S)-3-[5-Deoxy-5-(dimethylarsinoyl)-β-D-ribofuranosyloxy]-2-hydroxypropyl hydrogen sulfate**
(previously known)

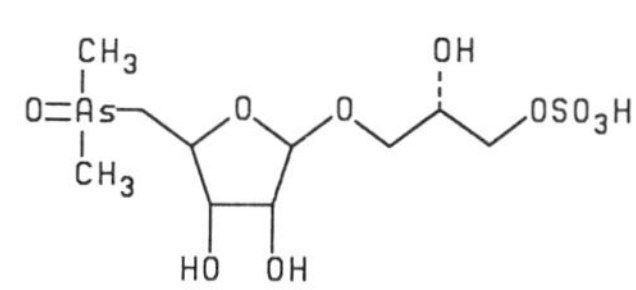

Mol. Wt.: 408
Melting Point: Syrup
Organism: *Hizikia fusiforme* (Harvey) Okamura
(Phaeophyta)
Location: Nakaminato, Japan
Reference: 255, 256

$C_{10}H_{22}AsNO_8S$ **2-Amino-3-[5-deoxy-5-(dimethylarsinoyl)-β-D-ribofuranosyloxy]propane-1-sulphonic acid**

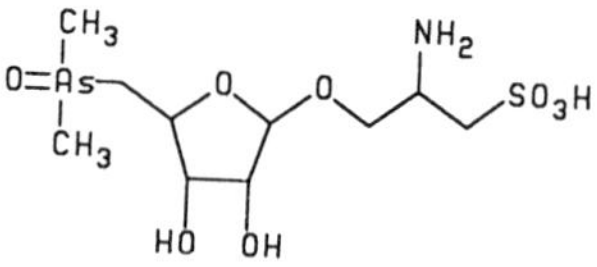

Mol. Wt.: 391
Melting Point: Syrup
Spectral Data: CMR, PMR
Organism: *Hizikia fusiforme* (Harvey) Okamura
Sphaerotrichia divaricata
(Phaeophyta)
Location: Nakaminato and Hokkaido, Japan
Reference: 256, 498

F. Phenols, Quinones, and Related Compounds

$C_7H_7BrO_3$	**3-Bromo-4,5-dihydroxybenzyl alcohol** (previously known)	
Mol. Wt.:	219	
Bioactivity:	KB: ID_{50} 8.9 μg/ml Antimicrobial activity	
Melting Point:	104-105°C	
Spectral Data:	PMR	
Organism:	*Avrainvillea nigricans* Decaisne (Chlorophyta)	
Location:	Isla Guayacan, Puerto Rico	
Reference:	193, 624, 872	

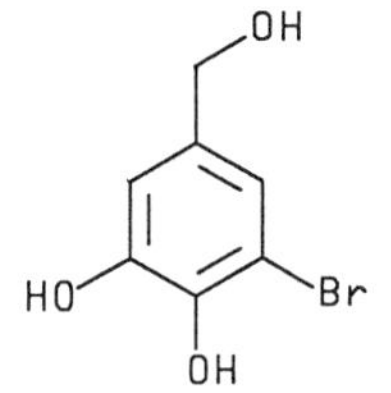

$C_9H_9Br_3O_2$	**3-Butyl-4-bromo-5-(dibromomethylidene)-2(5<u>H</u>)-furanone**	
Mol. Wt.:	389	
Melting Point:	Oil	
Spectral Data:	UV, IR, CMR, PMR, Mass Spec.	
Organism:	*Delisea elegans* *D. fimbriata* (Rhodophyta)	
Location:	New Zealand; Australia	
Reference:	535, 720	

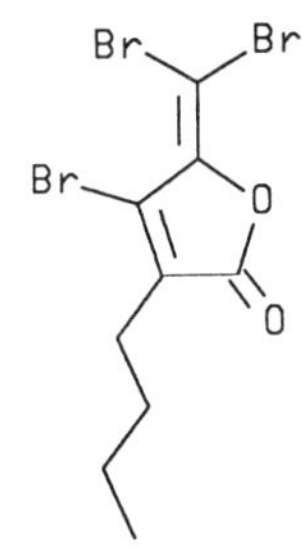

$C_9H_{11}Br_3O_3$	**3-Butyl-4-bromo-5-dibromomethyl-5-hydroxy-2(5<u>H</u>)-furanone**	
Mol. Wt.:	407	
Melting Point:	Oil	
Spectral Data:	UV, IR, CMR, PMR, Mass Spec.	
Organism:	*Delisea elegans* (Rhodophyta)	
Location:	New Zealand	
Reference:	720	

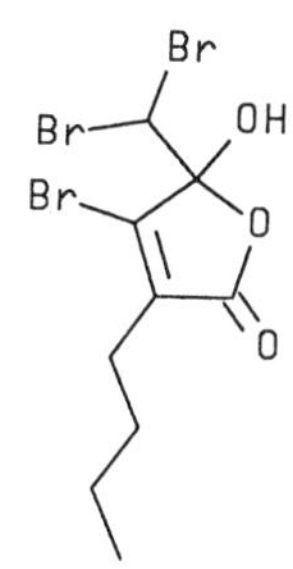

$C_{14}H_{12}Br_2O_4$ **Avrainvilleol**
(previously known)

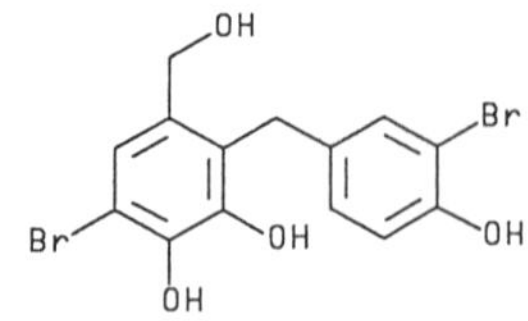

Mol. Wt.: 404
Bioactivity: Antimicrobial activity
Ichthyotoxicity
Melting Point: Oil
Organism: *Avrainvillea nigricans* Decaisne (Chlorophyta)
Location: Isla Guayacan, Puerto Rico
Reference: 193, 1048

$C_{14}H_{12}Br_2O_5$ **5'-Hydroxyisoavrainvilleol**

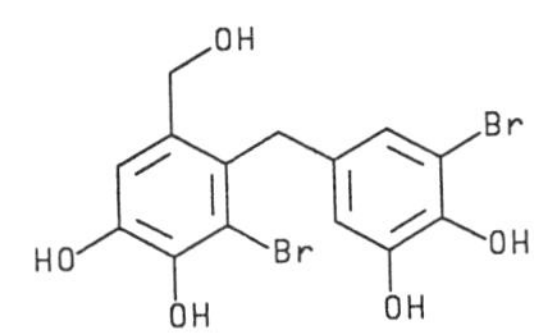

Mol. Wt.: 420
Bioactivity: Antibacterial activity against *Bacillus subtilis* and *Staphylococcus aureus*
Melting Point: Oil
Spectral Data: UV, IR, CMR, PMR, Mass Spec.
Organism: *Avrainvillea nigricans* Decaisne (Chlorophyta)
Location: Isla Guayacan, Puerto Rico
Reference: 193

$C_{18}H_{18}Br_4O_4$ **(Z,Z)-5,5'-(1,2-Dibromo-1,2-ethanediylidene)bis[4-bromo-3-butyl-2(5H)-furanone]**

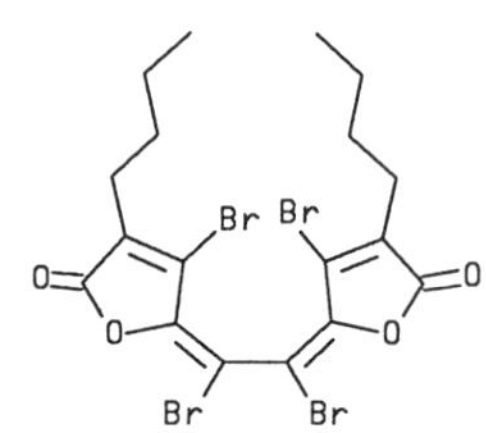

Mol. Wt.: 618
Spectral Data: UV, IR, CMR, x-ray c.s.
Organism: *Delisea elegans* (Rhodophyta)
Location: New Zealand
Reference: 720

$C_{18}H_{18}Br_4O_5$

cis-4,11,12,13-Tetrabromo-3,10-dibutyl-1,6,8-trioxadispiro[4.1.4.2]-trideca-3,10,12-triene-2,9-dione

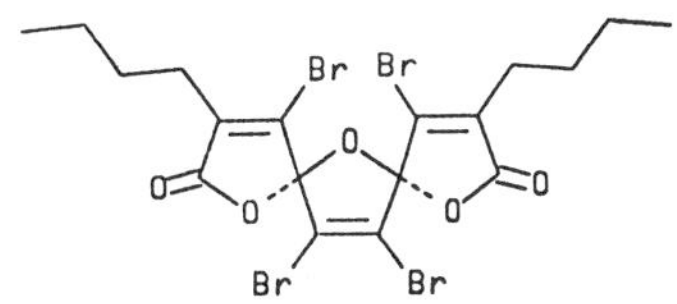

Mol. Wt.: 634
Spectral Data: Mass Spec., x-ray c.s.
Organism: *Delisea elegans* (Rhodophyta)
Location: New Zealand
Reference: 720

$C_{18}H_{18}Br_6O_4$

(±)-cis-4,10,11,11,12,12-Hexabromo-3,9-dibutyl-1,7-dioxadispiro[4.0.4.2]-dodeca-3,9-diene-2,8-dione

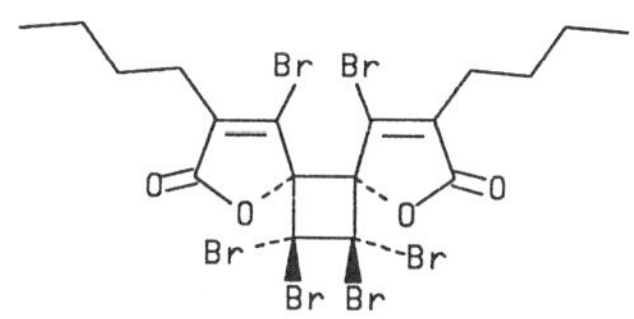

Mol. Wt.: 777
Melting Point: 153-154°C
Spectral Data: UV, IR, CMR, PMR, x-ray c.s.
Organism: *Delisea elegans* (Rhodophyta)
Location: New Zealand
Reference: 720

$C_{18}H_{18}Br_6O_4$

(±)-trans-4,10,11,11,12,12-Hexabromo-3,9-dibutyl-1,7-dioxadispiro[4.0.4.2]-dodeca-3,9-diene-2,8-dione

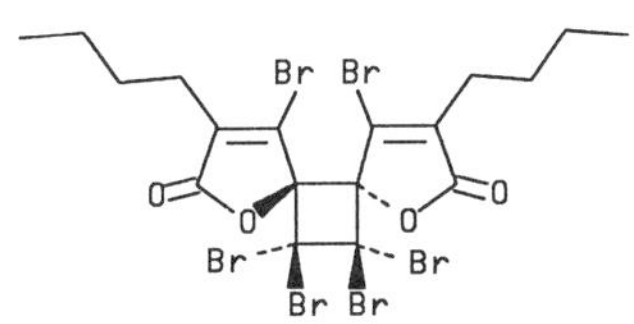

Mol. Wt.: 777
Melting Point: 102-104°C
Spectral Data: UV, IR, CMR, PMR, Mass Spec., x-ray c.s.
Organism: *Delisea elegans* (Rhodophyta)
Location: New Zealand
Reference: 720

$C_{18}H_{18}Br_6O_4$

3,5′,7′,7′-Tetrabromo-1′,4-dibutyl-4′-(dibromomethylene)spiro[furan-2(5H),6′-[3]oxabicyclo[3.2.0]heptane]-2′,5-dione

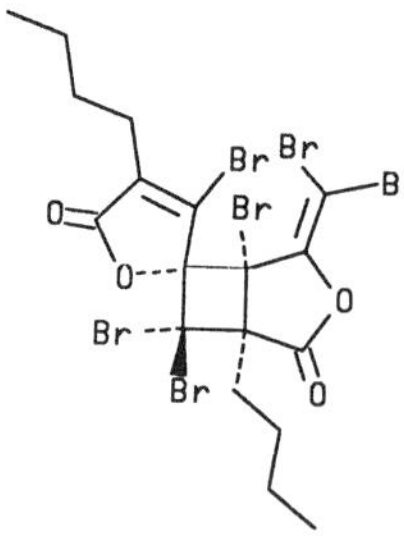

Mol. Wt.: 777
Melting Point: 105.5-106°C
Spectral Data: UV, IR, CMR, x-ray c.s.
Organism: *Delisea elegans* (Rhodophyta)
Location: New Zealand
Reference: 720

$C_{22}H_{26}Br_2O_3$

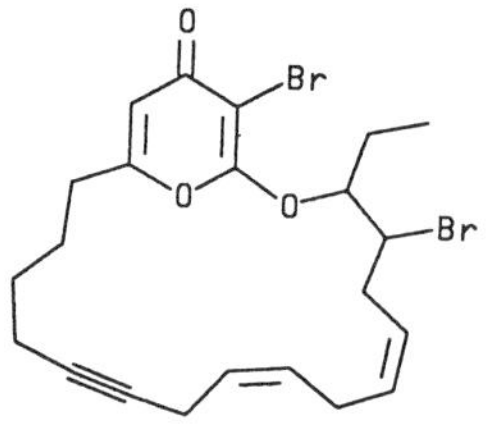

Mol. Wt. 498
$[\alpha]_D$: -41 Solvent: Chf
Spectral Data: UV, IR, CMR, PMR, Mass Spec.
Organism: *Phacelocarpus labillardieri* (Rhodophyta)
Location: Melbourne, Australia
Reference: 1010

$C_{22}H_{26}O_3$

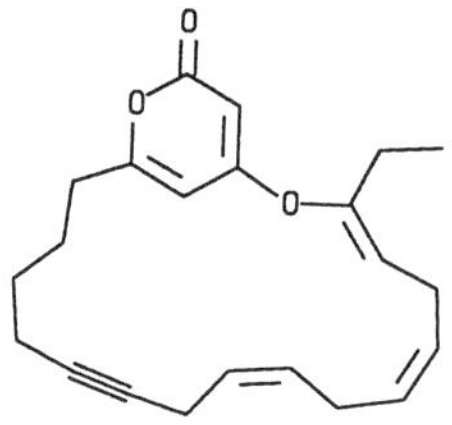

Mol. Wt.: 338
Spectral Data: UV, IR, CMR, PMR, Mass Spec.
Organism: *Phacelocarpus labillardieri* (Rhodophyta)
Location: Melbourne, Australia
Reference: 1010

$C_{22}H_{26}O_3$

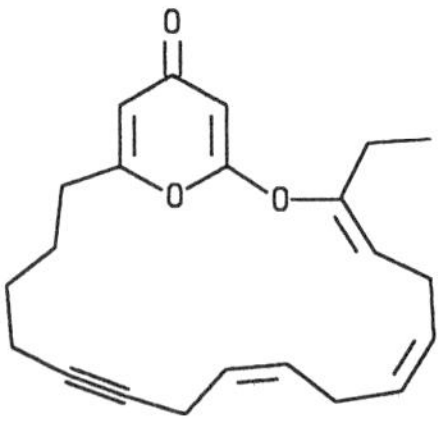

Mol. Wt.: 338
Spectral Data: UV, IR, CMR, PMR, Mass Spec.
Organism: *Phacelocarpus labillardieri* (Rhodophyta)
Location: Melbourne, Australia
Reference: 1010

$C_{22}H_{26}O_4$

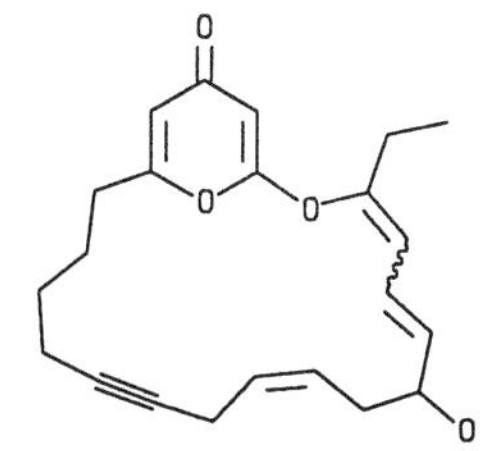

Mol. Wt.: 354
Spectral Data: UV, IR, CMR, PMR, Mass Spec.
Organism: *Phacelocarpus labillardieri* (Rhodophyta)
Location: Melbourne, Australia
Reference: 1010

$C_{27}H_{38}O_5$ **Amentadione**

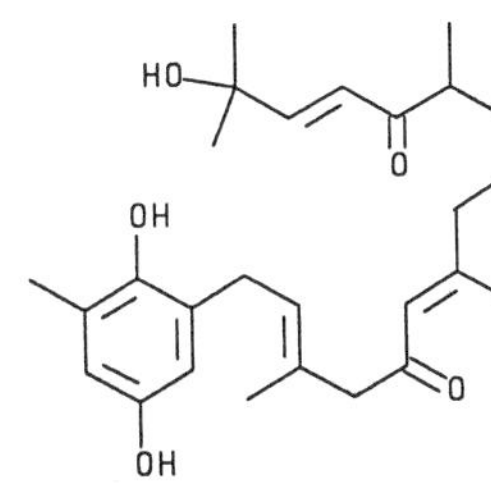

Mol. Wt.: 442
Melting Point: Oil
$[\alpha]_D^{20}$: -0.44 Solvent: Alc
Spectral Data: UV, IR, CMR, PMR, Mass Spec.
Organism: *Cystoseira stricta* var. *amentacea* Bory (Phaeophyta)
Location: Castelluccio, Sicily
Reference: 18

$C_{27}H_{38}O_5$ **Amentaepoxide**

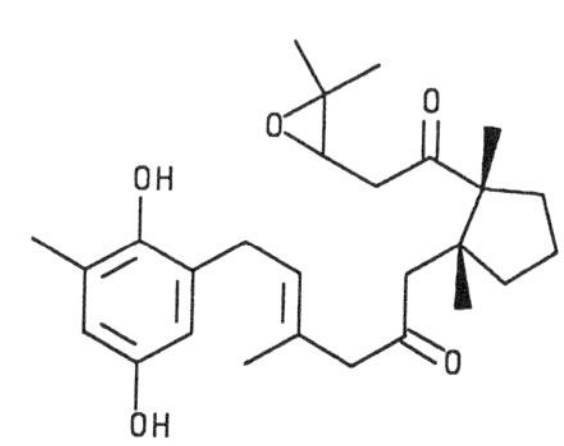

Mol. Wt.: 442
Melting Point: Oil
$[\alpha]_D^{20}$: +14.6 Solvent: Alc
Spectral Data: UV, IR, CMR, PMR, Mass Spec.
Organism: *Cystoseira stricta* var. *amentacea* Bory (Phaeophyta)
Location: Castelluccio, Sicily
Reference: 18

$C_{27}H_{38}O_5$	**trans-Bifurcarenone**	
Mol. Wt.:	442	
Melting Point:	Oil	
$[\alpha]_D^{20}$:	+5.5 Solvent: Alc	
Spectral Data:	UV, IR, CMR, PMR, Mass Spec.	
Organism:	*Cystoseira stricta* var. *amentacea* Bory (Phaeophyta)	
Location:	Castelluccio, Sicily	
Reference:	18	

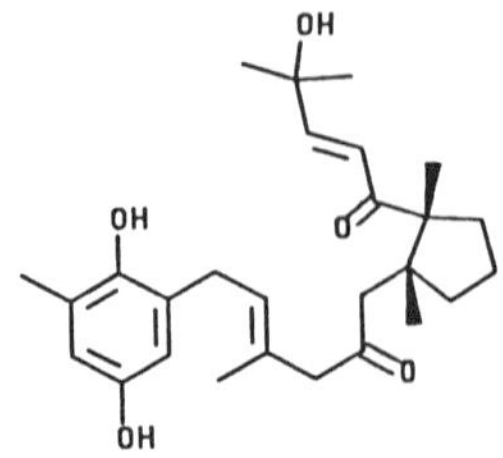

$C_{27}H_{42}O_4$	**(7'R*,8'S*)-6-Hydroxy-2,8-dimethyl-2-[(3'E)-4',8',12'-trimethyl-7',8'-dihydroxytrideca-3',11'-dien-1'-yl] chroman**	
Mol. Wt.:	430	
Melting Point:	Oil	
$[\alpha]_D$:	+12.6 Solvent: Alc	
Spectral Data:	UV, IR, CMR, PMR, Mass Spec.	
Organism:	*Cystoseira caespitosa* Sauv. (Phaeophyta)	
Location:	Sicily	
Reference:	19	

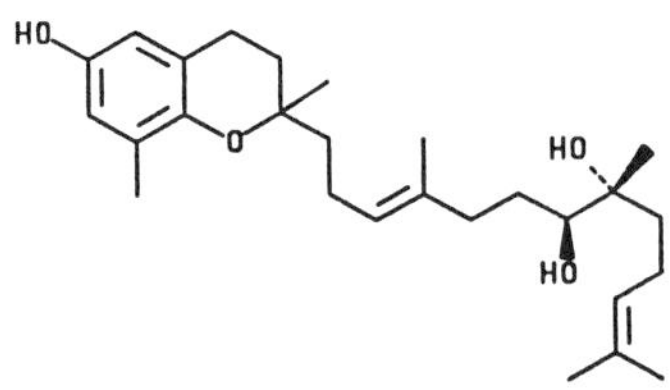

$C_{28}H_{34}O_4$		
Mol. Wt.:	434	
Melting Point:	45-46°C	
Spectral Data:	UV, IR, CMR, PMR, Mass Spec.	
Organism:	*Zonaria tournefortii* (Phaeophyta)	
Location:	Sicily	
Reference:	1105	

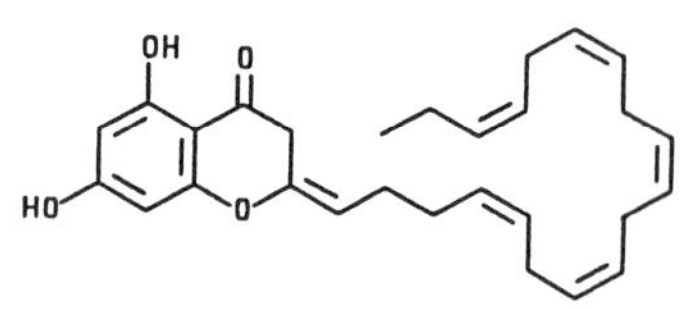

$C_{28}H_{40}O_5$ **1'-O-Methyl-trans-bifurcarenone**

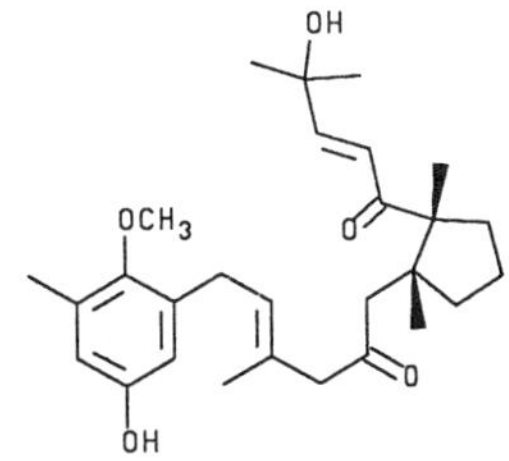

Mol. Wt.: 456
Melting Point: Oil
$[\alpha]_D^{20}$: +5.3 Solvent: Alc
Spectral Data: UV, IR, CMR, PMR, Mass Spec.
Organism: *Cystoseira stricta* var. *amentacea* Bory (Phaeophyta)
Location: Castelluccio, Sicily
Reference: 18

$C_{28}H_{40}O_5$ **Strictaketal**

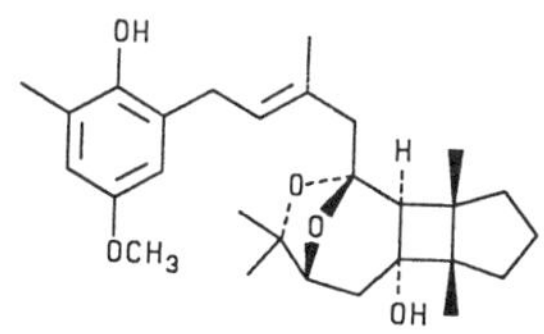

Mol. Wt.: 456
Melting Point: Oil
$[\alpha]_D^{20}$: +21.7 Solvent: Alc
Spectral Data: UV, IR, CMR, PMR, Mass Spec.
Organism: *Cystoseira stricta* (Mont.) Sauv. (Phaeophyta)
Location: Portopalo, Sicily
Reference: 17, 21

$C_{29}H_{42}O_4$ **Cystalgerone**

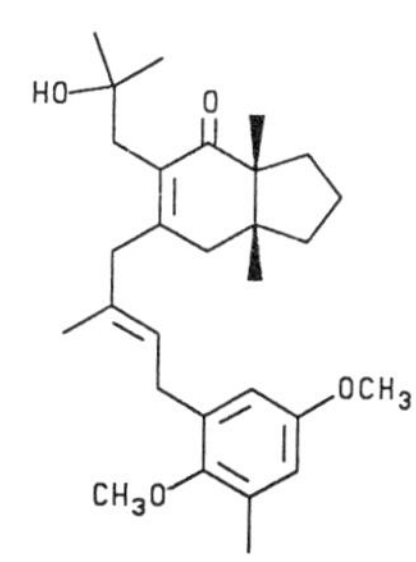

Mol. Wt.: 454
Melting Point: 75-76°C
$[\alpha]_D^{20}$: +75 Solvent: Alc
Spectral Data: UV, IR, CMR, PMR, Mass Spec.
Organism: *Cystoseira algeriensis* Feldm. (Phaeophyta)
Location: Pachino, Sicily
Reference: 20

G. Amines and Nitrogen Heterocyclic Compounds

$C_6H_{12}ClNO_2$ **Charamin**

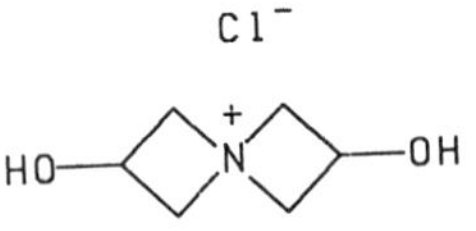

Mol. Wt.: 165
Bioactivity: Antibiotic activity toward a natural bacteria population
Spectral Data: IR, CMR, PMR; Mass Spec. of the synthetic sample
Organism: *Chara globularis* Thuillier (Chlorophyta)
Reference: 30

$C_6H_{12}N_4O_2$ **Carnosadine**

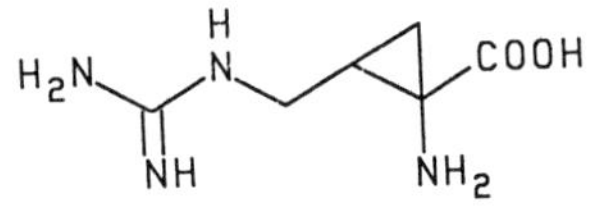

Mol. Wt.: 172
$[\alpha]_D^{19}$: -20.0 Solvent: HCl (1M)
Spectral Data: CMR, PMR, Mass Spec.; x-ray c.s. of derivative
Organism: *Grateloupia carnosa* (Rhodophyta)
Location: Wakayama, Japan
Reference: 1146, 1147

$C_7H_{11}NO_2$ **N,N-Dimethyl-Δ^2-pyrrolinio-3-carboxylate**

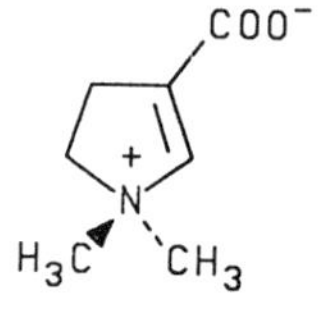

Mol. Wt.: 141
Spectral Data: PMR, Mass Spec.
Organism: *Pterocladia capillacea* (Rhodophyta)
Location: Sicily
Reference: 989

$C_7H_{13}NO_3$ **4-Hydroxy-N,N-dimethyl-pyrrolidinio-3-carboxylate**

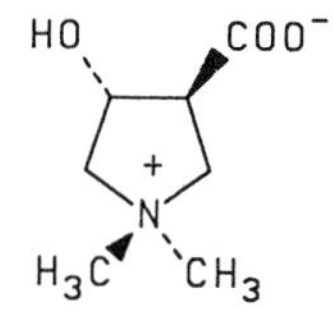

Mol. Wt.: 159
$[\alpha]_D^{25}$: +14.42 Solvent: Aq
Spectral Data: CMR, PMR, Mass Spec.
Organism: *Grateloupia proteus* (Rhodophyta)
Location: Sicily
Reference: 988

$C_7H_{15}NO_3S$ **5-Dimethylsulfonio-4-hydroxy-2-aminovalerate**

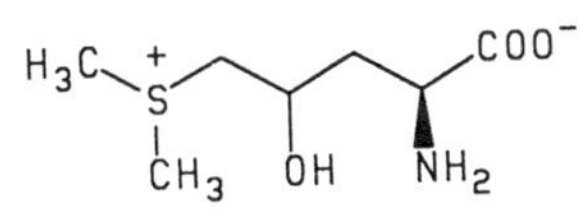

Mol. Wt.: 193
$[\alpha]_D^{25}$: +1.3; +12.6 Solvent: Aq; 5N HCl
Spectral Data: CMR, PMR, Mass Spec.
Organism: *Lophocladia lallemandi* (Rhodophyta)
Location: Sicily
Reference: 988

$C_8H_{13}NO_2$ **L-Baikiain betaine**

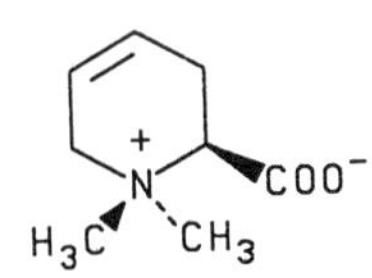

Mol. Wt.: 155
Melting Point: 184-186°C
$[\alpha]_D^{25}$: -103 Solvent: Aq
Spectral Data: CMR, PMR, Mass Spec.
Organism: *Pterocladia capillacea* (Rhodophyta)
Location: Sicily
Reference: 989

$C_{13}H_{17}NO$ **Aphanorphine**

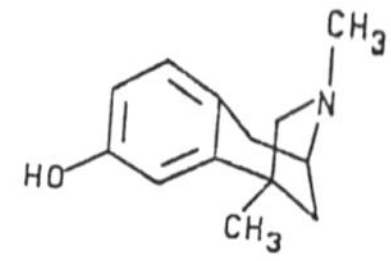

Mol. Wt.:	203
Melting Point:	223-229°C
$[\alpha]_D^{25}$:	-43.7 Solvent: Aq (HCl salt)
Spectral Data:	IR, CMR, PMR, Mass Spec. x-ray c.s.
Organism:	*Aphanizomenon flos-aquae* (Cyanophyta) Culture
Reference:	378

$C_{15}H_{21}NO_6$ **Isodomoic acid A**

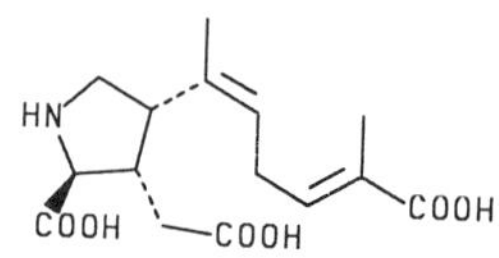

Mol. Wt.:	311
Bioactivity:	Insecticidal activity against *Periplaneta americana* (American cockroach)
Melting Point:	185-187°C (dec.)
$[\alpha]_D^{25}$:	-70.0 Solvent: Aq
Spectral Data:	UV, CD, IR, CMR, PMR, Mass Spec.
Organism:	*Chondria armata* (Rhodophyta)
Location:	Japan
Reference:	687

$C_{15}H_{21}NO_6$ **Isodomoic acid B**

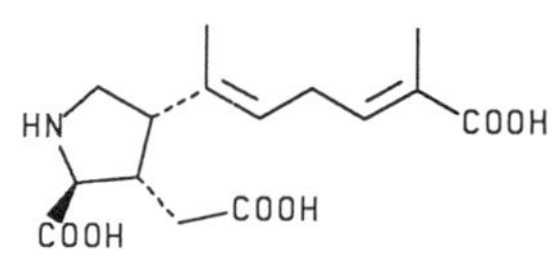

Mol. Wt.:	311
Bioactivity:	Insecticidal activity against *Periplaneta americana* (American cockroach)
Melting Point:	182-183°C (dec.)
$[\alpha]_D^{25}$:	-8.1 Solvent: Aq
Spectral Data:	UV, CD, IR, CMR, PMR, Mass Spec.
Organism:	*Chondria armata* (Rhodophyta)
Location:	Japan
Reference:	687

$C_{15}H_{21}NO_6$ **Isodomoic acid C**

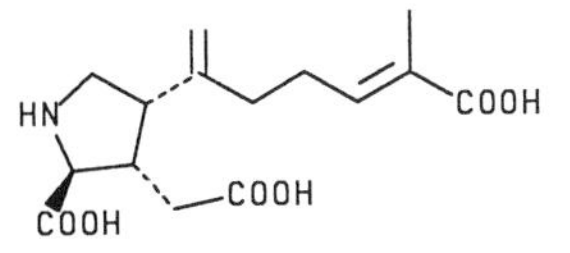

Mol. Wt.: 311
Bioactivity: Insecticidal activity against *Periplaneta americana* (American cockroach)
Melting Point: 257-260°C (dec.)
$[\alpha]_D^{25}$: -30.0 Solvent: Aq
Spectral Data: UV, CD, IR, PMR, Mass Spec.
Organism: *Chondria armata* (Rhodophyta)
Location: Japan
Reference: 687

$C_{15}H_{21}NO_7$ **Domoilactone A**

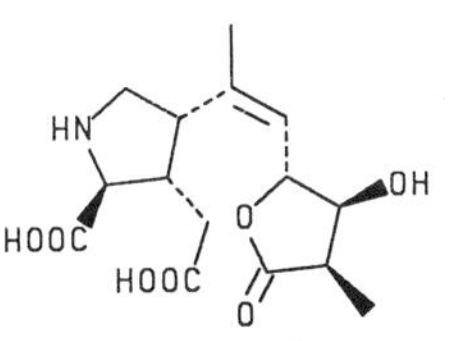

Mol. Wt.: 327
Spectral Data: UV, CD, IR, PMR, Mass Spec.
Organism: *Chondria armata* (Rhodophyta)
Location: Japan
Reference: 688

$C_{15}H_{21}NO_7$ **Domoilactone B**

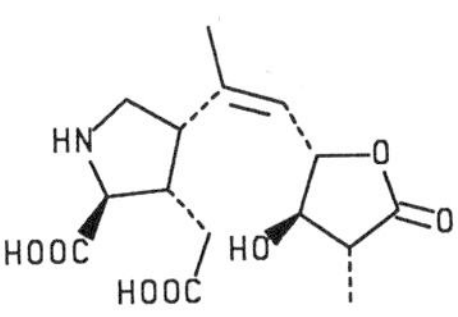

Mol. Wt.: 327
Spectral Data: UV, CD, IR, PMR, Mass Spec.
Organism: *Chondria armata* (Rhodophyta)
Location: Japan
Reference: 688

$C_{16}H_{22}N_2O_3S_2$ **(-)-Gliovictin**
(previously known)

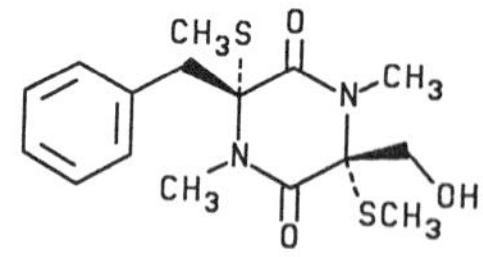

Mol. Wt.: 354
[α]D: -62 Solvent: Chf
Spectral Data: CMR
Organism: *Asteromyces cruciatus*
(Eumycophyta)
Culture of sample
Location: Chesapeake Bay
Reference: 243, 1009

$C_{20}H_{22}ClNO_2$ **Fontonamide**

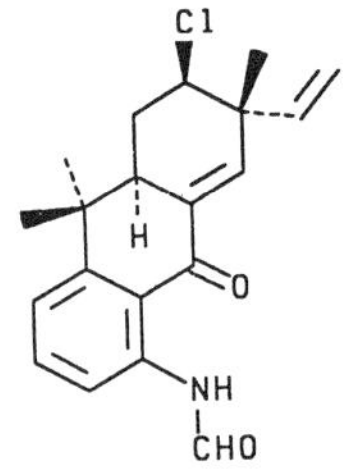

Mol. Wt.: 343
Melting Point: 156-157°C
[α]D: -141 Solvent: Chf
Spectral Data: UV, CMR, PMR, Mass Spec.
Organism: *Hapalosiphon fontinalis*
(Ag.) Bornet
(Cyanophyta)
Culture
Reference: 766

$C_{21}H_{21}ClN_2O$ **Anhydrohapaloxindole A**

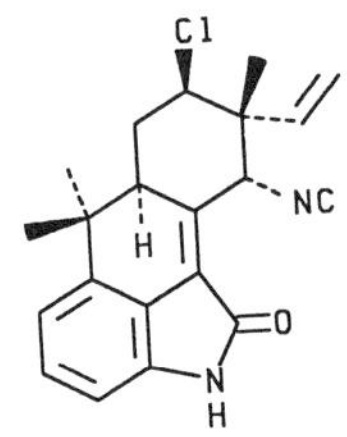

Mol. Wt.: 352
Melting Point: 123°C (dec.)
[α]D: +150 Solvent: Alc
Spectral Data: UV, CMR, PMR, Mass Spec.
Organism: *Hapalosiphon fontinalis*
(Ag.) Bornet
(Cyanophyta)
Culture
Reference: 766

$C_{41}H_{60}N_8O_{10}$ **Nodularin**

Mol. Wt.: 824
Bioactivity: Toxic to mice: LD_{50} 50 μg/kg
Hepatotoxicity
Spectral Data: UV, IR, CMR, PMR, Mass Spec.
Organism: *Nodularia spumigena*
(Cyanophyta)
Location: New Zealand; Baltic Sea
Reference: 274, 934

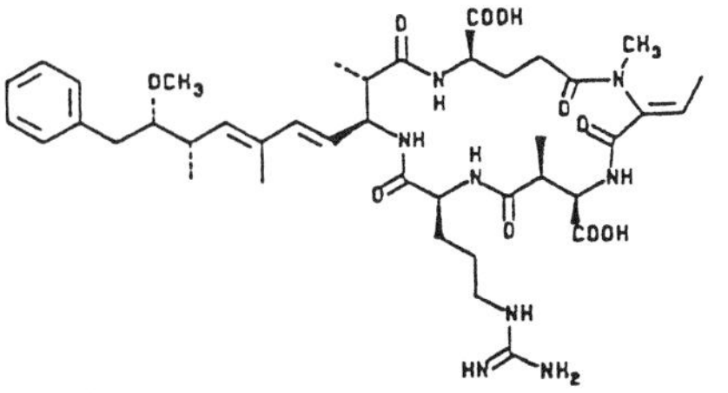

$C_{49}H_{75}N_{13}O_{12}$ Cyanoviridin RR

Mol. Wt.: 1039
Bioactivity: Toxin
Melting Point: 235°C (dec.)
$[\alpha]_D$: -95.2 Solvent: Aq
Spectral Data: UV, CMR, PMR, Mass Spec.
Organism: *Microcystis viridis*
(Cyanophyta)
Location: Japan
Reference: 628

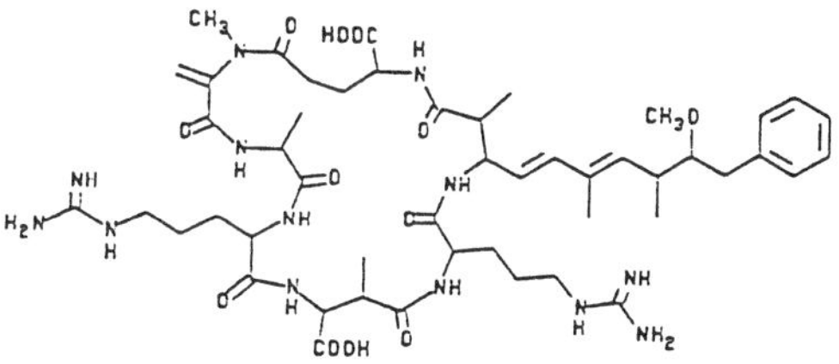

$C_{71}H_{106}N_{12}O_{21}$ Scytonemin A

Mol. Wt.: 1464
Bioactivity: Calcium antagonism
Mild cytotoxicity: CCRF-CEM
IC_{50} 2.9 μg/ml
Antibacterial and antifungal activity
$[\alpha]_D$: +38.8 Solvent: Me
Spectral Data: UV, IR, CMR, PMR, Mass Spec.; CD of degradation products
Organism: *Scytonema* sp.
(Cyanophyta)
Culture from soil sample
Location: Marshall Islands
Reference: 409

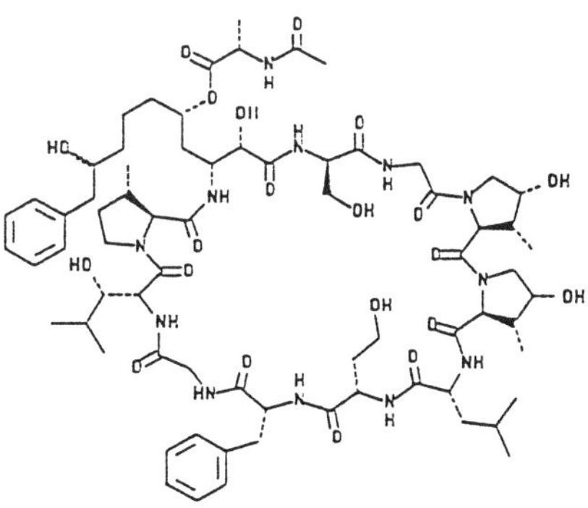

P-1
(Cyclic peptide)

Mol. Wt.:	994
Bioactivity:	Toxicity
Spectral Data:	CD, Mass Spec.
Organism:	*Microcystis aeruginosa* (strain M228) (Cyanophyta) Culture
Location:	Japan
Reference:	621

P-2
(Cyclic peptide)

Mol. Wt.:	1044
Bioactivity:	Toxicity: LD_{99} 70 μg/kg mice (i.p.)
Melting Point:	218°C (dec.)
$[\alpha]_D^{24}$:	-74.42 Solvent: Me
Spectral Data:	UV, CD, CMR, PMR, Mass Spec.
Organism:	*Microcystis aeruginosa* (strain M228) (Cyanophyta) Culture
Location:	Japan
Reference:	621

Thioredoxin I

Mol. Wt.:	12,000
Bioactivity:	Cytoplasmic thioredoxin
Organism:	*Scenedesmus obliquus* (strain D3) *Scenedesmus obliquus* (mutant C-2A') (Chlorophyta) Culture
Reference:	633

Thioredoxin II

Mol. Wt.:	12,000
Bioactivity:	Cytoplasmic thioredoxin
Organism:	*Scenedesmus obliquus* (strain D3)
	Scenedesmus obliquus (mutant C-2A')
	(Chlorophyta)
	Culture
Reference:	633

Thioredoxin III

Mol. Wt.:	12,000
Organism:	*Scenedesmus obliquus* (strain D3)
	Scenedesmus obliquus (mutant C-2A')
	(Chlorophyta)
	Culture
Reference:	633

Thioredoxin F

Mol. Wt.:	28,000
Bioactivity:	Cytoplasmic thioredoxin
Organism:	*Scenedesmus obliquus* (strain D3)
	(Chlorophyta)
	Culture
Reference:	633

SUBJECT INDEX

MOLECULAR WEIGHTS
(All weights are rounded up)

141 - 494

148 - 448

149 - 378

150 - 448

154 - 80,114

155 - 495

156 - 335

159 - 495

162 - 80

165 - 494

169 - 355

172 - 114,494

179 - 115,378

180 - 233

182 - 385

192 - 80,380

193 - 495

194 - 81,171,379,385,455

196 - 386

200 - 220

202 - 335

203 - 496

204 - 233,234

205 - 355

207 - 454

208 - 335

210 - 209

212 - 116,170,386

213 - 391

214 - 116,170,336

215 - 381

216 - 336,357,455

218 - 172,381,455

219 - 487

220 - 234,235

221 - 173,356

222 - 236,457

229 - 379

230 - 81,359

231 - 173,387,425,426

232 - 336,357

233 - 171

234 - 358

235 - 423

236 - 359,457

237 - 392,393,423

238 - 236

239 - 396,424

BIBLIOGRAPHY

1. P. H. Abelson. *Science* **237**, 473 (1987).

2. E. Abushanab and M. S. P. Sarma. *J. Med. Chem.* **32**, 76 (1989).

3. "Acrylonitrile Linked to Cancer in Workers." *C & E News*, May 30, 1977, p. 6.

4. M. Adamczeski, E. Quiñoà, and P. Crews. *J. Am. Chem. Soc.* **110**, 1598 (1988).

5. W. Adolf, E. H. Seip, E. Hecker, and S. F. Dossaji. *J. Nat. Prod.* **51**, 662 (1988).

6. S. S. Afiyatullov, L. Y. Tishchenko, V. A. Stonik, A. I. Kalinovskii, and G. B. Elyakov. *Chem. Nat. Compd.* **21**, 228 (1985).

7. A. Aiello, P. Ciminiello, E. Fattorusso, and S. Magno. *J. Nat. Prod.* **51**, 999 (1988).

8. A. Aiello, E. Fattorusso, and S. Magno. *J. Nat. Prod.* **50**, 191 (1987).

9. A. Aiello, E. Fattorusso, S. Magno, and L. Mayol. *Tetrahedron* **43**, 5929 (1987).

10. M. Alam, N. M. Trieff, S. M. Ray, and J. E. Hudson. *J. Pharm. Sci.* **64**, 865 (1975).

11. K. F. Albizati, J. R. Pawlik, and D. J. Faulkner. *J. Org. Chem.* **50**, 3428 (1985).

12. J. R. F. Allen and B. R. Holmstedt. *Phytochemistry* **19**, 1573 (1980).

13. H. Allgeier, Ek. Weiss, and T. Reichstein. *Helv. Chim. Acta* **50**, 431 (1967).

14. A. Almourabit, A. Ahond, A. Chiaroni, C. Poupat, C. Riche, P. Potier, P. Laboute, and J.-L. Menou. *J. Nat. Prod.* **51**, 282 (1988).

15. M. S. Al-Said, M. S. Hifnawy, A. T. McPhail, and D. R. McPhail. *Phytochemistry* **27**, 3245 (1988).

16. B. N. Ames, R. Magaw, and L. S. Gold. *Science* **236**, 271 (1987).

17. V. Amico, F. Cunsolo, M. Piattelli, G. Ruberto, and L. Mayol. *J. Nat. Prod.* **50**, 449 (1987).

18. V. Amico, G. Oriente, P. Neri, M. Piattelli, and G. Ruberto. *Phytochemistry* **26**, 1715 (1987).

19. V. Amico, G. Oriente, M. Piattelli, and G. Ruberto. *Gazz. Chim. Ital.* **113**, 217 (1983).

20. V. Amico, G. Oriente, M. Piattelli, and G. Ruberto. *Gazz. Chim. Ital.* **114**, 169 (1984).

21. V. Amico, M. Piattelli, P. Neri, and G. Ruberto. *J. Nat. Prod.* **51**, 191 (1988).

22. D. Anaise, R. Steinitz, and N. Ben Hur. *Cancer* **42**, 299 (1978).

23. H. N. Ananthaswamy, J. E. Price, L. H. Goldberg, and E. S. Bales. *Cancer Res.* **48**, 3341 (1988).

24. L. Andersson, S. Bano, L. Bohlin, R. Riccio, and L. Minale. *J. Chem. Res. (S)* 366 (1985).

25. L. Andersson, A. Nasir, L. Bohlin, and L. Kenne. *J. Nat. Prod.* **50**, 944 (1987).

26. L. J. G. Angenot, C. A. Coune, M. J. G. Tits, and K. Yamada. *Phytochemistry* **17**, 1687 (1978).

27. L. Angenot, O. Dideberg, and L. Dupont. *Tetrahedron Lett.* 1357 (1975).

28. U. Anthoni, K. Bock, L. Chevolot, C. Larsen, P. H. Nielsen, and C. Christophersen. *J. Org. Chem.* **52**, 5638 (1987).

29. U. Anthoni, L. Chevolot, C. Larsen, P. H. Nielsen, and C. Christophersen. *J. Org. Chem.* **52**, 4709 (1987).

30. U. Anthoni, P. H. Nielsen, L. Smith-Hansen, S. Wium-Andersen, and C. Christophersen. *J. Org. Chem.* **52**, 694 (1987).

31. K. Anzai, G. Nakamura, and S. Suzuki. *J. Antibiotics* **A10**, 201 (1957).

32. L. Arabshahi and F. J. Schmitz. *J. Org. Chem.* **52**, 3584 (1987).

33. L. Arabshahi and F. J. Schmitz. *Tetrahedron Lett.* **29**, 1099 (1988).

34. V. E. Archer. *Cancer* **39**, 1802 (1977).

35. J. C. Arcos. *American Laboratory*, June 1978, p. 65.

36. M. Arisawa, A. Fujita, M. Saga, T. Hayashi, N. Morita, N. Kawano, and S. Koshimura. *J. Nat. Prod.* **49**, 298 (1986).

37. M. Arisawa, A. D. Kinghorn, G. A. Cordell, C. H. Phoebe, and N. R. Farnsworth. *Planta Med.* 544 (1985).

38. M. Arisawa, M. Nimura, A. Fujita, T. Hayashi, N. Morita, and S. Koshimura. *Planta Med.* 297 (1986).

39. M. Arisawa, M. Nimura, A. Ikeda, T. Hayashi, N. Morita, Y. Momose, R. Takeda, and S. Nakanishi. *Planta Med.* 38 (1986).

40. B. G. Armstrong and G. Kazantzis. *Lancet* **I**, 1425 (1983).

41. H. R. Arthur, W. H. Hui, and Y. L. Ng. *J. Chem. Soc.* 1840 (1959).

42. Y. Asakawa. *Rev. Latinoamer. Quim.* **14-3**, 109 (1984).

43. K. Asano, K. Takahashi, F. Tomita, and I. Kawamoto. *J. Antibiotics* **39**, 619 (1986).

44. O. Auerbach and L. Garfinkel. *Cancer* **64**, 983 (1989).

45. M. M. Badawi, S. S. Handa, A. D. Kinghorn, G. A. Cordell, and N. R. Farnsworth. *J. Pharm. Sci.* **72**, 1285 (1983).

46. B. Baker, L. Ratnapala, M. P. D. Mahindaratne, E. D. de Silva, L. M. V. Tillekeratne, J. H. Jeong, P. J. Scheuer, and K. Seff. *Tetrahedron* **44**, 4695 (1988).

47. B. J. Baker, P. J. Scheuer, and J. N. Shoolery. *J. Am. Chem. Soc.* **110**, 965 (1988).

48. J. T. Baker, R. J. Wells, W. E. Oberhänsli, and G. B. Hawes. *J. Am. Chem. Soc.* **98**, 4010 (1976).

49. M. Balerna, W. Keller-Schierlein, C. Martius, H. Wolf, and H. Zähner. *Arch. Mikrobiol.* **65**, 303 (1969).

50. J. J. Barchi, Jr., T. R. Norton, E. Furusawa, G. M. L. Patterson, and R. E. Moore. *Phytochemistry* **22**, 2851 (1983).

51. C. J. Barrow, J. W. Blunt, M. H. G. Munro, and N. B. Perry. *J. Nat. Prod.* **51**, 275 (1988).

52. K. Bartik, J.-C. Braekman, D. Daloze, C. Stoller, J. Huysecom, G. Vandevyver, and R. Ottinger. *Can. J. Chem.* **65**, 2118 (1987).

53. R. Bassleer, M.-Cl. Depauw-Gillet, Br. Massart, J.-M. Marnette, Ph. Wiliquet, M. Caprasse, and L. Angenot. *Planta Med.* **45**, 123 (1982).

54. F. J. Baur. *J. Am. Oil Chem. Soc.* **52**, 263 (1975).

55. A. Bavoso, F. Cafieri, L. De Napoli, B. Di Blasio, E. Fattorusso, V. Pavone, and C. Santacroce. *Gazz. Chim. Ital.* **117**, 87 (1987).

56. S. Beers, J. Brownell, and R. Vince. "Prodrugs of Carbovir, A Selective Inhibitor of HIV: Synthesis and Enzymatic Activation," 199th ACS Division of Medicinal Chemistry Meeting, Boston, MA, April, 1990

57. S. A. Beers, Y. Imakura, H.-J. Dai, D.-H. Li, Y.-C. Cheng, and K.-H. Lee. *J. Nat. Prod.* **51**, 901 (1988).

58. G. Bennett, S. Chapman, and F. Bray. *Med. J. Aust.* **151**, 314 (1989).

59. L. Bensley. *Oncology Times* **11**, 1 (1989).

60. A. F. Benslimane, Y. F. Pouchus, J. Le Boterff, J. F. Verbist, C. Roussakis, and F. Monniot. *J. Nat. Prod.* **51**, 582 (1988).

61. V. Beral, T. A. Peterman, R. L. Berkelman, and H. W. Jaffe. *Lancet* **335**, 123 (1990).

62. A. Bernard and R. Lauwerys. *Experientia* **40**, 143 (1984).

63. M. Bernart and W. H. Gerwick. *Tetrahedron Lett.* **29**, 2015 (1988).

64. A. W. Bernheimer and C. Y. Lai. *Toxicon* **23**, 791 (1985).

65. F. Besson and G. Michel. *J. Antibiotics* **41**, 282 (1988).

66. K. C. Bible, M. Buytendorp, P. D. Zierath, and K. L. Rinehart. *Proc. Natl. Acad. Sci. USA* **85**, 4582 (1988).

67. I. R. C. Bick, J. H. Bowie, and G. K. Douglas. *Aust. J. Chem.* **20**, 1403 (1967).

68. I. R. C. Bick, P. S. Clezy, and W. D. Crow. *Aust. J. Chem.* **9**, 111 (1956).

69. L. W. Bieber, Á. A. da Silva Filho, R. M. O. Corrêa Lima, A. de Andrade Chiappeta, S. C. do Nascimento, I. A. de Souza, J. F. de Méllo, and H. J. Veith. *Phytochemistry* **25**, 1077 (1986).

70. M. Bittner, F. Gonzalez, H. Valdebenito, M. Silva, V. J. Paul, W. Fenical, M. H. M. Chen, and J. Clardy. *Tetrahedron Lett.* **28**, 4031 (1987).

71. A. J. Blackman, B. F. Bowden, J. C. Coll, B. Frick, M. Mahendran, and S. J. Mitchell. *Aust. J. Chem.* **35**, 1873 (1982).

72. A. J. Blackman and R. D. Green. *Aust. J. Chem.* **40**, 1655 (1987).

73. A. J. Blackman, T. W. Hambley, K. Picker, W. C. Taylor, and N. Thirasasana. *Tetrahedron Lett.* **28**, 5561 (1987).

74. A. J. Blackman and D. J. Matthews. *Heterocycles* **23**, 2829 (1985).

75. A. J. Blackman, D. J. Matthews, and C. K. Narkowicz. *J. Nat. Prod.* **50**, 494 (1987).

76. A. Blair. *J. Natl. Cancer Inst.* **82**, 544 (1990).

77. A. Blair, D. J. Grauman, J. H. Lubin, and J. F. Fraumeni, Jr. *J. Natl. Cancer Inst.* **71**, 31 (1983).

78. A. Blair, P. Stewart, M. O'Berg, W. Gaffey, J. Walrath, J. Ward, R. Bales, S. Kaplan, and D. Cubit. *J. Natl. Cancer Inst.* **76**, 1071 (1986).

79. S. J. Bloor and F. J. Schmitz. *J. Am. Chem. Soc.* **109**, 6134 (1987).

80. A. Blum and B. N. Ames. *Science* **195**, 17 (1977).

81. R. S. Blumberg, T. J. Paradis, D. Crawford, R. E. Byington, M. S. Hirsch, and R. T. Schooley. *Aids Res. & Human Retroviruses* **3**, 303 (1987).

82. J. W. Blunt, R. J. Lake, and M. H. G. Munro. *Phytochemistry* **23**, 1951 (1984).

83. P. Bogovski. *J. Tox. Environ. Health* **6**, 921 (1980).

84. F. Bohlmann, N. Ates (Gören), J. Jakupovic, R. M. King, and H. Robinson. *Phytochemistry* **23**, 1180 (1984).

85. J. D. Boice, Jr., M. Blettner, R. A. Kleinerman, M. Stovall, W. C. Moloney, G. Engholm, D. F. Austin, A. Bosch, D. L. Cookfair, E. T. Krementz, H. B. Latourette, L. J. Peters, M. D. Schulz, M. Lundell, F. Pettersson, H. H. Storm, C. M. J. Bell, M. P. Coleman, P. Fraser, M. Palmer, P. Prior, N. W. Choi, T. G. Hislop, M. Koch, D. Robb, D. Robson, R. F. Spengler, D. von Fournier, R. Frischkorn, H. Lochmüller, V. Pompe-Kirn, A. Rimpela, K. Kjørstad, M. H. Pejovic, K. Sigurdsson, P. Pisani, H. Kucera, and G. B. Hutchison. *J. Natl. Cancer Inst.* **79**, 1295 (1987).

86. J. D. Boice, Jr., M. H. Greene, J. Y. Killen, Jr., S. S. Ellenberg, R. J. Keehn, E. McFadden, T. T. Chen, and J. F. Fraumeni, Jr. *N. Engl. J. Med.* **309**, 1079 (1983).

87. W. Boland and D. G. Müller. *Tetrahedron Lett.* **28**, 307 (1987).

88. S. Bonassi, F. Merlo, N. Pearce, and R. Puntoni. *Int. J. Cancer* **44**, 648 (1989).

89. V. P. Bond and L. D. Hamilton. *J. Am. Med. Assoc.* **244**, 1610 (1980).

90. C. Boni, G. Cocconi, G. Bisagni, G. Ceci, and G. Peracchia. *Cancer* **63**, 638 (1989).

91. J. Borges, M. T. Manresa, J. L. Martín Ramón, C. Pascual, and A. Rumbero. *Tetrahedron Lett.* **34**, 3197 (1979).

92. M. Bortolotto, J. C. Braekman, D. Daloze, and B. Tursch. *Bull. Soc. Chim. Belg.* **87**, 539 (1978).

93. B. A. M. Botros, D. M. Watts, A. K. Soliman, A. W. Salib, M. I. Moussa, H. Mursal, C. Douglas, and M. Farah. *J. Med. Virol.* **29**, 79 (1989).

94. B. Botta, F. Delle Monache, G. Delle Monache, and K. Kabangu. *Phytochemistry* **25**, 766 (1986).

95. B. Botta, F. Delle Monache, G. Delle Monache, G. B. Marini Bettolo, and J. D. Msonthi. *Phytochemistry* **24**, 827 (1985).

96. B. Botta, F. Delle Monache, G. Delle Monache, G. B. Marini Bettolo, and J. U. Oguakwa. *Phytochemistry* **22**, 539 (1983).

97. B. F. Bowden, J. C. Coll, L. M. Engelhardt, A. Heaton, and A. H. White. *Aust. J. Chem.* **40**, 1483 (1987).

98. B. F. Bowden, J. C. Coll, L. M. Engelhardt, G. V. Meehan, G. G. Pegg, D. M. Tapiolas, A. H. White, and R. H. Willis. *Aust. J. Chem.* **39**, 123 (1986).

99. B. F. Bowden, J. C. Coll, L. M. Engelhardt, D. M. Tapiolas, and A. H. White. *Aust. J. Chem.* **39**, 103 (1986).

100. B. F. Bowden, J. C. Coll, J. M. Gulbis, M. F. Mackay, and R. H. Willis. *Aust. J. Chem.* **39**, 803 (1986).

101. B. F. Bowden, J. C. Coll, A. Heaton, G. König, M. A. Bruck, R. E. Cramer, D. M. Klein, and P. J. Scheuer. *J. Nat. Prod.* **50**, 650 (1987).

102. B. F. Bowden, J. C. Coll, S. J. Mitchell, and G. J. Stokie. *Aust. J. Chem.* **31**, 1303 (1978).

103. B. F. Bowden, J. C. Coll, S. J. Mitchell, G. J. Stokie, and J. F. Blount. *Aust. J. Chem.* **31**, 2039 (1978).

104. B. F. Bowden, J. C. Coll, W. Patalinghug, B. W. Skelton, I. Vasilescu, and A. H. White. *Aust. J. Chem.* **40**, 2085 (1987).

105. B. F. Bowden, J. C. Coll, and R. H. Willis. *Aust. J. Chem.* **39**, 1717 (1986).

106. P. R. Boyd and G. J. Mark. *Cancer* **40**, 1765 (1977).

107. G. L. Boyer and S. S. Dougherty. *Phytochemistry* **27**, 1521 (1988).

108. J. C. Braekman, D. Daloze, B. Moussiaux, and R. Riccio. *J. Nat. Prod.* **50**, 994 (1987).

109. D. J. Braver, M. Modan, A. Chêtrit, A. Lusky, and Z. Braf. *J. Natl. Cancer Inst.* **78**, 437 (1987).

110. B. Bridges. *Jpn. J. Cancer Res. (Gann)* **81**, 105 (1990).

111. G. Bronson. "Chemical Acrylonitrile Linked to Cancer in Workers Exposed to It, Agency Says," *Wall Street Journal*, June 30, 1977, p. 4.

112. I. Bross and N. Natarajan. *Invest. Radiol.* **15**, 52 (1980).

113. R. C. Bruening, E. M. Oltz, J. Furukawa, K. Nakanishi, and K. Kustin. *J. Am. Chem. Soc.* **107**, 5298 (1985).

114. R. C. Bruening, E. M. Oltz, J. Furukawa, K. Nakanishi, and K. Kustin. *J. Nat. Prod* **49**, 193 (1986).

115. R. A. Brumback, J. E. Gerber, D. G. Hicks, and J. A. Strauchen. *Cancer* **54**, 994 (1984).

116. M. Bruneteau, I. Fabre, J. Perret, G. Michel, P. Ricci, J.-P. Joseleau, J. Kraus, M. Schneider, W. Blaschek, and G. Franz. *Carbohydr. Res.* **175**, 137 (1988).

117. M. A. Buchanan and E. E. Dickey. *J. Org. Chem.* **25**, 1389 (1960).

118. D. D. Buechter and D. E. Thurston. *J. Nat. Prod.* **50**, 360 (1987).

119. J. D. Burch, G. R. Howe, A. B. Miller, and R. Semenciw. *J. Natl. Cancer Inst.* **67**, 1219 (1981).

120. H. Burger, A. L. Belman, R. Grimson, A. Kaell, K. Flaherty, J. Gulla, R. A. Gibbs, P.-N. Nguyun, and B. Weiser. *Lancet* **336**, 134 (1990).

121. W. F. Busby, Jr. and G. N. Wogan. "Aflatoxins" In Chemical Carcinogens, Second Edition, Revised and Expanded, Vol. 2, Chap. 16, C. E. Searle, Ed., Amer. Chem. Soc., Washington, D.C., 1984, p. 945.

122. J. A. Bush, B. H. Long, J. J. Catino, W. T. Bradner, and K. Tomita. *J. Antibiotics* **40**, 668 (1987).

123. S. Caccamese, A. Compagnini, R. M. Toscano, F. Nicolo, and G. Chapuis. *Tetrahedron* **43**, 5393 (1987).

124. S. Caccamese and R. M. Toscano. *Gazz. Chim. Ital.* **116**, 177 (1986).

125. F. Cafieri, L. de Napoli, E. Fattorusso, and C. Santacroce. *Phytochemistry* **26**, 471 (1987).

126. F. Cafieri, L. de Napoli, E. Fattorusso, and C. Santacroce. *Phytochemistry* **27**, 621 (1988).

127. F. Cafieri, B. Di Blasio, E. Fattorusso, and C. Pedone. *Tetrahedron Lett.* **22**, 4123 (1981).

128. F. Cafieri, E. Fattorusso, M. Gavagnin, and C. Santacroce. *J. Nat. Prod.* **48**, 944 (1985).

129. F. Cafieri, E. Fattorusso, L. Mayol, and C. Santacroce. *Tetrahedron* **42**, 4273 (1986).

130. L. Caglioti, G. Cainelli, and G. Maina. *Tetrahedron* **19**, 1057 (1963).

131. G. G. Caldwell, D. B. Kelley, and C. W. Heath, Jr. *J. Am. Med. Assoc.* **244**, 1575 (1980).

132. R. C. Cambie, P. R. Bergquist, and P. Karuso. *J. Nat. Prod.* **51**, 1014 (1988).

133. R. C. Cambie, P. A. Craw, P. R. Bergquist, and P. Karuso. *J. Nat. Prod.* **50**, 948 (1987).

134. R. C. Cambie, P. A. Craw, P. R. Bergquist, and P. Karuso. *J. Nat. Prod.* **51**, 331 (1988).

135. R. C. Cambie, P. A. Craw, M. J. Stone, and P. R. Bergquist. *J. Nat. Prod.* **51**, 293 (1988).

136. A. K. Campbell and P. J. Herring. *Comp. Biochem. Physiol.* **86B**, 411 (1987).

137. *Cancer Lett.* **5**, 5 (1979).

138. *Cancer Lett.* **13**, 4 (1987).

139. Cancer Possibility Remains in Hair Dyes: U.S. Food and Drug Administration Proposal, January 1978.

140. K. P. Cantor, R. Hoover, T. J. Mason, and L. J. McCabe. *J. Natl. Cancer Inst.* **61**, 979 (1978).

141. R. J. Capon and J. K. Macleod. *Tetrahedron* **41**, 3391 (1985).

142. R. J. Capon and J. K. MacLeod. *J. Nat. Prod.* **50**, 225 (1987).

143. R. J. Capon and J. K. MacLeod. *J. Nat. Prod.* **50**, 1136 (1987).

144. R. J. Capon and J. K. MacLeod. *Aust. J. Chem.* **40**, 1327 (1987).

145. R. J. Capon, J. K. MacLeod, and P. J. Scammells. *Tetrahedron* **42**, 6545 (1986).

146. R. J. Capon, J. K. MacLeod, and A. C. Willis. *J. Org. Chem.* **52**, 339 (1987).

147. J. H. Cardellina II, R. L. Hendrickson, K. P. Manfredi, S. A. Strobel,

147. J. H. Cardellina II, R. L. Hendrickson, K. P. Manfredi, S. A. Strobel, and J. Clardy. *Tetrahedron Lett.* **28**, 727 (1987).

148. J. H. Cardellina II, D. Nigh, and B. C. Van Wagenen. *J. Nat. Prod.* **49**, 1065 (1986).

149. R. W. Carey, R. M. Linggood, W. Wood, and P. H. Blitzer. *Cancer* **54**, 2234 (1984).

150. S. Carmely, M. Cojocaru, Y. Loya, and Y. Kashman. *J. Org. Chem.* **53**, 4801 (1988).

151. S. Carmely and Y. Kashman. *J. Org. Chem.* **51**, 784 (1986).

152. G. T. Carter. *J. Org. Chem.* **51**, 4264 (1986).

153. S. K. Carter. *Cancer Chemother. Pharmacol.* **12**, 67 (1984).

154. R. A. Cartwright. "Cancer Epidemiology" In Chemical Carcinogens, Second Edition, Revised and Expanded, Vol. 1, Chap. 1, C. E. Searle, Ed., Amer. Chem. Soc., Washington, D.C., 1984, p. 1.

155. N. Cascinelli and R. Marchesini. *Photochem. Photobiol.* **50**, 497 (1989).

156. P. J. Casey, P. A. Solski, C. J. Der, and J. E. Buss. *Proc. Natl. Acad. Sci. USA* **86**, 8323 (1989).

157. M. P. Cassidy, E. L. Ghisalberti, P. R. Jefferies, B. W. Skelton, and A. H. White. *Aust. J. Chem.* **38**, 1187 (1985).

158. G. Cassinelli, C. Geroni, B. Botta, G. delle Monache, and F. delle Monache. *J. Nat. Prod.* **49**, 929 (1986).

159. C. L. Casterline, P. F. Casterline, and D. A. Jaques. *Cancer* **39**, 1686 (1977).

160. R. E. Chaisson, P. Bacchetti, D. Osmond, B. Brodie, M. A. Sande, and A. R. Moss. *J. Am. Med. Assoc.* **261**, 561 (1989).

161. S. K. Chambers, R. L. Chopyk, J. T. Chambers, P. E. Schwartz, and T. P. Duffy. *Cancer* **64**, 2459 (1989).

162. W. R. Chan, W. F. Tinto, P. S. Manchand, and L. J. Todaro. *J. Org. Chem.* **52**, 3091 (1987).

163. C. W. J. Chang, A. Patra, J. A. Baker, and P. J. Scheuer. *J. Am. Chem. Soc.* **109**, 6119 (1987).

164. C. W. J. Chang, A. Patra, D. M. Roll, P. J. Scheuer, G. K. Matsumoto, and J. Clardy. *J. Am. Chem. Soc.* **106**, 4644 (1984).

165. D. J. Chapman. *Phytochemisty* **5**, 1331 (1966).

166. B. Charles, J. Bruneton, and Ad. Cavé. *J. Nat. Prod.* **49**, 303 (1986).

167. K. Chebaane and M. Guyot. *Tetrahedron Lett.* **27**, 1495 (1986).

168. K. T. K. Chen, K. D. Hoffman, and E. J. Hendricks. *Cancer* **44**, 2044 (1979).

169. Y.-P. Chen and C. A. Squier. *J. Natl. Cancer Inst.* **82**, 861 (1990).

170. J.-F. Cheng, Y. Ohizumi, M. R. Wälchli, H. Nakamura, Y. Hirata, T. Sasaki, and J. Kobayashi. *J. Org. Chem.* **53**, 4621 (1988).

171. J. Chin and J. Mann. *Bull. World Health Org.* **67**, 1 (1989).

172. J. Chin, P. A. Sato, and J. M. Mann. *Bull. World Health Org.* **68**, 1 (1990).

173. J.-H. Cho and C. Djerassi. *J. Chem. Soc., Perkin Trans. 1* 1307 (1987).

174. J.-H. Cho and C. Djerassi. *J. Org. Chem.* **52**, 4517 (1987).

175. Y.-H. Choi, J. Kim, J. M. Pezzuto, A. D. Kinghorn, N. R. Farnsworth, H. Lotter, and H. Wagner. *Tetrahedron Lett.* **27**, 5795 (1986).

176. Y.-H. Choi, J. M. Pezzuto, A. D. Kinghorn, and N. R. Farnsworth. *J. Nat. Prod.* **51**, 110 (1988).

177. H.-N. Chou, Y. Shimizu, G. Van Duyne, and J. Clardy. *Tetrahedron Lett.* **26**, 2865 (1985).

178. M. C. Chu, E. J. O'Rourke, and D. W. Trent. *J. Gen. Virol.* **70**, 1701 (1989).

179. P. Ciminiello, E. Fattorusso, S. Magno, and L. Mayol. *Experientia* **42**, 625 (1986).

180. P. Ciminiello, S. Magno, L. Mayol, and V. Piccialli. *J. Nat. Prod.* **50**, 217 (1987).

181. G. Cimino, A. Crispino, S. De Rosa, S. De Stefano, M. Gavagnin, and G. Sodano. *Tetrahedron* **43**, 4023 (1987).

182. G. Cimino, A. Crispino, A. Spinella, and G. Sodano. *Tetrahedron Lett.* **29**, 3613 (1988).

183. G. Cimino, A. De Giulio, S. De Rosa, S. De Stefano, R. Puliti, C. A. Mattia, and L. Mazzarella. *J. Nat. Prod.* **48**, 523 (1985).

184. G. Cimino, S. De Rosa, S. De Stefano, and G. Sodano. *Pure Appl. Chem.* **58**, 375 (1986).

185. G. Cimino, S. De Stefano, and A. Di Luccia. *Experientia* **35**, 1277 (1979).

186. G. Cimino, S. De Stefano, and G. Strazzullo. *J. Nat. Prod.* **50**, 1171 (1987).

187. G. Cimino, M. Gavagnin, G. Sodano, R. Puliti, C. A. Mattia, and L. Mazzarella. *Tetrahedron* **44**, 2301 (1988).

188. G. Cimino, M. Gavagnin, G. Sodano, A. Spinella, G. Strazzullo, F. J. Schmitz, and G. Yalamanchili. *J. Org. Chem.* **52**, 2301 (1987).

189. J. Clardy, G. Van Duyne, A. G. González, E. Manta, J. D. Martin, C. Pérez, J. L. Ravelo, and G. K. Schulte. *J. Chem. Soc., Chem. Commun.* 767 (1987).

190. D. Coggon, D. J. P. Barker, R. B. Cole, and M. Nelson. *J. Natl. Cancer Inst.* **81**, 1178 (1989).

191. J. C. Coll and A. D. Wright. *Aust. J. Chem.* **40**, 1893 (1987).

192. K. W. Collingwood, B. S. Pasternack, and R. E. Shore. *J. Natl. Cancer Inst.* **78**, 1127 (1987).

193. M. Colon, P. Guevara, W. H. Gerwick, and D. Ballantine. *J. Nat. Prod.* **50**, 368 (1987).

194. T. A. Connors. "Carcinogenicity of Medicines" In Chemical Carcinogens, Second Edition, Revised and Expanded, Vol. 2, Chap. 20, C. E. Searle, Ed., Amer. Chem. Soc., Washington, D.C., 1984, p. 1241.

195. T. P. Cooley, L. M. Kunches, C. A. Saunders, J. K. Ritter, C. J. Perkins, C. McLaren, M. R. C. Path, R. P. McCaffrey, and H. A. Liebman. *N. Engl. J. Med.* **322**, 1340 (1990).

196. N. M. Cooray, P. J. Scheuer, L. Parkanyi, and J. Clardy. *J. Org. Chem.* **53**, 4619 (1988).

197. S. Cordier, M. Poisson, M. Gerin, J. Varin, F. Conso, and D. Hemon. *Br. J. Indust. Med.* **45**, 705 (1988).

198. E. J. Corey and P. A. Magriotis. *J. Am. Chem. Soc.* **109**, 287 (1987).

199. D. G. Corley, R. Herb, R. E. Moore, P. J. Scheuer, and V. J. Paul. *J. Org. Chem.* **53**, 3644 (1988).

200. D. G. Corley, R. E. Moore, and V. J. Paul. *J. Am. Chem. Soc.* **110**, 7920 (1988).

201. D. G. Corley, G. E. Rottinghaus, J. K. Tracy, and M. S. Tempesta. *Tetrahedron Lett.* **27**, 4133 (1986).

202. P. Cottagnoud, K. A. Neftel, M. Hany, and R. M. Zinkernagel. *Antiviral Res.* **10**, 59 (1988).

203. Council on Scientific Affairs. *J. Am. Med. Assoc.* **262**, 380 (1989).

204. S. J. Coval, S. Cross, G. Bernardinelli, and C. W. Jefford. *J. Nat. Prod.* **51**, 981 (1988).

205. S. J. Coval, P. J. Scheuer, G. K. Matsumoto, and J. Clardy. *Tetrahedron* **40**, 3823 (1984).

206. G. M. Cragg and M. Suffness. "The Development of the Anticancer Drug, Taxol," Pharmacog. Soc. Meeting, Utah, July 1988.

207. T. Creagh-Kirk, P. Doi, E. Andrews, S. Nusinoff-Lehrman, H. Tilson, D. Hoth, and D. W. Barry. *J. Am. Med. Assoc.* **260**, 3009 (1988).

208. K. J. Cremer, S. B. Spring, and J. Gruber. *J. Natl. Cancer Inst.* **82**, 1016 (1990).

209. P. Crews and P. Bescansa. *J. Nat. Prod.* **49**, 1041 (1986).

210. P. Crews, L. V. Manes, and M. Boehler. *Tetrahedron Lett.* **27**, 2797 (1986).

211. R. Crohare, H. A. Priestap, M. Fariña, M. Cedola, and E. A. Rúveda. *Phytochemistry* **13**, 1957 (1974).

212. J. Cuzick. *N. Engl. J. Med.* **304**, 204 (1981).

213. R. Dagani. *C & E News*, Feb. 5, 1990, p. 5.

214. M. D'Ambrosio, A. Guerriero, and F. Pietra. *Helv. Chim. Acta* **70**, 612 (1987).

215. M. D'Ambrosio, A. Guerriero, and F. Pietra. *Helv. Chim. Acta* **70**, 2019 (1987).

216. M. D'Ambrosio, A. Guerriero, and F. Pietra. *Helv. Chim. Acta* **71**, 964 (1988).

217. S. J. Danishefsky, N. B. Mantlo, D. S. Yamashita, and G. Schulte. *J. Am. Chem. Soc.* **110**, 6890 (1988).

218. M. C. Das and S. B. Mahato. *Phytochemistry* **21**, 2069 (1982).

219. M. V. D'Auria, L. Minale, C. Pizza, R. Riccio, and F. Zollo. *Gazz. Chim. Ital.* **114**, 469 (1984).

220. M. V. D'Auria, L. Minale, R. Riccio, and E. Uriarte. *Experientia* **44**, 719 (1988).

221. M. V. D'Auria, R. Riccio, L. Minale, S. La Barre, and J. Pusset. *J. Org. Chem.* **52**, 3947 (1987).

222. F. G. Davis, J. D. Boice, Jr., Z. Hrubec, and R. R. Monson. *Cancer Res.* **49**, 6130 (1989).

223. R. D. Dawe and J. L. C. Wright. *Tetrahedron Lett.* **27**, 2559 (1986).

224. M. De Bernardi, L. Garlaschelli, G. Gatti, G. Vidari, and P. Vita-Finzi. *Tetrahedron* **44**, 235 (1988).

225. K. M. De Cock, B. Barrere, L. Diaby, M.-F. Lafontaine, E. Gnaore, A. Porter, D. Pantobe, G. C. Lafontant, A. Dago-Akribi, M. Ette, K. Odehouri, and W. L. Heyward. *Science* **249**, 793 (1990).

226. M. L. Deinzer, P. A. Thomson, D. M. Burgett, and D. L. Isaacson. *Science* **195**, 497 (1977).

227. F. Delle Monache, B. Botta, G. Delle Monache, and G. B. Marini Bettolo. *Phytochemistry* **24**, 1855 (1985).

228. F. Delle Monache, F. Ferrari, G. B. Marini Bettolo, and L. E. Cuca Suarez. *Planta Med.* **40**, 340 (1980).

229. F. Delle Monache, F. Ferrari, G. B. Marini Bettolo, P. Maxfield, S. Cerrini, W. Fedeli, E. Gavuzzo, and A. Vaciago. *Gazz. Chim. Ital.* **109**, 301 (1979).

230. N. Demattè, A. Guerriero, F. Lafargue, and F. Pietra. *Comp. Biochem. Physiol.* **84B**, 11 (1986).

231. T. Demirer, F. Icli, O. Uzunalimoglu, and O. Kucuk. *Cancer* **65**, 2344 (1990).

232. G. de Nanteuil, A. Ahond, J. Guilhem, C. Poupat, E. Tran Huu Dau, P. Potier, M. Pusset, J. Pusset, and P. Laboute. *Tetrahedron* **41**, 6019 (1985).

233. S. De Rosa, S. De Stefano, R. Puliti, C. A. Mattia, and L. Mazzarella. *J. Nat. Prod.* **50**, 876 (1987).

234. S. De Rosa, S. De Stéfano, P. Scarpelli, and N. Zavodnik. *Phytochemistry* **27**, 1875 (1988).

235. S. De Rosa, S. De Stefano, and N. Zavodnik. *J. Org. Chem.* **53**, 5020 (1988).

236. L. B. De Silva, W. H. M. W. Herath, R. C. Jennings, M. Mahendran, and G. E. Wannigama. *Phytochemistry* **21**, 1173 (1982).

237. F. De Simone, A. Dini, E. Finamore, L. Minale, C. Pizza, R. Riccio, and F. Zollo. *J. Chem. Soc., Perkin Trans 1*, 1855 (1981).

238. P. De Waard, J. P. Kamerling, H. Van Halbeek, J. F. G. Vliegenthart, and J. J. S. Broertjes. *Eur. J. Biochem.* **168**, 679 (1987).

239. P. Dickson and G. Beardmore. *Med. J. Aust.* 396 (1983).

240. C. Djerassi, H. Budzikiewicz, J. M. Wilson, J. Gosset, J. Le Men, and M.-M. Janot. *Tetrahedron Lett.* 235 (1962).

241. L. A. Dolak and C. DeBoer. *J. Antibiotics* **33**, 83 (1980).

242. R. Doll and R. Peto. *J. Natl. Cancer Inst.* **66**, 1192 (1981).

243. F. Dorn and D. Arigoni. *Experientia* **30**, 134 (1974).

244. K. Dornberger. *Pharmazie* **41**, 265 (1986).

245. G. A. Doss and C. Djerassi. *J. Am. Chem. Soc.* **110**, 8124 (1988).

246. P. E. Driedger and P. M. Blumberg. *Proc. Natl. Acad. Sci. USA* **77**, 567 (1980).

247. M.-A. Dubois, R. Higuchi, T. Komori, and T. Sasaki. *Liebigs Ann. Chem.* 845 (1988).

248. M.-A. Dubois, Y. Noguchi, R. Higuchi, and T. Komori. *Liebigs Ann. Chem.* 495 (1988).

249. C.-Y. Duh, J. M. Pezzuto, A. D. Kinghorn, S. L. Leung, and N. R. Farnsworth. *J. Nat. Prod.* **50**, 63 (1987).

250. C.-Y. Duh, C. H. Phoebe, Jr., J. M. Pezzuto, A. D. Kinghorn, and N. R. Farnsworth. *J. Nat. Prod.* **49**, 706 (1986).

251. D. F. Easton, J. Peto, and R. Doll. *Br. J. Indust. Med.* **45**, 652 (1988).

252. "Ebola Virus Infection in Imported Primates--United States." *Can. Dis. Wkly. Rep.* **16**, 17 (1990).

253. J. S. Edmonds and K. A. Francesconi. *Nature* **289**, 602 (1981).

254. J. S. Edmonds and K. A. Francesconi. *J. Chem. Soc., Perkin Trans 1* 2375 (1983).

255. J. S. Edmonds, K. A. Francesconi, P. C. Healy. and A. H. White. *J. Chem. Soc., Perkin Trans 1* 2989 (1982).

256. J. S. Edmonds, M. Morita, and Y. Shibata. *J. Chem. Soc., Perkin Trans 1* 577 (1987).

257. K. Edo, M. Mizugaki, Y. Koide, H. Seto, K. Furihata, N. Ōtake, and N. Ishida. *Tetrahedron Lett.* **26**, 331 (1985).

258. K. Edo, K. Saito, Y. Akiyama-Murai, M. Mizugaki, Y. Koide, and N. Ishida. *J. Antibiotics* **41**, 554 (1988).

259. E. Eich, C. Becker, K. Mayer, A. Maidhof, and W. E. G. Müller. *Planta Med.* 290 (1986).

260. E. Eich, C. Becker, R. Sieben, A. Maidhof, and W. E. G. Müller. *J. Antibiotics* **39**, 804 (1986).

261. E. Eich, R. Sieben, and C. Becker. *Arch. Pharm.* **318**, 214 (1985).

262. A. Elgsaeter, J. D. Tauber, and S. Liaaen-Jensen. *Biochim. Biophys. Acta* **530**, 402 (1978).

263. M. M. Elkind. *Cancer* **65**, 2165 (1990).

264. R. C. Elliott, R. S. Konya, and K. Vickneshwara. *Toxicon* **24**, 117 (1986).

265. J. M. Elwood, R. P. Gallagher, J. Davison, and G. B. Hill. *Br. J. Cancer* **51**, 543 (1985).

266. G. O. Emerole, A. O. Uwaifo, M. I. Thabrew, and E. A. Bababunmi. *Cancer Lett.* **15**, 123 (1982).

267. R. Endean. *Toxicon* **25**, 483 (1987).

268. A. Endo, S. S. Khora, M. Murata, H. Naoki, and T. Yasumoto. *Tetrahedron Lett.* **29**, 4127 (1988).

269. K. Endo and H. Hikino. *Can. J. Chem.* **62**, 2011 (1984).

270. M. Endo, M. Nakagawa, Y. Hamamoto, and M. Ishihama. *Pure Appl. Chem.* **58**, 387 (1986).

271. M. Endo, M. Nakagawa, Y. Hamamoto, and T. Nakanishi. *J. Chem. Soc., Chem. Commun.* 322 (1983).

272. M. Endo, M. Nakagawa, Y. Hamamoto, and T. Nakanishi. *J. Chem. Soc., Chem. Commun.* 980 (1983).

273. P. E. Enterline and G. M. Marsh. *J. Natl. Cancer Inst.* **68**, 925 (1982).

274. J. E. Eriksson, J. A. O. Meriluoto, H. P. Kujari, K. Österlund, K. Fagerlund, and L. Hällbom. *Toxicon* **26**, 161 (1988).

275. L. Ettlinger, E. Gäumann, R. Hütter, W. Keller-Schierlein, F. Kradolfer, L. Neipp, V. Prelog, and H. Zähner. *Helv. Chim. Acta* **41**, 216 (1958).

276. I. A. Evans. "Bracken Carcinogenicity" In Chemical Carcinogens, Second Edition, Revised and Expanded, Vol. 2, Chap. 18, C. E. Searle, Ed., Amer. Chem. Soc., Washington, D.C., 1984, p. 1171.

277. L. A. Evans, J. Moreau, K. Odehouri, D. Seto, G. Thomson-Honnebier, H. Legg, A. Barboza, C. Cheng-Mayer, and J. A. Levy. *Lancet* **II**, 1389 (1988).

278. E. Fahy, R. J. Andersen, G. D. Van Duyne, and J. Clardy. *J. Org. Chem.* **51**, 57 (1986).

279. E. Fahy, R. J. Andersen, C. Xu, and J. Clardy. *J. Org. Chem.* **51**, 5145 (1986).

280. E. Fahy, T. F. Molinski, M. K. Harper, B. W. Sullivan, D. J. Faulkner, L. Parkanyi, and J. Clardy. *Tetrahedron Lett.* **29**, 3427 (1988).

281. T. Y. Fan, J. Morrison, D. P. Rounbehler, R. Ross, D. H. Fine, W. Miles, and N. P. Sen. *Science* **196**, 70 (1977).

282. A. A. Fantini, N. A. Kuck, R. E. Wallace, J. P. Thomas, J. D. Korshalla, and R. T. Testa. "LL-D05139β, A New Antitumor Antibiotic: Fermentation and Biological Properties of the Producing Culture," Program and Abstracts of The 24th Intersci. Conf. on Antimicrob. Agents Chemother., No. 1143, Washington D.C., October, 1984, p. 292.

283. D. C. Farrow and S. Davis. *Int. J. Cancer* **45**, 816 (1990).

284. C. F. Farthing, A. G. Dalgleish, A. Clark, M. McClure, A. Chanas, and B. G. Gazzard. *AIDS* 1, 21 (1987).

285. R. Fathi-Afshar and T. M. Allen. *Can. J. Chem.* **66**, 45 (1988).

286. E. Fattorusso, V. Lanzotti, S. Magno, and E. Novellino. *J. Nat. Prod.* **48**, 924 (1985).

287. E. Fattorusso, S. Magno, and L. Mayol. *Gazz. Chim. Ital.* **109**, 589 (1979).

288. E. Fattorusso, S. Magno, L. Mayol, C. Santacroce, D. Sica, V. Amico, G. Oriente, M. Piattelli, and C. Tringali. *J. Chem. Soc., Chem. Commun.* 575 (1976).

289. D. J. Faulkner, B. N. Ravi, J. Finer, and J. Clardy. *Phytochemistry* **16**, 991 (1977).

290. S. A. Fedoreyev, N. K. Utkina, S. G. Ilyin, M. V. Reshetnyak, and O. B. Maximov. *Tetrahedron Lett.* **27**, 3177 (1986).

291. H. W. Fehlhaber, H. Kogler, T. Mukhopadhyay, E. K. S. Vijayakumar, and B. N. Ganguli. *J. Am. Chem. Soc.* **110**, 8242 (1988).

292. H.-W. Fehlhaber, H. Kogler, T. Mukhopadhyay, E. K. S. Vijayakumar, K. Roy, R. H. Rupp, and B. N. Ganguli. *J. Antibiotics* **41**, 1785 (1988).

293. W. Fenical. *J. Nat. Prod.* **50**, 1001 (1987).

294. V. J. Feron, J. P. Bruyntjes, R. A. Woutersen, H. R. Immel, and L. M. Appelman. *Cancer Lett.* **39**, 101 (1988).

295. M. Fiebig, C.-Y. Duh, J. M. Pezzuto, A. D. Kinghorn, and N. R. Farnsworth. *J. Nat. Prod.* **48**, 981 (1985).

296. S. Findlay and J. Silberner. "The Worsening Spread of the AIDS Crisis," *U. S. News and World Rept.*, Jan. 29, 1990, p. 28.

297. M. Fischl, J. E. Galpin, J. D. Levine, J. E. Groopman, D. H. Henry, P. Kennedy, S. Miles, W. Robbins, B. Starrett, R. Zalusky, R. I. Abels, H. C. Tsai, and S. A. Rudnick. *N. Engl. J. Med.* **322**, 1488 (1990).

298. P. V. Fish, G. Pattenden, and S. T. Hodgson. *Tetrahedron Lett.* **29**, 3857 (1988).

299. S. Fogle. *J. NIH Res.* **2**, 35 (1990).

300. D. Fontenille. *Arch. Inst. Pasteur Madagascar* **55**, 1 (1989).

301. C. J. R. Fookes, M. J. Garson, J. K. MacLeod, B. W. Skelton, and A. H. White. *J. Chem. Soc., Perkin Trans 1* 1003 (1988).

302. S. Forenza, L. Minale, R. Riccio, and E. Fattorusso. *J. Chem. Soc., Chem. Commun.* 1129 (1971).

303. P. Foss, R. R. L. Guillard, and S. Liaaen-Jensen. *Phytochemistry* **23**, 1629 (1984).

304. P. Foss, T. Skjetne, and S. Liaaen-Jensen. *Acta Chem. Scand.* **B40**, 172 (1986).

305. R. M. Fourney, C. L. Hew, S. B. Joshi, and G. L. Fletcher. *Comp. Biochem. Physiol.* **78B**, 791 (1984).

306. J. L. Fox, *C & E News*, Dec. 12, 1977, p. 34.

307. C. Francisco, B. Banaigs, M. Rakba, J. Teste, and A. Cave. *J. Org. Chem.* **51**, 2707 (1986).

308. J. F. Fraumeni, Jr. *Cancer Res.* **39**, 2851 (1979).

309. G. Freund. *Cancer Res.* **39**, 2899 (1979).

310. K. Fujii and K-I. Nomoto. *Cancer Lett.* **18**, 321 (1983).

311. H. Fujiki, M. Suganuma, and T. Sugimura. *Envir. Carcino. Revs. (J. Envir. Sci. Hlth.)* **C7**, 1 (1989).

312. K. Fujimoto, T. Oka, and M. Morimoto. *Cancer Res.* **47**, 1516 (1987).

313. M. Fujioka, K. Biemann, A. Miyamae, K. Nakashima, I. Sumino, M. Shigi, M. Mera, S. Koda, S. Atarashi, and Y. Morimoto. 28th Symposium on The Chemistry of Natural Products, Symposium Papers, Sendai, 1986, p. 167.

314. M. Fujioka, S. Koda, Y. Morimoto, and K. Biemann. *J. Org. Chem.* **53**, 2820 (1988).

315. A. Fujita, T. Hayashi, M. Arisawa, M. Shimizu, N. Morita, T. Kikuchi, and Y. Tezuka. *J. Nat. Prod.* **51**, 708 (1988).

316. T. Fujita, Y. Takeda, H-D. Sun, Y. Minami, T. Marunaka, S. Takeda, Y. Yamada, and T. Togo. *Planta Med.* **54**, 414 (1988).

317. T. Fujita, Y. Takeda, and T. Shingu. *J. Chem. Soc., Chem. Commun.* 205 (1980).

318. T. Fujita, Y. Takeda, T. Shingu, and A. Ueno. *Chem. Lett.* 1635 (1980); *Chem. Abstr.* **94**, 61697v (1981).

319. N. Fukamiya and K.-H. Lee. *J. Nat. Prod.* **49**, 348 (1986).

320. N. Fukamiya, M. Okano, T. Aratani, K. Negoro, Y.-M. Lin, and K.-H. Lee. *Planta Med.* **53**, 140 (1987).

321. N. Fukamiya, M. Okano, T. Aratani, K. Negoro, A. T. McPhail, M. Ju-ichi, and K.-H. Lee. *J. Nat. Prod.* **49**, 428 (1986).

322. N. Fukamiya, M. Okano, K. Tagahara, T. Aratani, and K.-H. Lee. *J. Nat. Prod.* **51**, 349 (1988).

323. N. Fukamiya, M. Okano, K. Tagahara, T. Aratani, Y. Muramoto, and K.-H. Lee. *J. Nat. Prod.* **50**, 1075 (1987).

324. A. Fukuzawa, Y. Kumagai, T. Masamune, A. Furusaki, T. Matsumoto, and C. Katayama. *Chem. Lett.* 1389 (1982).

325. A. Fukuzawa and T. Masamune. *Tetrahedron Lett.* **22**, 4081 (1981).

326. A. Fukuzawa, M. Miyamoto, Y. Kumagai, A. Abiko, Y. Takaya, and T. Masamune. *Chem. Lett.* 1259 (1985).

327. K. Funaishi, K. Kawamura, Y. Sugiura, N. Nakahori, E. Yoshida, M. Okanishi, I. Umezawa, S. Funayama, and K. Komiyama. *J. Antibiotics* **40**, 778 (1987).

328. C. J. Fürst, M. Lundell, L.-E. Holm, and C. Silfverswärd. *J. Natl. Cancer Inst.* **80**, 1387 (1988).

329. A. Furusaki, T. Matsumoto, A. Nakagawa, and S. Ōmura. *J. Antibiotics* **33**, 781 (1980).

330. N. Fusetani, M. Asano, S. Matsunaga, and K. Hashimoto. *Tetrahedron Lett.* **28**, 5837 (1987).

331. N. Fusetani, Y. Kato, K. Hashimoto, T. Komori, Y. Itakura, and T. Kawasaki. *J. Nat. Prod.* **47**, 997 (1984).

332. N. Fusetani, Y. Kato, S. Matsunaga, and K. Hashimoto. *Tetrahedron Lett.* **24**, 2771 (1983).

333. N. Fusetani, T. Shiragaki, S. Matsunaga, and K. Hashimoto. *Tetrahedron Lett.* **28**, 4313 (1987).

334. N. Fusetani, M. Sugano, S. Matsunaga, and K. Hashimoto. *Experientia* **43**, 1234 (1987).

335. N. Fusetani, M. Sugano, S. Matsunaga, and K. Hashimoto. *Tetrahedron Lett.* **28**, 4311 (1987).

336. N. Fusetani, M. Sugano, S. Matsunaga, K. Hashimoto, H. Shikama, A. Ohta, and H. Nagano. *Experientia* **43**, 1233 (1987).

337. N. Fusetani, K. Yasukawa, S. Matsunaga, and K. Hashimoto. *Tetrahedron Lett.* **26**, 6449 (1985).

338. N. Fusetani, K. Yasukawa, S. Matsunaga, and K. Hashimoto. *Comp. Biochem. Physiol.* **83B**, 511 (1986).

339. N. Fusetani, K. Yasukawa, S. Matsunaga, and K. Hashimoto. *Tetrahedron Lett.* **28**, 1187 (1987).

340. E. E. Garcia, L. E. Benjamin, and R. I. Fryer. *J. Chem. Soc., Chem. Commun.* 78 (1973).

341. F. C. Garland, D. L. Mayers, T. M. Hickey, M. R. Miller, E. K. Shaw, E. D. Gorham, L. R. Bigbee, and M. M. McNally. *J. Am. Med. Assoc.* **262**, 3161 (1989).

342. L. Garmon. *Science News* **123**, 359 (1983).

343. J. Gaub, C. Pedersen, A.-G. Poulsen, L. R. Mathiesen, K. Ulrich, B. O. Lindhardt, V. Faber, J. Gerstoft, B. Hofmann, J.-O. Lernestedt, C. M. Nielsen, J. O. Nielsen, and P. Platz. *AIDS* **1**, 27 (1987).

344. T. Gebreyesus and C. Djerassi. *Tetrahedron Lett.* **23**, 4427 (1982).

345. T. Gebreyesus, T. Yosief, S. Carmely, and Y. Kashman. *Tetrahedron Lett.* **29**, 3863 (1988).

346. B. Gerbert, B. Maguire, V. Badner, D. Altman, and G. Stone. *J. Am. Med. Assoc.* **260**, 3481 (1988).

347. W. H. Gerwick, A. Lopez, R. Davila, and R. Albors. *J. Nat. Prod.* **50**, 1131 (1987).

348. W. H. Gerwick, A. Lopez, G. D. Van Duyne, J. Clardy, W. Ortiz, and A. Baez. *Tetrahedron Lett.* **27**, 1979 (1986).

349. C. Glidewell. *Chem. Brit.* 137 (1990).

350. S. E. Glushakova and I. S. Lukashevich. *Arch. Virol.* **104**, 157 (1989).

351. J. J. Goedert, C. M. Kessler, L. M. Aledort, R. J. Biggar, W. A. Andes, G. C. White II, J. E. Drummond, K. Vaidya, D. L. Mann, M. E. Eyster, M. V. Ragni, M. M. Lederman, A. R. Cohen, G. L. Bray, P. S. Rosenberg, R. M. Friedman, M. W. Hilgartner, W. A. Blattner, B. Kroner, and M. H. Gail. *N. Engl. J. Med.* **321**, 1141 (1989).

352. T. E. Goffman, E. A. McKeen, R. E. Curtis, and P. S. Schein. *Cancer* **52**, 1808 (1983).

353. J. Golik, G. Dubay, G. Groenewold, H. Kawaguchi, M. Konishi, B. Krishnan, H. Ohkuma, K.-I. Saitoh, and T. W. Doyle. *J. Am. Chem. Soc.* **109**, 3462 (1987).

354. R. W. Goodgame. *N. Engl. J. Med.* **323**, 383 (1990).

355. D. Gouiffès, S. Moreau, N. Helbecque, J. L. Bernier, J. P. Hénichart, Y. Barbin, D. Laurent, and J. F. Verbist. *Tetrahedron* **44**, 451 (1988).

356. T. R. Govindachari, N. Viswanathan, and H. Fuhrer. *Indian J. Chem.* **10**, 272 (1972).

357. J. Grabiec and D. A. Owen. *Cancer* **56**, 388 (1985).

358. J. D. Graham, L. C. Green, and M. J. Roberts. "In Search of Safety: Chemicals and Cancer Risk," Harvard Univ. Press, Cambridge, MA, 1988, 260 pages.

359. P. Grasso. "Carcinogens in Food" In Chemical Carcinogens, Second Edition, Revised and Expanded, Vol. 2, Chap. 19, C. E. Searle, Ed., Amer. Chem. Soc., Washington, D.C., 1984, p. 1205.

360. M. H. Greene, J. D. Boice, Jr., B. E. Greer, J. A. Blessing, and A. J. Dembo. *N. Engl. J. Med.* **307**, 1416 (1982).

361. H. Greim and T. Wolff. "Carcinogenicity of Organic Halogenated Compounds" In Chemical Carcinogens, Second Edition, Revised and Expanded, Vol. 1, Chap. 9, C. E. Searle, Ed., Amer. Chem. Soc., Washington, D.C., 1984, p. 525.

362. P. A. Grieco, Y. S. Hon, and A. Perez-Medrano. *J. Am. Chem. Soc.* **110**, 1630 (1988).

363. S. H. Grode, T. R. James, and J. H. Cardellina II. *Tetrahedron Lett.* **24**, 691 (1983).

364. S. H. Grode, T. R. James, Jr., J. H. Cardellina, II, and K. D. Onan. *J. Org. Chem.* **48**, 5203 (1983).

365. A. Groweiss, W. Fenical, C.-H. He, J. Clardy, Z. Wu, Z. Yiao, and K. Long. *Tetrahedron Lett.* **26**, 2379 (1985).

366. A. Groweiss, S. A. Look, and W. Fenical. *J. Org. Chem.* **53**, 2401 (1988).

367. H. W. Grünwald and F. Rosner. *Cancer* **50**, 676 (1982).

368. G. Guella, I. Mancini, and F. Pietra. *J. Chem. Soc., Chem. Commun.* 77 (1986).

369. G. Guella, I. Mancini, and F. Pietra. *Helv. Chim. Acta* **70**, 621 (1987).

370. G. Guella, I. Mancini, and F. Pietra. *Helv. Chim. Acta* **70**, 1050 (1987).

371. G. Guella, I. Mancini, and F. Pietra. *Helv. Chim. Acta* **70**, 1400 (1987).

372. G. Guella and F. Pietra. *Helv. Chim. Acta* **71**, 62 (1988).

373. A. Guerriero, M. D'Ambrosio, V. Cuomo, F. Vanzanella, and F. Pietra. *Helv. Chim. Acta* **71**, 57 (1988).

374. A. Guerriero, M. D'Ambrosio, and F. Pietra. *Helv. Chim. Acta* **70**, 984 (1987).

375. A. Guerriero, B. Dematté, M. D'Ambrosio, and F. Pietra. *J. Nat. Prod.* **49**, 608 (1986).

376. A. Guerriero, P. Traldi, and F. Pietra. *J. Chem. Soc., Chem. Commun.* 40 (1986).

377. N. K. Gulavita, E. D. de Silva, M. R. Hagadone, P. Karuso, P. J. Scheuer, G. D. Van Duyne, and J. Clardy. *J. Org. Chem.* **51**, 5136 (1986).

378. N. Gulavita, A. Hori, Y. Shimizu, P. Laszlo, and J. Clardy. *Tetrahedron Lett.* **29**, 4381 (1988).

379. G. P. Gunawardana, S. Kohmoto, S. P. Gunasekera, O. J. McConnell, and F. E. Koehn. *J. Am. Chem. Soc.* **110**, 4856 (1988).

380. K. Gustafson, R. J. Anderson, C.-H. He, and J. Clardy. *Tetrahedron Lett.* **26**, 2521 (1985).

381. K. R. Gustafson, J. H. Cardellina II, R. W. Fuller, O. S. Weislow, R. F. Kiser, K. M. Snader, G. M. L. Patterson, and M. R. Boyd. *J. Natl. Cancer Inst.* **81**, 1254 (1989).

382. M. Guyot, M. Durgeat, and E. Morel. *J. Nat. Prod.* **49**, 307 (1986).

383. T. B. T. Ha, W. C. M. C. Kokke, J. R. Proudfoot, C. Djerassi, and J. Thompson. *Steroids* **45**, 263 (1985).

384. A. M. Habib, D. K. Ho, S. Masuda, T. McCloud, K. S. Reddy, M. Aboushoer, A. McKenzie, S. R. Byrn, C.-J. Chang, and J. M. Cassady. *J. Org. Chem.* **52**, 412 (1987).

385. I. H. Hall, K. H. Lee, and H. C. Sykes. *Planta Med.* **53**, 153 (1987).

386. J. G. Hall and J. A. Reiss. *Aust. J. Chem.* **39**, 1401 (1986).

387. W. H. Hallenbeck. *Experientia* **40**, 136 (1984).

388. W. E. Halperin, M. Goodman, L. Stayner, L. J. Elliott, R. A. Keenlyside, and P. J. Landrigan. *J. Am. Med. Assoc.* **249**, 510 (1983).

389. T. Hamamoto, S. Gunji, H. Tsuji, and T. Beppu. *J. Antibiotics* **36**, 639 (1983).

390. T. Hamamoto, H. Seto, and T. Beppu. *J. Antibiotics* **36**, 646 (1983).

391. T. W. Hambley, A. Poiner, and W. C. Taylor. *Tetrahedron Lett.* **27**, 3281 (1986).

392. S. S. Handa, A. D. Kinghorn, G. A. Cordell, and N. R. Farnsworth. *J. Nat. Prod.* **46**, 248 (1983).

393. D. G. Hangauer. *Tetrahedron Lett.* **27**, 5799 (1986).

394. N. H. Harley. *N. Engl. J. Med.* **310**, 1525 (1984).

395. A. Harris, L. A. Anderson, J. D. Phillipson, and R. T. Brown. *Planta Med.* 151 (1985).

396. C. C. Harris. *J. Natl. Cancer Inst.* **63**, 275 (1979).

397. N. K. Hart, S. R. Johns, J. A. Lamberton, H. Suares, and R. I. Willing. *Aust. J. Chem.* **29**, 1295 (1976).

398. N. K. Hart, S. R. Johns, J. A. Lamberton, H. Suares, and R. I. Willing. *Aust. J. Chem.* **29**, 1319 (1976).

399. E. B. Harvey, J. D. Boice, Jr., M. Honeyman, and J. T. Flannery. *N. Engl. J. Med.* **312**, 541 (1985).

400. E. B. Harvey, C. Shairer, L. A. Brinton, R. N. Hoover, and J. F. Fraumeni, Jr. *J. Natl. Cancer Inst.* **78**, 657 (1987).

401. C. A. Harvis, M. T. Burch, and W. Fenical. *Tetrahedron Lett.* **29**, 4361 (1988).

402. C. Hashida, K. Nagayama, and N. Takemura. *Cancer Lett.* **17**, 101 (1982).

403. K. Hatanaka, T. Yoshida, T. Uryu, O. Yoshida, H. Nakashima, N. Yamamoto, T. Mimura, and Y. Kaneko. *Jpn. J. Cancer Res. (Gann)* **80**, 95 (1989).

404. R. D. Haworth and D. Woodcock. *J. Chem. Soc.* 1054 (1939).

405. Y. Hayakawa, K. Adachi, and N. Komeshima. *J. Antibiotics* **40**, 1349 (1987).

406. T. Hayashi, J. Koyama, A. T. McPhail, and K.-H. Lee. *Phytochemistry* **26**, 1065 (1987).

407. T. Hayashi, F. T. Smith, and K.-H. Lee. *J. Med. Chem.* **30**, 2005 (1987).

408. R. B. Hayes, J. W. Raatgever, A. de Bruyn, and M. Gerin. *Int. J. Cancer* **37**, 487 (1986).

409. G. L. Helms, R. E. Moore, W. P. Niemczura, G. M. L. Patterson, K. B. Tomer, and M. L. Gross. *J. Org. Chem.* **53**, 1298 (1988).

410. B. E. Henderson, B. Benton, J. Jing, M. C. Yu, and M. C. Pike. *Int. J. Cancer* **23**, 598 (1979).

411. R. L. Hendrickson and J. H. Cardellina II. *Tetrahedron* **42**, 6565 (1986).

412. T. Henne and D. Schmähl. *Cancer Treatment Reviews* **12**, 77 (1985).

413. H. Hennings, P. M. Blumberg, G. R. Pettit, C. L. Herald, R. Shores, and S. H. Yuspa. *Carcinogenesis* **8**, 1343 (1987).

414. H. Hennings, R. A. Shores, M. C. Poirier, E. Reed, R. E. Tarone, and S. H. Yuspa. *J. Natl. Cancer Inst.* **82**, 836 (1990).

415. E. Hietanen. *J. Tox. Environ. Health* **6**, 963 (1980).

416. T. Higa, T. Fujiyama, and P. J. Scheuer. *Comp. Biochem. Physiol.* **65B**, 525 (1980).

417. T. Higa, T. Ichiba, and R. K. Okuda. *Experientia* **41**, 1487 (1985).

418. T. Higa, R. K. Okuda, R. M. Severns, P. J. Scheuer, C.-H. He, X. Changfu, and J. Clardy. *Tetrahedron* **43**, 1063 (1987).

419. J. Higginson. *J. Tox. Environ. Health* **6**, 941 (1980).

420. J. Hilfrich, S. S. Hecht, and D. Hoffmann. *Cancer Lett.* **2**, 169 (1977).

421. M. W. Hinds and L. N. Kolonel. *Cancer* **45**, 811 (1980).

422. O. Hirai, K. Shimomura, T. Mizota, S. Matsumoto, J. Mori, and H. Kikuchi. *J. Antibiotics* **40**, 607 (1987).

423. Y. Hirata and D. Uemura. *Pure Appl. Chem.* **58**, 701 (1986).

424. I. Hirono, K. Yamada, H. Niwa, Y. Shizuri, M. Ojika, S. Hosaka, T. Yamaji, K. Wakamatsu, H. Kigoshi, K. Niiyama, and Y. Uosaki. *Cancer Lett.* **21**, 239 (1984).

425. M. Hirota, M. Suttajit, H. Suguri, Y. Endo, K. Shudo, V. Wongchai, E. Hecker, and H. Fujiki. *Cancer Res.* **48**, 5800 (1988).

426. S. Hirsch and Y. Kashman. *J. Nat. Prod.* **51**, 1243 (1988).

427. S. Hirsh, S. Carmely, and Y. Kashman. *Tetrahedron* **43**, 3257 (1987).

428. M. Hirst, D. G. Mills, S. Tse, L. Levin, and D. F. White. *Lancet* **I**, 186 (1984).

429. Y. Hitotsuyanagi, H. Fujiki, M. Suganuma, N. Aimi, S.-I. Sakai, Y. Endo, K. Shudo, and T. Sugimura. *Chem. Pharm. Bull.* **32**, 4233 (1984).

430. S. K. Hoar, A. Blair, F. F. Holmes, C. D. Boysen, R. J. Robel, R. Hoover, and J. F. Fraumeni, Jr. *J. Am. Med. Assoc.* **256**, 1141 (1986).

431. J. E. Hochlowski, Ph.D. Thesis, U. of Calif., San Diego, 1983.

432. C. Hogstedt, N. Malmqvist, and B. Wadman. *J. Am. Med. Assoc.* **241**, 1132 (1979).

433. C. H. Hoke, A. Nisalak, N. Sangawhipa, S. Jatanasen, T. Laorakapongse, B. L. Innis, S.-O. Kotchasenee, J. B. Gingrich, J. Latendresse, K. Fukai, and D. S. Burke. *N. Engl. J. Med.* **319**, 608 (1988).

434. M. Honda and T. Komori. *Tetrahedron Lett.* **27**, 3369 (1986).

435. T. Honda, M. Kato, M. Inoue, T. Shimamoto, K. Shima, T. Nakanishi, T. Yoshida, and T. Noguchi. *J. Med. Chem.* **31**, 1295 (1988).

436. H. Hori, G.-M. Pang, K. Harimaya, Y. Iitaka, and S. Inayama. *Chem. Pharm. Bull.* **35**, 2125 (1987).

437. Y. Hori, M. Hino, Y. Kawai, S. Kiyoto, H. Terano, M. Kohsaka, H. Aoki, M. Hashimoto, and H. Imanaka. *J. Antibiotics* **39**, 12 (1986).

438. Y. Horiuchi, S. Kondo, T. Ikeda, D. Ikeda, K. Miura, M. Hamada, T. Takeuchi, and H. Umezawa. *J. Antibiotics* **32**, 762 (1979).

439. S. B. Horwitz, L. Lothstein, J. J. Manfredi, W. Mellado, J. Parness, S. N. Roy, P. B. Schiff, L. Sorbara, and R. Zeheb. *Ann. N. Y. Acad. Sci.* **466**, 733 (1986).

440. M. Hoshijima, A. Kikuchi, T. Tanimoto, K. Kaibuchi, and Y. Takai. *Cancer Res.* **46**, 3000 (1986).

441. A. G. Howard, R. A. Pizzie, and J. W. Whitehouse. *Water Res.* **18**, 735 (1984).

442. G. R. Howe, D. Fraser, J. Lindsay, B. Presnal, and S. Z. Yu. *J. Natl. Cancer Inst.* **70**, 1015 (1983).

443. J. W. Huggins. *Rev. Infect. Dis.* **11**, Suppl. 4, S750 (1989).

444. Y. H. Hui, C. J. Chang, J. L. McLaughlin, and R. G. Powell. *J. Nat. Prod.* **49**, 1175 (1986).

445. S. Huneck and J.-M. Lehn. *Bull. Soc. Chim. Fr.* 1702 (1963).

446. T. R. Hurley, R. H. Bunge, N. E. Willmer, G. C. Hokanson, and J. C. French. *J. Antibiotics* **39**, 1651 (1986).

447. S. F. Hussain, A. J. Freyer, H. Guinaudeau, M. Shamma, and M. T. Siddiqui. *J. Nat. Prod.* **49**, 494 (1986).

448. T. Ichiba and T. Higa. *J. Org. Chem.* **51**, 3364 (1986).

449. T. Ichiba, R. Sakai, S. Kohmoto, G. Saucy, and T. Higa. *Tetrahedron Lett.* **29**, 3083 (1988).

450. M. Ichimura, K. Muroi, K. Asano, I. Kawamoto, F. Tomita, M. Morimoto, and H. Nakano. *J. Antibiotics* **41**, 1285 (1988).

451. K. Iguchi, S. Kaneta, K. Mori, and Y. Yamada. *Chem. Pharm. Bull.* **35**, 4375 (1987).

452. K. Iguchi, S. Kaneta, K. Mori, Y. Yamada, A. Honda, and Y. Mori. *J. Chem. Soc., Chem. Commun.* 981 (1986).

453. K. Iguchi, K. Mori, M. Suzuki, H. Takahashi, and Y. Yamada. *Chem. Lett.* 1789 (1986).

454. D. T. Imagawa, M. H. Lee, S. M. Wolinsky, K. Sano, F. Morales, S. Kwok, J. J. Sninsky, P. G. Nishanian, J. Giorgi, J. L. Fahey, J. Dudley, B. R. Visscher, and R. Detels. *N. Engl. J. Med.* **320**, 1458 (1989).

455. S. Imre, A. Öztunc, T. Çelik, and H. Wagner. *J. Nat. Prod.* **50**, 1187 (1987).

456. "Inosine Pranobex--Is a Single Positive Trial Enough?." *N. Engl. J. Med.* **322**, 1807 (1990).

457. Y. Inouye, H. Uchida, T. Kusumi, and H. Kakisawa. *J. Chem. Soc., Chem. Commun.* 346 (1987).

458. H. L. Ioachim. *Cancer Res.* (Suppl.) **50**, 5612s (1990).

459. M. Iorizzi, L. Minale, R. Riccio, M. Debray, and J. L. Menou. *J. Nat. Prod.* **49**, 67 (1986).

460. M. Iorizzi, L. Minale, R. Riccio, J.-S. Lee, and T. Yasumoto. *J. Nat. Prod.* **51**, 1098 (1988).

461. R. E. Ireland, S. Thaisrivongs, and P. H. Dussault. *J. Am. Chem. Soc.* **110**, 5768 (1988).

462. K. Irie, N. Hagiwara, A. Funaki, H. Hayashi, M. Arai, H. Tokuda, and K. Koshimizu. *Agric. Biol. Chem.* **52**, 3193 (1988).

463. H. Irschik, W. Trowitzsch-Kienast, K. Gerth, G. Höfle, and H. Reichenbach. *J. Antibiotics* **41**, 993 (1988).

464. M. Ishibashi, R. E. Moore, G. M. L. Patterson, C. Xu, and J. Clardy. *J. Org. Chem.* **51**, 5300 (1986).

465. M. Ishibashi, Y. Ohizumi, J.-F. Cheng, H. Nakamura, Y. Hirata, T. Sasaki, and J. Kobayashi. *J. Org. Chem.* **53**, 2855 (1988).

466. M. Ishibashi, Y. Ohizumi, M. Hamashima, H. Nakamura, Y. Hirata, T. Sasaki, and J. Kobayashi. *J. Chem. Soc., Chem. Commun.* 1127 (1987).

467. M. Ishibashi, Y. Ohizumi, T. Sasaki, H. Nakamura, Y. Hirata, and J. Kobayashi. *J. Org. Chem.* **52**, 450 (1987).

468. T. Ishida, M. Inoue, Y. Hamada, S. Kato, and T. Shiori. *J. Chem. Soc., Chem. Commun.* 370 (1987).

469. H. Ishii, Y.-I. Ichikawa, E. Kawanabe, M. Ishikawa, T. Ishikawa, K. Kuretani, M. Inomata, and A. Hoshi. *Chem. Pharm. Bull.* **33**, 4139 (1985).

470. H. Ishii, T. Ishikawa, Y.-I. Ichikawa, M. Sakamoto, M. Ishikawa, and T. Takahashi. *Chem. Pharm. Bull.* **32**, 2984 (1984).

471. M. O. Ishitsuka, T. Kusumi, and H. Kakisawa. *J. Org. Chem.* **53**, 5010 (1988).

472. M. Ishitsuka, T. Kusumi, H. Kakisawa, Y. Kawakami, Y. Nagai, and T. Sato. *Tetrahedron Lett.* **27**, 2639 (1986).

473. S. Ishizeki, M. Ohtsuka, K. Irinoda, K.-I. Kukita, K. Nagaoka, and T. Nakashima. *J. Antibiotics* **40**, 60 (1987).

474. M. Ishizuka, T. Masuda, S. Mizutani, M. Osono, H. Kumagai, T. Takeuchi, and H. Umezawa. *J. Antibiotics* **39**, 1736 (1986).

475. K. Isshiki, T. Sawa, K. Miura, B. Li, H. Naganawa, M. Hamada, T. Takeuchi, and H. Umezawa. *J. Antibiotics* **39**, 1013 (1986).

476. K. Isshiki, T. Tamamura, Y. Takahashi, T. Sawa, H. Naganawa, T. Takeuchi, and H. Umezawa. *J. Antibiotics* **38**, 1819 (1985).

477. Y. Itakura and T. Komori. *Liebigs Ann. Chem.* 359 (1986).

478. Y. Itakura and T. Komori. *Liebigs Ann. Chem.* 499 (1986).

479. A. Itoh, K. Iizuka, and S. Natori. *Jpn. J. Cancer Res. (Gann)* **76**, 1027 (1985).

480. H. Itokawa, H. Morita, I. Katou, K. Takeya, A. J. Cavalheiro, R. C. B. de Oliveira, M. Ishige, and M. Motidome. *Planta Med.* **54**, 311 (1988).

481. H. Itokawa, N. Totsuka, K. Nakahara, K. Takeya, J.-P. Lepoittevin, and Y. Asakawa. *Chem. Pharm. Bull.* **35**, 3016 (1987).

482. H. Itokawa, N. Totsuka, K. Takeya, K. Watanabe, and E. Obata. *Chem. Pharm. Bull.* **36**, 1585 (1988).

483. H. Itokawa, S. Tsuruoka, K. Takeya, N. Mori, T. Sonobe, S. Kosemura, and T. Hamanaka. *Chem. Pharm. Bull.* **35**, 1660 (1987).

484. H. Itokawa, J. Xu, and K. Takeya. *Chem. Pharm. Bull.* **35**, 4524 (1987).

485. H. Itokawa, J. Xu, and K. Takeya. *Chem. Pharm. Bull.* **36**, 2084 (1988).

486. H. Itokawa, J. Xu, K. Takeya, K. Watanabe, and J. Shoji. *Chem. Pharm. Bull.* **36**, 982 (1988).

487. Y. Iwai, A. Nakagawa, N. Sadakane, S. Ōmura, H. Ōiwa, S. Matsumoto, M. Takahashi, T. Ikai, and Y. Ochiai. *J. Antibiotics* **33**, 1114 (1980).

488. M. Iwami, Y. Kawai, S. Kiyoto, H. Terano, M. Kohsaka, H. Aoki, and H. Imanaka. *J. Antibiotics* **39**, 6 (1986).

489. M. Iwami, S. Kiyoto, H. Terano, M. Kohsaka, H. Aoki, and H. Imanaka. *J. Antibiotics* **40**, 589 (1987).

490. M. Iwamoto, T. Matsuo, K. Uchino, Y. Tonosaki, and A. Fukuchi. *Planta Med.* **54**, 422 (1988).

491. S. Iwasaki, H. Kobayashi, J. Furukawa, M. Namikoshi, S. Okuda, Z. Sato, I. Matsuda, and T. Noda. *J. Antibiotics* **37**, 354 (1984).

492. G. A. Jacobs, J. A. Tino, and R. Zahler. *Tetrahedron Lett.* **30**, 6955 (1989).

493. P. B. Jahrling, T. W. Geisbert, D. W. Dalgard, E. D. Johnson, T. G. Ksiazek, W. C. Hall, and C. J. Peters. *Lancet* **335**, 502 (1990).

494. S. C. Jain and M. Purohit. *Chem. Pharm. Bull.* **34**, 5154 (1986).

495. B. B. Jarvis, S. N. Cömezoglu, H. L. Ammon, C. K. Breedlove, R. W. Miller, M. K. Woode, D. R. Streelman, A. T. Sneden, R. G. Dailey, Jr., and S. M. Kupchan. *J. Nat. Prod.* **50**, 815 (1987).

496. B. B. Jarvis and C. S. Yatawara. *J. Org. Chem.* **51**, 2906 (1986).

497. C. Jiménez, E. Quiñoá, L. Castedo, and R. Riguera. *J. Nat. Prod.* **49**, 905 (1986).

498. K. Jin, Y. Shibata, and M. Morita. *Agric. Biol. Chem.* **52**, 1965 (1988).

499. S. R. Johns, J. A. Lamberton, H. Suares, and R. I. Willing. *Aust. J. Chem.* **38**, 1091 (1985).

500. G. R. N. Jones. *Human Toxicol.* **4**, 75 (1985).

501. R. R. Jones. *Lancet* **II**, 443 (1987).

502. A. Jordan, L. M. DuPlessis, and V. P. Joynt. *J. S. Afr. Chem. Inst.* **21**, 22 (1968).

503. H. Joseph, J. Gleye, C. Moulis, L. J. Mensah, C. Roussakis, and C. Gratas. *J. Nat. Prod.* **51**, 599 (1988).

504. G. C. Kabat, G. S. Dieck, and E. L. Wynder. *Cancer* **57**, 362 (1986).

505. G. C. Kabat and E. L. Wynder. *Int. J. Cancer* **43**, 190 (1989).

506. Y. Kakou, P. Crews, and G. J. Bakus. *J. Nat Prod.* **50**, 482 (1987).

507. T. Kameyama, A. Takahashi, S. Kurasawa, M. Ishizuka, Y. Okami, T. Takeuchi, and H. Umezawa. *J. Antibiotics* **40**, 1664 (1987).

508. M. Kanaoka, C. Kawanaka, T. Negoro, Y. Fukita, K. Taya, and H. Agui. *Agric. Biol. Chem.* **51**, 2641 (1987).

509. H. Kanayama, N. Adachi, Y. Fukai, I. Takeuchi, and M. Togami. *Yakugaku Zasshi* **106**, 199 (1986).

510. H. Kanayama, N. Adachi, Y. Fukai, I. Takeuchi, and M. Togami. *Yakugaku Zasshi* **106**, 206 (1986).

511. H. Kanayama, M. Togami, N. Adachi, Y. Fukai, and T. Okumoto. *Yakugaku Zasshi* **106**, 307 (1986).

512. P. Karuso, P. R. Bergquist, J. S. Buckleton, R. C. Cambie, G. R. Clark, and C. E. F. Rickard. *Tetrahedron Lett.* **27**, 2177 (1986).

513. P. Karuso, P. R. Bergquist, R. C. Cambie, J. S. Buckleton, G. R. Clark, and C. E. F. Rickard. *Aust. J. Chem.* **39**, 1643 (1986).

514. P. Karuso and P. J. Scheuer. *Tetrahedron Lett.* **28**, 4633 (1987).

515. P. Karuso, B. W. Skelton, W. C. Taylor, and A. H. White. *Aust. J. Chem.* **37**, 1081 (1984).

516. P. Karuso and W. C. Taylor. *Aust. J. Chem.* **39**, 1629 (1986).

517. H. Kasai, Z. Yamaizumi, S. Nishimura, K. Wakabayashi, M. Nagao, T. Sugimura, N. E. Spingarn, J. H. Weisburger, S. Yokoyama, and T. Miyazawa. *J. Chem. Soc., Perkin Trans 1* 2290 (1981).

518. H. Kasai, Z. Yamaizumi, K. Wakabayashi, M. Nagao, T. Sugimura, S. Yokoyama, T. Miyazawa, and S. Nishimura. *Chem. Lett.* 1391 (1980).

519. R. Kasai, M. Miyakoshi, K. Matsumoto, R.-L. Nie, J. Zhou, T. Morita, and O. Tanaka. *Chem. Pharm. Bull.* **34**, 3974 (1986).

520. Y. Kashman, A. Groweiss, and U. Shmueli. *Tetrahedron Lett.* **21**, 3629 (1980).

521. Y. Kashman, S. Hirsch, F. Koehn, and S. Cross. *Tetrahedron Lett.* **28**, 5461 (1987).

522. T. Kato, M. Aoki, and T. Uyehara. *J. Org. Chem.* **52**, 1803 (1987).

523. Y. Kato, N. Fusetani, S. Matsunaga, and K. Hashimoto. *Tetrahedron Lett.* **26**, 3483 (1985).

524. Y. Kato, N. Fusetani, S. Matsunaga, and K. Hashimoto. *Experientia* **42**, 1299 (1986).

525. Y. Kato, N. Fusetani, S. Matsunaga, K. Hashimoto, S. Fujita, and T. Furuya. *J. Am. Chem. Soc.* **108**, 2780 (1986).

526. Y. Kato, N. Fusetani, S. Matsunaga, K. Hashimoto, S. Fujita, T. Furuya, and K. Koseki. 28th Symposium on The Chemistry of Natural Products, Symposium Papers, Sendai, 1986, p. 175.

527. Y. Kato, N. Fusetani, S. Matsunaga, K. Hashimoto, and K. Koseki. *J. Org. Chem.* **53**, 3930 (1988).

528. Y. Kato, N. Fusetani, S. Matsunaga, K. Hashimoto, R. Sakai, T. Higa, and Y. Kashman. 29th Symposium on The Chemistry of Natural Products, Symposium Papers, Sapporo, 1987, p. 308.

529. Y. Kato, N. Fusetani, S. Matsunaga, K. Hashimoto, R. Sakai, T. Higa, and Y. Kashman. *Tetrahedron Lett.* **28**, 6225 (1987).

530. H. Kawai, Y. Hayakawa, M. Nakagawa, K. Furihata, K. Furihata, A. Shimazu, H. Seto, and N. Ōtake. *J. Antibiotics* **40**, 1266 (1987).

531. H. Kawai, Y. Hayakawa, M. Nakagawa, K. Furihata, H. Seto, and N. Ōtake. *J. Antibiotics* **40**, 1273 (1987).

532. M. Kawai, R. S. Pottorf, and D. H. Rich. *J. Med. Chem.* **29**, 2409 (1986).

533. Y. Kawai, K. Furihata, H. Seto, and N. Otake. *Tetrahedron Lett.* **26**, 3273 (1985).

534. Y. Kawano, R. Higuchi, R. Isobe, and T. Komori. *Liebigs Ann. Chem.* 19 (1988).

535. R. Kazlauskas, P. T. Murphy, R. J. Quinn, and R. J. Wells. *Tetrahedron Lett.* 37 (1977).

536. R. Kazlauskas, P. T. Murphy, R. G. Warren, R. J. Wells, and J. F. Blount. *Aust. J. Chem.* **31**, 2685 (1978).

537. R. Kazlauskas, P. T. Murphy, R. J. Wells, and J. F. Blount. *Tetrahedron Lett.* **21**, 315 (1980).

538. P. A. Keifer, K. L. Rinehart, Jr., and I. R. Hooper. *J. Org. Chem.* **51**, 4450 (1986).

539. P. Keil, E. G. Nielsen, U. Anthoni, and C. Christophersen. *Acta Chem. Scand.* **B40**, 555 (1986).

540. C. Keller-Juslén, M. Kuhn, A. von Wartburg, and H. Stähelin. *J. Med. Chem.* **14**, 936 (1971).

541. T. R. Kelly, S. H. Bell. N. Ohashi, and R. J. Armstrong-Chong. *J. Am. Chem. Soc.* **110**, 6471 (1988).

542. T. R. Kelly, N. Ohashi, R. J. Armstrong-Chong, and S. H. Bell. *J. Am. Chem. Soc.* **108**, 7100 (1986).

543. A. S. Kende and C. A. Smith. *Tetrahedron Lett.* **29**, 4217 (1988).

544. R. S. Kerbel and A. J. S. Davies. *Lancet* **II**, 977 (1982).

545. D. L. Kern, J. P. Schaumberg, G. C. Hokanson, and J. C. French. *J. Antibiotics* **39**, 469 (1986).

546. M. R. Kernan and D. J. Faulkner. *J. Org. Chem.* **53**, 4574 (1988).

547. M. R. Kernan, D. J. Faulkner, and R. S. Jacobs. *J. Org. Chem.* **52**, 3081 (1987).

548. M. R. Kernan, T. F. Molinski, and D. J. Faulkner. *J. Org. Chem.* **53**, 5014 (1988).

549. R. F. Khabbaz, W. W. Darrow, T. M. Hartley, J. Witte, J. B. Cohen, J. French, P. S. Gill, J. Potterat, R. K. Sikes, R. Reich, J. E. Kaplan, and M. D. Lairmore. *J. Am. Med. Assoc.* **263**, 60 (1990).

550. M. P. Khare, S. S. Bhatnagar, O. Schindler, and T. Reichstein. *Helv. Chim. Acta* **45**, 1515 (1962).

551. A. A. Kicha, A. I. Kalinovskii, P. V. Andrischenko, and E. V. Lenina. *Khim. Prir. Soedin.* 592 (1986).

552. A. A. Kicha, A. I. Kalinovskii, É. V. Levina, and P. V. Andriyashchenko. *Chem. Nat. Compd.* **21**, 760 (1985).

553. A. A. Kicha, A. I. Kalinovskii, É. V. Levina, Ya. B. Rashkes, V. A. Stonik, and G. B. Elyakov. *Chem. Nat. Compd.* **21**, 332 (1985).

554. H. Kigoshi, Y. Imamura, H. Niwa, and K. Yamada. *J. Am. Chem. Soc.* **111**, 2302 (1989).

555. H. Kigoshi, M. Ojika, Y. Shizuri, H. Niwa, and K. Yamada. *Tetrahedron Lett.* **23**, 5413 (1982).

556. H. Kigoshi, M. Ojika, Y. Shizuri, H. Niwa, and K. Yamada. *Tetrahedron* **42**, 3789 (1986).

557. E. D. Kilbourne. *J. Am. Med. Assoc.* **264**, 68 (1990).

558. Y. Kimura, T. Matsumoto, M. Suzuki, and S. Terashima. *J. Antibiotics* **38**, 1277 (1985).

559. M. M. King, P. B. McCay, and S. D. Kosanke. *Cancer Lett.* **14**, 219 (1981).

560. L. A. Kingsley, C. R. Rinaldo, D. W. Lyter, R. O. Valdiserri, S. H. Belle, and M. Ho. *J. Am. Med. Assoc.* **264**, 230 (1990).

561. K. F. Kinzer and J. H. Cardellina II. *Tetrahedron Lett.* **28**, 925 (1987).

562. I. Kitagawa, Z. Cui, Y. Cai, M. Kobayashi, and Y. Kyogoku. *Chem. Pharm. Bull.* **34**, 4641 (1986).

563. I. Kitagawa, Z. Cui, B. W. Son, M. Kobayashi, and Y. Kyogoku. *Chem. Pharm. Bull.* **35**, 124 (1987).

564. I. Kitagawa, M. Kobayashi, Z. Cui, Y. Kiyota, and M. Ohnishi. *Chem. Pharm. Bull.* **34**, 4590 (1986).

565. I. Kitagawa, M. Kobayashi, N. K. Lee, H. Shibuya, C. Kamba, and M. Yoshikawa. 28th Symposium on The Chemistry of Natural Products, Symposium Papers, Sendai, 1986, p. 151.

566. I. Kitagawa, M. Kobayashi, N. K. Lee, H. Shibuya, Y. Kawata, and F. Sakiyama. *Chem. Pharm. Bull.* **34**, 2664 (1986).

567. I. Kitagawa, M. Kobayashi, Y. Okamoto, M. Yoshikawa, and Y. Hamamoto. 29th Symposium on The Chemistry of Natural Products Symposium Papers, Sapporo, 1987, p. 575.

568. I. Kitagawa, M. Kobayashi, Y. Okamoto, M. Yoshikawa, and Y. Hamamoto. *Chem. Pharm. Bull.* **35**, 5036 (1987).

569. I. Kitagawa, N. Yoshioka, C. Kamba, M. Yoshikawa, and Y. Hamamoto. *Chem. Pharm. Bull.* **35**, 928 (1987).

570. S. Kiyoto, Y. Kawai, T. Kawakita, E. Kino, M. Okuhara, I. Uchida, H. Tanaka, M. Hashimoto, H. Terano, M. Kohsaka, H. Aoki, and H. Imanaka. *J. Antibiotics* **39**, 762 (1986).

571. S. Kiyoto, T. Shibata, M. Yamashita, T. Komori, M. Okuhara, H. Terano, M. Kohsaka, H. Aoki, and H. Imanaka. *J. Antibiotics* **40**, 594 (1987).

572. R. A. Kleinerman, R. E. Curtis, J. D. Boice, Jr., J. T. Flannery, and J. F. Fraumeni, Jr. *J. Natl. Cancer Inst.* **69**, 1027 (1982).

573. H. Kloos. *Soc. Sci. Med.* **30**, 643 (1990).

574. H. Kobayashi, S. Iwasaki, E. Yamada, and S. Okuda. *J. Chem. Soc., Chem. Commun.* 1702 (1986).

575. J. Kobayashi, J.-F. Cheng, M. Ishibashi, H. Nakamura, Y. Ohizumi, Y. Hirata, T. Sasaki, H. Lu, and J. Clardy. *Tetrahedron Lett.* **28**, 4939 (1987).

576. J. Kobayashi, J.-F. Cheng, H. Nakamura, Y. Ohizumi, Y. Hirata, T. Sasaki, T. Ohta, and S. Nozoe. *Tetrahedron Lett.* **29**, 1177 (1988).

577. J. Kobayashi, J.-F. Cheng, T. Ohta, H. Nakamura, S. Nozoe, Y. Hirata, Y. Ohizumi, and T. Sasaki. *J. Org. Chem.* **53**, 6147 (1988).

578. J. Kobayashi, J.-F. Cheng, M. R. Wälchli, H. Nakamura, Y. Hirata, T. Sasaki, and Y. Ohizumi. *J. Org. Chem.* **53**, 1800 (1988).

579. J. Kobayashi, M. Ishibashi, H. Nakamura, Y. Ohizumi, Y. Hirata, M. R. Wälchli, and T. Sasaki. 29th Symposium on The Chemistry of Natural Products, Symposium Papers, Sapporo, 1987, p. 324.

580. J. Kobayashi, M. Ishibashi, H. Nakamura, Y. Ohizumi, T. Yamasu, T. Sasaki, and Y. Hirata. *Tetrahedron Lett.* **27**, 5755 (1986).

581. J. Kobayashi, M. Ishibashi, M. R. Wälchli, H. Nakamura, Y. Hirata, T. Sasaki, and Y. Ohizumi. *J. Am. Chem. Soc.* **110**, 490 (1988).

582. J. Kobayashi, H. Nakamura, and Y. Ohizumi. *Toxicon* **23**, 783 (1985).

583. J. Kobayashi, H. Nakamura, Y. Ohizumi, and Y. Hirata. *Tetrahedron Lett.* **27**, 1191 (1986).

584. J. Kobayashi, Y. Ohizumi, H. Nakamura, and Y. Hirata. *Tetrahedron Lett.* **27**, 2113 (1986).

585. K. Kobayashi, C. Nishino, J. Ohya, S. Sato, T. Mikawa, Y. Shiobara, and M. Kodama. *J. Antibiotics* **41**, 502 (1988).

586. K. Kobayashi, C. Nishino, J. Ohya, S. Sato, T. Mikawa, Y. Shiobara, and M. Kodama. *J. Antibiotics* **41**, 741 (1988).

587. K. Kobayashi, C. Nishino, J. Ohya, S. Sato, T. Mikawa, Y. Shiobara, M. Kodama, and N. Nishimoto. *J. Antibiotics* **40**, 1053 (1987).

588. M. Kobayashi. *Chem. Pharm. Bull.* **36**, 488 (1988).

589. M. Kobayashi, T. Ishizaka, N. Miura, and H. Mitsuhashi. *Chem. Pharm. Bull.* **35**, 2314 (1987).

590. M. Kobayashi, B. W. Son, Y. Kyogoku, and I. Kitagawa. *Chem. Pharm. Bull.* **34**, 2306 (1986).

591. M. Kodama, Y. Shiobara, H. Sumitomo, K. Matsumura, M. Tsukamoto, and C. Harada. *J. Org. Chem.* **53**, 72 (1988).

592. S. Kohmoto, Y. Kashman, O. J. McConnell, K. L. Rinehart, Jr., A. Wright, and F. Koehn. *J. Org. Chem.* **53**, 3116 (1988).

593. S. Kohmoto, O. J. McConnell, and A. Wright. *Experientia* **44**, 85 (1988).

594. H. I. Kohn and R. J. M. Fry. *N. Engl. J. Med.* **310**, 504 (1984).

595. Y. Koide, F. Ishii, K. Hasuda, Y. Koyama, K. Edo, S. Katamine, F. Kitame, and N. Ishida. *J. Antibiotics* **33**, 342 (1980).

596. T. Kojima, K. Tabata, W. Itoh, and T. Yanaki. *Agric. Biol. Chem.* **50**, 231 (1986).

597. L. N. Kolonel, T. Hirohata, B. V. Chappell, F. V. Viola, and D. E. Harris. *J. Natl. Cancer Inst.* **64**, 739 (1980).

598. N. Komeshima, T. Tsuruo, and H. Umezawa. *J. Antibiotics* **41**, 548 (1988).

599. K. Komiyama, K. Okada, Y. Hirokawa, K. Masuda, S. Tomisaka, and I. Umezawa. *J. Antibiotics* **38**, 224 (1985).

600. K. Komiyama, K. Okada, H. Oka, S. Tomisaka, T. Miyano, S. Funayama, and I. Umezawa. *J. Antibiotics* **38**, 220 (1985).

601. M.-L. Kondracki and M. Guyot. *Tetrahedron Lett.* **28**, 5815 (1987).

602. M. Konishi, K. Sugawara, F. Kofu, Y. Nishiyama, K. Tomita, T. Miyaki, and H. Kawaguchi. *J. Antibiotics* **39**, 784 (1986).

603. F.-H. Kong, D.-Y. Zhu, R.-S. Xu, Z.-C. Fu, L.-Y. Zhou, T. Iwashita, and H. Komura. *Tetrahedron Lett.* **27**, 5765 (1986).

604. T. Konoshima and K.-H. Lee. *J. Nat. Prod.* **49**, 650 (1986).

605. T. Konoshima and K.-H. Lee. *J. Nat. Prod.* **49**, 1117 (1986).

606. T. Konoshima, T. Matsuda, M. Takasaki, J. Yamahara, M. Kozuka, T. Sawada, and T. Shingu. *J. Nat. Prod.* **48**, 683 (1985).

607. T. Konoshima, E. Okamoto, M. Kozuka, H. Nishino, H. Tokuda, and M. Tanabe. *J. Nat. Prod.* **51**, 1266 (1988).

608. T. Konoshima, M. Takasaki, M. Kozuka, and H. Tokuda. *J. Nat. Prod.* **50**, 1167 (1987).

609. T. Kosuge, K. Tsuji, K. Wakabayashi, T. Okamoto, K. Shudo, Y. Iitaka, A. Itai, T. Sugimura, T. Kawachi, M. Nagao, T. Yahagi, and Y. Seino. *Chem. Pharm. Bull.* **26**, 611 (1978).

610. W. Krick, F.-J. Marner, and L. Jaenicke. *Z. Naturforsch.* **38c**, 179 (1983).

611. C. A. Krone, S. M. J. Yeh, and W. T. Iwaoka. *Environ. Health Perspectives* **67**, 75 (1986).

612. F. H. Kruszewski, C. J. Conti, and J. DiGiovanni. *Cancer Res.* **47**, 3783 (1987).

613. M. B. Ksebati and F. J. Schmitz. *J. Org. Chem.* **50**, 5637 (1985).

614. M. B. Ksebati and F. J. Schmitz. *Bull. Soc. Chim. Belg.* **95**, 835 (1986).

615. M. B. Ksebati and F. J. Schmitz. *J. Org. Chem.* **52**, 3766 (1987).

616. M. B. Ksebati and F. J. Schmitz. *J. Nat. Prod.* **51**, 857 (1988).

617. M. B. Ksebati and F. J. Schmitz. *J. Org. Chem.* **53**, 3926 (1988).

618. M. B. Ksebati, F. J. Schmitz, and S. P. Gunasekera. *J. Org. Chem.* **53**, 3917 (1988).

619. I. Kubo, T. Kamikawa, T. Isobe, and T. Kubota. *Bull. Chem. Soc. Jpn.* **47**, 1277 (1974).

620. M. Kumagai, M. Murata, J. S. Lee, and T. Yasumoto. 29th Symposium on The Chemistry of Natural Products, Symposium Papers, Sapporo, 1987, p. 607.

621. A. Kungsuwan, T. Noguchi, S. Matsunaga, M. F. Watanabe, S. Watabe, and K. Hashimoto. *Toxicon* **26**, 119 (1988).

622. E. Kunz, J. Ševc, and V. Plaček. *Health Physics* **35**, 579 (1978).

623. I. Kurane, A. Meager, and F. A. Ennis. *J. Exp. Med.* **170**, 763 (1989).

624. K. Kurata and T. Amiya. *Bull. Chem. Soc. Jpn.* **53**, 2020 (1980).

625. M. Kuratsune, M. Ikeda, and T. Hayashi. *Environ. Health Perspectives* **67**, 143 (1986).

626. T. Kusumi, D. Muanza-Nkongolo, M. Goya, M. Ishitsuka, T. Iwashita, and H. Kakisawa. *J. Org. Chem.* **51**, 384 (1986).

627. T. Kusumi, D. Muanza-Nkongolo, M. Ishitsuka, Y. Inouye, and H. Kakisawa. *Chem. Lett.* 1241 (1986).

628. T. Kusumi, T. Ooi, M. M. Watanabe, H. Takahashi, and H. Kakisawa. *Tetrahedron Lett.* **28**, 4695 (1987).

629. T. Kusumi, H. Uchida, Y. Inouye, M. Ishitsuka, H. Yamamoto, and H. Kakisawa. *J. Org. Chem.* **52**, 4597 (1987).

630. R. Kuttan, P. Bhanumathy, K. Nirmala, and M. C. George. *Cancer Lett.* **29**, 197 (1985).

631. R. J. Lake, M. M. Brennan, J. W. Blunt, M. H. G. Munro, and L. K. Pannel. *Tetrahedron Lett.* **29**, 2255 (1988).

632. J. S. Lambert, M. Seidlin, R. C. Reichman, C. S. Plank, M. Laverty, G. D. Morse, C. Knupp, C. McLaren, C. Pettinelli, F. T. Valentine, and R. Dolin. *N. Engl. J. Med.* **322**, 1333 (1990).

633. P. Langlotz, W. Wagner, and H. Follmann. *Z. Naturforsch.* **41C**, 979 (1986).

634. J. Langone. *Discover* **11**, 62 (1990).

635. B. A. Larder and S. D. Kemp. *Science* **246**, 1155 (1989).

636. C. La Vecchia, A. Decarli, S. Franceschi, S. Pampallona, and G. Tognoni. *J. Natl. Cancer Inst.* **75**, 61 (1985).

637. P. D. Lawley. "Carcinogenesis by Alkylating Agents" **In** Chemical Carcinogens, Second Edition, Revised and Expanded, Vol. 1, Chap. 7, C. E. Searle, Ed, Am. Chem. Soc., Washington, D.C., 1984, p. 325.

638. M. V. Laycock, J. L. C. Wright, J. A. Findlay, and A. D. Patil. *Can. J. Chem.* **64**, 1312 (1986).

639. F. J. Leary, L. J. Resseguie, L. T. Kurland, P. C. O'Brien, R. F. Emslander, and K. L. Noller. *J. Am. Med. Assoc.* **252**, 2984 (1984).

640. J. Leclercq, M.-C. De Pauw-Gillet, R. Bassleer, and L. Angenot. *J. Ethnopharmacol.* **15**, 305 (1986).

641. J. Lederberg. *J. Am. Med. Assoc.* **260**, 684 (1988).

642. J. A. H. Lee. *Photochem. Photobiol.* **50**, 493 (1989).

643. K.-H. Lee, T. Ibuka, D. Sims, O. Muraoka, H. Kiyokawa, I. H. Hall, and H. L. Kim. *J. Med. Chem.* **24**, 924 (1981).

644. K.-H. Lee, Y.-M. Lin, T.-S. Wu, D.-C. Zhang, T. Yamagishi, T. Hayashi, I. H. Hall, J.-J. Chang, R.-Y. Wu, and T.-H. Yang. *Planta Med.* **54**, 308 (1988).

645. K.-H. Lee, G. K. Rice, I. H. Hall, and V. Amarnath. *J. Med. Chem.* **30**, 586 (1987).

646. M. D. Lee and D. B. Borders. "LL-D05139β, A New Antitumor Antibiotic: Isolation and Structure Determination," Program and Abstracts of the 24th Intersci. Conf. on Antimicrob. Agents Chemother., No. 1144, Washington, D.C., 1984, p. 293.

647. M. D. Lee, T. S. Dunne, C. C. Chang, G. A. Ellestad, M. M. Siegel, G. O. Morton, W. J. McGahren, and D. B. Borders. *J. Am. Chem. Soc.* **109**, 3466 (1987).

648. M. D. Lee, T. S. Dunne, M. M. Siegel, C. C. Chang, G. O. Morton, and D. B. Borders. *J. Am. Chem. Soc.* **109**, 3464 (1987).

649. M. D. Lee, A. A. Fantini, N. A. Kuck, M. Greenstein, R. T. Testa, and D. B. Borders. *J. Antibiotics* **40**, 1657 (1987).

650. H. Lelong, A. Ahond, A. Chiaroni, C. Poupat, C. Riche, P. Potier, J. Pusset, M. Pusset, P. Laboute, and J. L. Menou. *J. Nat. Prod.* **50**, 203 (1987).

651. G. F. Lemp, S. F. Payne, D. Neal, T. Temelso, and G. W. Rutherford. *J. Am. Med. Assoc.* **263**, 402 (1990).

652. D. Lester. *Cancer Res.* **39**, 2891 (1979).

653. M.-H. Li, S.-H. Lu, C. Ji, M.-Y. Wang, S.-J. Cheng, and C.-L. Jin. *Sci. Sinica* **22**, 471 (1979).

654. J.-Y. Liang, Z.-D. Min, M. Iinuma, T. Tanaka, and M. Mizuno. *Chem. Pharm. Bull.* **35**, 2613 (1987).

655. G. Lidgren, L. Bohlin, and J. Bergman. *Tetrahedron Lett.* **27**, 3283 (1986).

656. W. Lijinsky. *Cancer Res.* **39**, 2887 (1979).

657. W. Lijinsky, M. D. Reiber, and B. N. Blackwell. *Science* **209**, 817 (1980).

658. J.-Y. Lin and S.-Y. Liu. *Toxicon* **24**, 757 (1986).

659. L. T. Lin, C. C. Sung, and J. S. Hsu. *K'o Hsueh T'ung Pao (Chin. Ed.)* **24**, 478 (1979).

660. L.-Z. Lin, G. Blaskó, and G. A. Cordell. *J. Nat. Prod.* **51**, 1161 (1988).

661. N. Lindquist, W. Fenical, D. F. Sesin, C. M. Ireland, G. D. Van Duyne, C. J. Forsyth, and J. Clardy. *J. Am. Chem. Soc.* **110**, 1308 (1988).

662. N. Lindquist, W. Fenical, G. D. Van Duyne, and J. Clardy. *J. Org. Chem.* **53**, 4570 (1988).

663. G. S. Linz, R. Sanduja, A. J. Weinheimer, M. Alam, and G. E. Martin. *Tetrahedron Lett.* **27**, 4833 (1986).

664. M. B. Lipsett. *J. Am. Med. Assoc.* **237**, 1112 (1977).

665. M. B. Lipsett. *Cancer* **51**, 2426 (1983).

666. M. Litaudon and M. Guyot. *Tetrahedron Lett.* **27**, 4455 (1986).

667. C. Litchfield and S. Liaaen-Jensen. *Comp. Biochem. Physiol.* **66B**, 359 (1980).

668. J.-S. Liu, M.-F. Huang, and Y. Tao. *Can. J. Chem.* **66**, 414 (1988).

669. S. A. Look, M. T. Burch, W. Fenical, Q.-T. Zheng, and J. Clardy. *J. Org. Chem.* **50**, 5741 (1985).

670. S. A. Look and W. Fenical. *Tetrahedron* **43**, 3363 (1987).

671. S. A. Look, W. Fenical, R. S. Jacobs, and J. Clardy. *Proc. Natl. Acad. Sci. USA* **83**, 6238 (1986).

672. S. A. Look, W. Fenical, G. K. Matsumoto, and J. Clardy. *J. Org. Chem.* **51**, 5140 (1986).

673. A. Lopez and W. H. Gerwick. *Tetrahedron Lett.* **29**, 1505 (1988).

674. J. F. Loutit and E. L. Lloyd. *Nature* **266**, 355 (1977).

675. "Low Level Radioactive Waste." **In Brief** A Triannual Newsletter on Environmental Law, Sierra Club, March 1984, p. 1.

676. A. B. Lowenfels and M. E. Anderson. *Cancer* **39**, 1809 (1977).

677. A. B. Lowenfels, C. G. Lindström, M. J. Conway, and P. R. Hastings. *J. Natl. Cancer Inst.* **75**, 77 (1985).

678. S.-H. Lu, A.-M. Camus, L. Tomatis, and H. Bartsch. *J. Natl. Cancer Inst.* **66**, 33 (1981).

679. L. Lumonadio and M. Vanhaelen. *Phytochemistry* **23**, 453 (1984).

680. Z. Luo, D. Meksuriyen, C. A. J. Erdelmeier, H. H. S. Fong, and G. A. Cordell. *J. Org. Chem.* **53**, 2183 (1988).

681. S. F. Lyons and B. D. Schoub. *So. Afr. J. Sci.* **82**, 403 (1986).

682. N. E. MacDonald, G. A. Wells, W. A. Fisher, W. K. Warren, M. A. King, J.-A. A. Doherty, and W. R. Bowie. *J. Am. Med. Assoc.* **263**, 3155 (1990).

683. W. B. G. Macdonald, A. R. Tink, R. A. Ouvrier, M. A. Menser, L. M. de Silva, H. Naim, and R. A. Hawkes. *Med. J. Aust.* **150**, 334 (1989).

684. P. Maček and D. Lebez. *Toxicon* **26**, 441 (1988).

685. W. D. MacRae, J. B. Hudson, and G. H. N. Towers. *Planta Med.* **55**, 531 (1989).

686. W. D. MacRae and G. H. N. Towers. *Phytochemistry* **23**, 1207 (1984).

687. M. Maeda, T. Kodama, T. Tanaka, H. Yoshizumi, T. Takemoto, K. Nomoto, and T. Fujita. *Chem. Pharm. Bull.* **34**, 4892 (1986).

688. M. Maeda, T. Kodama, T. Tanaka, H. Yoshizumi, T. Takemoto, K. Nomoto, and T. Fujita. *Tetrahedron Lett.* **28**, 633 (1987).

689. K. Magnus. *Int. J. Cancer* **20**, 477 (1977).

690. P. Magnus and P. A. Carter. *J. Am. Chem. Soc.* **110**, 1626 (1988).

691. N. F. Magri and D. G. I. Kingston. *J. Nat. Prod.* **51**, 298 (1988).

692. J. C. Maize. *J. Am. Med. Assoc.* **237**, 1857 (1977).

693. A. K. Mallams, E. S. Waight, B. C. L. Weedon, D. J. Chapman, F. T. Haxo, T. W. Goodwin, and D. M. Thomas. *J. Chem. Soc., Chem. Commun.* 301 (1967).

694. S. W. Mamber, J. D. Mitulski, K. L. Hamelehle, J. C. French, G. C. Hokanson, J. L. Shillis, W. R. Leopold D. D. Von Hoff, and J. B. Tunac. *J. Antibiotics* **40**, 73 (1987).

695. I. Mancini, G. Guella, A. Guerriero, A. Boldrin, and F. Pietra. *Helv. Chim. Acta* **70**, 2011 (1987).

696. D. C. Manker and D. J. Faulkner. *Tetrahedron* **43**, 3677 (1987).

697. D. C. Manker, D. J. Faulkner, C.-F. Xe, and J. Clardy. *J. Org. Chem.* **51**, 814 (1986).

698. R. Marcus, K. Kay, and J. M. Mann. *Bull. World Health Org.* **67**, 577 (1989).

699. M. Markman, M. D. Pavy, and M. D. Abeloff. *Cancer* **50**, 672 (1982).

700. R. Marks, D. Jolley, S. Lectsas, and P. Foley. *Med. J. Aust.* **152**, 62 (1990).

701. A. C. Marriott, V. K. Ward, and P. A. Nuttall. *Virology* **169**, 341 (1989).

702. J. A. Marshall and B. S. DeHoff. *Tetrahedron* **43**, 4849 (1987).

703. J. A. Marshall, E. D. Robinson, and R. D. Adams. *Tetrahedron Lett.* **29**, 4913 (1988).

704. G. E. Martin, R. Sanduja, and M. Alam. *J. Nat. Prod.* **49**, 406 (1986).

705. J. L. Marx. *Science* **244**, 287 (1989).

706. K. Masuda, S. Funayama, K. Komiyama, I. Umezawa, and K. Ito. *J. Nat. Prod.* **50**, 958 (1987).

707. K. Masuda, T. Nakamura, T. Mizota, J. Mori, and K. Shimomura. *Cancer Res.* **48**, 5172 (1988).

708. N. Masuda, M. Fukuoka, K. Matsui, S. Negoro, M. Takada, N. Sakai, S. Ryu, N. Takifuji, K. Ito, S. Kudoh, and Y. Kusunoki. *Cancer* **65**, 2635 (1990).

709. J. H. Mathews and J. T. Roehrig. *J. Gen. Virol.* **70**, 2877 (1989).

710. C. C. Mathiot, D. Fontenille, A. J. Georges, and P. Coulanges. *Trans. R. Soc. Trop. Med. Hyg.* **83**, 407 (1989).

711. S. Matsueda, K. Shinpo, K. Abe, H. Karasawa, and Y. Katsukura. *Yakugaku Zasshi* **107**, 694 (1987).

712. S. Matsunaga, N. Fusetani, and K. Hashimoto. *Experientia* **42**, 84 (1986).

713. S. Matsunaga, N. Fusetani, K. Hashimoto, K. Koseki, and M. Noma. *J. Am. Chem. Soc.* **108**, 847 (1986).

714. S. Matsunaga, N. Fusetani, and S. Konosu. *Tetrahederon Lett.* **25**, 5165 (1984).

715. S. Matsunaga, N. Fusetani, and S. Konosu. *J. Nat. Prod.* **48**, 236 (1985).

716. S. Matsunaga, N. Fusetani, and S. Konosu. *Tetrahedron Lett.* **26**, 855 (1985).

717. L. Mayol, V. Piccialli, and D. Sica. *J. Nat. Prod.* **49**, 823 (1986).

718. L. Mayol, V. Piccialli, and D. Sica. *Tetrahedron* **42**, 5369 (1986).

719. M. O. McClure and T. F. Schulz. *Br. Med. J.* **298**, 1267 (1989).

720. J. D. McCombs, J. W. Blunt, M. V. Chambers, M. H. G. Munro, and W. T. Robinson. *Tetrahedron* 44, 1489 (1988).

721. G. D. McCoy and E. L. Wynder. *Cancer Res.* **39**, 2844 (1979).

722. C. McCrady, F. Lei, G. Pettit, and S. Grant. "Modulation of the Response of Highly Purified Human Hematopoietic Progenitor Cells (MY-10$^+$) to Hematopoietic Growth Factors by Bryostatin 1," The Intl. Soc. of Hematol. 23rd Congress, The Amer. Soc. of Hematol. 32nd Annual Meeting, Boston, MA, December 1990.

723. T. C. McKee and C. M. Ireland. *J. Nat. Prod.* **50**, 754 (1987).

724. A. J. McMichael, M. G. McCall, J. M. Hartshorne, and T. L. Woodings. *Int. J. Cancer* **25**, 431 (1980).

725. D. Mebs, I. Weiler, and H. F. Heinke. *Toxicon* **23**, 955 (1985).

726. B. Meier and C. Trost. *Wall Street Journal*, Feb. 14, 1985, p. 4.

727. L. Meijer, J. Maclouf, and R. W. Bryant. *Prostaglandins, Leukotrienes Med.* **23**, 179 (1986).

728. I. Messana, M. Sperandei, G. Multari, C. Galeffi, and G. B. Marini Bettolo. *Phytochemistry* **23**, 2617 (1984).

729. C. Mettlin. *Int. J. Cancer* **43**, 608 (1989).

730. P. Metzger and E. Casadevall. *Tetrahedron Lett.* **28**, 3931 (1987).

731. P. Metzger and E. Casadevall. *Tetrahedron Lett.* **29**, 2831 (1988).

732. Ts. S. Milkova, S. S. Popov, and St. N. Andreev. *Comp. Biochem. Physiol.* **87B**, 267 (1987).

733. B. R. Miller, T. P. Monath, W. J. Tabachnick, and V. I. Ezike. *Trop. Med. Parasitol.* **40**, 396 (1989).

734. J. Mills and H. Masur. *Scient. Amer.* 50 (1990).

735. H. Mimura, N. Ohno, I. Suzuki, and T. Yadomae. *Chem. Pharm. Bull.* **33**, 5096 (1985).

736. T. Mimura, S. Itoh, K. Tsujikawa, H. Nakajima, M. Satake, Y. Kohama, and M. Okabe. *Chem. Pharm. Bull.* **35**, 1144 (1987).

737. T. Mimura, K. Maeda, H. Hariyama, S. Aonuma, M. Satake, and T. Fujita. *Chem. Pharm. Bull.* 30, 1381 (1982).

738. T. Mimura, K. Maeda, Y. Oda, T. Terada, K. Yoshida, and S. Aonuma. *Chem. Pharm. Bull.* 33, 2061 (1985).

739. T. Mimura, K. Maeda, T. Terada, Y. Oda, K. Morishita, and S. Aonuma. *Chem. Pharm. Bull.* 33, 2052 (1985).

740. L. Minale, C. Pizza, A. Plomitallo, R. Riccio, F. Zollo, and F. A. Mellon. *Gazz. Chim. Ital.* **114**, 151 (1984).

741. L. Minale, C. Pizza, R. Riccio, and F. Zollo. *Experientia* **39**, 567 (1983).

742. J. P. Minton, H. Abou-issa, M. K. Foecking, and M. G. Sriram. *Cancer* **51**, 1249 (1983).

743. M. J. Mintzis, A. P. Berger, E. Greenwald, E. Greenwald, and F. Golomb. *Cancer* **42**, 804 (1978).

744. B. Mishu, W. Schaffner, J. M. Horan, L. H. Wood, R. H. Hutcheson, and P. C. McNabb. *J. Am. Med. Assoc.* **264**, 467 (1990).

745. R. Misra, R. C. Pandey, B. D. Hilton, P. P. Roller, and J. V. Silverton. *J. Antibiotics* **40**, 786 (1987).

746. D. Mitchell and L. S. Liebeskind. *J. Am. Chem. Soc.* **112**, 291 (1990).

747. H. Mitsuya, R. Yarchoan, and S. Broder. *Science* **249**, 1533 (1990).

748. T. Miyamoto, R. Higuchi, T. Komori, T. Fujioka, and K. Mihashi. *Tetrahedron Lett.* **27**, 1153 (1986).

749. K. Miyazawa, M. Higashiyama, K. Ito, T. Noguchi, O. Arakawa, Y. Shida, and K. Hashimoto. *Toxicon* **26**, 867 (1988).

750. J. Moan, A. Dahlback, T. Henriksen, and K. Magnus. *Cancer Res.* **49**, 5207 (1989).

751. J. Mokrý, I. Kompiš, L. Dúbravková, and P. Šefčovič. *Tetrahedron Lett.* 1185 (1962).

752. T. F. Molinski, E. Fahy, D. J. Faulkner, G. D. Van Duyne, and J. Clardy. *J. Org. Chem.* **53**, 1340 (1988).

753. T. F. Molinski and D. J. Faulkner. *J. Org. Chem.* **51**, 1144 (1986).

754. T. F. Molinski and D. J. Faulkner. *J. Org. Chem.* **51**, 2601 (1986).

755. T. F. Molinski and D. J. Faulkner. *J. Org. Chem.* **52**, 296 (1987).

756. T. F. Molinski and D. J. Faulkner. *Tetrahedron Lett.* **29**, 2137 (1988).

757. T. F. Molinski, D. J. Faulkner, C.-H. He, G. D. Van Duyne, and J. Clardy. *J. Org. Chem.* **51**, 4564 (1986).

758. T. F. Molinski, D. J. Faulkner, G. D. Van Duyne, and J. Clardy. *J. Org. Chem.* **52**, 3334 (1987).

759. T. F. Molinski and C. M. Ireland. *J. Org. Chem.* **53**, 2103 (1988).

760. T. P. Monath. *N. Engl. J. Med.* **319**, 641 (1988).

761. A. Mondon and K. Krohn. *Chem. Ber.* **105**, 3726 (1972).

762. A. Mondon and K. Krohn. *Chem. Ber.* **108**, 445 (1975).

763. M. R. Moore and P. A. Meredith. *Arch. Toxicol.* **42**, 87 (1979).

764. R. E. Moore, M. Ishibashi, G. M. L. Patterson, C. Xu, and J. Clardy. 28th Symposium on The Chemistry of Natural Products, Symposium Papers, Sendai, 1986, p. 191.

765. R. E. Moore, G. M. L. Patterson, J. S. Mynderse, J. Barchi, Jr., T. R. Norton, E. Furusawa, and S. Furusawa. *Pure Appl. Chem.* **58**, 263 (1986).

766. R. E. Moore, X.-Q. G. Yang, and G. M. L. Patterson. *J. Org. Chem.* **52**, 3773 (1987).

767. C. Moretti, S. Bhatnagar, J.-C. Beloeil, and J. Polonsky. *J. Nat. Prod.* **49**, 440 (1986).

768. K. Mori, K. Iguchi, N. Yamada, Y. Yamada, and Y. Inouye. *Tetrahedron Lett.* **28**, 5673 (1987).

769. K. Mori, K. Iguchi, N. Yamada, Y. Yamada, and Y. Inouye. 29th Symposium on The Chemistry of Natural Products, Symposium Papers, Sapporo, 1987, p. 294.

770. H. Morimoto, Y. Kawamatsu, and H. Sugihara. *Chem. Pharm. Bull.* **16**, 2282 (1968).

771. W. L. Morison. *Photochem. Photobiol.* **50**, 515 (1989).

772. H. Morita and H. Itokawa. *Planta Med.* **54**, 117 (1988).

773. M. Morita, A. Haji, A. Goto, N. Hattori (née Imaizumi), and Y. Hasegawa. *Folia Pharmacol. Japon.* **87**, 53 (1986).

774. J. C. Morrill, G. B. Jennings, A. J. Johnson, T. M. Cosgriff, P. H. Gibbs, and C. J. Peters. *Arch. Virol.* **110**, 195 (1990).

775. K. L. Mossman. *Cancer Invest.* **2**, 301 (1984).

776. R. Moura Pinheiro, M. Marquina Mac-Quhae, G. B. Marini Bettolo, and F. Delle Monache. *Phytochemistry* **23**, 1737 (1984).

777. B. Mukherji and H. T. Yamase. *Cancer Treatment Reports* **67**, 100 (1983).

778. K. Munakata, S. Marumo, K. Ohta, and Y.-L. Chen. *Tetrahedron Lett.* 4167 (1965).

779. M. Murakami, K. Makabe, K. Yamaguchi, S. Konosu, and M. R. Wälchli. 29th Symposium on The Chemistry of Natural Products, Symposium Papers, Sapporo, 1987, p. 316.

780. M. Murakami, K. Makabe, K. Yamaguchi, S. Konosu, and M. R. Wälchli. *Tetrahedron Lett.* **29**, 1149 (1988).

781. M. Murata, M. Kumagai, J. S. Lee, and T. Yasumoto. *Tetrahedron Lett.* **28**, 5869 (1987).

782. M. Murata, K. Miyagawa-Kohshima, K. Nakanishi, and Y. Naya. *Science* **234**, 585 (1986).

783. M. Murata, Y. Murakami, M. Kumagai, T. Yanagi, T. Yasumoto, T. Iwashita, and H. Naoki. 28th Symposium on The Chemistry of Natural Products, Symposium Papers, Sendai, 1986, p. 199.

784. M. Murata, M. Sano, T. Iwashita, H. Naoki, and T. Yasumoto. *Agric. Biol. Chem.* **50**, 2693 (1986).

785. E. L. Murphy, W. N. Gibbs, J. P. Figueroa, B. Bain, L. LaGrenade, B. Cranston, and W. A. Blattner. *J. Acq. Immune Def. Synd.* **1**, 143 (1988).

786. A. G. Myers, P. J. Proteau, and T. M. Handel. *J. Am. Chem. Soc.* **110**, 7212 (1988).

787. S. Mzengeza, C. M. Yang, and R. A. Whitney. *J. Am. Chem. Soc.* **109**, 276 (1987).

788. M. Nagao, Y. Fujita, K. Wakabayashi, H. Nukaya, T. Kosuge, and T. Sugimura. *Environ. Health Perspectives* **67**, 89 (1986).

789. K. Nagaoka, M. Matsumoto, J. Oono, K. Yokoi, S. Ishizeki, and T. Nakashima. *J. Antibiotics* **39**, 1527 (1986).

790. K. Nagasawa and T. W. Mak. *Proc. Natl. Acad. Sci. USA* **77**, 2964 (1980).

791. M. S. R. Nair, A. Mathur, K. Tabei, A. K. Bose, A. S. Goldberg, V. Koch, B. Hunt, V. K. Dayal, Y. S. Arkel, G. Obiedzinski, and M. A. van Allen. *J. Nat. Prod.* **51**, 184 (1988).

792. T. Najarian and T. Colton. *Lancet* **I**, 1018 (1978).

793. M. Nakagawa, M. Endo, Y. Hamamoto, M. Ishihama, and H. Kubota. The 1984 Intl. Chem. Congress of Pacific Basin Societies, Honolulu, Hawaii, Dec. 1984, Book of Abstracts, 10E69.

794. M. Nakagawa, Y. Hamamoto, M. Ishihama, S. Hamasaki, and M. Endo. *Tetrahedron Lett.* **28**, 431 (1987).

795. M. Nakagawa, M. Ishihama, Y. Hamamoto, and M. Endo. 28th Symposium on The Chemistry of Natural Products, Symposium Papers, Sendai, 1986, p. 207.

796. H. Nakamura, S. Deng, J. Kobayashi, Y. Ohizumi, and Y. Hirata. *Tetrahedron* **42**, 4197 (1986).

797. H. Nakamura, S. Deng, J. Kobayashi, Y. Ohizumi, Y. Tomotake, T. Matsuzaki, and Y. Hirata. *Tetrahedron Lett.* **28**, 621 (1987).

798. H. Nakamura, Y. Iitaka, M. Imoto, K. Isshiki, H. Naganawa, T. Takeuchi, and H. Umezawa. *J. Antibiotics* **39**, 314 (1986).

799. H. Nakamura, Y. Iitaka, and H. Umezawa. *J. Antibiotics* **32**, 765 (1979).

800. H. Nakamura, J. Kobayashi, Y. Nakamura, Y. Ohizumi, T. Kondo, and Y. Hirata. *Tetrahedron Lett.* **27**, 4319 (1986).

801. H. Nakamura, J. Kobayashi, Y. Ohizumi, and Y. Hirata. *J. Chem. Soc., Perkin Trans 1* 173 (1987).

802. H. Nakashima, T. Matsui, O. Yoshida, Y. Isowa, Y. Kido, Y. Motoki, M. Ito, S. Shigeta, T. Mori, and N. Yamamoto. *Jpn. J. Cancer Res. (Gann)* **78**, 767 (1987).

803. H. Nanba and H. Kuroda. *Chem. Pharm. Bull.* **35**, 1285 (1987).

804. M. Nasr, C. Litterst, and J. McGowan. *Antiviral Res.* **14**, 125 (1990).

805. Natl. Cancer Inst., DHEW Publ. No. (NIH) 79-837, Carcinogenesis Testing Program, Div. of Cancer Cause & Prevention, 1979.

806. Natl. Cancer Inst. Tech. Report, Series No. 55, U.S. Dept. of Health, Education & Welfare, 1978.

807. Natl. Cancer Program, Special Communication, Sept. 17, 1976.

808. D. F. Nelson, S. Cooper, M. G. Weston, and P. Rubin. *Cancer* **48**, 2386 (1981).

809. D. E. Nettleton, T. W. Doyle, B. Krishnan, G. K. Matsumoto, and J. Clardy. *Tetrahedron Lett.* **26**, 4011 (1985).

810. O. Neuhauer. *Br. J. Cancer* **1**, 192 (1947).

811. M. E. Newman. *J. Natl. Cancer Inst.* **81**, 1686 (1989).

812. News & Comment, "African AIDS: Whose Research Rules," *Science* **250**, 199 (1990).

813. F. Ngan, R. S. Chang, H. D. Tabba, and K. M. Smith. *Antiviral Res.* **10**, 107 (1988).

814. P. D. Nichols, J. K. Volkman, G. M. Hallegraeff, and S. I. Blackburn. *Phytochemistry* **26**, 2537 (1987).

815. W. J. Nicholson. *Cancer* **39**, 1792 (1977).

816. H. Nishimura, K. Katagiri, K. Sato, M. Mayama, and N. Shimaoka. *J. Antibiotics* **A9**, 60 (1956).

817. S. Nishimura. *Environ. Health Perspectives* **67**, 11 (1986).

818. C. Nishino, K. Kobayashi, and M. Fukushima. *J. Nat. Prod.* **51**, 1281 (1988).

819. H. Nishino, A. Nishino, J. Takayasu, T. Hasegawa, A. Iwashima, K. Hirabayashi, S. Iwata, and S. Shibata. *Cancer Res.* **48**, 5210 (1988).

820. Y. Nishio, T. Kakizoe, M. Ohtani, S. Sato, T. Sugimura, and S. Fukushima. *Science* **231**, 843 (1986).

821. H. Niwa, Y. Yoshida, and K. Yamada. *J. Nat. Prod.* **51**, 343 (1988).

822. Y. Noguchi, R. Higuchi, N. Marubayashi, and T. Komori. *Liebigs Ann. Chem.* 341 (1987).

823. F. Nohara, M. Nishii, K. Ogawa, K. Isono, M. Ubukata, T. Fujii, T. Itaya, and T. Saito. *Tetrahedron Lett.* **28**, 1287 (1987).

824. G.-I. Nonaka, I. Nishioka, M. Nishizawa, T. Yamagishi, Y. Kashiwada, G. E. Dutschman, A. J. Bodner, R. E. Kilkuskie, Y.-C. Cheng, and K.-H. Lee. *J. Nat. Prod.* **53**, 587 (1990).

825. S. Norell, H. Lipping, A. Ahlbom, and L. Österblom. *Lancet* **I**, 462 (1983).

826. T. Norseth. *J. Tox. Environ. Health* **6**, 1021 (1980).

827. M. Norte and J. J. Fernández. *Tetrahedron Lett.* **28**, 1693 (1987).

828. M. Norte, M. L. Rodriguez, J. J. Fernández, L. Eguren, and D. M. Estrada. *Tetrahedron* **44**, 4973 (1988).

829. P. T. Northcote and R. J. Andersen. *J. Nat. Prod.* **50**, 1174 (1987).

830. P. T. Northcote and R. J. Andersen. *Tetrahedron Lett.* **29**, 4357 (1988).

831. M. Nowak. *Nature* **347**, 522 (1990).

832. H. Nozaki, H. Suzuki, T. Hirayama, R. Kasai, R.-Y. Wu, and K.-H. Lee. *Phytochemistry* **25**, 479 (1986).

833. H. Nozaki, H. Suzuki, K.-H. Lee, and A. T. McPhail. *J. Chem. Soc., Chem. Commun.* 1048 (1982).

834. T. Nozoye. *Chem. Pharm. Bull.* **6**, 306 (1958).

835. M. Ochi, K. Asao, H. Kotsuki, I. Miura, and K. Shibata. *Bull. Chem. Soc. Jpn.* **59**, 661 (1986).

836. H. Ogawara, K. Uchino, T. Akiyama, and S.-I. Watanabe. *J. Antibiotics* **38**, 153 (1985).

837. H. Ogawara, K. Uchino, T. Akiyama, and S.-I. Watanabe. *J. Antibiotics* **38**, 587 (1985).

838. M. Ogura, G. A. Cordell, and N. R. Farnsworth. *Lloydia* **40**, 157 (1977).

839. K. Ohkura, S. Inoue, K. Ikeda, and K. Hayashi. *Biochim. Biophys. Acta* **954**, 148 (1988).

840. N. Ohno, K. Kurachi, and T. Yadomae. *Chem. Pharm. Bull.* **36**, 1016 (1988).

841. N. Ohno, I. Suzuki, and T. Yadomae. *Chem. Pharm. Bull.* **34**, 1362 (1986).

842. N. Ohno and T. Yadomae. *Carbohydr. Res.* **159**, 293 (1987).

843. S. Ohta and S. Kimoto. *Chem. Pharm. Bull.* **24**, 2977 (1976).

844. M. Ojika, K. Sugimoto, T. Okazaki, and K. Yamada. *J. Chem. Soc., Chem. Commun.* 1775 (1989).

845. M. Ojika, K. Wakamatsu, H. Niwa, and K. Yamada. *Tetrahedron* **43**, 5261 (1987).

846. T. Okabe, B. D. Yuan, F. Isono, I. Sato, H. Fukazawa, T. Nishimura, and N. Tanaka. *J. Antibiotics* **38**, 230 (1985).

847. T. Okamoto, Y. Torii, and Y. Isogai. *Chem. Pharm. Bull.* **16**, 1860 (1968).

848. K. Okano, N. Ohkawa, and S. Ikegami. *Agric. Biol. Chem.* **49**, 2823 (1985).

849. M. Okano, N. Fukamiya, T. Aratani, M. Juichi, and K.-H. Lee. *J. Nat. Prod.* **48**, 972 (1985).

850. M. Okigawa, T. Maeda, and N. Kawano. *Chem. Pharm. Bull.* **18**, 862 (1970).

851. M. Okigawa, T. Maeda, and N. Kawano. *Tetrahedron* **26**, 4301 (1970).

852. E. M. Oltz, R. C. Bruening, M. J. Smith, K. Kustin, and K. Nakanishi. *J. Am. Chem. Soc.* **110**, 6162 (1988).

853. S. Omar, C. Albert, T. Fanni, and P. Crews. *J. Org. Chem.* **53**, 5971 (1988).

854. T. Omori-Satoh, N. Izumi, T. Yamanaka, S. Kawaguchi, M. Takahashi, S. Takano, S. Sadahiro, S. Kondo, and H. Kondo. *Toxicon* **24**, 1045 (1986).

855. S. Ōmura, Y. Iwai, Y. Takahashi, N. Sadakane, A. Nakagawa, H. Ōiwa, Y. Hasegawa, and T. Ikai. *J. Antibiotics* **32**, 255 (1975).

856. S. Ōmura, A. Nakagawa, and N. Sadakane. *Tetrahedron Lett.* 4323 (1979).

857. B. E. Oppenheim. *J. Am. Med. Assoc.* **242**, 1390 (1979).

858. T. Otani, I. Yamawaki, H. Matsumoto, Y. Minami, Y. Yamada, T. Marunaka, C.-Q. Qi, T. Tian, R. Zhang, M.-Y. Xie, and J.-R. Lu. *J. Antibiotics* **41**, 275 (1988).

859. M. Païs, C. Fontaine, D. Laurent, S. La Barre, and E. Guittet. *Tetrahedron Lett.* **28**, 1409 (1987).

860. J. Palca. *Science* **247**, 1406 (1990).

861. J. Palca. *Science* **248**, 1484 (1990).

862. J. M. Palefsky, J. Gonzales, R. M. Greenblatt, D. K. Ahn, and H. Hollander. *J. Am. Med. Assoc.* **263**, 2911 (1990).

863. B. K. Park, M. Nakagawa, A. Hirota, and M. Nakayama. *J. Antibiotics* **41**, 751 (1988).

864. P.-U. Park, C. A. Broka, B. F. Johnson, and Y. Kishi. *J. Am. Chem. Soc.* **109**, 6205 (1987).

865. C. Pathirana and R. J. Anderson. *J. Am. Chem. Soc.* **108**, 8288 (1986).

866. A. Patra, C. W. J. Chang, P. J. Scheuer, G. D. Van Duyne, G. K. Matsumoto, and J. Clardy. *J. Am. Chem. Soc.* **106**, 7981 (1984).

867. V. J. Paul, P. Ciminiello, and W. Fenical. *Phytochemistry* **27**, 1011 (1988).

868. V. J. Paul and W. Fenical. *Phytochemistry* **24**, 2239 (1985).

869. L. A. Pavelka, F. A. Fuhrman, and H. S. Mosher. *Heterocycles* **17**, 225 (1982).

870. J. Pawlak, M. S. Tempesta, J. Golik, M. G. Zagorski, M. S. Lee, K. Nakanishi, T. Iwashita, M. L. Gross, and K. B. Tomer. *J. Am. Chem. Soc.* **109** 1144 (1987).

871. C. Pedersen, E. Sandström, C. S. Petersen, G. Norkrans, J. Gerstoft, A. Karlsson, K. Chr. Christensen, C. Hakansson, P.-O. Pehrson, J. O. Nielsen, H. J. Jürgensen, and The Scandinavian Isoprinosine Study Group. *N. Engl. J. Med.* **322**, 1757 (1990).

872. M. Pedersén, P. Saenger, and L. Fries. *Phytochemistry* **13**, 2273 (1974).

873. F. Perera and P. Boffetta. *J. Natl. Cancer Inst.* **80**, 1282 (1988).

874. N. B. Perry, J. W. Blunt, J. D. McCombs, and M. H. G. Munro. *J. Am. Chem. Soc.* **51**, 5476 (1986).

875. N. B. Perry, J. W. Blunt, and M. H. G. Munro. *Tetrahedron* **44**, 1727 (1988).

876. N. B. Perry, J. W. Blunt, M. H. G. Munro, T. Higa, and R. Sakai. *J. Org. Chem.* **53**, 4127 (1988).

877. N. B. Perry, J. W. Blunt, M. H. G. Munro, and L. K. Pannell. *J. Am. Chem. Soc.* **110**, 4850 (1988).

878. C. J. Peters, C.-T. Liu, G. W. Anderson, Jr., J. C. Morrill, and P. B. Jahrling. *Rev. Infect. Dis.* **11**, Suppl. 4, S743 (1989).

879. E. Petru and D. Schmähl. *TumorDiagnostik & Therapie* **7**, 99 (1986).

880. G. R. Pettit. "The Bryostatins" In Progress in the Chemistry of Organic Natural Products, No. 57, Founded by L. Zechmeister, Ed. by W. Herz, G. W. Kirby, W. Steglich, and Ch. Tamm, Springer-Verlag, New York, 1991, p. 153-195.

881. G. R. Pettit, G. M. Cragg, M. I. Suffness, D. Gust, F. E. Boettner, M. Williams, J. A. Saenz-Renauld, P. Brown, J. M. Schmidt, and P. D. Ellis. *J. Org. Chem.* **49**, 4258 (1984).

882. G. R. Pettit, V. Gaddamidi, D. L. Herald, S. B. Singh, G. M. Cragg, J. M. Schmidt, F. E. Boettner, M. Williams, and Y. Sagawa. *J. Nat. Prod.* **49**, 995 (1986).

883. G. R. Pettit, C. L. Herald, and C. R. Smith. Biosynthetic Products for Cancer Chemotherapy, Vol. 6, Elsevier Scientific Pub. Co., Amsterdam, 1989.

884. G. R. Pettit, M. Inoue, Y. Kamano, C. Dufresne, N. Christie, M. L. Niven, and D. L. Herald. *J. Chem. Soc., Chem. Commun.* 865 (1988).

885. G. R. Pettit, M. Inoue, Y. Kamano, D. L. Herald, C. Arm, C. Dufresne, N. D. Christie, J. M. Schmidt, D. L. Doubek, and T. S. Krupa. *J. Am. Chem. Soc.* **110**, 2006 (1988).

886. G. R. Pettit, Y. Kamano, and C. L. Herald. *J. Nat. Prod.* **49**, 661 (1986).

887. G. R. Pettit, Y. Kamano, and C. L. Herald. *J. Org. Chem.* **52**, 2848 (1987).

888. G. R. Pettit, Y. Kamano, C. L. Herald, J. M. Schmidt, and C. G. Zubrod. *Pure Appl. Chem.* **58**, 415 (1986).

889. G. R. Pettit, Y. Kamano, C. L. Herald, A. A. Tuinman, F. E. Boettner, H. Kizu, J. M. Schmidt, L. Baczynskyj, K. B. Tomer, and R. J. Bontems. *J. Am. Chem. Soc.* **109**, 6883 (1987).

890. G. R. Pettit, J. E. Leet, C. L. Herald, Y. Kamano, F. E. Boettner, L. Baczynskyj, and R. A. Nieman. *J. Org. Chem.* **52**, 2854 (1987).

891. G. R. Pettit and D. E. Schaufelberger. *J. Nat. Prod.* **51**, 1104 (1988).

892. G. R. Pettit, S. B. Singh, F. Hogan, P. Lloyd-Williams, D. L. Herald, D. D. Burkett, and P. J. Clewlow. *J. Am. Chem. Soc.* **111**, 5463 (1989).

893. G. R. Pettit, S. B. Singh, M. L. Niven, E. Hamel, and J. M. Schmidt. *J. Nat. Prod.* **50**, 119 (1987).

894. V. Piccialli and D. Sica. *J. Nat. Prod.* **49**, 779 (1986).

895. V. Piccialli and D. Sica. *J. Nat. Prod.* **50**, 915 (1987).

896. F. Piozzi, M. L. Marino, C. Fuganti, and A. Di Martino. *Phytochemistry* **8**, 1745 (1969).

897. C. Pizza, L. Minale, D. Laurent, and J.-L. Menou. *Gazz. Chim. Ital.* **115**, 585 (1985).

898. M. A. Portugal, H. C. Falkson, K. Stevens, and G. Falkson. *Cancer Treatment Reports* **63**, 177 (1979).

899. R. Preussmann. *Naturwissenschaften* **71**, 25 (1984).

900. R. Preussmann and B. W. Stewart. "*N*-Nitroso Carcinogens" **In** Chemical Carcinogens, Second Edition, Revised, and Expanded, Vol. 2, Chap. 12, C. E. Searle, Ed., Am. Chem. Soc., Washington, D.C., 1984, p. 643.

901. M. L. Price, M. J. Tidman, C. S. Ogg, and D. M. MacDonald. *N. Engl. J. Med.* **313**, 1420 (1985).

902. K. C. Pullaiah, R. K. Surapaneni, C. B. Rao, K. F. Albizati, B. W. Sullivan, D. J. Faulkner, C.-H. He, and J. Clardy. *J. Org. Chem.* **50**, 3665 (1985).

903. K. Purushothaman, R. Bhima Rao, and K. Kalyani. *Indian J. Chem.* **13**, 1357 (1975).

904. J. Qar, H. Schweitz, A. Schmid, and M. Lazdunski. *FEBS Lett.* **202**, 331 (1986).

905. E. Quiñoà, M. Adamczeski, P. Crews, and G. J. Bakus. *J. Org. Chem.* **51**, 4494 (1986).

906. E. Quiñoà and P. Crews. *Tetrahedron Lett.* **28**, 2467 (1987).

907. E. Quiñoà and P. Crews. *Tetrahedron Lett.* **28**, 3229 (1987).

908. E. Quiñoà and P. Crews. *Tetrahedron Lett.* **29**, 2037 (1988).

909. E. Quiñoà, Y. Kakou, and P. Crews. *J. Org. Chem.* **53**, 3642 (1988).

910. E. Quiñoà, E. Kho, L. V. Manes, P. Crews, and G. J. Bakus. *J. Org. Chem.* **51**, 4260 (1986).

911. O. G. Raabe, S. A. Book, and N. J. Parks. *Science* **208**, 61 (1980).

912. E. P. Radford and K. G. St. Clair Renard. *N. Engl. J. Med.* **310**, 1485 (1984).

913. J. E. Ranchalis, L. Gentry, Y. Ogawa, S. M. Seyedin, J. McPherson, A. Purchio, and D. R. Twardzik. *Biochem. Biophys. Res. Commun.* **148**, 783 (1987).

914. J. Rantanen. *J. Tox. Environ. Health* **6**, 971 (1980).

915. C. B. Rao, K. C. Pullaiah, R. K. Surapaneni, B. W. Sullivan, K. F. Albizati, D. J. Faulkner, C.-H. He, and J. Clardy. *J. Org. Chem.* **51**, 2736 (1986).

916. C. B. Rao, K. V. Ramana, D. V. Rao, E. Fahy, and D. J. Faulkner. *J. Nat. Prod.* **51**, 954 (1988).

917. S. M. Rappaport, M. C. McCartney, and E. T. Wei. *Cancer Lett.* **8**, 139 (1979).

918. E. Reed and M. K. Evans. *J. Natl. Cancer Inst.* **82**, 431 (1990).

919. A. E. Reif. *Amer. Scientist* **69**, 437 (1981).

920. R. S. Remis, K. D. Elmslie, D. Rylett, and G. Wells. *AIDS Update, Can. Med. Assoc. J.* **139**, 939 (1988).

921. J.-L. Reymond and P. Vogel. *Tetrahedron Lett.* **30**, 705 (1989).

922. G. Reznik, J. M. Hardisty, and A. Russefield. *J. Natl. Cancer Inst.* **63**, 205 (1979).

923. R. Riccio, M. V. D'Auria, M. Iorizzi, L. Minale, D. Laurent, and D. Duhet. *Gazz. Chim. Ital.* **115**, 405 (1985).

924. R. Riccio, M. V. D'Auria, and L. Minale. *Tetrahedron* **41**, 6041 (1985).

925. R. Riccio, M. V. D'Auria, and L. Minale. *J. Org. Chem.* **51**, 533 (1986).

926. R. Riccio, M. Iorizzi, O. Squillace Greco, L. Minale, D. Laurent, and Y. Barbin. *Gazz. Chim. Ital.* **115**, 505 (1985).

927. R. Riccio, L. Minale, S. Bano, and V. U. Ahmad. *Tetrahedron Lett.* **28**, 2291 (1987).

928. R. Riccio, L. Minale, S. Bano, N. Bano, and V. U. Ahmad. *Gazz. Chim. Ital.* **117**, 755 (1987).

929. R. Riccio, L. Minale, S. Pagonis, C. Pizza, F. Zollo, and J. Pusset. *Tetrahedron* **38**, 3615 (1982).

930. R. Riccio, O. Squillace Greco, and L. Minale. *J. Nat. Prod.* **51**, 989 (1988).

931. R. Riccio, O. Squillace Greco, L. Minale, D. Duhet, D. Laurent, J. Pusset, G. Chauviere, and M. Pusset. *J. Nat. Prod.* **49**, 1141 (1986).

932. R. Riccio, O. Squillace Greco, L. Minale, S. La Barre, and D. Laurent. *J. Nat. Prod.* **51**, 1003 (1988).

933. R. Riccio, O. Squillace Greco, L. Minale, D. Laurent, and D. Duhet. *J. Chem. Soc., Perkin Trans 1* 665 (1986).

934. K. L. Rinehart, K.-I. Harada, M. Namikoshi, C. Chen, C. A. Harvis, M. H. G. Munro, J. W. Blunt, P. E. Mulligan, V. R. Beasley, A. M. Dahlem, and W. W. Carmichael. *J. Am. Chem. Soc.* **110**, 8557 (1988).

935. K. L. Rinehart, Jr., J. Kobayashi, G. C. Harbour, J. Gilmore, M. Mascal, T. G. Holt, L. S. Shield, and F. Lafargue. *J. Am. Chem. Soc.* **109**, 3378 (1987).

936. S. J. Rinkus and M. S. Legator. *Cancer Res.* **39**, 3289 (1979).

937. J. Riondel, M. Jacrot, M.-F. Nissou, F. Picot, H. Bériel, C. Mouriquand, and P. Potier. *Anticancer Res.* **8**, 387 (1988).

938. A. P. Rivera, L. A. Astudillo, A. G. Gonzalez, E. Manta, and F. Cataldo. *J. Nat. Prod.* **50**, 965 (1987).

939. B. J. Roberts, K. L. Hamelehle, J. S. Sebolt, and W. R. Leopold. *Cancer Chemother. Pharmacol.* **16**, 95 (1986).

940. A. D. Rodriguez, R. K. Akee, and P. J. Scheuer. *Tetrahedron Lett.* **28**, 4989 (1987).

941. J. A. Roesener and P. J. Scheuer. *J. Am. Chem. Soc.* **108**, 846 (1986).

942. D. M. Roll, J. E. Biskupiak, C. L. Mayne, and C. M. Ireland. *J. Am. Chem. Soc.* **108**, 6680 (1986).

943. D. M. Roll, C. M. Ireland, H. S. M. Lu, and J. Clardy. *J. Org. Chem.* **53**, 3276 (1988).

944. D. M. Roll, P. J. Scheuer, G. K. Matsumoto, and J. Clardy. *J. Am. Chem. Soc.* **105**, 6177 (1983).

945. A. Roth, B. Kuballa, C. Bounthanh, P. Cabalion, T. Sévenet, J. P. Beck, and R. Anton. *Planta Med.* 450 (1986).

946. A. Roth, B. Kuballa, P. Cabalion, and R. Anton. *Planta Med.* 289 (1985).

947. M. Rothenberg and B. A. Chabner. *J. Am. Med. Assoc.* **263**, 2667 (1990).

948. A. L. Rothman, I. Kurane, Y.-M. Zhang, C.-J. Lai, and F. A. Ennis. *J. Virol.* **63**, 2486 (1989).

949. G. C. Roush, J. Walrath, L. T. Stayner, S. A. Kaplan, J. T. Flannery, and A. Blair. *J. Natl. Cancer Inst.* **79**, 1221 (1987).

950. J. M. Rovinski, G. L. Tewalt, and A. T. Sneden. *J. Nat. Prod.* **50**, 211 (1987).

951. E. K. Rowinsky, L. A. Cazenave, R. C. Donehower. *J. Natl. Cancer Inst.* **82**, 1247 (1990).

952. K. Roy, T. Mukhopadhyay, G. C. S. Reddy, K. R. Desikan, R. H. Rupp, and B. N. Ganguli. *J. Antibiotics* **41**, 1780 (1988).

953. N. Ruangrungsi, A. Rivepiboon, G. L. Lange, M. Lee, C. P. Decicco, P. Picha, and K. Preechanukool. *J. Nat. Prod.* **50**, 891 (1987).

954. A. Rudi, Y. Benayahu, I. Goldberg, and Y. Kashman. *Tetrahedron Lett.* **29**, 3861 (1988).

955. C. Rufer, H. Hoffmeister, H. Schairer, and M. Traut. *Chem. Ber.* **98**, 2383 (1965).

956. G. Ruffenach. "Study Links Silicone Gel to Cancer." *Wall Street Journal*, Nov. 10, 1988, p. B1.

957. R. M. Ruprecht, L. D. Bernard, T.-C. Chou, M. A. Gama Sosa, F. Fazely, J. Koch, P. L. Sharma, and S. Mullaney. *Cancer Res.* (Suppl.) **50**, 5618s (1990).

958. H. Saito, H. Yoshikawa, Y. Nishimura, S. Kondo, T. Takeuchi, and H. Umezawa. *Chem. Pharm. Bull.* **34**, 3733 (1986).

959. H. Saito, H. Yoshikawa, Y. Nishimura, S. Kondo, T. Takeuchi, and H. Umezawa. *Chem. Pharm. Bull.* **34**, 3741 (1986).

960. Y. Saito, H. Takizawa, S. Konishi, D. Yoshida, and S. Mizusaki. *Carcinogenesis* **6**, 1189 (1985).

961. K. Sakai, T. Ichikawa, K. Yamada, M. Yamashita, M. Tanimoto, A. Hikita, Y. Ijuin and K. Kondo. *J. Nat. Prod.* **51**, 845 (1988)

962. R. Sakai, T. Higa, C. W. Jefford, and G. Bernardinelli. *Helv. Chim. Acta* **69**, 91 (1986).

963. R. Sakai, T. Higa, C. W. Jefford, and G. Bernardinelli. *J. Am. Chem. Soc.* **108**, 6404 (1986).

964. R. Sakai, T. Higa, and Y. Kashman. *Chem. Lett.* 1499 (1986).

965. R. Sakai, S. Kohmoto, T. Higa, C. W. Jefford, and G. Bernardinelli. *Tetrahedron Lett.* **28**, 5493 (1987).

966. S.-I. Sakai, Y. Hitotsuyanagi, N. Aimi, H. Fujiki, M. Suganuma, T. Sugimura, Y. Endo, and K. Shudo. *Tetrahedron Lett.* **27**, 5219 (1986).

967. S.-I. Sakai, Y. Hitotsuyanagi, K. Yamaguchi, N. Aimi, K. Ogata, T. Kuramochi, H. Seki, R. Hara, H. Fujiki, M. Suganuma, T. Sugimura, Y. Endo, K. Shudo, and Y. Koyama. *Chem. Pharm. Bull.* **34**, 4883 (1986).

968. T. Sakaki, S. Yoshimura, T. Tsuyuki, T. Takahashi, and T. Honda. *Chem. Pharm. Bull.* **34**, 4447 (1986).

969. T. Sakaki, S. Yoshimura, T. Tsuyuki, T. Takahashi, T. Honda, and T. Nakanishi. *Tetrahedron Lett.* **27**, 593 (1986).

970. T. Sakaki, S. Yoshimura, T. Tsuyuki, T. Takahashi, T. Honda, and T. Nakanishi. *Bull. Chem. Soc. Jpn.* **59**, 3541 (1986).

971. S. Sakemi, T. Higa, U. Anthoni, and C. Christophersen. *Tetrahedron* **43**, 263 (1987).

972. S. Sakemi, T. Ichiba, S. Kohmoto, G. Saucy, and T. Higa. *J. Am. Chem. Soc.* **110**, 4851 (1988).

973. J. M. Samet, D. M. Kutvirt, R. J. Waxweiler, and C. R. Key. *N. Engl. J. Med.* **310**, 1481 (1984).

974. P. S. Sarma and J. Gruber. *J. Natl. Cancer Inst.* **82**, 1100 (1990).

975. T. Sasaki, N. Abiko, K. Nitta, N. Takasuka, and Y. Sugino. *Eur. J. Cancer* **15**, 211 (1979).

976. W. R. Schafer, R. Kim, R. Sterne, J. Thorner, S.-H. Kim, and J. Rine. *Science* **245**, 379 (1989).

977. A. Schatzkin, D. Y. Jones, R. N. Hoover, P. R. Taylor, L. A. Brinton, R. G. Ziegler, E. B. Harvey, C. L. Carter, L. M. Licitra, M. C. Dufour, and D. B. Larson. *N. Engl. J. Med.* **316**, 1169 (1987).

978. J. P. Schaumberg, G. C. Hokanson, and J. C. French. *J. Chem. Soc., Chem. Commun.* 1450 (1984).

979. D. Schlenk and W. H. Gerwick. *Phytochemistry* **26**, 1081 (1987).

980. D. Schmähl. *J. Cancer Res. Clin. Oncol.* **109**, 260 (1985).

981. I. Schmeltz, S. Abidi, and D. Hoffmann. *Cancer Lett.* **2**, 125 (1977).

982. F. J. Schmitz and S. J. Bloor. *J. Org. Chem.* **53**, 3922 (1988).

983. F. J. Schmitz and J. C. Chang. *J. Nat. Prod.* **51**, 745 (1988).

984. F. J. Schmitz, S. P. Gunasekera, G. Yalamanchili, M. B. Hossain, and D. van der Helm. *J. Am. Chem. Soc.* **106**, 7251 (1984).

985. F. J. Schmitz, M. B. Ksebati, S. P. Gunasekera, and S. Agarwal. *J. Org. Chem.* **53**, 5941 (1988).

986. P. A. Schulte, K. Ringen, G. P. Hemstreet, E. B. Altekruse, W. H. Gullen, S. Tillett, W. C. Allsbrook, Jr., J. H. Crosby, R. Witherington, W. Stringer, and M. M. Brubaker. *Cancer* **58**, 2156 (1986).

987. "Scientists Changing Therapy Outlook for AIDS Patients." *J. Natl. Cancer Inst.* **82**, 992 (1990).

988. S. Sciuto, R. Chillemi, R. Morrone, A. Patti, and M. Piattelli. *J. Nat. Prod.* **51**, 1017 (1988).

989. S. Sciuto, R. Chillemi, and M. Piattelli. *J. Nat. Prod.* **51**, 322 (1988).

990. C. E. Searle. *Chem. Brit.* 211 (1986).

991. M. Segawa, N. Enoki, M. Ikura, K. Hikichi, R. Ishida, H. Shirahama, and T. Matsumoto. *Tetrahedron Lett.* **28**, 3703 (1987).

992. A. B. Segelman, F. P. Segelman, J. Karliner, and R. D. Sofia. *J. Am. Med. Assoc.* **236**, 477 (1976).

993. M. Seidlin, K. Krasinski, D. Bebenroth, V. Itri, A. M. Paolino, and F. Valentine. *J. Acq. Immune Def. Synd.* **1**, 150 (1988).

994. A. M. Seldes, E. G. Gros, A. Suarez, J. Rovirosa, and A. San-Martín. *Tetrahedron* 44, 1359 (1988).

995. V. Sénilh, S. Blechert, M. Colin, D. Guénard, F. Picot, P. Potier, and P. Varenne. *J. Nat. Prod.* **47**, 131 (1984).

996. C. Sevcik, F. Alvarez-Vasquez, J. A. Saavedra, and G. Cordovez. *Toxicon* **24**, 851 (1986).

997. C. P. Sharma and H. Gehring. *Biochem. Biophys. Res. Commun.* **139**, 1243 (1986).

998. P. Sharma and M. Alam. *J. Chem. Soc., Perkin Trans 1* 2537 (1988).

999. K. Shibata, S. Satsumabayashi, A. Nakagawa, and S. Ōmura. *J. Antibiotics* **39**, 1630 (1986).

1000. K. Shibata, S. Satsumabayashi, H. Sano, K. Komiyama, A. Nakagawa, and S. Ōmura. *J. Antibiotics* **39**, 415 (1986).

1001. S. Shibata, T. Murata, and M. Fujita. *Chem. Pharm. Bull.* **11**, 382 (1963).

1002. Y. Shibata, M. Morita, and J. S. Edmonds. *Agric. Biol. Chem.* **51**, 391 (1987).

1003. S. Shimada, O. Yano, H. Inoue, E. Kuramoto, T. Fukuda, H. Yamamoto, T. Kataoka, and T. Tokunaga. *J. Natl. Cancer Inst.* **74**, 681 (1985).

1004. T. Shimizu, T. Watanabe, M. Kirihara, S. Hiranuma, Y. Fujimoto, and H. Yoshioka. 29th Symposium on The Chemistry of Natural Products, Symposium Papers, Sapporo, 1987, p. 503.

1005. Y. Shimizu, H.-N. Chou, H. Bando, G. Van Duyne, and J. C. Clardy. *J. Am. Chem. Soc.* **108**, 514 (1986).

1006. K. Shimomura, O. Hirai, T. Mizota, S. Matsumoto, J. Mori, F. Shibayama, and H. Kikuchi. *J. Antibiotics* **40**, 600 (1987).

1007. K. Shimomura, T. Manda, S. Mukumoto, K. Masuda, T. Nakamura, T. Mizota, S. Matsumoto, F. Nishigaki, T. Oku, J. Mori, and F. Shibayama. *Cancer Res.* **48**, 1166 (1988).

1008. A. Shimosaka, H. Kawai, Y. Hayakawa, N. Komeshima, M. Nakagawa, H. Seto, and N. Ōtake. *J. Antibiotics* **40**, 1283 (1987).

1009. J. Shin and W. Fenical. *Phytochemistry* **26**, 3347 (1987).

1010. J. Shin, V. J. Paul, and W. Fenical. *Tetrahedron Lett.* **27**, 5189 (1986).

1011. H. Shinohara, N. Ohno, and T. Yadomae. *Chem. Pharm Bull.* **36**, 819 (1988).

1012. K. Shiomi, M. Aoyama, H. Yamanaka, and T. Kikuchi. *Comp. Biochem. Physiol.* **90C**, 361 (1988).

1013. K. Shiomi, E. Tanaka, H. Yamanaka, and T. Kikuchi. *Toxicon* **23**, 865 (1985).

1014. S. M. Sieber and R. H. Adamson. "V. Carcinogenic Potential of Antineoplastic Agents in the Human--Toxicity of Antineoplastic Agents in Man: Chromosomal Aberrations, Antifertility Effects, Congenital Malformations, and Carcinogenic Potential," In Advances in Cancer Research, Vol. 22, 1975, p. 571.

1015. S. M. Sieber and R. H. Adamson. *Cancer* **40**, 1950 (1977).

1016. N. Simon. *J. Am. Med. Assoc.* **237**, 789 (1977).

1017. N. Simon and S. M. Silverstone. *Bull. N. Y. Acad. Med.* **52**, 741 (1976).

1018. B. K. Simpson and N. F. Haard. *Comp. Biochem. Physiol.* **79B**, 613 (1984).

1019. E. E. Sisskin and J. C. Barrett. *Cancer Res.* **41**, 346 (1981).

1020. J. Slavík. *Collect. Czech. Chem. Commun.* **20**, 198 (1955).

1021. J. Slavík and L. Slavíková. *Collect. Czech. Chem. Commun.* **20**, 21 (1955).

1022. H.-R. Sliwka, O. W. Nokleby, and S. Liaaen-Jensen. *Acta Chem. Scand.* **B41**, 245 (1987).

1023. W. A. Slusarchyk, M. G. Young, G. S. Bisacchi, D. R. Hockstein, and R. Zahler. *Tetrahedron Lett.* **30**, 6453 (1989).

1024. T. A. Smitka, R. H. Bunge, J. H. Wilton, G. C. Hokanson, J. C. French, C.-H. He, and J. Clardy. *J. Antibiotics* **39**, 800 (1986).

1025. T. A. Smitka, J. B. Deeter, A. H. Hunt, F. P. Mertz, R. M. Ellis, L. D. Boeck, and R. C. Yao. *J. Antibiotics* **41**, 726 (1988).

1026. G. Sodano and A. Spinella. *Tetrahedron Lett.* **27**, 2505 (1986).

1027. Y. Sone, R. Okuda, N. Wada, E. Kishida, and A. Misaki. *Agric. Biol. Chem.* **49**, 2641 (1985).

1028. P. A. Southorn and G. Powis. *Mayo Clinic Proceed.* **63**, 381 (1988).

1029. P. A. Southorn and G. Powis. *Mayo Clinic Proceed.* **63**, 390 (1988).

1030. N. E. Spingarn, H. Kasai, L. L. Vuolo, S. Nishimura, Z. Yamaizumi, T. Sugimura, T. Matsushima, and J. H. Weisburger. *Cancer Lett.* **9**, 177 (1980).

1031. J. P. Springer, J. Clardy, R. H. Cox, H. G. Cutler, and R. J. Cole. *Tetrahedron Lett.* 2737 (1975).

1032. B. V. Stadel. *Lancet* **I**, 890 (1976).

1033. W. Stevens, D. C. Thomas, J. L. Lyon, J. E. Till, R. A. Kerber, S. L. Simon, R. D. Lloyd, N. A. Elghany, and S. Preston-Martin. *J. Am. Med. Assoc.* **264**, 585 (1990).

1034. J. B. Stewart, V. Bornemann, J. L. Chen, R. E. Moore, F. R. Caplan, H. Karuso, L. K. Larsen, and G. M. L. Patterson. *J. Antibiotics* **41**, 1048 (1988).

1035. I. L. Stoilov, J. E. Thompson, J.-H. Cho, and C. Djerassi. *J. Am. Chem. Soc.* **108**, 8235 (1986).

1036. C. Stoller, J. C. Braekman, D. Daloze, and G. Vandevyver. *J. Nat. Prod.* **51**, 383 (1988).

1037. M. Šturdíková, J. Fuska, E. Grossmann, and Z. Votický. *Pharmazie* **41**, 270 (1986).

1038. J. Su, K. Long, T. Pang, C.-H. He, and J. Clardy. *J. Am. Chem. Soc.* **108**, 177 (1986).

1039. M. Suganuma, H. Fujiki, H. Suguri, S. Yoshizawa, M. Hirota, M. Nakayasu, M. Ojika, K. Wakamatsu, K. Yamada, and T. Sugimura. *Proc. Natl. Acad. Sci. USA* **85**, 1768 (1988).

1040. K. Sugawara, M. Ohbayashi, K. Shimizu, M. Hatori, H. Kamei, M. Konishi, T. Oki, and H. Kawaguchi. *J. Antibiotics* **41**, 862 (1988).

1041. K. Sugawara, M. Tsunakawa, M. Konishi, H. Kawaguchi, B. Krishnan, C.-H. He, and J. Clardy. *J. Org. Chem.* **52**, 996 (1987).

1042. T. Sugimura. *Environ. Health Perspectives* **67**, 5 (1986).

1043. B. Sullivan, P. Djura, D. E. McIntyre, and D. J. Faulkner. *Tetrahedron* **37**, 979 (1981).

1044. B. W. Sullivan, D. J. Faulkner, G. K. Matsumoto, C.-H. He, and J. Clardy. *J. Org. Chem.* **51**, 4568 (1986).

1045. B. W. Sullivan, D. J. Faulkner, K. T. Okamoto, M. H. M. Chen, and J. Clardy. *J. Org. Chem.* **51**, 5134 (1986).

1046. H.-D. Sun, Z.-W. Lin, Y.-L. Xu, Y. Minami, T. Marunaka, T. Togo, Y. Takeda, and T. Fujita. *Heterocycles* **24**, 1 (1986).

1047. H.-D. Sun, X.-C. Sun, Z.-W. Lin, Y.-L. Xu, Y. Minami, T. Muranaka, and T. Fujita. *Chem. Lett.* 753 (1981).

1048. H. H. Sun, V. J. Paul, and W. Fenical. *Phytochemistry* **22**, 743 (1983).

1049. N.-J. Sun, M. Antoun, C.-J. Chang, and J. M. Cassady. *J. Nat. Prod.* **50**, 843 (1987).

1050. N.-J. Sun, C.-J. Chang, and J. M. Cassady. *Phytochemistry* **27**, 951 (1988).

1051. "Sunburn." *Oncology Times*, June 1986, p. 3.

1052. P. H. Sureau. *Rev. Infect. Dis.* **11**, Suppl. 4, S790 (1989).

1053. K. Suri, H. M. Goldman, and H. Wells. *Nature* **230**, 383 (1971).

1054. K. Suwanborirux, C.-J. Chang, and J. M. Cassady. *J. Nat. Prod.* **50**, 102 (1987).

1055. M. Suzuki and E. Kurosawa. *Tetrahedron Lett.* 2503 (1978).

1056. M. Suzuki and E. Kurosawa. *Phytochemistry* **24**, 1999 (1985).

1057. M. Suzuki and E. Kurosawa. *Bull. Chem. Soc. Jpn.* **60**, 3791 (1987).

1058. M. Suzuki, E. Kurosawa, and K. Kurata. *Bull. Chem. Soc. Jpn.* **60**, 3793 (1987).

1059. M. Suzuki, E. Kurosawa, and K. Kurata. *Bull. Chem. Soc. Jpn.* **60**, 3795 (1987).

1060. M. Suzuki, M. Segawa, H. Kikuchi, T. Suzuki, and E. Kurosawa. *Phytochemistry* **24**, 2011 (1985).

1061. N. Suzuki, K.-I. Yoshino, M. Kurita, K. Nomura, and M. Yamaguchi. *Comp. Biochem. Physiol.* **90C**, 305 (1988).

1062. S. Suzuki and S. Marumo. *J. Antibiotics* **13**, 360 (1960).

1063. T. Suzuki, M. Suzuki, and E. Kurosawa. *Tetrahedron Lett.* 3057 (1975).

1064. T. Suzuki, S. Takeda, M. Suzuki, and E. Kurosawa. 29th Symposium on The Chemistry of Natural Products, Symposium Papers, Sapporo, 1987, p. 583.

1065. T. Suzuki, S. Takeda, M. Suzuki, E. Kurosawa, A. Furusaki, T. Matsumoto, Y. Imanaka, and A. Kato. 28th Symposium on The Chemistry of Natural Products, Symposium Papers, Sendai, 1986, p. 215.

1066. K. Tachibana and S. H. Gruber. *Toxicon* **26**, 839 (1988).

1067. K. Tachibana, P. J. Scheuer, Y. Tsukitani, H. Kikuchi, D. Van Engen, J. Clardy, Y. Gopichand, and F. J. Schmitz. *J. Am. Chem. Soc.* **103**, 2469 (1981).

1068. H. Tada, T. Tozyo, and M. Shiro. *J. Org. Chem.* **53**, 3366 (1988).

1069. H. Tada and F. Yasuda. *Chem. Lett.* 779 (1984).

1070. A. Takahashi, H. Nakamura, T. Kameyama, S. Kurasawa, H. Naganawa, Y. Okami, T. Takeuchi, H. Umezawa, and Y. Iitaka. *J. Antibiotics* **40**, 1671 (1987).

1071. I. Takahashi, K. Takahashi, K. Asano, I. Kawamoto, T. Yasuzawa, T. Ashizawa, F. Tomita, and H. Nakano. *J. Antibiotics* **41**, 1151 (1988).

1072. K. Takahashi, I. Takahashi, M. Morimoto, and F. Tomita. *J. Antibiotics* **39**, 624 (1986).

1073. M. Takahashi, S. Iwasaki, H. Kobayashi, S. Okuda, T. Murai, Y. Sato, T. Haraguchi-Hiraoka, and H. Nagano. *J. Antibiotics* **40**, 66 (1987).

1074. Y. Takeda, T. Fujita, and A. Ueno. *Chem. Lett.* 1229 (1981).

1075. Y. Takeda, T. Ichihara, Y. Takaishi, T. Fujita, T. Shingu, and G. Kusano. *J. Chem. Soc., Perkin Trans 1* 2403 (1987).

1076. S. Takenaka, H. Oldiges, H. König, D. Hochrainer, and G. Oberdörster. *J. Natl. Cancer Inst.* **70**, 367 (1983).

1077. T. Tamamura, T. Sawa, K. Isshiki, T. Masuda, Y. Homma, H. Iinuma, H. Naganawa, M. Hamada, T. Takeuchi, and H. Umezawa. *J. Antibiotics* **38**, 1664 (1985).

1078. I. Tanaka, K. Osaki, and K. Takahashi. *Yakugaku Zasshi* **95**, 1388 (1975).

1079. J. Tanaka and T. Higa. *Tetrahedron* **44**, 2805 (1988).

1080. Y. Tanaka and T. Katayama. *Bull. Jap. Soc. Sci. Fish.* **42**, 801 (1976).

1081. S. Tanida, M. Muroi, and T. Hasegawa. *Chem. Abstr.* **101**, 108940z (1984).

1082. S. R. Tannenbaum, M. C. Archer, J. S. Wishnok, and W. W. Bishop. *J. Natl. Cancer Inst.* **60**, 251 (1978).

1083. N. M. Targett and W. S. Keeran. *J. Nat. Prod.* **47**, 556 (1984).

1084. D. L. Taylor, L. E. Fellows, G. H. Farrar, R. J. Nash, D. Taylor-Robinson, M. A. Mobberley, T. A. Ryder, D. J. Jeffries, and A. S. Tyms. *Antiviral Res.* **10**, 11 (1988).

1085. D. R. Taylor, J. M. Warner, and J. A. Wright. *J. Chem. Soc., Perkin Trans 1* 397 (1977).

1086. V. L. Teixeira, T. Tomassini, B. G. Fleury, and A. Kelecom. *J. Nat. Prod.* **49**, 570 (1986).

1087. V. L. Teixeira, T. Tomassini, and A. Kelecom. *Bull. Soc. Chim. Belg.* **95**, 263 (1986).

1088. G. Thériault, S. Cordier, C. Tremblay, and S. Gingras. *Lancet* **I**, 947 (1984).

1089. D. K. Thompson, F. P. Li, and J. R. Cassady. *Cancer* **44**, 2362 (1979).

1090. S. A. Thompson, K. Tachibana, K. Nakanishi, and I. Kubota. *Science* **233**, 341 (1986).

1091. L. S. Thurston, H. Irie, S. Tani, F.-S. Han, Z.-C. Liu, Y.-C. Cheng, and K.-H. Lee. *J. Med. Chem.* **29**, 1547 (1986).

1092. L. M. V. Tillekeratne and F. J. Schmitz. *Phytochemistry* **23**, 1331 (1984).

1093. M. Tischler, S. W. Ayer, and R. J. Andersen. *Comp. Biochem. Physiol.* **84B**, 43 (1986).

1094. M. Tits, C. Desaive, J.-M. Marnette, R. Bassleer, and L. Angenot. *J. Ethnopharmacol.* **12**, 287 (1984).

1095. M. A. Tius and A. H. Fauq. *J. Am. Chem. Soc.* **108**, 1035 (1986).

1096. H. Tokuda, T. Konoshima, M. Kozuka, and T. Kimura. *Cancer Lett.* **40**, 309 (1988).

1097. M. Tokunaga, J. E. Norman, Jr., M. Asano, S. Tokuoka, H. Ezaki, I. Nishimori, and Y. Tsuji. *J. Natl. Cancer Inst.* **62**, 1347 (1979).

1098. L. Tomatis, A. Aitio, J. Wilbourn, and L. Shuker. *Jpn. J. Cancer Res. (Gann)* **80**, 795 (1989).

1099. P. Toniolo, E. Riboli, F. Protta, M. Charrel, and A. P. M. Cappa. *Cancer Res.* **49**, 5203 (1989).

1100. K. Torigoe, M. Murata, T. Yasumoto, and T. Iwashita. *J. Am. Chem. Soc.* **110**, 7876 (1988).

1101. W. Torjussen, L. A. Solberg, and A. Chr. Høgetveit. *Cancer* **44**, 963 (1979).

1102. N. Touchette. *J. NIH Res.* **2**, 61 (1990).

1103. D. W. Trent, J. A. Grant, T. P. Monath, C. L. Manske, M. Corina, and G. E. Fox. *Virology* **172**, 523 (1989).

1104. D. Trichopoulos, G. Ouranos, N. E. Day, A. Tzonou, O. Manousos, Ch. Papadimitriou, and A. Trichopoulos. *Int. J. Cancer* **36**, 291 (1985).

1105. C. Tringali and M. Piattelli. *Gazz. Chim. Ital.* **112**, 465 (1982).

1106. C. Tringali, M. Piattelli, and G. Nicolosi. *J. Nat. Prod.* **49**, 236 (1986).

1107. J. Trojánek, J. Hoffmannová, O. Štrouf, and Z. Čekan. *Collect. Czech. Chem. Commun.* **24**, 526 (1959).

1108. W. Trowitzsch-Kienast, H. Irschik, H. Reichenbach, V. Wray, and G. Höfle. *Liebigs Ann. Chem.* 475 (1988).

1109. E. R. Trumbull, E. Bianchi, D. J. Eckert, R. M. Wiedhopf, and J. R. Cole. *J. Pharm. Sci.* **65**, 1407 (1976).

1110. S. Tsujii, K. L. Rinehart, S. P. Gunasekera, Y. Kashman, S. S. Cross, M. S. Lui, S. A. Pomponi, and M. C. Diaz. *J. Org. Chem.* **53**, 5446 (1988).

1111. M. A. Tucker, J. A. Shields, P. Hartge, J. Augsburger, R. N. Hoover, and J. F. Fraumeni, Jr. *N. Engl. J. Med.* **313**, 789 (1985).

1112. M. J. Turell and P. V. Perkins. *Am. J. Trop. Med. Hyg.* **42**, 185 (1990).

1113. A. J. Tuyns. *Cancer Res.* **39**, 2840 (1979).

1114. A. J. Tuyns, G. Péquignot, and J. S. Abbatucci. *Int. J. Cancer* **23**, 443 (1979).

1115. T. Uchida, M. Imoto, Y. Takahashi, A. Odagawa, T. Sawa, K. Tatsuta, H. Naganawa, M. Hamada, T. Takeuchi, and H. Umezawa. *J. Antibiotics* **41**, 404 (1988).

1116. K. Uchino, T. Matsuo, M. Iwamoto, Y. Tonosaki, and A. Fukuchi. *Planta Med.* **54**, 419 (1988).

1117. K. Uchino, H. Ogawara, T. Akiyama, A. Fukuchi, S. Shibata, K. Takahashi, and T. Narui. *J. Antibiotics* **38**, 157 (1985).

1118. K. Uchino, H. Ogawara, T. Akiyama, A. Fukuchi, S. Shibata, K. Takahashi, and T. Narui. *J. Antibiotics* **38**, 592 (1985).

1119. Y. Uchio, S. Eguchi, M. Nakayama, and T. Hase. *Chem. Lett.* 277 (1982).

1120. Y. Uchio, S. Eguchi, M. Nakayama, and T. Hase. 27th Symposium on the Chemistry of Terpenes, Essential Oils, and Aromatics, Abstracts of Papers, Kanazawa, Japan, 1984, p. 59.

1121. D. Uemura, K. Takahashi, T. Yamamoto, C. Katayama, J. Tanaka, Y. Okumura, and Y. Hirata. *J. Am. Chem. Soc.* **107**, 4796 (1985).

1122. Y. Umeda, M. Moriguchi, K. Ikai, H. Kuroda, T. Nakamura, A. Fujii, T. Takeuchi, and H. Umezawa. *J. Antibiotics* **40**, 1316 (1987).

1123. Y. Umeda, M. Moriguchi, H. Kuroda, T. Nakamura, A. Fujii, H. Iinuma, T. Takeuchi, and H. Umezawa. *J. Antibiotics* **40**, 1303 (1987).

1124. Y. Umeda, M. Moriguchi, H. Kuroda, T. Nakamura, H. Iinuma, T. Takeuchi, and H. Umezawa. *J. Antibiotics* **38**, 886 (1985).

1125. K. Umehara, K. Nakahara, S. Kiyoto, M. Iwami, M. Okamoto, H. Tanaka, M. Kohsaka, H. Aoki, and H. Imanaka. *J. Antibiotics* **36**, 478 (1983).

1126. H. Umezawa, M. Imoto, T. Sawa, K. Isshiki, N. Matsuda, T. Uchida, H. Iinuma, M. Hamada, and T. Takeuchi. *J. Antibiotics* **39**, 170 (1986).

1127. I. Umezawa, K. Komiyama, H. Oka, K. Okada, S. Tomisaka, T. Miyano, and S. Takano. *J. Antibiotics* **37**, 706 (1984).

1128. A. C. Upton. *Scient. Amer.* **246**, 41 (1982).

1129. A. C. Upton. *Cancer Invest.* **7**, 267 (1989).

1130. A. C. Upton. *J. Natl. Cancer Inst.* **82**, 448 (1990).

1131. F. Urbach. *Photochem. Photobiol.* **50**, 507 (1989).

1132. "U.S. Scientists Warn of Exposure to Solvent Tied to Cancer in Rats." *Wall Street Journal*, April 28, 1977.

1133. J. Valisolalao, L. Bang, J.-P. Beck, and G. Ourisson. *Bull. Soc. Chim. Fr.* II-473 (1980).

1134. R. Valls, B. Banaigs, C. Francisco, L. Codomier, and A. Cave. *Phytochemistry* **25**, 751 (1986).

1135. I. A. van Altena. *Aust. J. Chem.* **41**, 49 (1988).

1136. D. A. Vanden Berghe, A. J. Vlietinck, and L. Van Hoff. *Bull. Inst. Pasteur (Paris)* **84**, 101 (1986).

1137. L. A. G. M. van den Broek, R. M. J. Liskamp, J. H. Colstee, P. Lelieveld, M. Remacha, D. Vázquez, J. P. G. Ballesta, and H. C. J. Ottenheijm. *J. Med. Chem.* **30**, 325 (1987).

1138. B. L. Van Duuren, G. Loewengart, I. Seidman, A. C. Smith, and S. Melchionne. *Cancer Res.* **38**, 3236 (1978).

1139. F. J. van Schooten, F. E. van Leeuwen, M. J. X. Hillebrand, M. E. de Rijke, A. A. M. Hart, H. G. van Veen, S. Oosterink, and E. Kriek. *J. Natl. Cancer Inst.* **82**, 927 (1990).

1140. J. T. Vázquez, M. Chang, K. Nakanishi, E. Manta, C. Pérez, and J. D. Martín. *J. Org. Chem.* **53**, 4797 (1988).

1141. M. P. Veares, L. J. Goad, and J. W. ApSimon. *Comp. Biochem. Physiol.* **90B**, 25 (1988).

1142. C. G. Victora, N. Muñoz, N. E. Day, L. B. Barcelos, D. A. Peccin, and N. M. Braga. *Int. J. Cancer* **39**, 710 (1987).

1143. "Vinylidene Chloride Linked to Cancer." *C & E News*, Feb. 28, 1977, p. 6.

1144. M. von Glehn, R. Norrestam, P. Kierkegaard, L. Maron, and L. Ernster. *FEBS Lett.* **20**, 267 (1972).

1145. S. Wahidulla, L. D'Souza, and J. Patel. *Phytochemistry* **26**, 2864 (1987).

1146. T. Wakamiya, H. Nakamoto, and T. Shiba. *Tetrahedron Lett.* **25**, 4411 (1984).

1147. T. Wakamiya, Y. Oda, H. Fujita, and T. Shiba. *Tetrahedron Lett.* **27**, 2143 (1986).

1148. E. A. Walker, M. Castegnaro, L. Garren, G. Toussaint, and B. Kowalski. *J. Natl. Cancer Inst.* **63**, 947 (1979).

1149. R. P. Walker and D. J. Faulkner. *J. Org. Chem.* **46**, 1098 (1981).

1150. *Wall Street Journal*, June 11, 1990.

1151. M. E. Wall, M. C. Wani, B. N. Meyer, and H. Taylor. *J. Nat. Prod.* **50**, 1152 (1987).

1152. M. E. Wall, M. C. Wani, S. M. Natschke, and A. W. Nicholas. *J. Med. Chem.* **29**, 1553 (1986).

1153. M. E. Wall, M. C. Wani, and H. Taylor. *J. Nat. Prod.* **50**, 1095 (1987).

1154. C. L. Walters. *Chem. Brit.* 140 (1977).

1155. J.-X. Wang, J. D. Boice, Jr., B.-X. Li, J.-Y. Zhang, and J. F. Fraumeni, Jr., *J. Natl. Cancer Inst.* **80**, 344 (1988).

1156. J.-X. Wang, P. D. Inskip, J. D. Boice, Jr., B.-X. Li, J.-Y. Zhang, and J. F. Fraumeni, Jr. *Int. J. Cancer* **45**, 889 (1990).

1157. Y. Y. Wang, S. M. Rappaport, R. F. Sawyer, R. E. Talcott, and E. T. Wei. *Cancer Lett.* **5**, 39 (1978).

1158. Z.-W. Wang, W.-W. Ma, J. L. McLaughlin, and M. P. Gupta. *J. Nat. Prod.* **51**, 382 (1988).

1159. M. C. Wani, A. W. Nicholas, and M. E. Wall. *J. Med. Chem.* **30**, 2317 (1987).

1160. M. Wani, H. L. Taylor, M. E. Wall, P. Coggon, and A. T. McPhail. *J. Amer. Chem. Soc.* **93**, 2325 (1971).

1161. M. A. Warpehoski. *Tetrahedron Lett.* **27**, 4103 (1986).

1162. M. A. Warpehoski, R. C. Kelly, J. P. McGovren, and W. Wierenga. *Proc. Am. Assoc. Cancer Res.* **26**, 870 (1985).

1163. J. M. Wasylyk, A. J. Weinheimer, and M. I. Alam., 191st American Chemical Society Meeting, New York, April, 1986.

1164. P. G. Waterman. *Phytochemistry* **15**, 347 (1976).

1165. D. M. Watts, M. A. Ussery, D. Nash, and C. J. Peters. *Am. J. Trop. Med. Hyg.* **41**, 581 (1989).

1166. A. J. Weinheimer, J. A. Matson, D. van der Helm, and M. Poling. *Tetrahedron Lett.* 1295 (1977).

1167. I. B. Weinstein. *Cancer. Res.* **48**, 4135 (1988).

1168. E. K. Weisburger. *Cancer* **40**, 1935 (1977).

1169. E. K. Weisburger. "Carcinogenic Halogenated Aliphatic Compounds" **In** Chemical Carcinogens, Activation Mechanisms, Structural and Electronic Factors, and Reactivity, Eds. P. Politzer & F. J. Martin, Jr., Elsevier, The Netherlands, Vol. 5, Bioactive Molecules, Chap. 4, 1988, p. 91.

1170. O. S. Weislow, R. Kiser, D. L. Fine, J. Bader, R. H. Shoemaker, and M. R. Boyd. *J. Natl. Cancer Inst.* **81**, 577 (1989).

1171. R. J. Wells. *Tetrahedron Lett.* 2637 (1976).

1172. G. Wenke and D. Hoffmann. *Carcinogenesis* **4**, 169 (1983).

1173. R. R. West and J. H. Cardellina, II. *J. Org. Chem.* **53**, 2782 (1988).

1174. D. A. Whiting. *S. Afr. Med. J.* **53**, 131 (1978).

1175. D. A. Whiting. *S. Afr. Med. J.* **53**, 134 (1978).

1176. D. A. Whiting. *S. Afr. Med. J.* **53**, 162 (1978).

1177. D. A. Whiting. *S. Afr. Med. J.* **53**, 166 (1978).

1178. W. C. Willett, M. J. Stampfer, G. A. Colditz, B. A. Rosner, C. H. Hennekens, and F. E. Speizer. *N. Engl. J. Med.* **316**, 1174 (1987).

1179. D. E. Williams and R. J. Andersen. *Can. J. Chem.* **65**, 2244 (1987).

1180. D. E. Williams, R. J. Andersen, L. Parkanyi, and J. Clardy. *Tetrahedron Lett.* **28**, 5079 (1987).

1181. D. Williams, R. J. Andersen, G. D. Van Duyne, and J. Clardy. *J. Org. Chem.* **52**, 332 (1987).

1182. D. E. Williams, S. W. Ayer, and R. J. Andersen. *Can. J. Chem.* **64**, 1527 (1986).

1183. R. R. Williams. *Lancet* I, 996 (1976).

1184. R. R. Williams, P. D. Sorlie, M. Feinleib, P. M. McNamara, W. B. Kannel, and T. R. Dawber. *J. Am. Med. Assoc.* **245**, 247 (1981).

1185. T. H. Williams. *J. Antibiotics* **28**, 85 (1975).

1186. S. G. Winslow and H. B. Gerstner. *Drug and Chem. Toxicol.* **1**, 259 (1978).

1187. S.-M. Wong, Y. Oshima, J. M. Pezzuto, H. H. S. Fong, and N. R. Farnsworth. *J. Pharm. Sci.* **75**, 317 (1986).

1188. A. E. Wright, O. J. McConnell, S. Kohmoto, M. S. Lui, W. Thompson, and K. M. Snader. *Tetrahedron Lett.* **28**, 1377 (1987).

1189. A. E. Wright, S. A. Pomponi, O. J. McConnell, S. Kohmoto, and P. J. McCarthy. *J. Nat. Prod.* **50**, 976 (1987).

1190. H. Wu, H. Nakamura, J. Kobayashi, M. Kobayashi, Y. Ohizumi, and Y. Hirata. *Bull. Chem. Soc. Jpn.* **59**, 2495 (1986).

1191. H. Wu, H. Nakamura, J. Kobayashi, Y. Ohizumi, and Y. Hirata. *Experientia* **42**, 855 (1986).

1192. R.-Y. Wu, L.-M. Yang, T. Yokoi, and K.-H. Lee. *J. Antibiotics* **41**, 481 (1988).

1193. Y.-C. Wu, S.-T. Lu, J.-J. Chang, and K.-H. Lee. *Phytochemistry* **27**, 1563 (1988).

1194. Z. Wu, Z. Yiao, and K. Long. *Zhongshan Daxue Xuebao, Ziran Kexueban* **3**, 69 (1982); *Chem. Abstr.* **98**, 68827d (1983).

1195. E. L. Wynder. *J. Am. Diet. Assoc.* **71**, 385 (1977).

1196. E. L. Wynder and R. Goldsmith. *Cancer* **40**, 1246 (1977).

1197. S. Yamada, K. Ando, S. Koike, and K. Isono. *Jpn. J. Cancer Res. (Gann)* **81**, 112 (1990).

1198. T. Yamagishi, X.-Z. Yan, R.-Y. Wu, D. R. McPhail, A. T. McPhail, and K.-H. Lee. *Chem. Pharm. Bull.* **36**, 1615 (1988).

1199. T. Yamagishi, D.-C. Zhang, J.-J. Chang, D. R. McPhail, A. T. McPhail, and K.-H. Lee. *Phytochemistry* **27**, 3213 (1988).

1200. M. Yamato, K. Hashigaki, N. Kokubu, and Y. Nakato. *J. Chem. Soc., Perkin Trans 1* 1301 (1984).

1201. M. Yamato, K. Hashigaki, N. Kokubu, T. Tashiro, and T. Tsuruo. *J. Med. Chem.* **29**, 1202 (1986).

1202. M. Yamato, K. Hashigaki, N. Kokubu, T. Tsuruo, and T. Tashiro. *J. Med. Chem.* **27**, 1749 (1984).

1203. T. Yamauchi, F. Abe, Y. Nishishita, H. Okabe, K. Shima, and S. Nishibe. *Phytochemistry* **18**, 1240 (1979).

1204. L.-M. Yang, R.-Y. Wu, A. T. McPhail, T. Yokoi, and K.-H. Lee. *J. Antibiotics* **41**, 488 (1988).

1205. K. Yano. *J. Agric. Food Chem.* **27**, 456 (1979).

1206. T. Yasumoto, N. Seino, Y. Murakami, and M. Murata. *Biol. Bull.* **172**, 128 (1987).

1207. T. Yasumoto, M. Yotsu, M. Murata, and H. Naoki. *J. Am. Chem. Soc.* **110**, 2344 (1988).

1208. S. Yeh and G. A. Cordell. *J. Nat. Prod.* **50**, 195 (1987).

1209. K. Yokoi, K. Nagaoka, and T. Nakashima. *Chem. Pharm. Bull.* **34**, 4554 (1986).

1210. T. Yokoi, L.-M. Yang, T. Yokoi, R.-Y. Wu, and K.-H. Lee. *J. Antibiotics* **41**, 494 (1988).

1211. T. Yokota, S. K. Kim, Y. Fukui, N. Takahashi, Y. Takeuchi, and T. Takematsu. *Phytochemistry* **26**, 503 (1987).

1212. I. Yosioka, I. Kitagawa, K. Hino, A. Matsuda, and Y. Nakagawa. *Chem. Pharm. Bull.* **16**, 190 (1968).

1213. M. Yotsu, M. Murata, T. Yasumoto, and H. Naoki. 29th Symposium on The Chemistry of Natural Products, Symposium Papers, Sapporo, 1987, p. 247.

1214. W.-C. You, W. J. Blot, Y.-S. Chang, A. G. Ershow, Z.-T. Yang, Q. An, B. Henderson, G.-W. Xu, J. F. Fraumeni, Jr., and T.-G. Wang. *Cancer Res.* **48**, 3518 (1988).

1215. T. M. Zabriskie, J. A. Klocke, C. M. Ireland, A. H. Marcus, T. F. Molinski, D. J. Faulkner, C. Xu, and J. C. Clardy. *J. Am. Chem. Soc.* **108**, 3123 (1986).

1216. T. M. Zabriskie, C. L. Mayne, and C. M. Ireland. *J. Am. Chem. Soc.* **110**, 7919 (1988).

1217. L. H. Zalkow, S. Bonetti, L. Gelbaum, M. M. Gordon, B. B. Patil, A. Shani, and D. Van Derveer. *J. Nat. Prod.* **42**, 603 (1979).

1218. S. Zayed, W. Adolf, A. Hafez, and E. Hecker. *Tetrahedron Lett.* 3481 (1977).

1219. M. S. Zedeck. "Hydrazine Derivatives, Azo and Azoxy Compounds, and Methylazoxymethanol and Cycasin" In Chemical Carcinogens, Second Edition, Revised and Expanded, Vol. 2, Chap. 15, C. E. Searle, Ed., Amer. Chem. Soc., Washington, D.C., 1984, p. 915.

1220. R. Zelnik, M. Haraguchi, A. K. Matida, D. Lavie, F. Frolow, and A. L. Weis. *J. Chem. Soc., Perkin Trans 1* 2051 (1986).

1221. D. Zhang, M. Haruna, A. T. McPhail, and K.-H. Lee. *Phytochemistry* **25**, 899 (1986).

1222. L.-G. Zhuang, O. Seligmann, K. Jurcic, and H. Wagner. *Planta Med.* **45**, 172 (1982).

1223. J. Zielinski, W. C. M. C. Kokke, T. B. T. Ha, A. Y. L. Shu, W. L. Duax, and C. Djerassi. *J. Org. Chem.* **48**, 3471 (1983).

1224. F. Zollo, E. Finamore, and L. Minale. *Gazz. Chim. Ital.* **115**, 303 (1985).

1225. F. Zollo, E. Finamore, and L. Minale. *J. Nat. Prod.* **50**, 794 (1987).

1226. F. Zollo, E. Finamore, L. Minale, D. Laurent, and G. Bargibant. *J. Nat. Prod.* **49**, 919 (1986).

1227. M. B. Zurita, A. Ahond, C. Poupat, P. Potier, and J. L. Menou. *J. Nat. Prod.* **49**, 809 (1986).

1228. T. A. Zykova, E. P. Kozlovskaya, and G. B. Elyakov. *Bioorg. Khim.* **14**, 878 (1988).